APHASIA AND LANGUAGE

THE SCIENCE AND PRACTICE OF NEUROPSYCHOLOGY
A Guilford Series

Robert A. Bornstein, *Series Editor*

Aphasia and Language: Theory to Practice
Stephen E. Nadeau, Leslie J. Gonzalez Rothi, and Bruce Crosson, Editors

Pediatric Neuropsychology: Research, Theory, and Practice
Keith Owen Yeates, M. Douglas Ris, and H. Gerry Taylor, Editors

The Human Frontal Lobes: Functions and Disorders
Bruce L. Miller and Jeffrey L. Cummings, Editors

APHASIA AND LANGUAGE

Theory to Practice

Edited by

Stephen E. Nadeau
Leslie J. Gonzalez Rothi
Bruce Crosson

THE GUILFORD PRESS
New York London

© 2000 The Guilford Press
A Division of Guilford Publications, Inc.
72 Spring Street, New York, NY 10012
www.guilford.com

Printed in the United States of America

This book is printed on acid-free paper.

Last digit is print number: 9   8   7   6   5   4   3   2   1

Library of Congress Cataloging-in-Publication Data
Aphasia and language : theory to practice / [edited by] Stephen E. Nadeau, Leslie J.
    Gonzalez Rothi, Bruce Crosson.
        p. ; cm. — (The science and practice of neuropsychology)
    Includes bibliographical references and index.
    ISBN 1-57230-581-9
    1. Aphasic persons—Rehabilitation. 2. Brain damage—Complications. I. Nadeau,
Stephen E.   II. Rothi, Leslie J. (Leslie Janine), 1949– III. Crosson, Bruce. IV. Series.
    [DNLM: 1. Aphasia—rehabilitation. 2. Aphasia—diagnosis. 3. Aphasia—etiology.
4. Speech–Language Pathology. WL 340.5 A6403 2000]
    RC425 .A613 2000
    616.85'52—dc21   00-034097

To our teacher, mentor, colleague, and friend,
Kenneth M. Heilman

ABOUT THE EDITORS

Stephen E. Nadeau, MD, received his medical degree from the University of Florida and completed a behavioral neurology fellowship with Kenneth Heilman. He is currently Professor of Neurology at the University of Florida College of Medicine; staff neurologist at the Geriatric Research, Education, and Clinical Center; and Research Director of the Physiological and Behavioral Treatment Initiative of the VA RR&D Brain Rehabilitation Center at the Malcolm Randall DVA Medical Center in Gainesville, Florida. Dr. Nadeau's major research has been in the fields of cerebrovascular disease and behavioral neuroscience, and his chief interests are in language, attentional processes, and the explanation of higher neural functions on the basis of connectionist models. He runs a functional imaging program involving single photon emission computed tomography, is extensively involved in medical education, and is in the process of writing a textbook in medical neuroscience.

Leslie J. Gonzalez Rothi, PhD, received her doctoral degree in speech pathology, followed by a postdoctoral fellowship in behavioral neurology and neuropsychology in the Department of Neurology, from the University of Florida in Gainesville. For many years, Dr. Gonzalez Rothi worked clinically in the management of neurologically induced communication disorders, with her research focused on the study of the neuropsychological mechanisms of disorders of language and limb apraxia. Currently, she serves as the Program Director for the VA RR&D Brain Rehabilitation Research Center at the Malcolm Randall DVA Medical Center and as Professor of Neurology at the University of Florida in Gainesville, where she continues to focus on research regarding the neuropsychological mechanisms of and treatment of aphasia, apraxia, alexia, and agraphia.

Bruce Crosson, PhD, received his doctoral degree in psychology from Texas Tech University. Throughout his career, Dr. Crosson has maintained an interest in the interface between language disorders and attention systems, including the role of subcortical structures in these functions. Formerly, he was director of an outpatient brain trauma rehabilitation program at Washington University Medical Center in St. Louis, Missouri. At present, Dr. Crosson is Professor of Clinical and Health Psychology at the University of Florida Health Science Center, where he has received a University of Florida Research Foundation Professorship (2000–2002). Current research projects include a study, using functional magnetic resonance imaging, of how the medial frontal cortex participates in initiation of language and treatment of intention and attention in aphasia.

CONTRIBUTORS

Pelagie M. Beeson, PhD, Assistant Research Scientist at the National Center for Neurogenic Communication Disorders, Department of Speech and Hearing Sciences and the Department of Neurology, University of Arizona, Tucson, Arizona

Lee Xenakis Blonder, PhD, Associate Professor of the Department of Behavioral Science, Neurology, and Anthropology, and the Stroke Program of the Sanders-Brown Center on Aging, University of Kentucky College of Medicine, Lexington, Kentucky

Anjan Chatterjee, MD, Associate Professor of the Department of Neurology and Center for Cognitive Neuroscience, University of Pennsylvania, Philadelphia, Pennsylvania

H. Branch Coslett, MD, Professor of the Department of Neurology, University of Pennsylvania, and the Moss Rehabilitation Research Institute, Philadelphia, Pennsylvania

Bruce Crosson, PhD, Professor of the Department of Clinical and Health Psychology, University of Florida Health Science Center, Gainesville, Florida; Research Neuropsychologist of the VA RR&D Brain Rehabilitation Research Center, Malcolm Randall DVA Medical Center, Gainesville, Florida

Patrick J. Doyle, PhD, Director of the Aphasia Rehabilitation Research Laboratory and Clinics, VA Pittsburgh Healthcare System, Pittsburgh, Pennsylvania; Department of Communication Science and Disorders, University of Pittsburgh, Pittsburgh, Pennsylvania

Ira Fischler, PhD, Professor of the Department of Psychology, University of Florida, Gainesville, Florida

Margaret L. Greenwald, PhD, Assistant Professor of the Department of Audiology and Speech–Language Pathology, and Adjunct Assistant Professor of the Department of Neurology, Wayne State University, Detroit, Michigan

Kenneth M. Heilman, MD, Distinguished Professor of the Department of Neurology, University of Florida, Gainesville, Florida; System Chief of the Neurology Service and Medical Director of the VA RR&D Brain Rehabilitation Research Center, Malcolm Randall DVA Medical Center, Gainesville, Florida

Kevin P. Kearns, PhD, Professor and Director of the Department of Communication Sciences and Disorders, Massachusetts General Hospital Institute of Health Professions, Boston, Massachusetts

Lynn Maher, PhD, Assistant Professor of the Department of Educational Psychology and Special Education, Georgia State University, Atlanta, Georgia

Malcolm R. McNeil, PhD, Professor and Chair of the Department of Communication Science and Disorders, and Professor of the Department of Otolaryngology, University of Pittsburgh, Pittsburgh, Pennsylvania; Research Scientist at the VA Pittsburgh Healthcare System, Pittsburgh, Pennsylvania; Co-Director of the Pittsburgh Aphasia Treatment, Research, and Education Center (PATREC), Pittsburgh, Pennsylvania

Stephen E. Nadeau, MD, Staff Neurologist of the Geriatric Research, Education and Clinical Center and Research Director of the Physiological and Behavioral Treatment Initiative of the VA RR&D Brain Rehabilitation Research Center, Malcolm Randall DVA Medical Center, Gainesville, Florida; Professor of the Department of Neurology, University of Florida, Gainesville, Florida

Cynthia Ochipa, PhD, Speech Pathology Section Chief of the Audiology and Speech Pathology Service, James A. Haley VA Medical Center, Tampa, Florida

Steven Z. Rapcsak, MD, Associate Professor of the Departments of Neurology and Psychology, University of Arizona, Tucson, Arizona; Chief of the Neurology Section, VA Medical Center, Tucson, Arizona

Anastasia M. Raymer, PhD, Assistant Professor of the Department of Early Childhood, Speech–Language Pathology, and Special Education, Old Dominion University, Norfolk, Virginia

Heidi L. Roth, MD, Visiting Assistant Professor of the Department of Neurology, University of Florida, Gainesville, Florida

Leslie J. Gonzalez Rothi, PhD, Program Director of the VA RR&D Brain Rehabilitation Research Center, Malcolm Randall DVA Medical Center, Gainesville, Florida; Professor of the Department of Neurology, University of Florida, Gainesville, Florida

Julie Wambaugh, PhD, Assistant Professor of the Department of Communication Disorders, University of Utah, Salt Lake City, Utah; Research Speech Pathologist, Salt Lake City VA Medical Center, Salt Lake City, Utah

Carolyn E. Wilshire, PhD, Lecturer in the School of Psychology, Victoria University of Wellington, Wellington, New Zealand; Adjunct Scientist at the Moss Rehabilitation Research Institute, Philadelphia, Pennsylvania

SERIES EDITOR'S FOREWORD

Aphasia and Language: Theory to Practice, edited by Stephen E. Nadeau, Leslie J. Gonzalez Rothi, and Bruce Crosson, is the third volume in The Science and Practice of Neuropsychology series. The volume reflects the central role that the study of language and language disorders has held in the evolution of our understanding of brain–behavior relationships. The editors of the volume, as well as the exceptional group of contributing authors, epitomize the richness and diversity of the field of neuropsychology. The contributors include speech and language pathologists, neurologists, neuropsychologists, a cognitive psychologist, and an anthropologist. The vast majority of these individuals exemplify the integration of research and practice in their own work.

In this series, neuropsychology is defined broadly as the study of brain–behavior relationships, incorporating the perspectives of the full range of related disciplines. Although some volumes in the series will undoubtedly be of greater interest to specific subsets of readers, it is intended that the series be of interest to scientists and practitioners in all the disciplines that address the questions of brain and behavior in research and/or applied contexts. A wide range of topics will be covered, and will include reviews of emerging technologies and their potential impact on the science and clinical understanding of neuropsychology.

This timely volume reflects the importance of the study of language in its own right, and the inherent impact of language on many domains of higher cognitive function. Language disorders are among the most common and most debilitating consequences of brain injury and illness. Historically, these disorders have been vital in establishing the very essence of brain–behavior relationships. In the modern era, the study of language and its disorders is frequently the exemplar in the development of new technologies. This volume integrates contemporary theoretical models of cognitive neuroscience with a more sophisticated understanding of language disorders, associated conditions, and new concepts and innovations in therapy. The volume also demonstrates the important interrelationships between language and other evolving concepts and constructs in our appreciation of brain functions, and therefore provides a future-oriented view of the central role that the study of language will continue to play in our evolving understanding of brain–behavior relationships.

ROBERT A. BORNSTEIN, PhD

PREFACE

Aphasia is an acquired disorder of language form, language structure, verbal elaboration, or communicative intention resulting from dysfunction of the brain. It can be caused by stroke, diseases affecting brain substance and function, or traumatic injury. Worldwide, the annual incidence of stroke is estimated to be between 300 and 500 per 100,000 people (Sudlow & Warlow, 1997). Stroke is the leading health care problem requiring rehabilitation services in older Americans today (Lee, Huber, & Stetson, 1996). Twenty-five percent of strokes are associated with aphasia (Mayo, 1993; Paolucci et al., 1988). Add to these numbers the patients living with language disorders due to dementia caused by degenerative diseases or traumatic brain injury, and it is clear that aphasia is a health problem of staggering proportions. The work of Kertesz and McCabe (1977) tells us that aphasia after stroke is not only common but enduring: Only 21% of patients eventually recover normal language function. Furthermore, many aphasic patients never return to work, and many require restrictive living arrangements upon discharge from hospitals and rehabilitation facilities. Thus aphasia is a costly problem, not simply in dollars but also in human terms—such as poor functional outcomes, caregiver burden, and quality of life (Stineman, Maikslin, Fiedler, & Granger, 1997; Paolucci et al., 1988; Wyller, Sveen, Sodring, Pettersen, & Bautz-Holter, 1997).

That aphasia is common, enduring, and costly underscores the need for attending not only to its specification but also to its treatment. The purpose of this book is to review what is known about language impairment with brain damage, the inferences we can draw from the study of aphasia regarding the normal representation of language in the central nervous system, and (most importantly) what this information on normal and pathological processing might tell us about how to rehabilitate aphasia.

Part I of this book consists of a chapter by Roth and Heilman on the history of the study of aphasia, discussing not only the findings of early investigators but also the political and social issues influencing their work. We are reminded of the extraordinary insight of early investigators, and at times we are humbled by our failure to move much beyond them in many areas and our tendency to recapitulate old mistakes. The five chapters of Part II then review the major domains of language impairment in aphasia, what can be inferred about normal language from disordered language, the major principles of language rehabilitation in these domains, and the state of the scientific evidence on rehabilitation. Included are chapters on verbal fluency and generativity by Greenwald, Nadeau, and Rothi; on phonological processing by Nadeau; on word retrieval by Wilshire and Coslett; on the verbal semantic system by Raymer and Rothi; and on grammatical processing by Chatterjee and Maher. These reviews fully demonstrate the eclecticism that currently characterizes language research, including the richly detailed theoretical structure that has emerged from disciplined use of information-processing models by cognitive neuropsychologists, incisive investigations by experimental psychologists, current adaptations of ideas originally born of linguistic theory, insights derived from our increasingly sophisticated understanding of brain structure and function in general, and perspectives on language function reflecting insights into neural network function derived from work with connectionist models. Although we are very much in an era of transition, never before has there been so much promise of being able to relate a complex behavior such as language to processes occurring at the neuronal level.

Part III includes three chapters on disorders of functions directly linked to the neural substrate for spoken language: acquired dyslexias (Greenwald), agraphia (Rapcsak & Beeson), and apraxia of speech (McNeil, Doyle, & Wambaugh), and a chapter by Ochipa and Rothi on a dominant-hemisphere function—limb apraxia—that in many ways parallels language function and is often also impaired in aphasic patients. The chapters on acquired dyslexias and agraphia fully exemplify the sophistication of current cognitive-neuropsychological approaches to language function. The chapter on apraxia of speech focuses on the inscrutable interface between linguistic systems and the motor system, and gives us a particularly detailed review of rehabilitation research in this area. The chapter on limb apraxia elaborates on some provocative parallels between language function and complex motoric function, and reminds us that in many patients, limb apraxia, which nearly invariably affects the nonparetic hand, often seriously interferes with the development of potentially compensatory strategies in aphasic patients. In such patients, rehabilitation of apraxia is scarcely less important than rehabilitation of aphasia. Rounding out Part III is a chapter by Blonder on communication in natural settings by aphasic patients. For many this chapter will provide a rude awakening, confronting us with evidence that to a great extent, the theoretically motivated dimensions of language function that we tend to focus on in aphasia rehabilitation may be substantially orthogonal to the dimensions of language function that constrain communication in natural settings. The dimensions in natural settings often have less to do with symbolic exchange than they do with impairment of other behaviorally crucial brain functions in aphasic patients and with the sometimes functional, sometimes dysfunctional evolution of familial interpersonal relationships after brain damage.

Part IV consists of four chapters that deal with language in the context of several different neuroscientific perspectives. Because of the enormous advances of connectionist or parallel-distributed-processing models over the past 15 years, the degree to which these models successfully emulate brain structure and function, their ability to relate a complex behavior to the function of ensembles of neuron-like entities, and their success in recapitulating fine details of experimentally observed behavior in both normal and brain-impaired subjects, we consider a chapter on connectionist models and language to be essential. Nadeau briefly reviews this burgeoning field.

Fischler then reviews language function from the perspective of an experimental psychologist interested in constraints governing the allocation of brain resources to language. His employment of the term "attention" to denote the resource allocation device (reflecting a Jamesian perspective and common terminology in the discipline) may confuse those who understand attention as a behavior characterized by the direction of sensory resources to a particular stimulus. In fact, attention in Fischler's conceptualization corresponds to the selective engagement or bringing on line of the particular neuronal networks necessary at any given moment (what is often referred to as "working memory").

When this selective engagement involves networks in sensory association cortices, then it subserves attention as traditionally and behaviorally defined. However, when it involves supramodal cortices, such as those supporting language, it has nothing to do with attentional behavior except to the extent that the allocation of network resources to genuinely attentional processes by the damaged brain may constrain its ability to allocate resources to language function. Coslett and colleagues (Coslett, Schwartz, Goldberg, Hass, & Perkins, 1993; Coslett, 1999) have provided tentative evidence of such dysfunctional competition for limited resources in aphasic patients whose language function improves when examiners interact from the left hemispace, thus presumably allowing the right hemisphere to subsume much of the burden of attentional demands (or potentiating right-hemisphere language processing). Richards, Singletary, Koehler, Crosson, and Rothi (2000) have shown that language rehabilitation can be promoted by having the patient engage right-hemisphere intentional mechanisms by making complex movements and/or gestures with the left hand in left hemispace. Thus not only is the research Fischler reviews of great interest with respect to constraints on resource allocation in the normal brain, but it bears directly on behavioral rehabilitation in brain-injured patients.

Finally, Crosson reviews language function in relation to attentional processes and verbal working memory. These two chapters bear on precisely the domains reviewed by Fischler, but from completely different perspectives—those of neuropsychology and functional imaging. At the same time that we are reminded of the richness of the scientific data in these various fields, we are confronted with the disparity between them and the difficulty of bringing them together in a fruitful way.

In Part V, the concluding section of the book, Kearns's chapter provides a remarkably succinct and lucid update of his influential book on single-subject experimental design (McReynolds & Kearns, 1983). Single-subject experimental design, now a mature and highly sophisticated discipline, constitutes the bedrock for evidence-based medicine in language rehabilitation.

The authors of this book include speech pathologists (one now also an innovative statistician), neurologists, neuropsychologists, a cognitive psychologist, and even an anthropologist. We hope that this book fully demonstrates the value of intensive and extensive multidisciplinary collaboration. Many of the contributors are past students and present colleagues and friends of Kenneth M. Heilman. The disparate scientific fields represented and points of view expressed in this volume exemplify the scientific eclecticism that Ken has always enthusiastically endorsed. The diverse backgrounds of the authors, most of whom have spent time in Gainesville, bear strong testimony to Ken's commitment to including everyone in the fun of joint scientific inquiry and his implicit belief that investigative opportunities can only be enhanced by including yet another person with another point of view, however different. The names of many of the authors on large numbers of the studies reviewed reflect the gift for experimental design that Ken has been so successful in passing on to many of his students. The neuroscientific dimension that threads through this book honors Ken's constant efforts to relate behavior to neuroanatomy and principles of neural function. The commitment to rehabilitation expressed in this volume parallels Ken's constant concern for improving the lives of the patients he has cared for over many years. It is for these reasons that this work is dedicated to him.

STEPHEN E. NADEAU
LESLIE J. GONZALEZ ROTHI
BRUCE CROSSON

REFERENCES

Coslett, H. B. (1999). Spatial influences on motor and language function. *Neuropsychologia, 37,* 695–706.

Coslett, H. B., Schwartz, M. F., Goldberg, G., Hass, D., & Perkins, J. (1993). Multi-modal hemispatial deficits after left hemisphere stroke. *Brain, 116,* 527–554.

Kertesz, A., & McCabe, P. (1977). Recovery patterns and prognosis in aphasia. *Brain, 100,* 1–18.

Lee, A. J., Huber, J., & Stetson, W. B. (1996). Post stroke rehabilitation in older Americans: The Medicare experience. *Medical Care, 34,* 811–825.

Mayo, N. E. (1993). Epidemiology and recovery. In R. W. Teasell (Ed.), *Long term consequences of stroke: State of the art reviews in physical medicine* (pp. 1–25). Philadelphia: Hanley & Belfast.

McReynolds, L. V., & Kearns, K. P. (1983). *Single-subject experimental designs in communicative disorders.* Baltimore: University Park Press.

Paolucci, S., Antonucci, G., Gialloretti, L. E., Traballesi, M., Lubich, S., Pratesi, L., & Palombi, L. (1988). Predicting stroke inpatient rehabilitation outcome: The prominent role of neuropsychological disorders. *European Neurology, 36,* 385–390.

Richards, K., Singletary, F., Koehler, S., Crosson, B., & Rothi, L. J. G. (2000, February). *Treatment of nonfluent aphasia through the pairing of a non-symbolic movement sequence and naming.* Paper presented at the annual meeting of the International Neuropsychological Society, Denver, CO.

Stineman, M. G., Maikslin, G., Fiedler, R. C., & Granger, C. V. (1997). A prediction model for functional recovery in stroke. *Stroke, 28,* 550–556.

Sudlow, C. L. M., & Warlow, C. P. (1997). Comparable studies of the incidence of stroke and its pathological types: Results from an international collaboration. *Stroke, 28,* 491–499.

Wyller, T. B., Sveen, U., Sodring, K. M., Pettersen, A. M., & Bautz-Holter, E. (1997). Subjective well-being one year after stroke. *Clinical Rehabilitation, 11,* 139–145.

CONTENTS

APHASIA AND LANGUAGE

PART I

Beginnings

1

APHASIA: A HISTORICAL PERSPECTIVE

HEIDI L. ROTH
KENNETH M. HEILMAN

This chapter highlights how the concepts central to our understanding of aphasia today have developed since ancient times, and particularly over the last two centuries. Not only does the history of aphasia provide us with insight into our current understanding of aphasia; it also provides us with an opportunity to review the localization debates of the 19th century, which established some of the basic assumptions that have allowed scientists to continue to explore how higher mental functions relate to the brain. In addition, the history of aphasia is revealing of how methodologies influence the course of science, and how political and social milieus can change the reception of findings and shape efforts within a scientific field.

People have been aware since ancient times that brain injury can be associated with impairments of speech. The oldest recorded documentation is in an Egyptian surgical papyrus (see Breasted, 1930). The papyrus provides guidelines for how to treat victims of battle, depending on their injuries and symptoms, and includes two cases of head wounds to the temple that were associated with loss of speech. The papyrus was written in approximately 1600 B.C., but may be based on documents dating back as early as the 28th century B.C. Ancient Greek, Roman, and Hebrew writings also describe speech impairment associated with brain injury. Over the centuries since these writings, there have been continued reports of people who developed language impairments with brain injury. It was not, however, until the last two centuries that language impairment and its relation to the brain began to be studied more systematically.

EARLY VIEWS ON THE LOCALIZATION OF MENTAL FUNCTION, AND THE BACKGROUND AT THE BEGINNING OF THE 19TH CENTURY

The study of language in the 19th century developed in the context of a gradually changing view of how higher mental functions relate to the substance of the brain. The traditions that formed the backdrop for the different views on localization of mental functions during this time provide a perspective on how investigators in the 19th century broke with or were influenced by past conceptions. Several different views relating to the localization of higher mental functions were prevalent during this time. The medieval system of "faculty psychology," which originated with Namesius (4th century A.D.), had been the dominant model for the organization of psychological functions during medieval times (see Pagel, 1958; Clarke, 1962). It divided the mind into faculties, such as "perception," "reasoning," and "memory," which were each assigned to different locations in the ventricular system. The model was a modification and elaboration of the teaching of Herophilus of Alexandria (300 B.C.), who had also located mind functions in the ventricles. The ventricles seemed to ancient theorists to provide an especially attractive location for assignment of psychological functions, since, as cavities, they were regarded as not technically "material" in substance. The dynamic and space-filling characteristics of ventricular fluid seemed to better accommodate attributes often assigned to the mind, such as its ethereal nature and dynamic character. A well-respected anatomist of the 18th century, Soemmerring went so far as to try to use empirical evidence (by claiming that the nerves end at the edge of the ventricles) to locate the soul in the ventricular system (see Hagner, 1997, pp. 73–86).

On the basis of more careful experimental and anatomical work, anatomists of the 17th and 18th centuries built models locating mental functions more consistently in the substance of the brain (see Neuberger, 1897/1981). Thomas Willis (1621–1675) assigned the location of all mental functions to the cerebrum, of vegetative functions to the cerebellum, and of motor functions to the corpus striatum. Albrecht von Haller (1708–1777), who studied the excitability of the nervous system, suggested that the entire white matter might work as an integrated mass to support mental activity (Haller, 1755/1936). This extraordinary conclusion derived from his experiments in which he found that the white matter appeared to be "irritable," whereas the cortex was not. The medulla and basal ganglia were exceptions to Haller's communal system model of brain function. Based on his results, he came to view the medulla as dedicated to supporting the basic vital element for life, and the ganglia, as responsible for vegetative functions.

In the 19th century, the legacy of Descartes and religious doctrine worked against the localization concept (see Harrington, 1987; Hagner, 1997). Descartes's dualistic model of mind and body denied the mind any materializability or localizability. Descartes regarded the pineal gland as the location for the interface between the mind and the material world. In the pineal gland, sensory impressions were thought to be translated into behavior, and the soul could influence behavior at that point. However, the soul was still believed to exist somewhere beyond the pineal gland, since it was viewed as not material in nature or localizable. Religious leaders who confidently believed in immortality, the fundamental difference between animals and humans, and free will argued variously that the material concept of mind had to be faulty, since it could not be reconciled with these beliefs. These leaders regarded the soul or mind as of a different nature than the brain, because the brain, as a material substance, is subject to dissolution and decay, whereas they viewed the soul and mind as having the capacity for immortality. Religious doctrine posited important differences between animals and humans, related to immortality and the soul. The fact that evidence was accumulating that the brains of animals and humans are unexpectedly similar made some people believe it even less likely that the mind or the soul could be located in the brain. Localization of mental function in the brain was also seen as potentially jeopardizing free will. If the brain were to be accepted as the location of the mind, constraints on human behavior would not be as easily separable from laws governing the material world. Without free will, there could no longer be notions of responsibility or choice in decision making, and the basis of morality could be threatened.

THE EMERGENCE OF LOCALIZATION OF LANGUAGE
FUNCTION IN THE 19TH CENTURY: FROM GALL TO BROCA

Despite the dominant religious and philosophical views of the early 19th century, Franz Joseph Gall (1810–1819, 1822–1825, 1835) introduced a conception of psychology based on detailed localization of mental function in the brain, which later became known as "phrenology" (see Young, 1970/1990 for Gall's work and the legacy of phrenology; also Harrington, 1987; Hagner, 1997; Finger, 1994; Clarke & Jacyna, 1987). Gall's view went far beyond the localization of brain function advanced by other anatomists of the 18th and early 19th centuries. Many of Gall's claims seemed to be based on what we would now call pseudoscience and speculative conjecture, but his underlying assumption that all higher-level psychological faculties could be located within the specific structure of the brain was revolutionary and provided a framework that inspired scientists to look for the biology underlying mental function. Gall's basic assumptions were that all of psychology or individual personality could be divided into a certain core group of functions, located in different parts of the brain. This differed from previous attempts to link mental functions with regions of the brain, because in those attempts only the most general and basic faculties (such as "reasoning" and "perception") were localized. Gall posited that the mental capacities could be localized to different areas on the surface of the brain, and that the larger the size of the region corresponding to a particular function, the more developed that function would be. In addition, he claimed that the differences in protrusions on the skull between individuals could correspond to differences in the development of the underlying brain regions. Through the method of palpating the skull, one could determine which brain regions and corresponding faculties were most developed, and could thus explain an individual's personality.

Although Gall was an esteemed anatomist in his own right, and one of the first to distinguish between the gray and white matter of the brain, the evidence supporting his localization of higher mental functions to different regions on the surface of the brain and skull was criticized for its anecdotal and speculative nature. For example, he placed verbal memory in the anterior region of the brain, corresponding on the skull surface to protrusions in the region of the forehead, because he had noted that a childhood classmate who had bulging eyes and a protruding forehead had been very good at memorizing. Such observations were then reinforced over the course of his life by others of a similar nature. Gall was more tentative in his claims about whether the protruding portions on the average person's skull could always be understood to correspond to underlying anatomical differences. One of his students, Johann Caspar Spurzheim (1776–1832), developed a popularized version of the theory in which mostly positive psychological faculties were featured, and the skull bumps were advertised more confidently as reflections of the underlying brain organization associated with these faculties.

Gall's claims about the biological basis for the organization of mental functions in the brain directly influenced key figures of the 19th century, who were eventually to show that language could indeed be localized in the brain. (For this reason, the timeline we have provided in Figure 1.1 begins with Gall.) However, in the first half of the century there was great opposition to this view, originating mostly with those who believed that the mind could not be divided or localized, for the religious and philosophical reasons noted above. These sentiments were also strongly fueled by the political establishment in continental Europe, which had vested interests in the Catholic church, and in France by most thinkers' special allegiance to the philosophy of their countryman Descartes. Furthermore, the evidence for Gall's theory and for later claims made by those supporting localization of brain

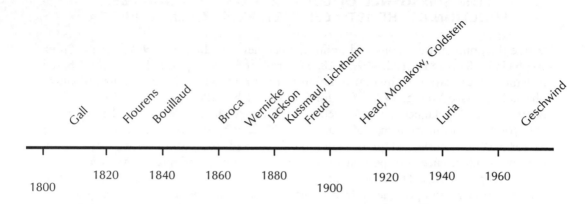

FIGURE 1.1. Timeline for the history of aphasiology.

Major contributors to aphasiology:

Early 1800s:	Gall, Flourens
Early to mid-1800s:	Bouillaud
Mid-1800s:	Broca
Mid- to later 1800s:	Wernicke
Late 1800s:	Jackson, Lichtheim, Kussmaul, Freud
Early 1900s:	Head, Monakow, Goldstein
Mid- to later 1900s:	Luria, Geschwind

Major events in neuroscience:

Magendie and Bell, 1822: Anterior and posterior nerve roots of the spinal cord have different functions.

Fritsch and Hitzig, 1870: Localized cortical stimulation of motor function.

functions during this time could not compete with the standards of evidence created by the new experimentalists in biology. This further undermined Gall's influence.

The work of Jean Pierre Flourens (1794–1867), who became the most important and influential figure to oppose Gall in France, exemplifies the manner in which political and religious forces, as well as methodological factors, worked to influence the acceptance of ideas in this time (see Harrington, 1987; Clarke & Jacyna, 1987; Young, 1970/1990; Finger, 1994; Hagner, 1997). Flourens, in his early career, spoke with admiration of Gall's ideas on localization. However, when Georges Cuvier, who opposed the views of Gall, became Flourens's patron, Flourens began to distinguish his work on localization from that of Gall. Throughout his career, Flourens's anatomical and experimental work was oriented toward exploring the localization of function in the nervous system. He eventually made important contributions to the characterization of the "vital node" in the medulla, and to the function of the cerebellum, to which he attributed all specific motor abilities (Flourens, 1851, 1824). When it came to higher-level mental functions, however, Flourens did not find evidence that they could be localized, at least not on the piecemeal basis suggested by Gall. In Flourens's experiments, which were mostly performed on birds, he successively removed portions of the birds' brains and did not find that their behavior was changed specifically in any way. As more and more of the brains of the birds were removed, they could still perform the same functions, but they had less spontaneous energy and gradually became less responsive. Flourens (1824) concluded that the function of the cerebrum (as distinguished from the medulla and cerebellum) was to perform mental functions as an integrated whole, and that there could be no division of mental capacities into separate locations or functions. Flourens (1845/1846) later specifically attacked Gall's view on localization of mental functions. One of his arguments relied heavily on introspective knowledge of the mind as a unified whole (i.e., on how one recognizes the *moi* or "self"). He also made arguments against Gall based on the problems Gall's theory posed for the notions of immortality and free will. Flourens's stature was secured not only because his ideas and observations accorded with the conservative political and religious notions of the day, but also because of the way in which his observations could be replicated by those of others, and met what were perceived as modern standards of science.

Gall had been forced early in his career to leave his home country of Austria, where in 1802 his lectures were banned, due to the potentially destabilizing political implications of his views. Many European countries at this time were especially wary of any views that might challenge authority or religion, since they wanted to protect themselves from the revolutionary activity that had begun in France over a decade earlier. After leaving Austria, Gall lectured widely in Europe, until deciding to settle in France in 1807. Unfortunately for Gall, Napoleon was attempting a reconciliation with the Catholic church, and religious doctrines had again become important to the government. The philosophical views of Descartes also held sway in the official philosophy in France, called "eclecticism," which relied heavily on rational reflection to determine which philosophical views should be considered valid. However, there were other philosophical movements in France that had more affinity with Gall's view. Specifically, the sensationalists, who were represented by such figures as Cabanis and de Tracy, viewed the mind as a product of material and natural substance and rejected the dualistic view. They regarded the mind as a product of the accumulation of sensations (or perceptions) from experiences in the outside world, impressed upon the material substance of the brain. Although Gall believed that the basis of mind was material, he differed from the sensationalists in that he viewed mental functions as innate, as products of the organization of the brain, and as independent of experience gained from accumulated sensations.

In academic circles Gall's teaching in France was strongly rejected, mostly for the reasons represented by Flourens. However, there were a few within the scientific establishment, chiefly from within the field of clinical medicine, who seemed to be able to ignore the dominant political and academic opinion and to present evidence in support of the view that mental functions could be specifically localized in the brain. Most notable among them was Jean Baptiste Bouillaud (1825, 1847–1848), who was one of the founding members of the Paris Phrenology Society, established 3 years after Gall's death in 1828. On the basis of clinical-pathological correlations, Bouillaud eventually accumulated over 100 clinical cases supporting the location of the control of speech in the anterior portion of the brain. Without much success, Bouillaud stubbornly continued to promote the concept of anterior brain localization of language function for over 35 years, long after Gall's death. In 1848, Bouillaud was so convinced of this localization that he went so far as to offer a reward to anyone who could show him a case of a person with a deep frontal lesion without a disturbance in the faculty of speech. Claims such as Bouillaud's were not received with much enthusiasm or interest in the French community, in part because they seemed to be associated with the teaching of Gall—whose ideas, especially in the scientific community, had fallen into general discredit. Bouillaud's findings, like Gall's, could also be criticized on the basis of what were considered to be the scientific standards for biology of the time. With the work of the new physiologists and Flourens, it seemed that one should be able to expect greater reliability, replicability, and precision than seemed to be possible for the clinical-pathological studies of Bouillaud. Even though Flourens's interpretation of his findings in birds might well have been questioned, his observations met the standards of the new experimentalist creed, because they could be replicated by others who followed his same experimental procedures. Bouillaud was working with clinical subjects, in whom variables could not be as completely controlled. Patients would not necessarily all have lesions in exactly the same location, and as a consequence, his findings could not show as perfect a correlation. Even physicians who used the clinical-pathological method of investigation, such as Andral, Cruvellier, and Lallemand, sided against Bouillaud's conclusions because they had observed too much variability among their patients with respect to language disturbance and brain localization to feel that such definite conclusions were warranted. Although Bouillaud had accumulated many cases of patients with language disturbance associated with anterior brain damage, these investigators could not ignore other cases that did not seem to fit the pattern.

Finally, in 1861, the tide turned toward those who were trying to localize language in the brain. In that year, Paul Broca published an article that drew widespread attention from the medical community in France and abroad. In this article he associated loss of the faculty of articulate speech with destruction of the posterior portions of the second and third frontal convolutions. Subsequently, after studying additional cases, he narrowed the localization to the third frontal convolution. In his 1861 article, he described the case of a patient, M. Leborgne, who had been nicknamed "Tan" by other patients because one of the few words he was able to utter was "Tan." Despite "Tan's" limited verbal repertoire and limited ability to write, he did not seem to have difficulty understanding what was said to him, which suggested to Broca and others that his "general intelligence" was intact despite his speech problem. He was also able to use gestures and speech intonation to communicate. This case was thought to provide a relatively clear-cut case of speech disturbance. "Tan" also had some motor impairment on the right side of his body, but this had developed 10 years after the onset of his speech impairment and was therefore thought to be somewhat independent of it. When Broca examined "Tan's" brain after he died, he found that it harbored a cystic lesion approximately the size of an egg in the anterior left hemisphere; the lesion involved the inferior portions of the frontal lobe, as well as portions of the insula, corpus striatum, and anterior superior temporal lobe. Although the affected brain areas were extensive, Broca argued that the injury to the third frontal convolution in the inferior frontal lobe was likely to have been most important for "Tan's" speech problem, since this area seemed to be the oldest area involved pathologically, and the patient's first problem had been with speaking. Six months later, Broca had the opportunity to examine the brain of a second patient with speech loss, M. Lelong, and to confirm his previous localization. In M. Lelong's case, the third frontal convolution was most affected, and there was less damage to other areas.

In his original articles, Broca (1861, 1863) referred to the impairment of speech production in these cases as "aphemia." He distinguished, as Bouillaud had, between a general capacity for internal language and the inability to use "external speech" or produce speech sounds. The faculty that had been damaged in these cases, according to Broca, was the ability to produce "articulate speech," which could occur in the absence of impairment in internal language. The term "aphemia" was later replaced by "aphasia," over Broca's protests, because a Greek physician who was assisting another influential neurologist, Armand Trousseau, had told Trousseau that in modern Greek *aphemia* meant "infamy" (Trosseau, 1864; Ryalls, 1984). According to Greek word roots, the term "aphemia" was a more accurate characterization, but the influential Trousseau's opinions held sway and the term "aphasia" subsequently prevailed. The language disturbance associated with the lesion in the third frontal convolution that was described by Broca, characterized by reduced verbal output, halting, effortful speech, impaired writing, and repetition, but spared comprehension, has subsequently been called "Broca's aphasia."

One might wonder why Broca's announcement was met with such enthusiasm while Bouillaud, who had promoted a similar view of language localization, was for so long ignored (Harrington, 1987). Among the reasons for this was the greater political liberalization that had occurred in France in the more than 30 years since Gall's death. Attesting to this liberalization was the fact that the Anthropological Society, which was headed and founded by Paul Broca in 1859, had emerged as a scientific society even while it was known for its left-wing and anticlerical views. Young scientists in the 1860s were also more committed to a positivistic scientific view of biology in which biological phenomena, like those of physics, were thought to be best understood through the division of material structure into parts. Successes in biology, such as that of the "cell theory" of Virchow, had bolstered the contention that the positivistic approach could provide insight into animate systems. A key discovery by Magendie (1822) and Bell (1811) played a crucial role in extending this line of thinking to the nervous system. In 1822, Magendie reported his experiments in dogs that established the existence of the sensory and motor divisions of spinal cord nerve roots. This discovery demonstrated quite dramatically that functional specialization in the nervous system can correspond directly to anatomical structures.

In this changed political, philosophical, and scientific climate, the search for material underpinnings to higher mental function seemed more acceptable, and those in the Anthropological Society, like Broca, found themselves in a community that was especially committed to materialistic explanations. Broca's investigation was actually prompted specifically by a debate that erupted on the floor of this society about whether specific intellectual functions could be localized to particular portions of the brain ("Discussion sur le volume et la forme du cerveau," 1861). The distinguished anatomist, Pierre Gratiolet, had been discussing how racial differences in cerebral volume might relate to differences in intellectual function. The question of whether particular intellectual functions might be localized in different regions of the brain was raised, and Gratiolet confessed his belief that different intellectual functions could not be separately localized. Ernest Aubertin, who was Bouillaud's son-in-law and was sympathetic to Bouillaud's persistent attempts to show that language was localized in frontal regions of the brain, spoke up against Gratiolet. In addition to making reference to Bouillaud's many cases, Aubertin, at a later session of the Anthropological Society, gave his own observation of a patient who had a skull lesion that exposed the brain. Whenever a metal implement was inserted into a cavity in the anterior brain, the patient lost his ability to speak. Aubertin argued that if a single intellectual capacity could be localized in the brain, it would establish the principle of localizability of mental function in the brain. In a gesture reminiscent of his father-in-law, he declared that he would abandon the claim for localization of language function in the brain if it were shown that a particular patient he had known did not have a lesion in the frontal lobes. Broca happened to have the patient "Tan" on his hospital service at the time. "Tan" had cellulitis of the leg. Broca contacted Aubertin, and they both agreed that "Tan" might be a good case to determine whether the claim about language localization was true. Broca was able to study the brain quite soon thereafter, because "Tan" died of gangrene only 6 days later.

Although there were several reasons why the reception of findings regarding localization of language might have been more favorable at the time of Broca's report, and several reasons why people might have been more willing to investigate these issues at this time, there were also several features of Broca's 1861 report that distinguished it from earlier reports. First, in contrast to previous reports, he paid much greater attention to describing the clinical deficits. Thus it was much clearer what particular aspects of language and intellectual function were at issue. In addition, he described with much greater precision the extent of the brain lesions (although Leborgne's brain was never sectioned). Broca's claim that it was not simply the anterior lobes in general that were responsible for speech production, but that speech could be localized to a specific area of the frontal lobes, further reinforced the impression that his study was more accurate and differed from previous reports. The legitimacy of Broca's study may also have been furthered by his careful efforts to dissociate his work from phrenology, which also localized verbal capacities to the anterior portion of the brain. For example, in the conclusion of his 1861 paper, Broca emphasized that his method of localization by convolution "cannot be reconciled by any system of bumps" (Broca 1861/1960, p. 147).

Shortly after Broca's initial case, reports began to accumulate suggesting that language function might be more often located in the left hemisphere. In 1863 Broca reported that eight cases of speech loss he had accumulated had all been associated with left-hemisphere lesions. Later the same year, a Parisian physician, Jules Parrot, reported a patient who had complete destruction of the third frontal convolution of the right hemisphere, but did not have any associated speech impairment (Atrophie, etc. 1863). Gustav Dax (1865/1974) reported to the Academy of Medicine that his deceased father, Marc Dax, who had been a country doctor, had collected over 40 cases of speech loss and that all had been associated with left-hemisphere damage. From today's point of view, the concept that language can be asymmetrically represented in the cerebral hemispheres seems a small step once the principle of localization is accepted. However, cerebral asymmetry represented a different challenge from localization to scientists of that day.

Gall (1822) had promoted the concept of localization of mental functions earlier, but believed that these mental functions were localized symmetrically on each side of the brain, so that if one side were injured the other side could compensate for the injury. Xaviar Bichat (1805) had argued that organs subserving interaction with the environment had to have a duplicate form, each component of the pair subserving interactions involving one side of the body. This provided a mechanism for the organism to integrate information from the two sides of the body in order to produce coordinated function. It would be especially important for the cerebral hemispheres, which were thought to house the soul and mind, to be able to interact equally with the different sides of the environment, and to be able to integrate information from both sides of the body. When the hemispheres were asymmetric, Bichat suggested, maladaptive behavior would be the result.

Broca and his contemporaries struggled to find an explanation for left-sided language dominance and generated a variety of hypotheses to explain the dominance (for a more detailed discussion of the history of concepts of cerebral asymmetry, see Harrington, 1987). Bouillaud, in defense of Dax's submission to the Academy of Medicine regarding hemispheric asymmetry in language function, raised the analogy with handedness ("Discussion sur la faculte," 1864–1865, p. 843). Baillarger more specifically suggested that handedness might be related to hemispheric dominance in language ("Discussion sur la faculte," 1864–1865, pp. 851–852). Gratiolet (1839–1857) had reported that the frontal portion of the left hemisphere develops before the right, and Baillarger suggested that dominance might be related to asymmetries of hemispheric development. Finally, in 1865, Broca published his formal reflections on the cerebral asymmetry associated with language. His thesis carefully preserved Bichat's principle of symmetry in the cerebral hemispheres, but he described this symmetry as extending only to the biological substrate of the hemispheres before development. Expanding upon the developmental hypothesis of Baillarger, and making reference to the findings of Gratiolet, Broca argued that language asymmetry could arise during development—an argument he also used to account for hand preference.

Whereas Broca suggested that people with left-hand preference might have language localized in the right hemisphere (because the right hemisphere might have developed earlier than the left in these cases), he also noted that language dominance was more variable in left-handers than in right-handers—an observation that has later been proven to be true. Elaborating on his thesis of developmental asymmetry, Broca suggested that in cases in which there was unilateral brain damage during development, speech capacity could develop on the remaining good side. Later in his life, Broca claimed hemispheric asymmetry to be a mark of advanced species. The asymmetry developing in response to the environment, he asserted, tends to occur in those species with greater adaptive ability. This adaptive ability allows humans to develop beyond their initial neurobiological symmetry (Harrington, 1987, pp. 63–67).

THE DEVELOPMENT OF INFORMATION-PROCESSING MODELS: WERNICKE AND THE GERMAN SCIENTIFIC CLIMATE

The next important event in the history of aphasia was the publication in 1874 of Carl Wernicke's paper "The Aphasia Symptom Complex: A Psychological Study on an Anatomical Basis" (Wernicke, 1874/1977). Wernicke's article represented a new stage in the integration of anatomical, physiological, and clinical observations.

The scientific climate in Germany at the time Wernicke published his paper was not conducive to clinical-pathological correlative studies, and therefore such studies were not met with much interest (see Hagner, 1997, for discussion of German scientific milieu). The Germans at that time were more focused on experimental physiology. Even Paul Broca's reports about language function had not been as influential as in France, partly for this reason. The dominance of a physiological approach can be attributed to the success of German physiologists, including Johannes Mueller and Hermann Helmholtz, who had made physiological studies the standard against which scientific biological research was measured. In addition to being easier to replicate, studies in experimental physiology seemed to provide a way to establish concrete principles with a more dynamic character, and thus a better basis for explaining biological phenomena. Clinical-pathological studies of language had also been criticized by German linguists and psychologists, who found the clinical descriptions of language deficits in these studies to be inadequate. In 1874, shortly before Wernicke's publication, the approaches to the study of aphasia were debated at a meeting of the Berlin Society for Anthropology, Ethnology, and Ancient History, under the direction of Rudolf Virchow (Hagner, 1997, 279–293). The limits of physiological experimentation, linguistic analysis, and clinical case reports were weighed against one another. Heymann Steinthal, a linguist, challenged clinicians to make more sophisticated distinctions in their descriptions of language problems. A prominent physician, Carl Westphal, agreed that physicians had not adequately considered the complexity of language disturbances in case descriptions, but he also criticized linguists' systems for understanding language. The linguists' systems, he charged, could not account for the complexity of language disturbances that were apparent clinically. In Germany, the bias against clinical-pathological studies of language came more from methodological concerns than in France, where philosophical forces played more of a role.

Wernicke's 1874 report satisfied the demands of both physiologists and psychologists, and established a more powerful framework for the clinical-pathological study of language. From the physiological side, Wernicke's report explained the development of the brain centers responsible for speech in terms of a reflex arc connecting sensory memory images to motor memories. Unlike the more primitive sensory–motor arcs operating as automatic reflexes, this higher-order arc could be controlled voluntarily. The particular anatomical principles that Wernicke used to support his model must be partly credited to Wernicke's mentor, the Viennese neuroanatomist Theodor Meynert. Meynert had been the first to distinguish between association and projection fibers in the brain, and had emphasized how the anatomical networks supported by the association fibers could provide the basis for higher mental function (Lesky, 1976). Wernicke had also familiarized himself with concepts developed in the field of linguistics. Wernicke's paper was a fusion of anatomy and function, and was hailed with great enthusiasm by the scientists of his time. Although the report by Fritsch and Hitzig (1870/1960) of the effects of electrical stimulation of the motor cortex in dogs was recognized internationally as a landmark discovery, and revealed that there is localization of elemental functions in the cerebrum, it was not until Wernicke's report that physiology and anatomy were brought together to help explain complex behaviors like language.

Wernicke's was the first in a series of information-processing models of language developed in Germany. These models mapped language functions onto interconnected brain structures, and succeeded in associating specific language deficits with localized brain damage to one part of the interconnected systems. Henry Head (1926), who was a proponent of a neurodynamic approach to aphasia, called the physicians who developed this influential approach "diagram makers." Head and others criticized this approach as too simplistic, but the information-processing approach has heuristic value and has proven of enormous utility in enabling investigators to generate a priori hypotheses and test them against observed behavior. To understand the origins of the modern classification scheme for aphasia, it is useful to review the models that were generated in this way and that even today provide good bases for understanding aphasic syndromes. Wernicke's paper was important, beyond the methodological breakthrough it represented, for establishing the classification of sensory aphasia or "Wernicke's aphasia." It also predicted the syndrome of conduction aphasia, and clearly distinguished both sensory and conduction aphasia from Broca's aphasia.

WERNICKE'S MODEL: WERNICKE'S APHASIA, BROCA'S APHASIA, AND CONDUCTION APHASIA

In Wernicke's model, there are two main language centers in the brain (see Figure 1.2, section i, left). In the anterior third frontal convolution there is the area identified by Broca, or Broca's area, which is responsible for the type of language disturbance described by Broca and his colleagues. With disruption in this area, also called the frontal operculum, patients have markedly impaired ability to produce words, and their speech production is effortful and halting. In general, comprehension of words is relatively spared. In the posterior region of the superior temporal gyrus, near the primary auditory cortex, is a second language center, described by Wernicke. Disruption of this center produces fluent speech, but the speech does not have meaningful communicative content. It is characterized by distortions of words, including paraphasic errors and neologisms. These patients are often unaware of their deficits, and in contrast to patients with Broca's aphasia, they have severely reduced ability to comprehend speech. This syndrome of aphasia later came to be referred to as "Wernicke's aphasia."

In addition to describing a new form of aphasia and a new center in the brain associated with language processes, Wernicke placed the aphasias in a more general explana-

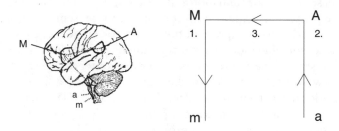

i.   **Wernicke's arc**

ii.   **Schematic of Lichtheim's model**

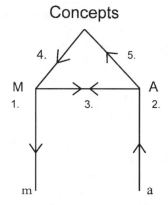

iii.   **Schematic of Kussmaul's model**

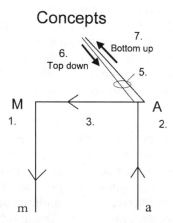

FIGURE 1.2. "A" represents the center for the memory of auditory images of words, also called the phonological lexicon, or "Wernicke's area." "M" represents the center for the memory of motor images of words, or the center for motor programs of speech, also called "Broca's area." The afferent branch, a → A, transmits acoustic impressions to A. The efferent branch, M → m, conducts impulses from M to the muscles for articulation. The "Concepts" center contains knowledge of the meaning of words and is also called the "semantic field." Disruption at 1 causes Broca's aphasia. Disruption at 2 causes Wernicke's aphasia. Disruption at 3 causes conduction aphasia. The integrity of Wernicke's arc, a → A, A → M, M → m, is necessary for repetition of words. Disruption at 4 in ii, Lichtheim's model, causes transcortical motor aphasia. Disruption at 5 causes transcortical sensory aphasia. Disruption at 6 in iii, Kussmaul's model, causes anomia. Disruption at 7 causes transcortical sensory aphasia with spared naming and spontaneous speech.

tory framework, based on sensory and motor divisions in the brain. According to Wernicke, the basic language-processing centers are more likely to represent basic functions related to elemental motor and sensory representations, and for language, these centers should represent the basic sensory and motor elements of language. Wernicke's area is the primary area responsible for storing the auditory representations of words, the auditory images, or the memory of how words sound. Wernicke's area is located adjacent to the primary auditory cortex, the location of which was identified by Meynert (1866). In contrast, Broca's area is postulated to contain representations of the motor images of words, or the memories of the motor operations necessary to produce sounds. Normal function of this language system requires the integrity of both the sensory and motor components, as well as the connections between them. In addition to providing a physiological explanation for the division of language into different centers, based on separation of sensory and motor components, Wernicke also introduced the concept that flow of information between centers can be important. From anatomical studies, Wernicke had seen fiber bundles running under the superior temporal gyrus. Phylogenetic and embryological studies suggested that the perisylvian gyri might come from a single gyrus. Wernicke therefore posited that these different centers in the perisylvian region might be connected and might all subserve a related function. The fiber bundle connecting the anterior Broca's region with the posterior Wernicke's region was subsequently identified as the arcuate fasciculus.

Patients with lesions in the posterior auditory association cortex or Wernicke's area, which stores the phonological representation of words (the phonological lexicon, sometimes now called the phonological input lexicon), cannot comprehend speech because they have lost their phonological lexical representations. Speech is fluent because Broca's area is still intact. Speech contains neologisms and phonemic paraphasic errors because output is unconstrained by lexical knowledge. Logorrhea (an increased tendency to speak) may be related to disinhibition of Broca's area and the impaired ability of the phonologic lexicon to monitor output. In addition, patients have impaired repetition and naming, presumably because both these tasks require processing involving the phonological lexicon.

Patients with Broca's type of aphasia understand speech because the phonologic lexicon is intact, but have great difficulty producing speech because they cannot convert the phonological lexical information stored in Wernicke's area into the correct speech sounds. Patients with Broca's aphasia, therefore, are nonfluent when attempting to speak spontaneously, and also have impaired repetition and naming because of their difficulty programming speech sounds.

Wernicke's model provided an explanation for the deficits associated with the observed syndromes and allowed him to predict a third type of aphasic syndrome, which would result if the flow of information between the two centers were disrupted. Wernicke predicted that patients with a disruption of the fibers connecting Wernicke's and Broca's areas should have a syndrome characterized by speech output that in certain respects resembles that seen with Wernicke's aphasia, but because the phonological lexicon is intact, the comprehension of auditory input should be preserved. Disruption of the connection between the phonological lexicon stored in Wernicke's area and the speech production center in Broca's area was postulated to result in the inaccurate transfer of phonological information to Broca's area, resulting in phonological paraphasic errors and inaccurate word forms. These patients, in contrast to patients with Wernicke's aphasia, should be aware of their speech errors because the intact phonological lexicon can monitor the speech produced. Patients should therefore be expected to try to correct their errors. After Wernicke predicted the deficits he expected to be associated with this disconnection, his predictions were supported by numerous reports. The term used for this aphasic syndrome is "conduction aphasia," or in the original German, *Leitungsaphasie*.

FURTHER CONTRIBUTIONS TO LOCALIZATION AND INFORMATION-PROCESSING THEORIES: KUSSMAUL'S AND LICHTHEIM'S MODELS

Later investigators were able to build on Wernicke's model. A few years after Wernicke's influential paper appeared, Adolf Kussmaul (1877) reported another language syndrome that could be fitted into Wernicke's scheme. This disorder, "pure word deafness," is characterized by an inability to understand speech with a preserved ability to read, speak, and name. Pure word deafness is caused by a lesion that isolates Wernicke's area from auditory input. These lesions often involve the left primary auditory cortex and projections from the right auditory cortex. These patients can read and name, because the visual system can still gain access to Wernicke's area (the phonological lexicon). And these patients can produce normal speech, because both Wernicke's area and Broca's area are intact and the connections between them are preserved.

Eleven years after Wernicke's publication, Ludwig Lichtheim (1885), in an influential paper published in *Brain*, reported two patients—one who could not comprehend and the other who was nonfluent, despite preserved repetition. Because Wernicke's language-processing model could not account for these symptom complexes, Lichtheim proposed a modification and expansion of Wernicke's model. Lichtheim's model contains at its core Wernicke's model, called "Wernicke's arc," which include's the following: the primary auditory cortex (which performs an auditory analysis of spoken words), the posterior superior temporal gyrus or Wernicke's area, the connection from Wernicke's area to the anterior perisylvian region, Broca's area, and projections from Broca's area to the primary motor cortex (for the generation of the muscle movements producing sound) (see Figure 1.2, section i, schematic at right). To this arc Lichtheim added a new module that stores the concepts or meaning of words, later called the "semantic field" (see Figure 1.2, section ii). This functional module was postulated to be anatomically distributed in the brain. The semantic field is connected to both Wernicke's and Broca's areas, but is outside the direct loop from Wernicke's to Broca's area. This modification and expansion of Wernicke's model provide an explanation for aphasias in which repetition is normal. When connections from Wernicke's area to the concept center are disrupted, comprehension is impaired, because a semantic analysis of words cannot be performed. However, repetition is spared, because auditory information can access Wernicke's area and be transmitted to Broca's area for production of speech. This disorder is called "transcortical sensory aphasia." In contrast, when connections between the concept center and Broca's area are disrupted, internally generated speech (spontaneous speech or naming) will be halting and effortful, as in Broca's aphasia. However, because Wernicke's arc is intact, repetition is normal. This type of aphasia is called "transcortical motor aphasia."

Lichtheim's model has been criticized for not being able to account for certain findings in aphasia—for example, the abnormal speech output seen in Wernicke's aphasia. In Lichtheim's model, a lesion of Wernicke's area should not disrupt spontaneous language, because the direct pathway from internal concepts (the semantic field) to Broca's area is preserved. Lichtheim explained the abnormal spontaneous language in Wernicke's aphasia by claiming that whenever Broca's area is activated, it automatically retrieves information form the phonological lexicon (Wernicke's area) when the connection between the two is intact. Therefore, disruption in the phonological lexicon will affect speech output even when speech originates from the semantic field and proceeds directly to Broca's area.

In Freud's (1891/1953) critical study of aphasia, he argued that Lichtheim's model cannot account for impaired repetition in conduction aphasia. In conduction aphasia, the direct connection between the phonological lexicon and Broca's area has been disrupted, but repetition should still be possible via the concept/semantic route. According to Lichtheim's model, repetition should be preserved—however, only for words with meaning. The repetition of nonwords or pseudowords (e.g., "flig," "blup"), which cannot be processed by the concept/semantic loop, should be impaired. The inability to repeat only nonwords had not been described in Freud's time, but patients with this specific inability have subsequently been identified. These patients cannot repeat nonwords but can repeat real words. When attempting to repeat nonwords, they may change them into real words. They can also make semantic errors when repeating real words. These symptoms can be explained if these patients are repeating using the concept/semantic loop, as Freud suggested, and as predicted by Lichtheim's model. This type of aphasia has been called "deep dysphasia" (Katz & Goodglass, 1990). According to Lichtheim's model, patients with deep dysphasia can repeat only real words because these can be processed through the concept route, whereas nonwords cannot be repeated because they are not represented in this route. The repetition of nonwords is dependent on the direct phonological route from Wernicke's to Broca's areas, which is disrupted. Patients with deep dysphasia do not make frequent phonological errors in repetition, because they are processing information through the concept route and therefore primarily make semantic errors.

Although there are problems with information-processing models, it is ironic that the one aspect of Lichtheim's model that Freud chose to highlight and criticize actually supports the model. Information-processing models have inherent problems, but they also have predictive power, can be useful for generating hypotheses, and can generate plausible explanations for syndromes observed.

Kussmaul (1877) proposed an alternative model to Lichtheim's (see Figure 1.2, section iii). Kussmaul's model does not explain transcortical motor aphasia but can explain other syndromes. In Kussmaul's model, the area of concepts can gain access to motor representations only via the phonological lexicon, or Wernicke's area. In Lichtheim's model (Figure 1.2, section ii), however, the concept semantic area is directly connected to Broca's area. In order for information to get from the concept area to the phonological lexicon, it must go through Broca's area. Kussmaul's model, in contrast, has a two-way connection between the concept/semantic area and Wernicke's area. Unlike Lichtheim's model, Kussmaul's model can account for an isolated naming disorder. While "anomia" is often a residual sign of many different forms of aphasia, it has also been demonstrated that anomia, in isolation, can occur after a discrete lesion. Patients with deficits in the concept/semantic field, in the phonological lexicon (Wernicke's area), or in the output production area (Broca's area) may be impaired at naming, but these patients also have deficits in other aspects of language, such as comprehension, repetition, or speech production. According to Kussmaul's model, isolated anomia should result when the concept/semantic field cannot activate the phonological lexicon (Wernicke's area) but the phonological lexicon can activate the concept/semantic area, thus enabling comprehension. It is the one-way disconnection or dissociation between semantic and phonological information that should specifically impair naming without affecting other aspects of speech. Kussmaul's model also predicts a complementary condition, in which the semantic field can access the phonological lexicon but the lexicon cannot access the semantic field. This prediction was confirmed by a report (Heilman,

Rothi, McFarling, & Rottman, 1981) describing a patient who had impaired comprehension, but intact repetition, naming, and spontaneous speech. Kussmaul's model, like Lichtheim's, can also explain transcortical sensory aphasia. This aphasia results when both pathways between Wernicke's area and the semantic field are disrupted, so that naming and spontaneous speech are affected as well as comprehension. In all these lexical–semantic access disorders, repetition is spared because Wernicke's arc remains intact.

Kussmaul and Lichtheim disagreed about whether the intactness of Broca's area and the connection between Broca's and Wernicke's areas are necessary for the activation of the phonological lexicon in spontaneous language. In Kussmaul's model, activation of the phonological lexicon by Broca's area is not necessary, because concepts can activate the phonological lexicon directly. However, for Lichtheim, the connection from Broca's area to Wernicke's area is vital for spontaneous speech, because there is no direct connection from the concept/semantic field to Wernicke's area and the phonological lexicon. In other words, in Lichtheim's model there is only a one-way, bottom-up connection from the phonological lexicon to the semantic field, so that in spontaneous speech originating from the semantic field, it is necessary for the phonological lexicon to be accessed from Broca's area. Lichtheim posited that if the concept/semantic field can directly access the phonological lexicon, contrary to his hypothesis, and does not require the detour through Broca's area, then a patient with Broca's aphasia should know how many syllables are in words that he or she is unable to produce. Lichtheim then studied patients with Broca's aphasia who were told to squeeze his hand for the number of syllables in words they were unable to produce. Because these patients could not correctly perform the task, Lichtheim felt that the results supported his view that access to the phonological lexicon is dependent on Broca's area. However, his interpretation of these results may have been incorrect. Syllable judgments may not be completely dependent on information contained in the phonological lexicon (Heilman, Tucker, & Valenstein, 1976). Knowledge about number of syllables in a word may depend upon articulation, and may be impaired when successful articulation of a word is impaired. A better test of the ability to access the phonological lexicon may be a test requiring homophone judgments. The judgment of homophones should more directly assess the knowledge contained in the phonological input lexicon. Such a homophone judgment test has been performed by patients with conduction aphasia, who have disruption of the pathway from Broca's area to the phonological lexicon (Feinberg, Rothi, & Heilman, 1986). In this study, patients were able to make correct judgments even when they were unable to vocalize words. According to Lichtheim's scheme, they should not be able to access the phonological lexicon because of the disruption of the connection between Broca's area and the phonological lexicon. This study provides more support for Kussmaul's model, in which the concept/semantic field can directly activate the phonological lexicon.

In contrast to Kussmaul's model, Lichtheim's model can account for transcortical motor aphasia, in which patients are nonfluent but comprehend and repeat normally. In Lichtheim's model the concept/semantic field is directly connected to Broca's speech production center, and transcortical motor aphasia may be explained by an inability of the concept/semantic field to access and activate Broca's area. Therefore, patients whose concepts cannot activate the speech production center should have difficulty initiating spontaneous speech. However, because the phonological lexicon can access the speech production system in Broca's area, repetition is intact, and because the lexicon can access the concept/semantic field, comprehension is also intact. In Kussmaul's model, the concept/semantic area is not directly connected to the production center, and is only connected by way of the phonological lexicon. Therefore, using Kussmaul's model, one cannot account for the person who has an intact Wernicke's arc and is able to comprehend and repeat but still has difficulty with production. Some investigators have suggested that transcortical motor aphasia is not a language impairment, but may be related to a deficit of the frontal intentional/motivational systems and the ability to activate concepts. However, in addition to being unable to provide an account for transcortical motor aphasia, Kussmaul's model cannot explain deep dysphasia with the impaired repetition of nonsense words. Lichtheim's model can account for deep dysphasia, because repetition can occur by an alternate route: Instead of Wernicke's area activating Broca's area directly, Wernicke's area accesses Broca's area indirectly through the concept/semantic field. This alternative route is impossible in Kussmaul's scheme, because the concept/semantic field is not directly connected to Broca's area.

Although there are problems with both Lichtheim's and Kussmaul's models, these diagrammatic information-processing models help explain clinical syndromes and guide research. Therefore, they should not be abandoned. The aphasia syndromes recognized today are often placed within the schematics provided by these early information-processing models, and the important distinctions between the different components of language assessed in modern neurological evaluation are based on the distinctions derived from these schemas. The perspectives of different models, despite their discrepancies, can work together to generate hypotheses that lead to modifications or more refined models with greater explanatory power.

THE ENGLISH SCIENTIFIC CLIMATE AND LATER FUNCTIONAL AND HOLISTIC APPROACHES

Broca, Wernicke, Lichtheim, Kussmaul, and other localizationists contributed much to our understanding of aphasia. In England, however, the study of aphasia was approached differently. To understand the English approach to the brain and neuropsychological function, it is important to consider the influence of philosophy and the reigning scientific paradigms (see Young, 1970). Like the continental Europeans, the English were influenced by the experimental success of physiologists, including Flourens, Magendie, Bell, and Mueller. They also initially based their models on the sensory–motor paradigm. Whereas continental neurologists developed increasingly complex models of speech and language processing based on their observations of aphasia, the English, in general, were more committed to how the reflex model fit in with the concepts of association or connectionist psychology. Association psychology had its philosophical roots in the English empiricist tradition. The English empiricist philosophers had argued that the mind is a product of sensory impressions derived from experience, rather than being composed of innate mental contents. According to philosophers such as John Locke, each person's mind starts out as a *tabula rasa* or "blank slate," and the sensory experiences that accumulate over one's lifetime combine to form the mental content. David Hartly, a strong proponent of this doctrine, tried to explain how all psychological faculties, including such capacities as imagination, understanding, will, and memory, could be reduced to the terms of repetitive associations between basic sensations and the memory of sensations. Alexander Bain, under the influence of Johannes Mueller, expanded this view to emphasize that not only sensory associations, but also connections between sensory inputs and motor outputs, are important. Evolutionary models, which were becoming increasingly popular in England in the latter part of the 19th century, also made use of the associationist doctrine. Many evolutionary models, including those of Darwin and especially Herbert Spencer, used association principles to explain how populations could acquire psychological characteristics (see, e.g., Darwin, 1871/1890, Ch. 3, and 1873). These models allowed for the mind to be a product both of experience gained through associations and of inherited structure.

The two Englishmen who most prominently contributed to aphasiology were John Hughlings Jackson (1835–1911) and Henry Head (1861–1940). Jackson briefly considered abandoning his medical career and neurology training to pursue philosophy. He was a contemporary of Broca and Wernicke, but had many differences of opinion with respect to how to approach the study of higher mental functions, including the study of aphasia. He was also aware of and admired Kussmaul's writings on aphasia. Jackson disagreed with Broca's and Wernicke's proposals that there are language centers. He was fundamentally averse to suggestions of discontinuity between basic processes and higher-level mental abilities. He was committed to referring to brain anatomy and mechanisms in terms of sensory and motor processes. This commitment was in large part generated and reinforced by the associationist principles of Alexander Bain and Herbert Spencer, to whom he acknowledged great intellectual debts.

In the journal *Brain*, which Jackson cofounded in 1878, he summarized many of his observations about aphasia in a series of reports entitled "On Affectations of Speech from Disease of the Brain" (Jackson 1878–1879/1915, 1879–1880/1915). Jackson emphasized the importance of the distinction between emotionally generated speech and propositional speech. He cited Baillarger and Broca as being the first to note that emotional speech may be preserved in patients who have otherwise very impaired verbal output, but in this article he elaborated on the implications of this for understanding the language system. Jackson rejected the view that specific brain centers are specialized for certain behaviors, and emphasized instead the complexity of motor system structure in the mediation of language. According to Jackson, it cannot be that aphasic patients have lost the ability to say certain words, because they can say these same words under different circumstances. For example, an aphasic person may not be able to answer simple questions with the words "yes" and "no," and yet spontaneously exclaim the word "no" when placed in an emotionally provocative situation. Jackson's observations led him to the conclusion that language and other behaviors are organized hierarchically in the brain. There is not necessarily a center responsible for all motor output for a particular behavior, but there may be various centers for different modes of this behavior. He distinguished the localization of "movements" in the brain from the more simplistic notion of localization of motor centers corresponding to activity in particular body parts. Jackson, influenced by Spencer's concepts of evolution and dissolution, suggested that the more sophisticated motor systems, which are higher on the evolutionary scale, are usually more closely associated with voluntary activity, and are generally damaged first in neurological disease. The higher motor centers are damaged first because, as the most evolutionarily advanced, they are the least well developed, incorporate the least redundancy, and therefore are the most susceptible to the effects of injury. Thus propositional speech, which is under more voluntary control, is damaged before emotional speech, which is more primitive and automatic. Jackson supported this concept with his observations on the organization of simpler motor behaviors. He noted that voluntary activation of a limb may not occur even while more automatic activity is still possible. Jackson influenced many subsequent investigators of biology–mind relationships. For example, the Russian neuropsychologist A. R. Luria (1973, 1962/1966) hailed Jackson's hierarchical approach to understanding the complexity of systems as an improvement over the concepts of the localizationists. Others influenced by Jackson include Henry Head, Sigmund Freud, and Kurt Goldstein.

Henry Head, who only became interested in Jackson's views on aphasia late in his career, began his work in neurology with study of the sensory system (Head, 1908, 1911, 1920). His approach to the study of the sensory system provides some insight into his later approach to the study of language. In his studies on sensation, he found that the commonly acknowledged divisions of sensation into cold, hot, light touch, and pin prick, could not always adequately account for the changes in sensation that occurred after injury, and he proposed two classes of sensation: "epicritic" and "protopathic." These designations have found further physiological support in subsequent investigations and are still in use today. His work on the sensory systems fostered his belief that it is not always expedient to think in terms of predefined or classical categories, and that sometimes it is important to consider the phenomenology afresh. In the field of language, Head (1926) strongly opposed the way in which the localizationists, with their information-processing models, divided language into particular language centers and functions. As noted earlier, he called them "diagram makers," and argued for a much broader view of language and its role in many types of mental function. In his studies, primarily of young soldiers injured in World War I, he did not find that symptoms fit well into the syndrome complexes described by Lichtheim and Wernicke. He therefore accused the localizationists of distorting their data to support their hypotheses. He was unaware, as was subsequently demonstrated, that young and old subjects with similar lesions may demonstrate different aphasic signs. Unhappy with the way language was tested in brain-damaged patients, he developed his own aphasia testing battery, which was more extensive and included testing of drawing skills and body orientation in space. Head divided aphasic disorders into four types: "verbal," "nominal," "syntactic," and "semantic." Three of these four types have features that map roughly onto the aphasia syndromes that have been described. For example, verbal aphasia has characteristics in common with Broca's aphasia, nominal aphasia has similarities to anomic aphasia, and syntactic aphasia is similar in some aspects to Wernicke's aphasia. The final type, semantic aphasia, was described by Head as a syndrome in which it is difficult for patients to understand the overall meaning of complex sentences and holistic spatial relationships. Head's overall theoretical schema was more linguistic than that of the localizationists, at the same time that he was less concerned about clinical-pathological correlations.

Henry Head is only one representative of a group of contributors to the study of aphasia in the late 1800s and early 1900s who placed more emphasis on the interdependency of speech and language dysfunction with other complex functions of the brain—a holistic approach. These investigators, although from many different countries, often acknowledged Jackson as a source of their inspiration.

One of the earliest figures who directly attacked the localizationists' view of aphasia was Sigmund Freud (1856–1939). From his psychoanalytic theories, one might have expected that Freud would have had very little interest in the biological basis of mental activities. However, early in his career he, like Wernicke, studied with Theodor Meynert and other neurologists who were attempting to understand the anatomical and physiological basis of the mind. He even devoted himself to something he called a "Project for a Scientific Psychology," in which he intended to establish a basis for all higher mental function using a model of sensory and motor units, which would interact according to laws of energy in physics. (For a discussion of Freud's early neuroscientific career, see Sulloway, 1979, 1992.) Although he was dissatisfied with the results of the project and later abandoned it, it attests to his early commitment to biologically based models. Freud's (1891/1953) monograph *On aphasia: A Critical Study*, which he wrote a few years prior to the time he became engaged in his ambitious scientific psychology project, carefully criticized the inadequacy of Wernicke's and Lichtheim's models of language, and outlined some of his own views about language organization and the brain. Freud claimed that Wernicke's and Lichtheim's models are internally inconsistent because they predict certain signs and symptoms that are not present in the clinical reports of the syndromes described. Although Freud did not fully abandon the aphasic classifications described by Wernicke and Lichtheim, in his alternative model of language he rejected the concept of speech centers and emphasized that language disturbances should always be understood as arising from disruption of connecting fibers. In Freud's model, the perisylvian area lying between Broca's area and Wernicke's area is designated as the speech area. Broca's area and Wernicke's area are significant because they are sources of connections to motor output and auditory input, respectively, but in themselves they do not contain specific "word memories." In Freud's model, connections to visual and tactile systems also border on the speech area. If any of the bordering regions of the speech area are disrupted, particular syndromes of language dysfunction occur that are related to the sensory or motor modality affected. As Freud saw it, the word, which is closely related to the idea of the concept, is the most important unit of language. This most basic aspect of language cannot be localized, but is constituted in complex connections in the speech area, in which kinesthetic, visual, somatosensory, and auditory elements all contributed. In addition to proposing a revised anatomical model to account for speech and language disturbances, Freud emphasized that certain types of language disturbance can only be understood according to a global hierarchical view of loss of function. According to Freud, when lesions incompletely disrupt connections to bordering areas, or when lesions are located in the center of the speech area, the language system responds in a hierarchical manner, in which first (with lesser degrees of damage), more voluntary aspects of speech are affected (spontaneous speech); second (with slightly more damage), stimulus-provoked aspects of speech are affected (repetition, object naming); and finally (with the most severe damage), all aspects of speech are affected. Freud was a great admirer of Jackson, who originally used hierarchical principles to understand brain injury. As Freud's theories in psychiatry developed, the role of language and hierarchical systems featured prominently, but he did not later attempt to make explicit connections to anatomical models. For this reason, among others, his view of aphasia and his interpretation of language as it relates to the brain, despite his worthy insights, have received less attention from later neurologists.

The views of Constantin von Monakow and Kurt Goldstein on brain organization also differed from those of the localizationists (see Harrington, 1996). Monakow, who was raised in Russia and moved as a 16-year-old to Switzerland, trained in neuroanatomy and engaged in neuroanatomical research in his early career. Monakow's careful early studies in the visual and auditory systems have been heralded by later investigators as providing a foundation for 20th-century thinking about the functional relations of the thalamus to the cerebral cortex. In his writings on higher mental function (Monakow, 1911/1960, 1914), his main contribution was to emphasize the importance of the interdependency of different regions in the nervous system. He introduced the term "diaschisis" to refer to the fact that damage in a localized area of the brain can change the balance in the interdependent brain systems, so that regions far away from the damaged location are also affected. In the process of recovery, the brain can achieve a new balance in which the areas that were remotely affected resume their ability to function in a new reorganized system. In a fashion reminiscent of Jackson's views, Monakow also posited that higher levels of brain organization are more vulnerable to disruption, whereas lower levels on the evolutionary or developmental scale are less susceptible to injury. This meant that information acquired more recently, on either the evolutionary or the developmental time scale, should be lost preferentially in the setting of injury, whereas information acquired in early life should be spared and may become relatively more prominent. Monakow's emphasis on how symptomatology can change over time, his explanation of this in terms of the function of areas remote from the location of damage, and his claim that certain aspects of function are more vulnerable (depending on their developmental and evolutionary history) provided perspectives on brain organization that could not be captured by the localizationists' information-processing models.

Kurt Goldstein was sympathetic to Monakow's ideas and promoted them later in his career. Like Jackson, he initially had to be dissuaded from a career in philosophy to enter medicine. He trained in neurology and worked with Carl Wernicke, with whom he maintained a lifelong friendship. Goldstein's ideas later in his life about the organization of language were not as closely tied to anatomy as were those of his mentor. After spending several years with patients injured in World War I, he became convinced that the manner in which neurological symptoms were categorized at that time did not capture the experience and struggle of patients. He was also interested in how these patients might be rehabilitated and recover from injury (Harrington, 1996). The period in which Goldstein was in Germany, under the Weimar government, was a time that was oriented toward reconciliation and the attempt to integrate older German traditions with newer ones. The time provided fertile ground for efforts oriented toward synthesis of romantic and mechanistic models. It was during this time that the Gestalt movement developed and, in turn, influenced Goldstein (see Harrington, 1996). Because Goldstein was Jewish, he was forced to flee Germany as the Nazis came to power in 1933, and later he moved to the United States. Like Monakow, Goldstein (1934/1995, 1948) emphasized that after local injury, the function of more widespread brain areas can be affected because of the interrelatedness of brain components. Goldstein also focused on how a person reacts to the loss of function and described what he called the "catastrophic reaction." Goldstein claimed that brain injury will often cause the loss of an ability to respond to the environment on an abstract level. In the absence of the ability to use the "abstract attitude" or produce "categorical behavior," patients will confront the environment on a concrete level and will tend to become stimulus-bound. According to Goldstein, when patients first encounter this failure to form the normal abstract attitude toward the environment, they experience a sense of anxiety or despair, which is the "catastrophic reaction." Goldstein argued that the language system is especially important for the ability to maintain an abstract attitude; therefore, its impairment causes the most widespread dysfunction and the most severe catastrophic reaction. Some of Goldstein's theory is reminiscent of Jackson's idea that brain injury most severely affects the highest-level, voluntary integrating or abstracting abilities. However, the concept of the "abstract attitude" emphasized by Goldstein did not seem useful to many clinicians and investigators, because it could be applied equally to any brain injury or brain system affected. Norman Geschwind (1964) was sympathetic to this view; he pointed out that Goldstein's more detailed analyses of particular syndromes used the localizationist approach, and that his actual descriptions of aphasic subtypes did not differ greatly from those of Wernicke and Lichtheim. Goldstein's original ideas regarding the "abstract attitude" and the process of recovery were better received in Germany than they were in the United States. Although not rejected outright, Goldstein's work, with its emphasis on subjective experience (the anxiety of the catastrophic reaction) and existentialist dilemmas, seemed less relevant to American scientists and practitioners of neurology of the time. This may have been partly due to the rising influence of behaviorism in America—a discipline that fundamentally eschewed consideration of subjective states.

THE MID-20TH CENTURY: WANING INTEREST IN APHASIA

Interest in aphasia, which had been prominent in neurology in the latter half of the 19th century and the first decades of the 20th century, waned in the middle of the 20th century. This may have been in part due to the shift in emphasis from anatomically grounded models toward more dynamic aspects of language dysfunction and language's role in more general mental operations, as emphasized by those who downplayed the importance of information-processing models (e.g., Head, Monakow, Goldstein). With the rise of these different approaches to language, localizationist models by default lost popularity, and were almost ignored for the 50 years from 1910 to 1960. It is important to note that those advocating a reorientation away from the localizationist models often ended up describing syndromes that fit into the categories promoted by these models. It might be more appropriate to understand this period as one in which there was a shift in perspective on aphasia. Aspects of aphasia were receiving consideration that were not explained by the localizationist models, including issues related to recovery, dynamic changes in remote parts of the brain, and patients' altered subjective experience. Norman Geschwind (1972) suggested that the new perspectives' downplaying the information-processing models' validity, combined with Henry Head's polemical attacks on the "diagram makers," left the impression on the scientific community that there was little consensus regarding the pathophysiology of language disturbances, even when in actuality many of these investigators agreed on basic anatomical explanations and classifications. Another factor that may have contributed to the decreased interest in aphasia research was the increased prominence of biochemical approaches in medical research. In contrast to the methods of biochemistry, the techniques used to study aphasia, such as clinical-pathological correlation and the generation of processing models, could seem technically less sophisticated and thus "unscientific." From the biochemical laboratory perspective, it seemed unlikely that higher-level aphasia research would lead to the discovery of important biological mechanisms. As Geschwind (1972) noted, aphasia research began to appear as "an exotic and unscientific activity suitable only for those with philosophical inclinations"(p. 755). Also reinforcing the disfavor surrounding the study of higher cognitive systems in neurology was the dominance of dynamic models in psychiatry, which promoted the view that biological and anatomical information was irrelevant to the understanding of behavior at the cognitive level. Finally, the models of behaviorist psychology of the time—which viewed the brain as a "black box" and emphasized the effects of the environment on behaviors—made neuroanatomically based explanations of behavior seem less important.

REKINDLING INTEREST IN APHASIA:
NORMAN GESCHWIND AND A. R. LURIA

In the 1960s, however, a resurgence of interest in aphasia occurred, in great part due to the efforts and contributions of Norman Geschwind and his colleagues Edith Kaplan, Harold Goodglass, and D. Frank Benson. About four decades ago, Geschwind and Kaplan evaluated a patient who had signs of callosal disconnection, including an inability to write or pantomime to command with the left hand or to name objects placed in the left hand. At the time they were evaluating this patient, Claude Quadfasel, a European-born and trained neurologist who had been a student of Kurt Goldstein, was working at the same hospital in the Boston area. Qaudfasel suggested to Geschwind that he review the classic European literature, which had already addressed callosal disconnection and provided localizationist and biologically based postulates for neurobehavioral disorders. Geschwind's review of this historical literature helped shape his career and his approach to aphasia. In 1962, Geschwind and Kaplan published the case of callosal disconnection, and in 1965 Geschwind published a two-part article, "Disconnexion Syndromes in Animals and Man." In these articles, Geschwind reviewed the historical contributions of the French, German, and English neurologists of the late 19th and 20th centuries, whose wealth of information and thoeries had been forgotten. In these articles and his later work, he demonstrated how higher levels of behavior could be analyzed in a systematic fashion. Geschwind's models in many cases were extensions of the 19th-century information-processing models, but they attempted to explain in a more differentiated way why particular aspects of language function may break down while others are preserved. For example, after reviewing Dejerine's original description of alexia without agraphia, Geschwind developed the model further and sought to explain how reading of numbers and naming of objects may be preserved, while the reading of words is impaired. In order to explain these dissociations, Geschwind discussed parallel systems and alternative pathways. He suggested that with brain injury, preserved functions may be mediated by alternative systems. Geschwind also used comparative anatomy to help explain the organization of language in humans. In Geschwind's view, one of the most basic requirements for language is the ability to name, which requires the association of objects or concepts with language symbols, specifically words. This corresponds to the association of perceptual representations (either unimodal or polymodal) with abstract, supramodal representations. Geschwind suggested that this capacity can be performed by humans because humans have greater capacity for supramodal representations in what are now referred to as "heteromodal association cortices." In animals, including subhuman primates, only the limbic system is capable of integrating information to create supramodal representations. Humans possess extralimbic supramodal association cortices, such as the dominant perisylvian cortex, that have the capacity for representation of abstract entities, such as words. Geschwind attempted to link function and anatomy closely, and thought that functional organization would be reflected in anatomical structure. Since the left posterior superior temporal lobe is dominant for language (storage of phonological lexical representations), Geschwind and Levitsky (1968) measured the size of the posterior portion of the superior temporal gyrus (the planum temporale or Wernicke's area). They found, in the majority of patients, that this area was larger on the left side than on the right side. This initiated an entire subfield of research oriented toward analyzing morphological–behavioral relationships. Geschwind's work initiated a renaissance in neuropsychology and behavioral neurology.

A second contemporary figure who played an important role in stimulating interest in aphasia and brain function was the Russian neuropsychologist and physician A. R. Luria. Luria's (1945/1970) book *Traumatic Aphasia* is filled with careful descriptions of a large number of World War II veterans who experienced language disturbances as a result of war-related injuries to the brain. Although the details of Luria's specific explanations of aphasic syndromes in most cases did not have as lasting an influence as those of the localizationists, he contributed methodological approaches to the study of aphasia and other neuropsychological disorders. In all of his major books, which include *Traumatic Aphasia* (1945/1970), *Higher Cortical Functions in Man* (1962/1966), and *The Working Brain* (1973), Luria emphasized the importance of understanding the modular structure of psychological functions. In order to determine how psychological functions are related to neuroanatomy, he advocated using a method based on the principle of double dissociation of function, initially introduced by Hans Teuber. The principle of double dissociation provides a way to determine whether functions are independent and whether they can be associated specifically with independent anatomical structures. When a focal lesion causes impairment in one function without affecting a second function, and another focal lesion impairs the second function without affecting the first, these functions can be considered to be independent. In Luria's view, it is generally the case that psychological functions at the phenomenological level (e.g., reading, writing, repetition, speech output, and comprehension) are not localized in a single location in the brain, but rather are distributed across a system of different modular subcomponents. A particular area in the brain usually only represents a subelement, or what Luria often called a "factor." One factor may subserve several different systems supporting different psychological functions. Luria's approach also emphasizes the importance of analyzing syndromes. It is by analyzing the constellation of functions produced by a lesion, and comparing it to the constellation of functions that is spared, that one can discern the factor that unites all of the disturbed functions. It is this factor that can be localized to a particular region of the brain. In order to understand the basis for a particular psychological function and the many factors that underlie it, one needs to recognize how lesions in different locations, representing different modules, can each induce some form of impairment in that psychological function. It should be noted that the localizationist information-processing models of aphasia also contain distributed subelements, such that a psychological function does not always directly correlate with a single location. For example, speech production in Wernicke's and Lichtheim's models requires both the element of phonological processing in Wernicke's area and articulatory motor programming in Broca's area. Luria, in a sense, extended the localizationist approach to a more complex level, more explicitly anticipating the concept of distributed representations of functions that is accepted today.

Luria's approach resulted in some alternative explanations of the brain mechanisms responsible for aphasia syndromes that differed from those of the localizationists. An example is the way in which Luria characterized what was called "transcortical motor aphasia" by localizationists. In Lichtheim's model, this aphasia is explained as a disconnection of the concept area from the speech production area. In Luria's model, this aphasia, which he called "frontal dynamic aphasia," is posited to result from impairment in premotor functions that initiate motor programs. Rather than a defect of an element or module that maps onto a psychological function within the system of language, Luria claimed that the speech problem is caused by disturbances related to motor initiation of speech. Another aphasia exemplifying Luria's approach is what he called "afferent (apraxic) aphasia." He argued that with lesions in the parietal lobe, near the sylvian fissure, there can be breakdown in afferent feedback so that it becomes difficult to discriminate between different articulatory positions for different phonemes. This leads to confusion of "articulemes" that have similar articulatory properties, even though they may have different acoustic properties. As Geschwind (1972) noted, at the same time that Luria provided brilliant descriptions of the phenomenology of neurological disturbances, "he is uncompromising throughout in his stress on attempting to understand how these relate to the changed physiology of the brain," and this led to his insistence on the factor type of analysis he advocated (p. 757). In addition to analyzing the functional antecedents of speech and language, such as motivation and attention, and coordinate processes such as sensory feedback, Luria investigated the role of language in controlling and regulating behavior.

Luria also contributed to the course of behavioral brain research by emphasizing the importance of analyzing the qualitative nature of disturbances that result from brain injury. Luria argued against the use of predesigned neuropsychological batteries, which quantify deficits but fail to characterize the specific neuropsychological attributes of neurological syndromes. Luria bequeathed to the scientific community a treasure trove of useful psychological tests specifically designed to demonstrate, at the bedside, qualitative psychological dysfunction that is often only poorly characterized by standardized batteries. In the case of language, Luria's interest in qualitative analysis led him to an approach in which he attempted to analyze the types of errors made in language disturbances. In this way, he introduced the experimental study of linguistic error—an approach that has proved extraordinarily fruitful in the investigation of aphasia, and has contributed fundamentally to the modern discipline of cognitive neuropsychology.

CONCLUSION

This chapter has attempted to provide a historical perspective on how our understanding of aphasia has developed over the past 200 years. It has highlighted how differences in philosophical backgrounds and political conditions, as well as commitments to certain methodologies, influenced aphasia research. The history of aphasiology provides an especially good opportunity to view how people gradually learned that mental functions can be separated and localized in the brain. Although localizationists' information-processing models continue to be productive for our understanding of brain organization and its relation to function, the merits of other models, which account for more dynamic features of brain injury, or which emphasize the more distributed nature of processing elements, have also been recognized. Historical studies can alert us to our own prejudices as we approach the study of brain–behavior relationships, provide us with important insights that have been forgotten, and serve to stimulate investigation and new developments in research. In a survey of the history of aphasia such as this, only the contributions of major figures can be considered, and then only briefly. We hope, however, that this review can serve as an introduction and provide a starting point for those who may be interested in more particular aspects of aphasia history.

REFERENCES

Atrophie complète du lobule de l'insula et de la troisième circonvulution du lobe frontale avec conservation de l'intelligence et de la faculté du langage articulé—Observation par M. le Dr. Parrot. (1863). *Bulletins de la Société Anatomique, 38*, 372–401.

Bell, C. (1811). *Idea of a new anatomy of the brain: Submitted for the observation of his friends.* London: Strahan and Preson. (Reprinted in *Medical Classics, 1*, 105–120)

Bichat, F.-X. (1978). Physiological researches on life and death (F. Gold, Trans.). In D. N. Robinson (Ed.), *Significant contributors to the history of psychology* (pp. i–334). Ser. E. *Physiological psychology: Vol 2, X. Bichat, J. G. Spurzheim, P. Flourens.* Washington, DC: University Publications of America. (Original work published 1805)

Bouillaud, J.-B. (1825). Recherches cliniques propre à dé montrer que la perte de la parole correspond à la lésion des lobules antérieurs du cerveau et a confirmer l'opinion de M. Gall sur la siège de l'organe du langage articulé. *Archives Génerale de Médicine, 8*, 25–45.

Bouillaud, J.-B. (1847–1848). Recherches cliniques propre à démontrer que le sens du langage articulé et le principe coordinateur des mouvements de la parole résident dans le lobules antérieur du cerveau. *Bulletin de l'Académie Royale de Médicine, XIII*, 699–710, 778–816.

Breasted, J. H. (1930). *The Edwin Smith surgical papyrus.* Chicago: University of Chicago Press.

Broca, P. (1863). Localisations des fonctions cérébrales: Siège du langage articulé. *Bulletins de la Société d' Anthropologie, 4*, 200–204.

Broca, P. (1865) Sur le siège de la faculté du langage articulé. *Bulletins de la Société d'Anthropologie, 6*, 377–393.

Broca, P. (1960). Remarks on the seat of the faculty of articulate language followed by an observation of aphemia. In G. von Bonin (Trans.), *Some papers on the cerebral cortex* (pp. 136–149). Springfield, MA: Thomas. (Original work published 1861)

Clarke, E. (1962). The early history of the cerebral ventricles. *Transactions and Studies of the College of Physicians of Philadelphia, 30*, 85–89.

Clarke, E., & Jacyna, L. S. (1987). *Nineteenth century origins of neuroscientific concepts.* Berkeley: University of California Press.

Darwin, C. (1873). *The expression of the emotions in man and animals.* New York: Appleton.

Darwin, C. (1890). *The descent of man.* New York: Merrill & Baker. (Original work published 1871)

Dax, G. (1865). Sur le même sujet. *Gazette Hebdomadaire, II*, 260–262.

Dax, M. (1865). Lésions de la moitié gauche de l'encephale coïncident avec l'oubli des signes del la pensée (Lu a Montpellier en 1836). *Gazette Hebdomadaire, II*, 259–260.

Dax, M. (1974). Lésion de la moitié gauche de l'encéphale coincident avec l'oubli des signes de la pensée. In S. Diamond (Ed. and Trans.), *The roots of psychology*. New York: Basic Books. (Original work published 1865)

Discussion sur la faculté du langage articulé. (1864–1865). *Bulletin de L'Académie Imperiale de Médicine, 30*, 575–600, 604–638, 647–675, 679–703, 713–718, 724–781, 787–803, 816–832, 840–868, 888–890.

Discussion sur le volume et la forme du cerveau. (1861). *Bulletin de la Société d'Anthropologie, II*, 66–81, 139–207, 209–326, 421–449.

Feinberg, T. E., Rothi, L. J. G., & Heilman, K. M. (1986). "Inner speech" in conduction aphasia. *Archives of Neurology, 43*(6), 591–593.

Finger, S. (1994). *Origins of neuroscience*. Oxford: Oxford University Press.

Flourens, J. P. M. (1824). *Recherches experimentales sur les propriétés et les fonctions du système nerveux, dans les animaux vertebres*. Paris: Crevot.

Flourens, J. P. M. (1846). *Phrenology examined*. Philadelphia: Hogan and Thompson. (Original work published 1845)

Flourens, J. P. M. (1851). Note sur le point vital de la medulla allongée. *Comptes Rendus Hebdomadaires des Séances de l'Académies des Sciences, 33*, 340–344.

Freud, S. (1953). *On aphasia: A critical study* (E. Stengel, Trans.). London: Imago. (Original work published 1891)

Fritsch, G., & Hitzig, E. (1960). On the electrical excitability of the cerebrum. In G. von Bonin (Ed. and trans.), English translation in *Some papers on the cerebral cortex* (pp. 73–96). Springfield, Il.: Thomas. (Orignial work published 1870).

Gall, F. J., & Spurzheim, J. C. (1835). *On the functions of the brain and of each of its parts: With observations on the possiblity of determining the instincts, propensities, and talents, or the moral and intellectual dispositions of men and animals, by the configuration of the brain and head* (W. Lewis, Jr., trans.). Boston: Marsh, Capen, and Lyon. (Original work, *Sur le Fonctions du Cerveau*, published 1822–1825)

Gall, F. J., & Spurzheim, J. (1810–1819). *Anatomie et physiologie du systême nerveux en général, et du cerveau en particulier*. Paris: F. Schoell.

Geschwind, N. (1964). The paradoxical position of Kurt Goldstein in the history of aphasia. *Cortex, 1*, 214–224.

Geschwind, N. (1965). Disconnexion syndromes in animals and man: Parts I and II. *Brain, 88*, 237–294, 585–644.

Geschwind, N. (1972). Review of *Traumatic aphasia* by A. R. Luria. *Language, 48*, 755–763.

Geschwind, N., & Kaplan, E. (1962). A human cerebral disconnection syndrome: A preliminary report. *Neurology, 12*, 675–685.

Geschwind, N., & Levitsky, W. (1968). Human brain: Left–right asymmetries in temporal speech region. *Science, 161*, 186–187.

Goldstein, K. (1995). *The organism: A holistic approach to biology derived from pathological data in man*. New York: Zone Books. (Original work published 1934)

Goldstein, K. (1948). *Language and language disturbances*. New York: Grune and Stratton.

Gratiolet, P., & Leuret, F. (1839–1857). *Anatomie comparée du système nerveux, considérée dans ses rapports avec l'intelligence*. J. B. Baillière et Fils. II.

Gratiolet, L. P. (1854). *Memoire sur les plis cerebraux de l'homme et de primates*. Paris: Bertrand.

Hagner, M. (1997). *Der Wandel von Seelenorgan zum Gehirn*. Berlin: Berlin Verlag.

Haller, A. V. (1936). A dissertation on the sensible and irritable parts of animals (S.A.A.D. Tissot, Trans.). *Bulletin of the History of Medicine, 4*, 651–699. (Original work published 1755)

Harrington, A. (1987). *Medicine, mind, and the double brain*. Princeton, NJ: Princeton University Press.

Harrington, A. (1996). *Reenchanted science: Holism in German culture from Wilhelm II to Hitler*. Princeton, NJ: Princeton University Press.

Head, H. (1920). *Studies in neurology*. London: Oxford University Press.

Head, H. (1926). *Aphasia and kindred disorders of speech* (2 vols). Cambridge, England: Cambridge University Press.

Head, H., & Holmes, G. (1911). Sensory disturbances from cerebral lesion. *Brain, 34*, 105–254.

Head, H., & Rivers, W. H. R. (1908). A human experiment in nerve division. *Brain, 34*, 323–450.

Heilman, K. M., Tucker, D. M., & Valenstein, E. (1976). A case of mixed transcortical aphasia with intact naming. *Brain, 99*, 415–525.

Heilman, K. M., Rothi, L. J. G., McFarling, D., & Rottmann, A. (1981). Transcortical sensory aphasia with relatively spared spontaneous speech and naming. *Archives of Neurology, 38*, 236–239.

Jackson, J. H. (1878–1879). On affectations of speech from disease of the brain. *Brain, 1,* 304–330. (Reprinted in *Brain, 38.*)

Jackson, J. H. (1879–1880). On affectations of speech from disease of the brain. *Brain, 2,* 203–222, 323–356.

Katz, R. B., & Goodglass, H. (1990). Deep dysphasia: Analysis of a rare form of repetition disorder. *Brain and Language, 39*(1), 153–185.

Kussmaul, A. (1877). *Die Störungen der Sprache.* Leipzig: Vogel.

Lesky, Erna. (1976). *The Vienna Medical School of the 19th century* (L. Williams & I. S. Levij, Trans.). Baltimore: Johns Hopkins University Press. (Original work published 1965)

Lichtheim, L. (1885). On aphasia. *Brain, 7,* 433–484.

Luria, A. R. (1966). *Higher cortical functions in man* (B. Haigh, Trans.). New York: Basic Books. (Original work published 1962)

Luria, A. R. (1970). *Traumatic aphasia: Its syndromes, psychology, and treatment* (D. Bowen, Trans.). The Hague: Mouton. (Original work published 1945)

Luria, A. R. (1973). *The working brain: An introduction to neuropsychology* (B. Haigh, Trans.). New York: Basic Books.

Magendie, F. (1822). Expériences sur les fonctions des racines des nerfs rachidiens. *Journal de Physiologies Expreimentale et Pathologie, 2,* 276–279. (Translated and reprinted in *Francois Magendie—Pioneer in experimental physiology and scientific medicine in 19th century France,* pp. 100–102, by J. M. D. Olmsted, Ed., 1944, New York: Schuman)

Meynert, T. (1866). Ein Fall von Sprachstörung, anatomisch begründet. *Mediziniische Jahrbücher, 12,* 152–189.

Monakow, C. von. (1960). Localization of brain functions. In G. von Bonin (Ed. and Trans.), *Some papers on the cerebral cortex* (pp. 231–250). Springfield, Il: Thomas. (Original work published 1911).

Monakow, C. von. (1914). *Die Localisation im Grosshirn und der Abbau der Funktion durch Kortikale Herde.* Vienna: Bergmann. (Excerpted and translated in *Mood, States and mind,* pp. 27–37, by K. H. Pribram, Ed., and G. Harris, Trans./excepter, 1969, London: Penguin Books)

Neuberger, M. (1981). *The historical development of experimental brain and spinal cord physiology before Flourens* (E. Clarke, Trans.). Baltimore: Johns Hopkins University Press. (Original work *Die Historische Entwicklung,* published 1897)

Pagel, W. (1958). Medieval and renaissance contributions to knowledge of the brain and its functions. In F. N. L. Poynter (Ed.), *The brain and its functions* (pp. 95–114). Oxford: Blackwell.

Ryalls, J. (1984). Where does the term "aphasia" come from. *Brain and Language, 21,* 358–363.

Sulloway, F. J. (1992). *Freud: Biologist of the mind* (2nd ed.). Cambridge, MA: Harvard University Press.

Trousseau, A. (1864). De l'aphasie, maladie décrite récemment sous le nom impropre d'aphémie. *Gazette Hôpitaux Civils Militaires, 37,* 13–14, 25–26, 37–39, 49–50.

Wernicke, C. (1977). The aphasia symptom complex: A psychological study on an anatomical basis. In G. E. Eggert (Ed. and Trans.), *Wernicke's works on aphasia: A source book and review* (pp. 91–144). The Hague: Mouton. (Original work published 1874)

Young, R. (1970). *Mind, brain, and adaptation in the nineteenth century.* Oxford: Oxford University Press.

PART II

Dimensions of
Language Dysfunction

2

FLUENCY

MARGARET L. GREENWALD
STEPHEN E. NADEAU
LESLIE J. GONZALEZ ROTHI

In 1868 John Hughlings Jackson characterized two qualitative types of verbal output in aphasic patients: "speechless or nearly so" and "plenty of words but mistakes in words" (p. 275). Fifty years later Wernicke (1908) recapitulated the distinction, referring to two forms of speech production, "fluent" and "nonfluent," in aphasic individuals. We continue to recognize this difference today (see Nathaniel-James, Fletcher, & Frith, 1997).

The practical problem of discriminating fluent from nonfluent output might seem to be a trivial one. Yet this distinction may not be so easy when it is put to the test (as discussed by Goodglass, Quadfasel, & Timberlake, 1964). For example, we have had the experience of presenting cases with aphasia to a group of behavioral neurologists, neuropsychologists, and speech pathologists (all of whom have vast experience with aphasia), who could not reach agreement as to fluency. The genesis of this confusion may lie in the fact that the fluency–nonfluency distinction is made on the basis not of a single dimension but of multiple dimensions of verbal production, and there is not always consensus as to which are the obligatory distinguishing features. Kussmaul (1887) referred to the multiplicity of factors contributing to fluent verbal production when he stated:

> [There are] . . . most essential points in the process of talking. In the first place, a thought is conceived, and then [there is] an impulse of feeling urging us to express it. Next, we choose and say the words which the acquired language in our memory places at our disposal. Finally, the reflex apparatuses are called into play [to] give outward utterance to the words. (p. 595)

Whereas multiple attributes of fluent or nonfluent aphasic verbal production commonly co-occur (Wagenaar, Snow, & Prins, 1975), in a minority of cases typically concurrent features may be dissociated, possibly because of the uniqueness of the patients' functional neuroanatomy or the geographic extent of the lesion (Basso, Lecours, Moraschini, & Vanier, 1985). Although reliance on a few dimensions of verbal production may permit adequate distinction of fluency from nonfluency in the majority of cases, possibly 30% of the time (Benson, 1967) it will yield a controversial classification. In this chapter we discuss the various elements of normal fluency, in hopes that with an expanded focus, a more accurate characterization of fluency in aphasia will result. We also discuss how these elements of fluency may break down in the context of brain injury or disease, as well as possible treatments for acquired fluency disorders. Fluency as discussed in this chapter is not to be confused with the aberrant rhythm patterns of "dysfluent" speech, commonly known as "stuttering" or "cluttering."

BEHAVIORAL DESCRIPTIONS AND NEUROANATOMICAL CORRELATES OF FLUENCY

Traditionally, behavioral descriptions of fluency have been closely tied to neuroanatomical theories, particularly to hypothesized functions of anterior and posterior brain regions (e.g., Broca, 1861; Wernicke, 1874; Luria, 1945/1970). The functional importance of this fluency distinction was originally discussed by Wernicke (1908) close to a century ago, and has been reiterated by many during the intervening years (Weisenberg & McBride, 1935; Goodglass et al., 1964; Benson, 1967). As noted by Goodglass et al. (1964), "the most significant difference between the major groups of patients resides in the character of their speech production and not . . . in the opposition between the functions of language intake and language output." The clinical importance of the distinction between fluent and nonfluent verbal output in aphasia was first noted by Benson (1967), who showed that this finding could assist in determining the location of a lesion within the left hemisphere of the brain. That is, right-handed persons with nonfluent aphasia were reliably found to have a lesion in the left hemisphere that involved the frontal lobe. In contrast, right-handed persons with fluent aphasia were reliably found to have a lesion in the left cerebral hemisphere that did not extend rostral to the rolandic fissure (central sulcus) into the frontal lobe. The value of Benson's finding was enhanced by the fact that it preceded the availability of neuroimaging techniques to define the localization and extent of a lesion. His conclusions were subsequently confirmed by Naeser and Hayward (1978) and Mohr (1968). Knopman et al. (1983) later suggested that the persistence of nonfluency correlated with the prerolandic extent of lesion.

Fluent aphasic speech associated with posteriorly placed lesions is commonly characterized by normal or excessive rate; normal phrase length, rhythm, melody, and articulatory agility; and either normal or paragrammatic form. In contrast, nonfluent aphasic speech associated with anteriorly placed lesions is characterized by slow rate, reduced phrase length, abnormal intonational contour, effortful articulation, and simplified syntax and/or absent grammar (e.g., Albert, Goodglass, Helm, Rubens, & Alexander, 1981; Goodglass & Kaplan, 1983). Naming ability is impaired in all aphasic patients and does not contribute to the distinction between fluency and nonfluency. Thus the dimensions of spoken production that enable the distinction between fluent and nonfluent aphasia include the quantity of speech (rate, phrase length, and thematic elaboration/communicative intent), articulatory agility, melody/prosody, and adequacy and variety of grammatical form/syntax. Each is discussed below.

Quantity of Speech

Rate

Howes (1964) advocated the use of "words per minute" as a measure of speaking rate. He found that the speaking rate in conversational speech by normal adults ranges from 100 to

175 words per minute, while in aphasic subjects the rate is much more variable, ranging between 12 and 220 words per minute. Kreindler, Mihailescu, and Fradis (1980) advocated the use of an expanded definition of speech rate that incorporates total speaking time to tell a story, as well as total number of words used. However, the use of words per minute has predominated in studies of fluency in aphasia.

Benson (1967) classified aphasic patients with speaking rates below 50 words per minute as "distinctly subnormal," those with rates between 51 and 149 words per minute as "normal," and those with rates of 150 words per minute or more as "supernormal." However, Kerschensteiner, Poeck, and Brunner (1972), in agreement with Howes (1964), found few if any aphasic patients who had rates greater than 175 words per minute; they suggested that fluent aphasic patients are not "hyperfluent."

The importance of this one fluency dimension has been emphasized by Kerschensteiner et al. (1972), who described speaking rate as a powerful discriminator between nonfluency and fluency. However, speaking rate itself has never been studied as a predictor of lesion locus or extent.

Phrase Length

Goodglass et al. (1964) and Benson (1967), when studying fluency in aphasia, did not examine number of words produced per minute; rather, they examined the speech sample in terms of the lengths of word groupings and the number of word groupings of each length. Goodglass et al. (1964) found particularly high interrater reliability in judgment of phrase length. They formulated a ratio of number of utterances of five or more words to number of utterances of one or two words (thus the larger the ratio, the more common longer phrases were). Almost half the aphasic patients, but no normal subject, had a ratio of less than 0.31. They suggested that aphasic patients with low phrase length ratios were nonfluent.

Kerschensteiner et al. (1972) used distinct interruptions in speech production as a way of determining phrase length, which they defined as the number of utterances a patient produced between two such interruptions. They found that this factor strongly discriminated fluent from nonfluent aphasic patients. Wagenaar et al. (1975) found that the combination of shorter "mean length of utterance" (which might be considered similar to phrase length) and slowed "speech tempo" (number of words per minute) was the best measure of nonfluency in aphasia.

Thematic Elaboration

We define "thematic elaboration" as intention to communicate verbally with others in conjunction with desire and ability to elaborate on the theme of a communication. Kussmaul (1887) touched on this concept when he stated:

> The intellectual contents of our being slumbers unconscious in our memory until thrown into vibration by some vigorous shock from without or within. . . . If conceptions . . . be called upon, the extent to which they were set in motion will reflect back with such force of feeling upon the being as to awaken its interest and produce a readiness to follow up the thoughts; and to clothe them in words. (pp. 624–625)

Disinclination to speak or to elaborate on themes can be associated with nonfluent aphasia. Several mechanisms have been proposed, including deficits in activation of the semantic field by internal or self-generated motives (Rothi, 1997), a dissociation of lexical and conceptual strategy formation (Gold et al., 1997), or an inability to select between competing verbal response possibilities (Robinson, Blair, & Cipolotti, 1998).

Loss or diminution of inclination to speak or elaborate on themes in conversation is not always associated with reduced phrase length, impaired articulatory agility (i.e., effortful articulation), or impaired grammar. Isolated or nearly isolated loss of inclination to speak or thematically elaborate is characteristic of the group of disorders classified as "transcortical motor aphasia" (TCMA) (Freedman, Alexander, & Naeser, 1984; Ardila & Lopez, 1984; McCarthy & Warrington, 1984; Benson, 1993). TCMA is caused variously by infarcts in the distribution of the left anterior cerebral artery; cortical border zone infarcts involving the frontal convexity; and lesions of frontal subcortical white matter, most particularly the anterior limb of the internal capsule, as well as the midline thalamus. The heterogeneity of lesions associated with this syndrome suggests multiple mechanisms of speech impairment, none of which are well understood. These mechanisms may include deficits in the endogenous generation of concept representations (as in adynamic aphasia); bradyphrenia; akinesia/hypokinesia; loss of ability to generate complex syntax (as in Broca's aphasia); and anomia related to lesions of the temporo-frontal pathways that enable the translation of concept representations into articulatory word forms, or, less often, to damage to the semantic field from postrolandic lesions (as in "nonoptic aphasia"; Shuren & Heilman, 1993).

Articulatory Agility

We define "articulatory agility" as the facility and accuracy with which one produces the motoric aspects of speech (see McNeil, Doyle, & Wambaugh, Chapter 10, this volume). Some authors exclude quality of articulation as a parameter of fluency, reasoning that patients who have severe impairment of articulatory agility in conversation may demonstrate excellent articulation in reciting automatized verbal sequences, such as the letters of the alphabet (nonpropositional language) (e.g., Damasio, 1981). Others place great emphasis on articulatory agility as a defining feature of fluency. For example, Goodglass et al. (1964) found that scales of articulatory agility correlated strongly with their scale of phrase length and were reasonable discriminators between fluent and nonfluent speech production.

It is now possible to reconcile these disparate points of view. As a rule, patients with large, left perisylvian lesions involving the frontal operculum (and, typically, much of the frontal convexity cortex) will initially present with features of global aphasia and will be substantially mute. Ultimately, most will exhibit the features of Broca's aphasia, which include impaired articulatory agility and diminished phrase length (as observed by Goodglass et al., 1964), generally reflecting nondominant-hemisphere language capabilities. In some patients, nondominant-hemispheric substrates for motoric aspects of speech production are sufficiently well elaborated to support normal articulation, despite the left-hemisphere opercular lesion (Nadeau, 1988). Such patients will typically demonstrate excellent articulation during nonpropositional language, even during the acute phases of their stroke, reflecting the fact that mechanisms underlying nonpropositional language are frequently well represented in the nondominant hemisphere (Speedie, Wertman, Ta'ir, & Heilman, 1993). To the extent that the neural substrate for inclination to speak and thematic elaboration is represented exclusively in the dominant hemisphere and is implicated in the lesion, there will be loss of fluency, even in the presence of preserved articulatory agility.

Melody/Prosody

"Prosody," described as the "melodious aspect of speech" and particularly including stress (inflection), pitch (tone), timbre, and rhythm, was a term introduced by Monrad-Krohn (1947). Those with fluent aphasia are said to display normal prosody, while those with nonfluent aphasia are said to display halting and uneven rhythm, equal or absent inflection, and an amelodious speech pattern. Goodglass et al. (1964) found that "melodic line" was the best discriminator between fluent and nonfluent speakers—a conclusion subsequently independently confirmed by others (Benson, 1967; Kerschensteiner et al., 1972).

In aphasic patients, stressed syllables are less likely to be omitted (Pate, Saffran, & Martin, 1987; Goodglass, Fodor, & Schulhoff, 1967). In normal subjects, phoneme exchanges in slips of the tongue tend to involve syllables of equal stress (see Nadeau, Chapter 3, this volume). Furthermore, isolated stress errors (e.g., "económist," "differénces") and mixed stress–morphological errors (e.g., "proféssoral" for "professórial") may be observed in the speech of normal subjects (Shattuck-Hufnagel, 1983). These observations suggest that mechanisms underlying the definition of melodic line tend to be represented in inferior left frontal cortex, and normally operate in parallel and to some extent independently of mechanisms defining morphology.

Adequacy and Variety of Grammatical Form and Syntax

Goodglass et al. (1964) found that variety of grammatical form in language production was a reasonably good discriminator between fluent and nonfluent speech. Impoverishment of grammar is such a frequent concomitant of nonfluent aphasia that it would be quite natural to suppose that it contributes to nonfluency. This view is reinforced by conceptualizations of language production as a linear, stage-by-stage process (e.g., Levelt, 1989). In a linear process, processing deficits at any one stage will tend to impede the entire process. While it would be very premature to say that this matter is settled, limited clinical observations suggest that fluency can be preserved in the presence of impaired grammar, and insights born of computational neuroscience suggest that because language production involves multiple parallel processes, impairment of grammatical function does not necessarily impose a bottleneck that will affect fluency.

Grammatical function may be roughly divided into the ordering of words and phrases at the sentence and clause level, which we refer to as "syntax," and the ordering of words and grammatical morphemes at the phrase and word levels, which we will refer to as "grammatical morphology." Patients with Broca's aphasia commonly exhibit impairment in both aspects of grammatical function. However, impairment in the two aspects may be dissociated. One of us has reported patients with isolated impairment in syntax (Nadeau, 1988), and there have been reports of a number of patients with isolated impairment in grammatical morphology (Nadeau & Rothi, 1993). Patients with such isolated impairments are frequently fluent; this suggests that grammatical impairment is not what impairs fluency in patients with Broca's aphasia, but rather concurrent impairment in other aspects of language production, as discussed earlier.

The literature on grammatical function in aphasia has almost uniformly posited the existence of a grammatical processor, which represents in a neural machine the rules of grammar, presumably as elaborated in the field of linguistics. Much debate has revolved around whether this processor is damaged or simply rendered inaccessible in patients with grammatical impairment. However, work with parallel-distributed-processing (connectionist) models of language has shown that in general, the "rules" of language are not discretely encoded in neural structure, but are emergent properties of the interaction of large ensembles of neurons in neural networks supporting language (see Nadeau, Chapter 12, this volume). This is likely to be the case in the domain of grammatical function as well. In this view, simple declarative sentences represent the generation and incremental modification of one or two concept representations, depending on whether or not there is a patient or theme to the sentence. This facility is most specifically impaired in adynamic aphasia. Complex sentences, involving one or more embedded clauses, require more or less simultaneous generation of more than two concept representations in a specific relationship to one another. Inability to perform this more complex task may lead to poverty of syntax, but so long as the ability to generate concept representations is substantially intact, language fluency may be preserved, as it demonstrably has been in patients with isolated syntactic impairment. Grammatical morphology involves knowledge of morpheme sequence at the word and phrase level that may be computationally analogous to knowledge of phoneme sequence within words. It is now well established that connectionist models, and by inference neural structure, have enormous capability for representing sequence knowledge (e.g., Plaut, McClelland, Seidenberg, & Patterson, 1996). Loss of sequence knowledge underlying grammatical morphology might be expected to produce agrammatism or paragrammatism, but this should not be expected to impair fluency, any more than loss of sequence knowledge underlying phonology impairs fluency in patients with Wernicke's aphasia.

These are provocative notions. We offer them because they follow naturally from neural network conceptualizations of brain function, because we believe that some new perspectives are needed in the domain of grammatical function, because this new conceptualization accounts in a cogent fashion for clinical observations that are at odds with more traditional formulations, and because it sheds some light on the potential relationships of fluency and grammatical function in aphasia.

Summary

The "fluency" of an aphasic patient's verbal output can reflect function along a number of dimensions, including kinesis, thematic elaboration, semantic access, articulatory agility, prosody, and grammatical form. Each of these factors must be considered in determining the causes of a patient's loss of fluency and in defining treatment approaches.

TREATMENT

Because disorders of fluency can emanate from a variety of causes, the nature of treatment will need to be tailored to each patient's unique needs. Treatments for the motor aspects of speech production are described by McNeil et al. (Chapter 10, this volume). The reader is also referred to Chatterjee and Maher (Chapter 6, this volume) for a description of treatments appropriate to sentence production deficits.

Both behavioral and pharmacological treatments for disinclination to speak or to elaborate on conversational themes have been reported. Behavioral treatments have tended to be ineffective. For example, Huntley and Rothi (1988) trained their patient, through a series of self-managed cues, to elaborate on a defined concept and to report verbally on that elaboration. Generalization was negligible. In a few case reports (e.g., Albert, Bachman, Morgan, & Helm-Estabrooks, 1988; Stewart, Leadon, & Rothi, 1990), some improvements in quantity of output or thematic elaboration have been observed following administration of bromocriptine, a dopamine receptor agonist. The patient of Albert et al. (1988) had recovered from an intracerebral hemorrhage and had residual damage apparently involving the suprasylvian convexity cortex, hemispheric white matter, and insula, and largely sparing the caudate and putamen. These investigators speculated that bromocriptine treatment compensated interruption of mesocortical dopamine pathways. Similar findings have been reported with the administration of d-amphetamine (Walker-Batson, Devous, Curtis, Unwin, & Greenlee, 1990; Walker-Batson et al., 1992). The mechanism of action of d-amphetamine in these cases is uncertain. It could act to potentiate the effects of ascending dopaminergic, serotonergic, and noradrenergic projections on cortical function. Alternative possibilities include potentiation of axonal sprouting (Stroemer, Kent, & Hulsebosch, 1998), facilitation of long-term potentiation (i.e., memory formation), counteracting diaschisis (remote, physiologically mediated effects of acute infarction), and correction of the widespread cerebral hypometabolism typically seen after stroke (Feeney, 1998a, 1998b). Further research into the use of pharmacological management, possibly in conjunction with behavioral treatments, may provide an option for effective management of disinclination to communicate or elaborate on conversational themes. At this point, there is little evidence of an effective method for managing this aspect of nonfluent aphasia (Huntley & Rothi, 1988), other than training caregivers to provide external cueing that allows a nonfluent speaker to increase language production by elaborating verbally on the cues.

REFERENCES

Albert, M. L., Bachman, D. L., Morgan, A., & Helm-Estabrooks, N. (1988). Pharmacotherapy for aphasia. *Neurology, 38,* 877–879.

Albert, M. L., Goodglass, H., Helm, N. A., Rubens, A. B., & Alexander, M. P. (1981). *Clinical aspects of dysphasia.* New York: Springer-Verlag.

Ardila, A., & Lopez, M. V. (1984). Transcortical motor aphasia: One or two aphasias? *Brain and Language, 22,* 350–353.

Basso, A., Lecours, A. R., Moraschini, S., & Vanier, M. (1985). Anatomoclinical correlations of the aphasia as defined through computerized tomography: Exceptions. *Brain and Language, 26,* 201–229.

Benson, D. F. (1967). Fluency in aphasia: Correlation with radioactive scan localization. *Cortex, 3,* 373–394.

Benson, D. F. (1993). Aphasia. In K. M. Heilman & E. Valenstein (Eds.), *Clinical neuropsychology* (3rd ed., pp. 19–36). New York: Oxford University Press.

Broca, P. (1861). Remarques sur le siège de la faculté du langage articulé, suivies d'une observation d'aphémie. *Bulletins Société de la Anatomique, 2,* 330–357.

Damasio, A. (1981). The nature of aphasia: Signs and syndromes. In M. T. Sarno (Ed.), *Acquired aphasia* (pp. 57–73). New York: Academic Press.

Feeney, D. M. (1998a). Mechanisms of noradrenergic modulation of physical therapy: Effects on functional recovery after cortical injury. In L. B. Goldstein (Ed.), *Restorative neurology: Advances in pharmacotherapy for recovery after stroke* (pp. 35–78). Armonk, NY: Futura.

Feeney, D. M. (1998b). Rehabilitation pharmacology: Noradrenergic enhancement of physical therapy. In M. D. Ginsberg & J. Bogousslavsky (Eds.), *Cerebrovascular disease: Vol. 1. Pathophysiology, diagnosis and management* (pp. 620–636). Oxford: Blackwell.

Freedman, M., Alexander, M. P., & Naeser, M. A. (1984). The anatomical basis of transcortical motor aphasia. *Neurology, 34,* 409–417.

Gold, M., Nadeau, S. E., Jacobs, D. H., Adair, J. C., Rothi, L. J. G., & Heilman, K. M. (1997). Adynamic aphasia: A transcortical motor aphasia with defective semantic strategy formation. *Brain and Language, 57,* 374–393.

Goodglass, H., Fodor, I., & Schulhoff, C. (1967). Prosodic factors in grammar: Evidence from aphasia. *Journal of Speech and Hearing Research, 10,* 5–20.

Goodglass, H., & Kaplan, E. (1983). *The assessment of aphasia and related disorders* (2nd ed.). Philadelphia: Lea & Febiger.

Goodglass, H., Quadfasel, F. A., & Timberlake, W. H. (1964). Phrase length and the type of severity of aphasia. *Cortex, 1*, 133–153.

Howes, D. (1964). Application of word-frequency concept to aphasia. In A. V. S. de Reuch & M. O'Conner (Eds.), *Disorders of language* (pp. 47–62). London: Churchill.

Huntley, R. A., & Rothi, L. J. G. (1988). Treatment of verbal akinesia in a case of transcortical motor aphasia. *Aphasiology, 2*, 55–66.

Jackson, J. H. (1868, September 5). On the physiology of language. *Medical Times and Gazette*, p. 275.

Kerschensteiner, M., Poeck, K., & Brunner, E. (1972). The fluency–nonfluency dimension in the classification of aphasic speech. *Cortex, 8*, 233–247.

Knopman, D. S., Selnes, O. A., Niccum, N., Rubens, A. B., Yock, D., & Larson, D. (1983). A longitudinal study of speech fluency in aphasia: CT correlates of recovery and persistent nonfluency. *Neurology, 33*, 1170–1178.

Kreindler, A., Mihailescu, L., & Fradis, A. (1980). Speech fluency in aphasics. *Brain and Language, 9*, 199–205.

Kussmaul, A. (1887). Disturbances of speech: An attempt in the pathology of speech. In H. V. Ziemssen (Ed.), *Cyclopedia of the practice of medicine*. New York: Wood.

Levelt, W. J. M. (1989). *Speaking: From intention to articulation*. Cambridge, MA: MIT Press.

Luria, A. R. (1970). *Traumatic aphasia: Its syndromes, psychology, and treatment* (D. Bowen, Trans.). The Hague: Mouton. (Original work published 1945)

McCarthy, R., & Warrington, E. K. (1984). A two-route model of speech production: Evidence from aphasia. *Brain, 107*, 463–485.

Mohr, J. P. (1968). Cerebral control of speech. *New England Journal of Medicine, 279*, 107.

Monrad-Krohn, G. H. (1947). Dysprosody or altered 'melody of language'. *Brain, 70*, 405–415.

Nadeau, S. E. (1988). Impaired grammar with normal fluency and phonology. Implications for Broca's aphasia. *Brain, 111*, 1111–1135.

Nadeau, S. E., & Rothi, L. J. G. (1993). Morphologic agrammatism following a right hemisphere stroke in a dextral patient. *Brain and Language, 43*, 642–667.

Naeser, M. A., & Hayward, R. W. (1978). Lesion localization in aphasia with cranial computed tomography and the Boston Diagnostic Aphasia Exam. *Neurology, 28*, 545–551.

Nathaniel-James, D. A., Fletcher, P., & Frith, C. D. (1997). The functional anatomy of verbal initiation and suppression using the Hayling Test. *Neuropsychologia, 35*, 559–565.

Pate, D. S., Saffran, E. M., & Martin, N. (1987). Specifying the nature of the production impairment in a conduction aphasic. *Language and Cognitive Processes, 2*, 43–84.

Plaut, D. C., McClelland, J. L., Seidenberg, M. S., & Patterson, K. (1996). Understanding normal and impaired word reading: Computational principles in quasi-regular domains. *Psychological Review, 103*, 56–115.

Robinson, G., Blair, J., & Cipolotti, L. (1998). Dynamic aphasia: An inability to select between verbal responses? *Brain, 121*, 77–89.

Rothi, L. J. G. (1997). Transcortical motor, sensory, and mixed aphasias. In L. L. LaPointe (Ed.), *Aphasia and related neurogenic language disorders* (pp. 91–111). New York: Thieme.

Shattuck-Hufnagel, S. (1983). Sublexical units and suprasegmental structure in speech production planning. In P. F. MacNeilage (Ed.), *The production of speech* (pp. 109–136). New York: Springer-Verlag.

Shuren, J., & Heilman, K. M. (1993). Non-optic aphasia. *Neurology, 43*, 1900–1907.

Speedie, L. J., Wertman, E., Ta'ir, J., & Heilman, K. M. (1993). Disruption of automatic speech following a right basal ganglia lesion. *Neurology, 43*, 1768–1774.

Stewart, J. T., Leadon, M., & Rothi, L. J. G. (1990). Treatment of a case of akinetic mutism with bromocriptine. *Journal of Neuropsychiatry and Clinical Neurosciences, 2*(4), 462–463.

Stroemer, R. P., Kent, T. A., & Hulsebosch, C. E. (1998). Enhanced neocortical neural sprouting, synaptogenesis, and behavioral recovery with D-amphetamine therapy after neocortical infarction in rats. *Stroke, 29*, 2381–2395.

Wagenaar, E., Snow, C., & Prins, R. (1975). Spontaneous speech of aphasic patients: A psycholinguistic analysis. *Brain and Language, 2*, 281–303.

Walker-Batson, D., Devous, M. D., Curtis, S., Unwin, H., & Greenlee, P. (1990). Use of amphetamine to facilitate recovery from aphasia subsequent to stroke. *Clinical Aphasiology, 20*, 137–144.

Walker-Batson, D., Unwin, H., Curtis, S., Allan, E., Wood, M., Devous, M., & Greenlee, R. (1992). Use of amphetamine in the treatment of aphasia. *Restorative Neurology and Neuroscience, 4,* 47–50.

Weisenberg, T. H., & McBride, K. E. (1935). *Aphasia.* New York: Commonwealth Fund.

Wernicke, C. (1874). *Der Aphasische Symptomenkomplex.* Breslau: Cohn & Weigart.

Wernicke, C. (1908). The symptom complex of aphasia. In E. D. Church (Ed.), *Modern clinical medicine: Disease of the nervous system.* New York: Appleton.

3

PHONOLOGY

STEPHEN E. NADEAU

"Phonology" is the subfield of linguistics concerned with the structure and systematic patterning of sounds in language (Akmajian, Demers, & Harnish, 1984). The essential unit of phonology is the "phoneme," which corresponds to the smallest definable unit of language. To a large degree, phonemes, as they are normally produced in language, can be captured by single letters ("graphemes")—for example, /b/, /a/, /t/ (the representation /b/ indicates that we mean the actual sound produced as we begin to say the word "bat," and not the letter sound "bee"). However, there are phonemes that cannot be captured by a single letter, such as /sh/, /zh/, or /th/. Although phonemes were originally conceived as a denomination of language currency, it is the good fortune of neurolinguists that they also appear to represent a denomination of brain currency, defined as discrete entities by neural networks within language cortex.

The study of phonology employs many sources of data. In this chapter, I focus on studies of acquired language disorders and slip-of-the-tongue collections (e.g., "spoonerisms") in normal subjects. Although the data from aphasia and slip-of-the-tongue collections are considered in similar fashion, it is important to keep in mind the peculiarities of these data sources. Data from aphasia reflect the effects of damage to the phonological processor of nearly infinite variety; at the same time, most of our knowledge of this area comes from intensive studies of single patients, which potentially limit generalizability. Slip-of-the-tongue data, on the other hand, reflect the behavior of an intact phonological processor without lesion-induced variability in function; in contrast to data from aphasia, slip-of-the-tongue data reported in any one study are collected from many individuals. This provides a good basis for generalizability in normal subjects, but it does not necessarily predict the full spectrum of phonological dysfunction associated with lesions.

Abnormalities of phonological processing are seen exclusively with the perisylvian disorders: Broca's, conduction, and Wernicke's aphasias, and the rare syndrome of pure word deafness. The hallmarks of phonological impairment in these disorders are impaired repetition and the presence of phoneme errors in spoken output (paraphasias) and written output (paragraphias). The perisylvian aphasias have particular significance for the neurologist, because the cortex involved is always supplied by cortical branches of the middle cerebral artery. Therefore, any right-handed stroke patient with impaired repetition or phonemic paraphasias must have had a stroke in the distribution of a large vessel, the middle cerebral artery. This indicates that the clot causing the stroke must have originated in this artery (rarely), the carotid artery, the aorta (uncommonly), or the heart. Such a patient would consequently be a potential candidate for major therapeutic interventions, such as carotid endarterectomy or chronic systemic anticoagulation, to reduce the likelihood of stroke recurrence. No other attribute of aphasic language has such specificity for localization or such clear-cut implications for medical management.

As behavioral neuroscientists, our primary interest in phonology has to do with the nature and organization of brain systems supporting phonological function. There are not yet clearly definable links between rehabilitation strategies and the neuroscience of phonology. Nevertheless, the recent course of both science and practice suggests a need to forge such links. In this chapter, I begin with a model of phonological function (Figure 3.1). I proceed through this model several times—beginning simply with a definition of terms, subsequently discussing the organization of the model and the working principle (parallel distributed processing or PDP; McClelland, Rumelhart, & the PDP Research Group, 1986; Rumelhart, McClelland, & the PDP Research Group, 1986; see also Nadeau, Chapter 12, this volume), and concluding with a brief overview of the evidence supporting the model. I then discuss the spectrum of conduction aphasia in the context of the model, because the most essential attribute of conduction aphasia is impairment in phonological processing. The anatomy of phonological processing is then considered. I conclude with implications of the model for rehabilitation.

A MODEL OF PHONOLOGICAL PROCESSING

Definition of Terms

The core of language processing is the concept representation (Figure 3.1). A particular concept corresponds to a particular pattern of activity in the "semantic field"—the linked network of association cortices throughout the brain that enables a person to define the visual, somatosensory, auditory, functional, and emotional attributes of that concept. A concept can be translated into an articulatory motor form through its links to the "articulatory hierarchy" (Figure 3.1, pathway 1). The articulatory hierarchy translates the concept representation into the sequential pattern of contractions of oral, lingual, and pharyngeal muscles that will ultimately produce it as a spoken word. During speaking, activity spreads from the semantic field down through the articulatory hierarchy to articulatory motor representations at the bottom.

A concept representation can also be translated into an acoustic word form through its links to the "acoustic hierarchy" (Figure 3.1, pathway 2). The acoustic hierarchy translates a concept representation into a pattern of sound sequences that corresponds to the heard form of the word. When a person is listening to speech, activity spreads upward from acoustic representations to concept representations.

The articulatory hierarchy (concept representation $\rightarrow$ articulatory motor representations; Figure 3.1, pathway 1) is characterized in this model by a number of levels. Articulatory word forms are sequences of phonemes devoid of meaning that correspond to words. "Morphemes" constitute the major subsegments of words. For example, the word "passed" consists of two morphemes, a stem "pass" and an affix "ed." Stems are linked to the essential meaning of the word. Inflectional affixes modify the grammatical meaning of the word; in the example just provided, the affix "ed" indicates the past tense. Derivational affixes modify the semantic meaning of the word (e.g., "govern"/"government"). Words can be broken down further into syllables. Syllables are made up of still smaller segments: The syllable "bot" consists of

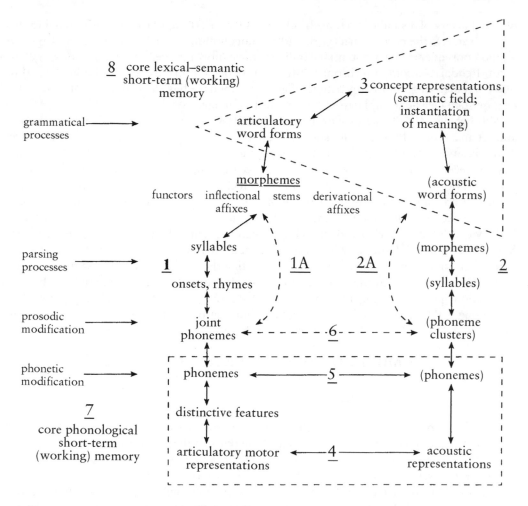

FIGURE 3.1. A composite model of phonological processing. See text for details.

Lesion effects: A lesion of pathway 1 is posited as the explanation for phonological aphasia. The hierarchy continues to function but in a noisy fashion, generating phonemic paraphasias in spontaneous language and naming. Repetition is preserved. A complete lesion at lower levels of pathway 2 should lead to pure word deafness. A lesion at higher levels of pathway 2 should lead to word meaning deafness (Ellis, 1984; Kohn & Friedman, 1986). A complete lesion of pathways 4 and 5 should lead to impaired phonetic discrimination, rhyme and homophone judgment, repetition of nonlinguistic sounds, and reduction in auditory–verbal recent memory seen in repetition conduction aphasia, and necessitate the use of an acoustic → concept representation → articulatory route of repetition. When such a lesion is combined with damage to the levels of concept representation and articulatory word forms, semantic paraphasias should be observed during repetition—the signature of deep dysphasia. Partial lesions of pathway 5, variably implicating pathway 4 (e.g., McCarthy & Warrington, 1984), should lead to reproduction conduction aphasia. Partial lesions of pathways 1 and 5 should lead to what I have defined as "combination conduction aphasia," generally referred to as "reproduction conduction aphasia" or simply "conduction aphasia" in the literature.

The network provides at least two major routes for repetition, as originally recognized by Wernicke (1874) and more recently expounded by Coslett, Roeltgen, Rothi, and Heilman (1987). Patients with damage to pathways 4 and 5 and repeating via the concept representation route (acoustic representation → concept representation → articulatory representation) will exhibit difficulty with nonwords. Patients with damage to the concept route and repeating via pathways 4 and 5 will fail to correct grammatically incorrect sentences, because the grammatical access that mediates this is acquired via the concept route.

an onset "b" and a rhyme "ot," which in turn consists of a nucleus or peak "o" and a coda "t." Within syllables, certain phonemes display a tendency to stick together as a consonant cluster; for example, the "str" of "stream" is defined as a "joint phoneme." Distinctive features correspond to the discrete dynamic properties of the vocal apparatus observable during speech that serve to distinguish phonemes (Akmajian et al., 1984). All phonemes in human language can be defined in terms of approximately 16 different distinctive features. Those most important in English are listed and exemplified below:

vowel → consonant	/a/ → /k/
→ nasal	/d/ → /n/
acute → grave	/d/ → /b/
diffuse → compact	/d/ → /g/
voice (tense → lax)	/t/ → /d/
→ continuant	/p/ → /f/
mellow → strident	/θ/ → /s/

The relative differences between phonemes can be measured in terms of the number of distinctive features that separate them—something Lecours and Lhermitte (1969) termed the "paradigmatic distance." For example, in their scheme, the phoneme pairs listed above are one distinctive feature apart, while /p/ and /m/ are separated by two distinctive features (nasality and voice) and /d/ and /f/ are separated by three distinctive features (voice, acute → grave, and continuance). Articulatory motor representations define the actual motoric patterns needed to translate abstract representations of distinctive features into the pattern of oral, pharyngeal, and laryngeal muscle contractions that produces speech.

I assume that the acoustic hierarchy (acoustic representations → concept representations; Figure 3.1, pathway 2) consists of a hierarchy of language sound structures analogous to the levels in the articulatory hierarchy, as shown in Figure 3.1. Unfortunately, the details of this hierarchy are more open to speculation, because processing in the acoustic hierarchy is largely hidden from us.

Processing in the articulatory hierarchy is affected by a number of additional processes, including grammar, parsing (the segmentation of a phonemic stream into clumps corresponding to words), prosody (accenting the stressed syllable), and a process I refer to simply as "phonetic modification." Phonemes may be modified in a variety of ways. For example, initial stop consonants are aspirated—compare the aspirated /p/ of "put" with the nonaspirated /p/ of "stop" (Akmajian et al., 1984). Phonemes are coarticulated, meaning that they are processed in parallel, such that the articulation of a sound is altered by neighboring sounds (Liberman, Cooper, Shankweiler, & Studdert-Kennedy, 1967). For example, the lips are rounded in producing the /p/ of "pool," but not the /p/ of "pit" (Caplan, 1993). There is also a wide variety of contractive modifications that occur after phonemes are selected (e.g., "want to" → "wanta" or "wanna"; see Levelt, 1989).

Finally, the phonological processor provides the substrate not only for core language function but also for memory, as will be discussed at somewhat greater length below.

Organization of the Model

The labels in Figure 3.1 characterize the classes of entities that are instantiated at various levels of the hierarchies. These entities are not actually stored at these locations. Rather, information is stored throughout the network; that is, it is "distributed."[1] For example, the articulatory lexicon is stored in the articulatory hierarchy, not in articulatory word forms. The labels reflect the nature of the differentiation of the hierarchies at these points in the model. They may fruitfully be viewed as labels on bundles of neural wires, rather than labels on storage sites. For example, at the phoneme level the hundreds of thousands of "wires" at higher levels (corresponding to articulatory word forms, syllables, etc.) project to just 35 discrete clumps corresponding to the phonemes available to us. Higher structures in the hierarchy correspond to various permutations and combinations of these phonemes.

A full representation of the model would include all possible representations at each level (e.g., all possible morphemes). Each representation is assumed to be distributed as well (e.g., the word form "cat" corresponds to a unique pattern of activity of neurons in the network, not activation of "cat" neurons). In general, linkages are all assumed to be bidirectional as indicated by the arrows. That is, neural activity can spread both upward and downward, as is the case both in PDP models (to be discussed below) and in the brain itself. However, some influences (grammar, prosody, phonetic modification, parsing) that are not discussed in detail in this chapter have been denoted by unidirectional arrows simply to indicate an influence, without making any presumptions about details. Also, to simplify this diagram further, I have not indicated potential nondominant-hemisphere components either.

The numbers in the following discussion correspond to the pathway numbers in Figure 3.1.

1. *The phonological articulatory hierarchy* (concept representations → articulatory motor representations). In this hierarchy, all representations are abstract. They are only defined in concrete terms by the pattern of neural activity elicited in articulatory motor representations, which will produce a particular word or sublexical entity, or in concept representations, which define meaning. Thus, if articulatory motor representations, acoustic representations, and concept representations were destroyed, all the intervening units would cease to have any meaning. The integrity of the phonological articulatory pathway can be probed with spontaneous language and naming.

1A, 2A. The direct influence of neural representations at any one level of a hierarchy may extend beyond levels immediately below and immediately above.

2. *The phonological acoustic hierarchy* (acoustic representations → concept representations). All representations are abstract, and they are only defined in concrete terms by the pattern of neural activity elicited in primary and association auditory cortices ("the mind's ear"), or by the pattern of activity elicited in semantic cortex (which defines meaning). A number of entities are given in parentheses in Figure 3.1 because their existence is assumed only by analogy with the articulatory processor, as I have noted. The definitive method for probing the integrity of this pathway is auditory lexical decision (indicating whether or not heard sound sequences are words).

3. *The concept representation.* This not only provides the core representation of the language processor, but is also presumably a major point of interface with other language-related word form systems, such as graphemic word forms and inscriptional word forms (the engrams for hand movements required to write words). These other word form systems may also have a more direct interface with other components of the phonological system (e.g., orthographic representations with articulatory motor representations) (Coltheart & Byng, 1989; Plaut, McClelland, Seidenberg, & Patterson, 1996).

4. *The acoustic–articulatory link.* This pathway directly translates sound representations into articulatory representations. This is likely to be a system and not a compact fiber bundle susceptible to simple disconnection. The optimal probes of the integrity of this

pathway are phonetic discrimination (are /gat/ and /gap/ the same or different?) and rhyme judgment (do "moan" and "bone" sound alike?).

5. *The phoneme-instantiating acoustic–articulatory linkage.* This link achieves the same end as pathway 4, but in the process it actually instantiates discrete patterns of neural activity corresponding to phonemes. Like pathway 4, this is likely to be a system rather than a discrete fiber bundle. The best probe of the integrity of this pathway is nonword repetition.

6. Linkages between higher levels of the acoustic and articulatory hierarchies may exist.

7. *Phonological short-term (working) memory.* This corresponds to activation of those portions of the composite network that actually represent and process phonemes, whether in acoustic or articulatory form (included within broken lines in Figure 3.1). These two forms are linked directly by pathway 4 and indirectly by pathway 5. Whereas short-term memory corresponds to a transiently sustained pattern of activation, and as such is working memory, the connection strengths between the neurons in these same networks provide the basis for long-term memory. To the extent that phonological representations in either hierarchy engage higher sublexical forms, core phonological working memory may expand to include these levels of the network.

8. *Lexical–semantic short-term (working) memory.* This corresponds to the current pattern of activation of those portions of the composite network that actually represent and process word forms and meaning (included within broken lines in Figure 3.1). Just as for phonological memory, the connection strengths provide the basis for long-term memory. The two phonological hierarchies provide the basis for interaction between phonological and lexical–semantic short-term memory.

The network depicted may not be homogeneous in structure. Most of it represents discrete variables—symbolic entities that are either present or absent at any one time, implying some kind of threshold phenomenon that defines "on" and "off" states. On the other hand, the lowest portions of the hierarchies instantiate continuous variables. For example, articulatory motor representations instantiate movements that, like limb movements, are infinitely adaptable (within physical limitations). Each discrete component of both articulatory and limb movements must be accommodated to other components of the movement as the movement is being designed. This type of process presumably accounts for such things as phonetic modification.

The Working Principle of the Model: Parallel Distributed Processing

It is easy to lull oneself into the notion that a model is a neutral vehicle that simply serves to organize the available data and facilitate predictions. However, models develop their own momentum, and they have the ability to mislead. The information-processing models introduced by Wernicke and Lichtheim (see Figure 1.2 in Roth & Heilman, Chapter 1, this volume) have distinguished themselves as extraordinarily powerful heuristic devices; they have made major contributions to the wealth of psycholinguistic data that have emerged over the past 20 years. However, information-processing and linguistic models are limited by their failure to take advantage of our knowledge of the principles of neural organization. Confusion often results from attempts to map these models onto brain structure. It is in this respect that PDP models have much to offer, because it is now clear that despite the limitations of any specific PDP model, PDP in general captures the essential architecture and principles of function of the brain (see Nadeau, Chapter 12, this volume). Thus PDP models are not simply further heuristic devices that should be expected to compete on equal terms with other linguistic models.

Linguistic theories have not yet provided a satisfactory account for the phonological processing disorders observed either in aphasic patients or in normal subjects demonstrating slips of the tongue. Two major reasons can be identified. First, linguistic theories have been founded on the concept of serial processing (a succession of processing steps performed, one at a time, in a fixed order), whereas abundant data (to be reviewed in part below) suggest that language production incorporates parallel processing (simultaneous performance of multiple processes at multiple levels) (Stemberger, 1985). Second, linguistic theories have difficulty capturing effects that are easily explained by bottom-up and top-down processing interactions within the phonological articulatory hierarchy, such as the occurrence of paraphasic errors that have both semantic and phonological similarity to the target (Dell & Reich, 1981; Dell, Schwartz, Martin, Saffran, & Gagnon, 1997; Harley, 1984).

PDP (connectionist) models offer an alternative approach. PDP models are neural-like in that they incorporate large arrays of simple units that are heavily interconnected with each other, like neurons in the brain. Their processing sophistication stems from the simultaneous interaction of large numbers of units (hundreds or even thousands). PDP models incorporate explicitly defined assumptions that are "wired" into them in the mathematical details of their computer implementation. They produce large numbers of predictions that can be (and have been) empirically tested through observations of normal subjects and patients. When damaged or fed noisy input, they do not produce novel or bizarre output unachievable by an intact network with good input; rather, they tend to produce output that may not be so reliably correct but is rule-bound—a characteristic of phonological selection errors. This property of graceful degradation with probabilistic selection obviates the need to postulate "error correction devices" in normal subjects and aphasic patients that filter out bizarre constructions (e.g., Buckingham, 1980; Garrett, 1975; Shattuck-Hufnagel, 1979). In PDP models, the memories (e.g., phonemes, joint phonemes, syllables, rhymes, morphemes, and sentence constituents) are represented in the same neural nets that support processing. In this way, a PDP model is able to accommodate the movements and exchanges of phonemes observed in abnormal language without the need for postulating the separate identity of linguistic units and time slots into which those units are placed, as is frequently done in the psycholinguistic literature (e.g., Shattuck-Hufnagel, 1979). The temporally shifting pattern of activity in the hierarchical system of neural nets supporting language automatically defines, at any one instant, both a temporal interval of opportunity and a repertoire of variously suitable lexical or sublexical candidates to fill that temporal interval. The latency of activity pattern shifts, related ultimately to the slowness of neural physiology, provides the potential basis for the sequential aspect of language in general and phonological processing in particular. The instantiation of short- and long-term memory in the same neural nets that are responsible for processing, in conjunction with processes underlying the engagement of working memory (Goldman-Rakic, 1990), also eliminates the need to posit buffers. Finally, PDP models are particularly appealing in the context of phonological processing because they involve simultaneous processing at a number of levels and locations, apparently mimicking what is going on in the brain.

I plan to consider in some detail a PDP model of phonological processing developed by Dell (1986). This model has achieved considerable success in accounting for human subject data and, in its transparency, provides singular insight into the processes that must underlie phonological processing.

Dell's model explicitly incorporates the hierarchy of aggregations of distinctive features and phonemes evident in slip-of-the-tongue errors. A small portion of that model is represented in Figure 3.2. Each unit or node in this model corresponds to a single linguistic element—something referred to as "local representation" in the PDP literature. In reality, we would expect a linguistic unit to correspond to a particular pattern of neural activity distributed over many neural elements (distributed representation). However, for practical reasons (the size of computer programs and the time it takes to run them), PDP models are generally designed to focus on one aspect of a problem and to make simplifying assumptions or arrangements to deal with other aspects. Dell was interested in behavior wrought of interactions between the linguistic units, and the assumption of local representations vastly simplified the exploration of this without significant risk to the validity of the results.

An absolutely correct model would be analog in nature, and processing would go on simultaneously throughout. However, because the model, like PDP models in general, was actually built and tested on a digital computer, this process has to be simulated by cycling once through every unit of the model each time step. At each time step, a level of activation is computed for each node (circle) according to a mathematical formula.

The running of the model is organized around clock cycles, each of which is divided into r time steps (range = 2–8). At the beginning of each clock cycle, the next morpheme in the input sequence is given an arbitrary level of activation (say, 100). With each time step, the activation level of each node is calculated as a function of its own prior activation level and the activation level of all of its neighbors above it and below it in the network. Thus

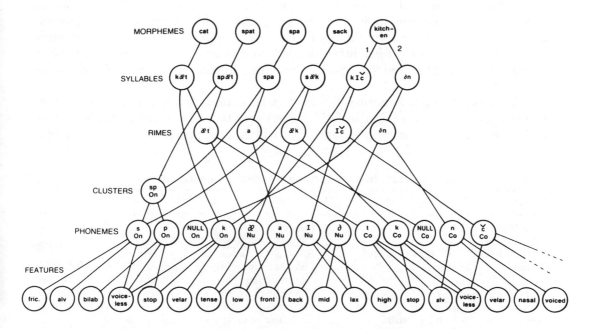

FIGURE 3.2. A portion of the PDP network developed by Dell (1986, 1988) to emulate phonological processing. Single-phoneme, phoneme cluster, and null nodes (representing absent initial or final consonants in a syllable) are labeled as to whether they are potential (on)sets, (nu)clei, or (co)das. All connections are both bottom-up and top-down. From Dell, G. S. (1986). A spreading-activation theory of retrieval in sentence production. *Psychological Review, 93,* 283–321. Copyright © 1986 by the American Psychological Association. Reprinted with permission.

the exclusive initial activation of the "cat" node (Figure 3.1) quickly spreads through a large portion of the network. With each time step, the activation level of each activated node also spontaneously declines. At each clock cycle, not only is a new morpheme (the next morpheme in the input stream) "flagged" with an activation level set to 100, but a syllable (consisting of onset, nucleus, and coda) is extracted from the most active nodes at the bottom of the network and flagged as the "output" of the network at that particular time. Once constituent nodes have been flagged, at the next time step their activity is set to 0. However, they quickly regain much of their original activity in subsequent time steps because of spreading activation from neighbors. Most of the simulations run with the model have employed phonemes rather than distinctive features as the output level of the network, but the distinctive-feature level has been retained in the computations, with the net effect of creating a tendency to erroneously exchange similar phonemes with each other. Increases in speaking rate are simulated by reducing the number of time steps per clock cycle.

Table 3.1 illustrates some of the errors produced by Dell's model. The phonemic errors produced clearly have substantial face validity, in that they strongly resemble errors observed in slip-of-the-tongue collections. The model also reasonably recapitulates the distribution of error substrates and error types that have been observed in such collections amassed from both Dutch (Nooteboom, 1969) and English (Shattuck-Hufnagel, 1983; Dell, 1986) (Table 3.2). Finally, the model demonstrates a number of phenomena that have been demonstrated in slip-of-the-tongue studies of experimental subjects:

1. *Lexical bias*. The model exhibits a preference for slips that result in other words in its vocabulary, as opposed to nonwords. This is because activation from selected syllables, rhymes, and phonemes spreads up to related morphemes, which in turn provide top-down activation of only those syllables, rhymes, or phonemes that are component parts. The model acts as if there were a built-in editor that tends to prevent nonword strings from being encoded, precluding the need for a special editor that scans the output and vetoes nonword outcomes.

2. *Similarity effects*. Repeated phonemes tend to induce misordering of sounds around them (MacKay, 1970; Wickelgren, 1969). For example, the repeated /ae/ in the phrase "hat pad" could induce either an exchange ("pat had"), an anticipation ("pat pad"), or a

TABLE 3.1. Examples of Errors from Phonological Encoding Simulation

Error	Error type
"kinsman" → "minsman"	Phoneme anticipation
"Infant" → "anfint"	Phoneme exchange (metathesis)
"ensign mercy" → "mensign mercy"	Anticipatory addition
"crackle" → "cackrel"	Phoneme/joint-phoneme metathesis (/kr/ ↔ /k/), with subsequent phonetic modification (/l/ ↔ /el/)
"topsail" → "topsay"	Phoneme deletion
"topsail" → "topsop"	Perseveration of rhyme
"typist figure" → "typig fisture"	Exchange of cluster and single phoneme
"seaman woman" → "seaman moman"	Phoneme anticipation/perseveration
"content convict" → "con con convict"	Syllable anticipation/perseveration
"topsail beggar" → "boptail beggar"	Multiple-site error

Note. Adapted from Dell, G. S. (1986) A spreading-activation theory of retrieval in sentence production. *Psychological Review*, 93, 283–321, Copyright © 1986 by the American Psychological Association. Adapted with permission.

TABLE 3.2. Distribution of Error Substrates and Error Types Produced by Model and in Slip-of-the-Tongue Corpora

	Simulation: Speech rate			Collection	
	$r = 3$	$r = 4$	$r = 8$	Nooteboom (1969)—Dutch	Shattuck-Hufnagel (1983)—English
	Unit size				
Phoneme	66	81	90	89	70
Cluster	6	6	2	7	16
Vowel–consonant	20	10	5	2	6
Consonant–vowel	1	1	2	0.5	2
Feature	0	0	0	0	1
Syllable	2	0	1	1.5	3
Other	5	2	0		2
Total	100	100	100	100	100
	Error type				
Anticipation	19	48	67	57	
Perseveration	49	25	6	13	
Exchange	5	2	0	5	
Total substitution	73	75	73	75	
Deletion	19	19	19	3	
Addition	5	6	8	21	
Shift	3	0	0	1	
Total nonsubstitution	27	25	27	25	

Note. Adapted from Dell, G. S. (1986). A spreading-activation theory of retrieval in sentence production. *Psychological Review*, 93, 283–321. Copyright © 1986 by the American Psychological Association. Adapted with permission.

perseveration ("hat had"). The /ae/ gets double top-down activation, leading to particularly strong bottom-up activation of all syllables containing /ae/ (only /hat/ and /pad/ are in this particular model's vocabulary) throughout the time that these two syllables are being processed. These in turn provide top-down activation of all the contained consonants, which then compete. In this example, at any one given time, all four component consonants (/h/, /t/, /p/, and /d/) are similarly activated, leading to a significant probability that the wrong one will be selected at a particular instant.

3. *Speaking rate effects.* Lexical bias is greater at slow speaking rates, because there is a greater opportunity for activation to spread from phonemic representations to the various related morphemic representations and back down again. The similarity (repeated-phoneme) effect is greater at slow speaking rates for similar reasons. The ratio of anticipations to exchanges and perseverations, both in the model and in experimental subjects (Dell, 1990), increases as speech slows, because there is greater time for loss of activation of the first phoneme and for exertion of lexical influences on the second phoneme in the interacting pair. For example, the exchange error "pancake" → "canpake" can happen only if /p/ remains sufficiently activated and free of influence by top-down lexical input (from "cake") to be dominant by the time the second syllable is initiated. If, on the other hand, sufficient time has elapsed for the activity of /p/ to die out further, the result will be an anticipation error, "pancake" → "cancake." Kohn and Smith (1990) provided partial empirical evidence of this effect in their finding that in the halting, severely paraphasic speech of a patient with conduction aphasia, exchange errors were rare, in contrast to their higher frequency in slips of the tongue produced in the rapid speech of normal subjects. Schwartz, Saffran,

Bloch, and Dell (1994) contrasted phoneme anticipation–perseveration error ratios and lexical errors in a jargon-aphasic patient with a speech error corpus collected from normal subjects. They predicted from the Dell model that weakened neuronal interconnections in the aphasic patient should slow the spread of activation, leading to reduced lexical influence on errors (more nonwords produced), and therefore to relatively fewer anticipatory and more perseverative errors. Both predictions were supported. Error patterns were also examined in normal subjects learning tongue twisters (Dell et al., 1997; Schwartz et al., 1994). It was predicted that as connection strengths increased with learning, there should be increased lexicalization and both an increase in anticipatory errors relative to perseverative errors and a decline in nonword errors. Again, both predictions were borne out. Thus fast speaking rates in the Dell model and in experimental subjects, lesion-induced weakening of connection strengths in patients, and weak connection strengths due to lack of practice by normal subjects on a demanding task have the same tendency to reduce the lexical effect, and therefore the anticipation–perseveration ratio. All three situations apparently reflect reduced opportunity for the spread of activation to the morphemic representations, which would then, through further spread of activation, correct nonword forms and perseverative errors.

The purpose of this review of Dell's model has been simply to demonstrate its power and plausibility, and, indirectly, to suggest something about the nature of the neural instantiation of phonological processing. The reader interested in fully exploring this model's predictive capability, considering the extent to which its behavior follows from the setting of its parameters rather than its intrinsic design, or critically examining its simplifications and shortcomings is referred to the original paper (Dell, 1986). PDP (Elman & McClelland, 1988) and a variety of other models have also been applied to phonological perception (Klatt, 1989).

Empirical Support for the Model

In the previous two sections, I have described the organization and processes that are presumed to govern the function of the model of phonological function introduced at the beginning of this chapter. In this section, I briefly review some of the empirical evidence supporting this model, in the process providing the reader with some sense of the linguistic phenomena I have discussed so far in largely theoretical terms.

Phonemic Clumping

In the model (Figure 3.1), the various levels within the articulatory hierarchy (and by inference, within the acoustic hierarchy) incorporate aggregations or clumps of phonemes. What is the evidence for this?

Single-phoneme selection errors, whether in slips of the tongue in normal subjects or in phonemic paraphasic errors made by aphasic patients, may be characterized as substitutions, simplifications (deletions), additions, or environmentally related changes (changes influenced by nearby phonemes). Blumstein (1973a) provides these examples:

Substitution: /timz/ ("teams") → /kimz/
Simplification: /prIti/ ("pretty") → /pIti/

Addition: /papa/ ("papa") → /papra/
Environmental:
    Anticipation within a word: "Crete" → /trit/
    Anticipation across word boundaries: "roast beef" → /rof bif/
    Metathesis (exchange): "degrees" → /gedriz/

Many phonemic substitutions, additions, deletions, or metatheses involve a joint phoneme (e.g., a consonant cluster), a syllable, a rhyme, an affix, a stem, a word, or even a phrase (Blumstein, 1978; Buckingham, Avakian-Whitaker, & Whitaker, 1978; Dell, 1986; Fromkin, 1971; Lecours & Lhermitte, 1969; Shattuck-Hufnagel, 1979; Shewan, 1980; Stemberger, 1982). The following examples are slips of the tongue collected by Dell (1986) and Fromkin (1971):

Joint phoneme: "eerie stamp" → "steerie stamp," "blue bug" → "blue blug"
Syllable or rhyme: "couch is comfortable" → "comf is . . ."
Stem: "thinly sliced" → "slicely thinned"
Affix: "self-destruct instruction" → "self-instruct de . . . ," "and so in conclusion" → "and so in concludement"
Word: "writing a letter to my mother" → "writing a mother to my letter"
Phrase: "A fall in pitch occurs at the end of the sentence" → "An end of the sentence occurs at the fall in pitch"

Several other phenomena seem to reflect similar clumping. Malapropisms (in aphasic speech, often referred to as "formal," "form-related," or "verbal" paraphasias) represent substitutions at the word level that are driven by similarity in phonology, number of syllables, stress pattern, and grammatical form, and are unconstrained by meaning (unlike semantic paraphasias); they provide evidence that word representations exist independently of meaning (Blanken, 1990; Fay & Cutler, 1977). "Functors" or free grammatical morphemes (closed-class items such as articles, prepositions, and conjunctions) are, with few exceptions (Kohn & Smith, 1993), not involved in phonemic paraphasic errors, suggesting that they exist as relatively indissoluble clumps of phonemes (Blumstein, 1973a; Garrett, 1975; Kohn & Smith, 1990; Lecours, 1982; Stemberger, 1984).

The presence of neologisms in patients with thalamic aphasia also provides evidence of phonemic clumping. Thalamic aphasia is characterized predominantly by difficulty with anomia in spontaneous language, variable difficulty in naming to confrontation, usually mild impairment of comprehension, and completely normal repetition. The consistent normality of repetition suggests that the phonological processor is intact. Thus neologisms cannot be attributed to semantic paraphasias compounded by literal paraphasias; therefore, it is logical to relate them to the problem patients with thalamic aphasia have with lexical access. If this line of reasoning is correct, it suggests that sublexical items (syllables, affixes, stems, even phonemes) must be explicitly represented, either as part of the lexicon or as a sort of sublexicon (Buckingham, 1987; Nadeau & Crosson, 1997). When an attempt to engage the lexicon is not successful in raising one and only one entry above threshold, one or more of these sublexical items may achieve threshold instead. Alternatively, the attempt to engage two lexical items simultaneously may have the indirect result of raising two or more sublexical items above threshold, so that parts of each lexical item are combined into a new morpheme (Buckingham & Kertesz, 1974; Burns & Canter, 1977; Stemberger, 1985). Probable examples of the latter have been observed in slip-of-the-tongue data from normal subjects ("blends") (Fromkin, 1971; Harley, 1984; MacKay, 1972; Shattuck-Hufnagel, 1979, 1987; Stemberger, 1982):

"my data consists mownly—maistly"	(mainly–mostly)
"I swindged"	(switched–changed)
"Don't shell"	(shout–yell)
"himpede"	(hinder–impede)

They have also been observed in aphasia (*phonemic télescopages*) (Lecours, 1982):

"*sashk*"   *sac–sacoches* (bag–satchel)

Other Constraints on Phonemic Selection Errors

Sublexical Substitutions Obey Phonetic Rules. Rarely in either aphasic or slip-of-the-tongue errors is there evidence of a capability for producing phonemic sequences that are beyond the native speaker (Blumstein, 1973a, 1978; Buckingham, 1980; Buckingham & Kertesz, 1974; Butterworth, 1979; Fromkin, 1971; Garrett, 1975; MacKay, 1972). For example:

"plant the seed/z/" → "plan the seat/s/"
"*sph*inx in the moonlight" → "minx in the *sp*oonlight"

Failure to modify these selection errors would have resulted in the impermissible sequences "seat/z/" and "sphoonlight." Blumstein (1973a) found that only 2.6% of phonemic errors resulted in non-English sequences. Substitutions such as "blame" → "mlame" never occur, even though the change involves but a single distinctive feature—a very small error (see "Anatomical Influences," below). This phenomenon strongly suggests bottom-up followed by top-down flow of activation: Impermissible phoneme sequences partially activate a number of permissible syllables, morphemes, and words containing similar but not identical phoneme sequences. These partially activated sublexical elements then provide converging top-down activation of a permissible alternative to the impermissible sequence.

Phoneme and Joint-Phoneme Errors are Governed by Syllabic and Class Constraints. Almost always, comparable parts of syllables and words are involved in exchanges, anticipations, and perseverations in normal speech (Blumstein, 1973a; Buckingham, 1980; Fromkin, 1971; Kohn & Smith, 1990; Laubstein, 1987; Shattuck-Hufnagel, 1979) and in repetition (Ellis, 1980). Sublexical components interact almost exclusively with other members of their kind (e.g., onsets with onsets, stems with stems, affixes with affixes, rhymes with rhymes, but not stems with affixes or onsets with rhymes) (Fromkin, 1971; Garrett, 1975; MacKay, 1970; Shattuck-Hufnagel, 1979, 1987; Stemberger, 1982). For example:

"space food" → "face spood" (involving exchange of initial phoneme/joint phoneme, but not "space foosp," which would entail exchange of an initial with a final phoneme)
"pinch hit" → "pich hint" (involving a coda exchange, but not "pinch hip," entailing reiterative modification of a terminal phoneme by an initial phoneme) (slip-of-the-tongue error; Fromkin, 1971)
"D*a*n hates" → "Dan /haen/," "Chi*l*dren wear" → "Children /wIll/" (patient with conduction aphasia; Kohn & Smith, 1990).

This suggests horizontal but not vertical mobility within the hierarchy, and provides evidence that there is in fact a hierarchy and not just a poorly differentiated lexical/sublexical "soup." However, within-word errors, rare in normal subjects but quite common among aphasic patients, often do not reflect such constraining forces (Stemberger, 1982).

Lexical and Semantic Effects

As phonological processing proceeds, it continues to be influenced by lexical and semantic constraints, even in aphasia. This constitutes another line of evidence that phonemic selections at various levels within the articulatory hierarchy are communicated through spread of activity to the highest levels of the hierarchy, where activated words then exert top-down effects that further influence those phonemic selections. This is true whether words are introduced from the top of the hierarchy, as in naming, or from the bottom, as in repetition. There are three lines of evidence of lexical/semantic constraints on phonological processing.

First, phonemic selection errors are constrained by the lexical target, and both normal subjects and aphasic patients make more phonological errors while repeating nonsense than real words (Alajouanine & Lhermitte, 1973; Brener, 1940; Martin & Rigrodsky, 1974). Patients with aphasias characterized by relatively good access to lexical targets (e.g., Broca's and conduction aphasias) demonstrate continuous improvement in their phonemic approximations during *conduite d'approche* (an effort to zero in on the target through successive attempts), whereas patients with aphasias characterized by poor lexical access (e.g., Wernicke's aphasia) tend not to improve (Butterworth, 1979; Gandour, Akamanon, Dechongkit, Khunadorn, & Boonklam, 1994; Joanette, Keller, & Lecours, 1980; Miller & Ellis, 1987; Valdois, Joanette, & Nespoulous, 1989). The phonological improvement noted during *conduite d'approche* is seen only with real words and not with nonwords. Mistakes in patients who make errors only during nonword repetition tend to reflect lexicalization (Bub, Black, Howell, & Kertesz, 1987). Normal subjects are more likely to produce real-word spoonerisms (e.g., "barn door" → "darn boor") than nonword spoonerisms (e.g., "dart board" → "bart doard") (Baars, Motley, & MacKay, 1975; Dell & Reich, 1981; Garrett, 1976). The likelihood of such real-word spoonerisms can be enhanced by semantic priming. For example, Motley and Baars (1976) found that "get one" is more likely to slip to "wet gun" if preceded by "damp rifle." When subjects produce semantic paraphasias or word blends (e.g., "taxi" and "cab" → "tab"), there is evidence of both semantic and phonological similarity between the interacting words, suggesting competing influences from separate neurological substrates for meaning and phonological representation (Dell & Reich, 1981).

Second, abstruse neologisms (neologisms without evident relationship to a plausible target) suggest the influence of lexical and sublexical selection by phonological as opposed to purely semantic constraints. Neologisms in jargon aphasia have the same number of syllables as the targets up to 80% of the time, and they share a greater than chance number of phonemes with the targets; these findings suggest substantial sublexical access from semantics, perhaps through the target lexical items, even when the targets are not sufficiently resolved to assure correct output (Ellis, Miller, & Sin, 1983; Miller & Ellis, 1987; Valdois et al., 1989). Butterworth (1979) found that 57% of neologisms in patients with jargon aphasia were phonologically linked to other neologisms as opposed to being semantically determined, suggesting that because of the brain lesion, phonological associations within the lexicon and its sublexical components substantially replace semantic constraints as the factors that elevate a particular morpheme above the threshold for production (an observation also made by Luria, 1974).

Third, in experiments in which normal subjects are given the definition of low-frequency words and develop the "tip-of-the-tongue" (TOT) phenomenon (i.e., they have a sense they know the word but cannot actually produce it), there is evidence of sublexical access from semantics despite unsuccessful lexical access. Despite anomia, subjects are able to guess the number of syllables in the target word with high accuracy; show knowledge of letters within the word (e.g., guessing the first letter with 57% accuracy); and show knowledge of which syllable in the target is accented (Brown, 1991; Brown & McNeill, 1966; Burke, MacKay, Worthley, & Wade, 1991; Koriat & Lieblich, 1974; Yarmey, 1973). Aphasic patients are also able to guess the first letter and the number of syllables with far greater than chance accuracy when they develop the TOT phenomenon; however, patients with conduction or Broca's aphasia do far better at this than patients with Wernicke's or anomic aphasia (Barton, 1971; Goodglass, Kaplan, Weintraub, & Ackerman, 1976; Laine & Martin, 1996). These data suggest that neural activity representing meaning engages phonemes and sublexical clumps of phonemes, even when the word itself is not sufficiently engaged to elevate it above the threshold for production.

Bottom-Up and Top-Down Effects

Phonemic and sublexical paraphasic errors and *conduite d'approche* in patients with dominant perisylvian lesions are similar, whether the task is spontaneous language, reading, repetition, or naming (Kohn & Smith, 1990). This observation and the data reviewed above suggest that a word and its entire hierarchy of sublexical components, together with phonologically similar associates of that word and its components, are routinely engaged from the top down (e.g., in spontaneous language). The various constraints on phonological selection errors, most particularly those that are nearly absolute (e.g., immunity of functors to phonemic paraphasias, the absence of paraphasias that violate phonetic rules [phonotactic constraints]) also strongly suggest that there is routine bottom-up access within this hierarchy. Thus the chance development of errors at lower levels that would violate these constraints is transmitted to higher levels, which in turn suppress these violations via subsequent top-down feedback (Dell, 1985, 1986; Stemberger, 1985). The repeated-phoneme effect (e.g., "left hemisphere" → "heft lemisphere"), and the tendency for malapropisms (formal verbal paraphasias) to have a greater number of phonemic substitutions than neologisms (see "Conduction Aphasia," below) can also be accounted for only by bottom-up transmission in the hierarchy. Damage to dominant perisylvian cortex, and to a far lesser degree natural noise in the system (e.g., in slips of the tongue), may reduce the availability of a word or any of its sublexical components and increase the availability of various associates, leading to addition, omission, or misselection at any level of the hierarchy. The actual error produced at any one instant may best be explained as the result of the convergence of bottom-up and top-down influences within the multiple levels of the hierarchy.

Anatomical Influences

I have noted above that patients with impaired lexical access due to more posterior lesions exhibit less evidence of lexical–semantic effects on phonological processing. Various other effects of lesion locus or corresponding type of aphasia have been demonstrated. Patients with Broca's aphasia tend to replace consonant clusters with single consonants and rarely create consonant clusters in lieu of a single consonant. In contrast, whereas patients with conduction aphasia alter consonants and consonant clusters just as often, they are more likely to replace a cluster with a different cluster or to replace a single consonant with a cluster (Nespoulous, Joanette, Béland, Caplan, & Lecours, 1984). Phonemic substitution errors in aphasic patients in general tend to involve changes of a minimum number of distinctive features, usually one or two (Blumstein, 1973b; Burns & Canter, 1977; Caramazza, Miceli, & Villa, 1986; Green, 1969; Keller, 1978; Klich, Ireland, & Weidner, 1979; La Pointe & Johns, 1975; Lecours & Lhermitte, 1969; MacKay, 1970; Poncet, Degos, Deloche, & Lecours, 1972; Shinn & Blumstein, 1983; Valdois, Joanette, Nespoulous, & Poncet, 1988), but to the extent that errors involving two or three distinctive features occur, they are more common among patients with conduction and jargon aphasia than among patients with Broca's aphasia (Burns & Canter, 1977; Canter, Trost, & Burns, 1985; MacNeilage, 1982; Miller & Ellis, 1987; Nespoulous et al., 1984; Nespoulous, Joanette, Ska, Capland, & Lecours, 1987; Poncet et al., 1972; Trost & Canter, 1974; Valdois et al., 1988). On the other hand, sequential phonemic errors (errors that are influenced by the immediate phonemic environment) are less common in Broca's aphasia and apraxia of speech than in conduction aphasia, and less common in conduction aphasia than in jargon aphasia (Burns & Canter, 1977; Canter et al., 1985; La Pointe & Johns, 1975; MacNeilage, 1982; Miller & Ellis, 1987; Nespoulous et al., 1984, 1987; Poncet et al., 1972; Shewan, 1980; Trost & Canter, 1974; Valdois et al., 1988); these findings suggest that as the production of language nears the output phase, the number of phonemes in various phases of simultaneous activation becomes progressively smaller. As I show below, this observation is also consistent with the concept that as language approaches its output stages, influences from higher levels, such as words and syllables, becomes less important. On the other hand, at earlier stages, at which word- and even phrase-level effects are prominent and environmentally linked phoneme errors are generated, these errors will tend to reflect the properties of the words (such as word frequency and anticipation effects—see below) rather than the properties of the phoneme. In phoneme errors in which the change reflects the influence of nearby phonemes, and that occur within a morpheme, regressive (anticipatory) errors occur more frequently than progressive (reiterative/perseverative) errors in patients with Broca's or conduction aphasia or apraxia of speech, and the two types of errors occur with about equal frequency in patients with Wernicke's aphasia (Blumstein, 1973a; La Pointe & Johns, 1975). The occurrence of both regressive and progressive errors reinforces the concept that as the brain processes phonemes, a number are maintained in a similar state of activity for some time, notwithstanding that they occur sequentially in the output phonemic stream. Thus a given phoneme may have as much opportunity to influence phonemes later in the stream (reiterative errors) as there is opportunity for later phonemes to influence it (anticipatory errors). The relative occurrence of anticipatory and reiterative errors in different types of aphasia may be related in good part to speech rate (see "The Working Principle of the Model: Parallel Distributed Processing," above). Thus progressive (perseverative) errors are relatively more common in patients with Wernicke's aphasia, because in their more rapid speech, there is still enough residual activation of already spoken phonemes to induce substitutions in current phonemes. Finally, in aphasic patients, both the size of units involved in phonemic errors and the size of units constituting errors increase with the posterior extent of the lesion. Thus sequential phonemic and syllabic errors become progressively more common with posterior extent of lesions (jargon > conduction > Broca's). Patients with Broca's aphasia (anterior lesions) are most likely to exhibit literal paraphasias best characterized as single-phoneme or distinctive-feature alterations. Patients with posterior lesions, such as those with Wernicke's aphasia, and particularly jargon aphasia (Kertesz & Benson, 1970), are most likely to exhibit paraphasias best characterized as joint-phoneme, syllable, or morpheme alterations.

Interim Summary

Phonological selection errors in normal subjects and aphasic patients provide evidence of several essential properties of the cerebral system instantiating phonological processing: (1) hierarchical structure; (2) simultaneous top-down and bottom-up processing; (3) simultaneous influence by clumping effects, phonotactic constraints, syllabic and class constraints, lexical–semantic representations, grammar, prosody, and parsing effects (parallel processing); (4) simultaneous processing of a chunk of the language stream, such that lexical and sublexical elements influence other elements that both precede and follow them; (5) anatomical distribution, such that lesion locus has major effects on the pattern of breakdown observed; (6) substantial but not absolute similarity between the errors made by aphasic patients and errors made by normal subjects in slips of the tongue; (7) stochastic function, such that lesions are associated with a reduced probability of correct phonological selection with actual performance that is variable, and relative preservation of ability to distinguish correct from incorrect selection. The patterns of errors indicate that whereas both natural and lesion-induced noise may reduce the likelihood of correct output, they do not result in violation of the central constraints built into the network (graceful degradation). Any viable model of phonological processing must take into account these overarching constraint systems.

The Acoustic Hierarchy and the Acoustic–Articulatory Links

I have briefly reviewed the empirical evidence for the various properties of the articulatory hierarchy I have postulated. In this section, I consider the limited data that bear on the acoustic hierarchy, and I review evidence of the primacy of the articulatory hierarchy and the existence of acoustic–articulatory links (Figure 3.1, pathways 4 and 5).

Phonetic Discrimination. One would predict that patients with posterior lesions encroaching on auditory association cortex (e.g., patients with Wernicke's aphasia) would be most impaired on phonetic discrimination tasks. Blumstein, Baker, and Goodglass (1977) did find that patients with Broca's aphasia made fewer phonetic discrimination errors than patients with Wernicke's or anomic aphasia, but, surprisingly, patients with Broca's aphasia with impaired comprehension made the most errors. Gainotti, Miceli, Silveri, and Villa (1982) found that on a similar task, patients with Broca's, Wernicke's, or conduction aphasia had similar degrees of impairment, whereas those with anomic aphasia were least impaired, and those with global aphasia were most impaired; those with frontal lobe lesions were most severely impaired, and those with temporal lobe lesions least impaired. Zattore, Evans, Meyer, and Gjedde (1992) found that excision of a tumor in Broca's area impaired phonetic discrimination. Ojemann and Mateer (1979) found that electrocortical stimulation in portions of Broca's area during stimulus presentation impaired subsequent phonemic identification. Patients with phonetic disintegration (cortical dysarthria, apraxia of speech) frequently but not invariably exhibit impaired phonetic perception (Hoit-Dalgaard, Murry, & Kopp, 1983).

Errors in acoustic processing exhibit some of the same features as errors in articulatory processing. Patients in all groups do better with discriminations involving two or more distinctive features relative to discriminations involving a single distinctive feature (Blumstein et al., 1977; Miceli, Caltagirone, Gainotti, & Payer-Rigo, 1978; Miceli, Gainotti, Caltagirone, & Masullo, 1980). All patients make more errors with discriminations involving phonemes in nonwords than in real words, suggesting that the top-down influence of words aids in performing this task (Blumstein et al., 1977; see also Elman & McClelland, 1988).

Several studies (e.g., Carpenter & Rutherford, 1973) have attempted to define more precisely a disorder of acoustic cue discrimination that might underlie impairment of phonetic discrimination. Aphasic patients appear to have preserved ability to discriminate spectral cues (e.g., the different /i/ sounds in "fig" and "fib"), but are often very impaired in discriminating temporal cues (e.g., duration of the vowel preceding the stop consonant in "kid" and "hit"). Although one might predict that only patients with Wernicke's aphasia would be impaired by virtue of involvement of auditory association cortex, Carpenter and Rutherford (1973) and others have reported results paralleling the phonetic discrimination data: Patients with anterior aphasias are at least as severely impaired as those with posterior aphasias. This could indicate that correct discrimination is significantly aided by rehearsal via a linked acoustic–articulatory processor, or that reverberation of acoustic input through phonological output cortex (articulatory motor representations) is important for these types of acoustic discriminations. In either case, aphasic patients with anterior lesions might be significantly impaired.

The Motor Theory of Phonetic Perception Revisited. Phonetic perception may depend not just on an acoustically based process but also on the rapid, automatic conversion of acoustic patterns into patterns of neural activity in Broca's area and opercular areas 4 and 6, which define motor programs for phonemic production (the ultimate neural instantiation of phonemes), as described above. There is an extensive literature on motor theories of speech perception (see Liberman & Mattingly, 1985), which posits that the objects of speech perception are the intended articulatory gestures of the speaker. To perceive a speech utterance, one must perceive a specific pattern of intended gesture defined by the movements of the articulators. Normal subjects listening to closely related syllables (e.g., /pa/, /ta/) that are synchronized with silent video recordings of faces of people saying these syllables will tend to "hear" what they see when the auditory and visual stimuli conflict (e.g., "hearing" /pa/ in response to an auditory stimulus /ta/ and a simultaneous silent video featuring the pronunciation of /pa/)—the "McGurk effect" (McGurk & MacDonald, 1976). Functional imaging studies provide strong evidence that phonetic discrimination relies on the establishment of patterns of activity in anterior perisylvian cortex corresponding to the definition of phonemes in terms of distinctive features and motor engrams, and not simply the discrimination of sound patterns in auditory association cortex and Wernicke's area. Zatorre et al. (1992) compared a passive consonant–vowel–consonant syllable pair listening task to a task with similar stimuli in which subjects had to signal whether the final phoneme was the same or different. The phoneme discrimination task elicited differential increases in blood flow in dominant Broca's area, not posterior area 22 (auditory association cortex).

The Linkage between Input and Output Phonetic Processes. The research I have reviewed strongly supports the existence of a close link between cortices defining acoustic input (auditory association cortex, Wernicke's area) and anterior cortices defining phonological output. It suggests that this entire *linked* system is engaged in the detection of rapid temporal changes in the acoustic input stream that is crucial to phonetic perception. Acquired disorders of the crucial output segments of this system disrupt the acoustic-signal-to-articulatory-gesture conversion patterns learned in infancy and early childhood (Liberman & Mattingly, 1985), leading to difficulty in phonetic discrimination in adults as reviewed above, and also in children (Tallal & Piercy, 1975).

There exist patients who, by virtue of the locus of their lesions in posterior perisylvian cortex and their linguistic behavior, may have breaks (disconnections) within this acoustic to articulatory conversion system (Friedrich, Glenn, & Marin, 1984; Morton, 1980). In one type of aphasia, repetition conduction aphasia, impairment in phonetic discrimination and homophone judgments has been reported even when the output segments were intact (Allport, 1984a; Friedrich et al., 1984). In a related type of aphasia, deep dysphasia, there is absolute inability to repeat nonwords, relatively normal spontaneous language, relatively spared naming and comprehension of single words, and a strong propensity for semantic paraphasias during repetition and writing to dictation (e.g., "balloon" → "kite," "beggar" → "tramp," "roast" → "chicken") (Duhamel & Poncet, 1986; Howard & Franklin, 1987, 1988; Katz & Goodglass, 1990; Martin, Saffran, & Dell, 1996; Michel & Andreewsky, 1983). Although disruption of the acoustic–articulatory linkage apparently precludes repetition via this normal direct route, access from the acoustic hierarchy to concept representations enables repetition through the intact articulatory hierarchy. The presence of semantic paraphasias during repetition and writing to dictation suggests that there is coexistent damage to lexical–semantic (concept) representations (Morton, 1980). These patients' inability to make homophone judgments (do "kernel" and "colonel" sound alike?) or perform pseudohomophone tasks (which sounds like a real word, "stawn" or "stawk"?) suggests that the same lesion that disrupts acoustic-to-articulatory conversion also disrupts articulatory-to-acoustic conversion (Howard & Franklin, 1988). Presumably both tasks require conversion of orthographic into articulatory sequences, followed by conversion to acoustic sequences in order to define a match or mismatch in the "mind's ear" representation.

There is also evidence of a higher-level, phoneme-instantiating acoustic–articulatory link (Figure 3.1, pathway 5). Bub et al. (1987) reported a patient, initially with conduction aphasia and subsequently with anomic aphasia, who performed poorly on nonword repetition tasks (8 of 12 monosyllabic, 6 of 12 bisyllabic, and 2 of 12 trisyllabic items), and yet exhibited nearly perfect phonetic discrimination. This suggests that there is a very low-level pathway (4) that supports phonetic discrimination and the verbal imitation of sounds, and a somewhat higher-level pathway (5) that instantiates phonemes, supports nonword repetition, and was damaged in the patient of Bub et al. (1987). We have observed this pattern of aphasia quite often as a transient phenomenon during the first few days after acute strokes causing anomic aphasia.

CONDUCTION APHASIA

Conduction aphasia is characterized by impaired repetition, in most cases frequent phonemic paraphasias, occasional semantic and verbal paraphasias, variable lexical access in spontaneous language and naming to confrontation, and relative sparing of comprehension and grammar (Benson et al., 1973; Dubois, Hécaen, Angelergues, Maufras de Chatelier, & Marcie, et al., 1973; Green & Howes, 1977; Kohn, 1984). Patients are not anosognosic and characteristically make extensive attempts to correct their errors. Conduction aphasia is essentially a disorder of phonological processing, and it is caused by a lesion at the core of the neural substrate for phonological processing. On the other hand, because patients with conduction aphasia have relatively spared lexical access and normal articulation, they are able to produce voluminous output. For these reasons, conduction aphasia provides an ideal situation for the study of phonological processing.

The model I have described at the beginning of this chapter provides the basis for at least three fundamental types of aphasia that fall within the rubric of conduction aphasia as reported in the literature (Table 3.3):

1. *Repetition conduction aphasia*, caused by *complete* destruction of both the lower-level, direct acoustic–articulatory linkage (pathway 4) and the higher-level, phoneme-

TABLE 3.3. Conduction Aphasias

	Repetition	Reproduction	Phonological	Combination
Pathway lesion				
Pathway 1			Partial	Partial
Pathway 4	Complete	[a]		[a]
Pathway 5	Complete	Partial		Partial
Naming	Relatively normal	Relatively normal	Relatively normal	Relatively normal
Word repetition	Impaired	Normal	Normal	Impaired
Nonword repetition	Poor	Impaired	Normal	Impaired
Phonemic paraphasias in naming	None	None	Present	Present
Phonemic paraphasias in nonword repetition	N/A	Present	Absent	Present
Phonetic discrimination	Impaired	[a]	Presumably normal	[a]
Auditory–verbal short-term memory	Impaired	[a]	Presumably normal	[a]

[a]May be variably damaged, accounting for variability in phonetic discrimination and auditory–verbal short-term memory (see text).

instantiating route (pathway 5). It is characterized by relatively normal naming and spontaneous language, no phonemic paraphasias even in repetition, usually poor phonetic discrimination, impaired auditory–verbal short-term memory, and severely impaired repetition, as a result of both the disconnection and the associated memory impairment.

2. *Reproduction conduction aphasia*, caused by *partial* disruption of the higher-level, phoneme-instantiating acoustic–articulatory linkage (pathway 5). To what extent damage to the lower-level link contributes to the syndrome is not yet entirely clear. Damage could account for observed variability in auditory–verbal short-term memory (tested by repetition, among other means). Partial disruption of the higher-level link is posited because there is behavioral evidence of malfunction rather than complete loss of function. Reproduction conduction aphasia is characterized by relatively normal naming and spontaneous language, good phonetic discrimination, presumably spared auditory–verbal short-term memory, and severely impaired repetition of nonwords because of disruption of phonemic selection in the repetition process. The prototype is the patient of Bub et al. (1987).

3. *Phonological aphasia*, caused by damage exclusively to the phonological articulatory hierarchy, with sparing of both acoustic–articulatory links. It is characterized by phonemic paraphasias in naming and spontaneous language, normal repetition, and presumably normal phonetic discrimination and auditory–verbal short-term memory (Kohn & Smith, 1991, 1994).

Most cases of reproduction conduction aphasia reported in the literature and essentially all cases of conduction aphasia reported in the neurological literature probably represent a combination of types 2 and 3, frequently at the juncture between the acoustic–articulatory links and the phonological articulatory hierarchy; I designate these as "combination conduction aphasia." Reproduction conduction and phonological aphasia, as defined above, represent polar extremes of combination conduction aphasia. I expand on these aphasia types below—devoting the most attention to combination conduction aphasia, both because it appears to be the most common type, and because it provides us with the most extensive insight into the perisylvian language processor.

Repetition Conduction Aphasia

Warrington and Shallice (1969) first described the entity that has come to be known as repetition conduction aphasia. These patients have great difficulty with repetition, but make few sublexical paraphasic errors (in sharp contrast to those with reproduction or combination conduction aphasia); have maximum difficulty with phrases and sentences; and tend to omit whole words, particularly functors. Warrington and Shallice have suggested that the fundamental problem is one of auditory–verbal short-term memory, based on observations that these patients have auditory digit spans of one to three; fail to exhibit a recency effect in digit recall (thought to depend on phonological short-term memory stores; Brooks & Watkins, 1990); demonstrate a primacy effect and perform better with familiar, meaningful, and more slowly presented stimuli (suggesting reliance on lexical–semantic short-term memory stores; Posner, 1964; Watkins & Watkins, 1977); and perform poorly on the distraction condition of the Brown–Petersen procedure. In contrast, patients with combination conduction aphasia generally have relatively preserved digit spans (Damasio & Damasio, 1980). The auditory–verbal short-term memory hypothesis has been extensively debated in the literature (Caramazza, Basili, Koller, & Berndt, 1981; Friedrich et al., 1984; Saffran & Marin, 1975; Shallice & Vallar, 1990; Shallice & Warrington, 1977; Strub & Gardner, 1974; Vallar & Baddeley, 1984; Warrington, Logue, & Pratt, 1971; Warrington & Shallice, 1972). It can be addressed in the model I have introduced. There are two possible ways in which the neural substrate for phonological processing could support short-term memory: (1) through the transient sustained activation of the acoustic and articulatory phonological networks (phonological working memory), and (2) through use of the network for silent rehearsal. The lesions of pathways 4 and 5 that I have posited to cause repetition conduction aphasia are likely to disrupt both mechanisms. In neural network models, the neural substrates for memory and processing are one and the same (i.e., there are no physically separate memory stores). Functional imaging studies in humans also suggest that long-term memories are represented in the same cortices that process the substance of those memories, and single-neuron studies in monkeys indicate that the immediate or working memory of a cue corresponds to sustained activity of neurons representing that cue (Ungerleider, 1995). Thus damage to a processor will inevitably be associated with concomitant impairment in its immediate and long-term mnestic capabilities (Martin & Saffran, 1997; Martin et al., 1996). This impairment is most likely to be evident in the performance of nonrehearsal tasks such as the distraction condition of the Brown–Petersen consonant trigram test, on which patients with repetition conduction aphasia are impaired (Caramazza et al., 1981; Shallice & Warrington, 1977). The ability to use the phonological network for both recall and silent rehearsal is likely to be most important for comprehension of long, grammatically complex sentences and of correct order in word lists. Patients with repetition conduction aphasia also show impairment on such tasks (Shallice & Warrington, 1977).

To the extent that auditory–verbal short-term memory deficits reflect impaired ability to rehearse silently, they are a result rather than a cause of the behavior observed. However, to the extent that auditory–verbal short-term memory deficits reflect damage to the neurological substrate for phonological working memory (the phonological processor itself), it is reasonable to view them as indicative of a genuine deficit in immediate memory (Caramazza et al., 1981). Because damage to articulatory portions of the phonological hierarchical network impairs both silent rehearsal and the substrate for phonological working memory, one would expect auditory–verbal short-term memory deficits in patients with Broca's aphasia—something that has been shown (Cermak & Tarlow, 1978; Goodglass, Gleason, & Hyde, 1970; Heilman, Scholes, & Watson, 1976).

Patients with repetition conduction aphasia apparently do not have the extensive damage to the hierarchical phonological articulatory processor that is associated with phonemic paraphasias and neologisms in naming and spontaneous language. The exact distribution of damage within the phonological apparatus that prevents its engagement as the substrate for phonological working memory remains uncertain. Two types of repetition conduction aphasia have been identified, raising the possibility of at least two mechanisms. In one type, the necessary and sufficient lesion may be complete destruction of the acoustic–articulatory phonological linkage (Figure 3.1, pathways 4 and 5) (Morton, 1980). Several investigators have noted abundant semantic and derivational paraphasic errors in the repetition of these patients, which, together with other properties of their language and their short digit span, suggest that they may have a form of deep dysphasia. With further research in deep dysphasia, the concept that impaired phonological short-term memory is an essential contributory factor has become more widely accepted (Duhamel & Poncet, 1986; Howard & Franklin, 1988; Katz & Goodglass, 1990; Martin et al., 1996; Michel & Andreewsky, 1983; Trojano, Stanzione, & Grossi, 1992), and Martin and colleagues (Martin & Saffran, 1992; Martin et al., 1996) have suggested that deep dysphasia and repetition conduction aphasia are variants of the same fundamental disorder. According to the hypothesis discussed earlier, because of the damage to the acoustic–articulatory linkage, patients with deep dysphasia cannot use a direct repetition route or directly recruit articulatory portions of the phonological hierarchy. They thus must repeat via the concept representation route. The prominence of semantic and derivational paraphasias during repetition in patients with deep dysphasia may indicate greater damage to lexical–semantic representations in these patients than in patients with repetition conduction aphasia. The acoustic–articulatory disconnection denies access to the articulatory components of the phonological hierarchy that could both inhibit these verbal paraphasias and support phonological working memory and phonetic discrimination, which are also usually impaired in these patients (Allport, 1984a). In contrast, in patients with conduction aphasia in whom the low-level acoustic articulatory linkage is preserved, as indicated by normal phonetic discrimination, phonological working memory is relatively preserved (Bub et al., 1987).

The possibility of a second potential mechanism—or two extremes accounting for a range of deficits—is raised by (1) reports of patients with deep dysphasia with normal phonetic discrimination (Howard & Franklin, 1988; Martin & Saffran, 1992), and (2) reports of patients with repetition conduction aphasia with normal phonetic discrimination; ability to read nonwords, make rhyme judgments, and assign syllabic stress to words; and some evidence of a recency effect in repetition (Berndt & Mitchum, 1990; Shallice & Vallar, 1990; Vallar & Baddeley, 1984). These spared abilities strongly suggest that both components of the acoustic–articulatory link were substantially preserved. The hypothesis proposed in the preceding paragraph posits that phonological working memory is reduced because the extent of the phonological representation (acoustic plus articulatory) is reduced by an anterior–posterior disconnection. How then can patients with reduced auditory–verbal short-term memory but an intact acoustic–articulatory link be accounted for? The substrate for auditory–verbal short-term memory may include not just the dominant-hemisphere acoustic and articulatory representations, but also representations of some type in the nondominant hemisphere. In this conceptualization, the patients with repetition conduction aphasia just cited lost a large portion of their phonological representations, either because their left and right hemispheres were disconnected, or because they substantially lost all dominant-hemisphere representations and were reliant mainly on nondominant-hemisphere representations (particularly likely in the patient of Vallar & Baddeley, 1984, who had a very large left-hemisphere lesion). They thus had moderate impairment of auditory–verbal short-term memory even in the presence of an intact acoustic–articulatory link. The availability of some substrate for phonological working memory, however limited, in turn provided a limited basis for the recency effect characterizing phonological short-term memory stores (Berndt & Mitchum, 1990). In contrast, the majority of patients with repetition conduction aphasia and deep dysphasia may have disruption of the acoustic–articulatory links coupled with either disruption of connections between the two hemispheres or an absence of right-hemisphere phonological capacity; the combined effect is a dramatic reduction in the extent of cortex available to support phonological working memory, more severe behavioral deficits, and no recency effect.

It is often observed but little reported that there are patients, apparently with conduction aphasia, who have relatively little tendency to make phonemic and other sublexical paraphasias but have difficulty mainly in the repetition of meaningless strings of functors, such as "no ifs, ands, or buts." This sequence has become a standard bedside probe used by behavioral neurologists to ferret out conduction aphasia. This is quite ironic, because the basis for this behavior is not clear: The relative absence of sublexical paraphasias actually tends to rule out reproduction or combination conduction aphasia; repetition of sentences containing large numbers of functors may be better than sentences made up of substantives in combination conduction aphasia (Kohn, 1989); and the phenomenon is most consistent with repetition conduction aphasia, which has not won wide acceptance as a nosological entity in the behavioral-neurological community. The data I have reviewed and the neural model I have developed clearly define nonword repetition as the definitive probe for reproduction and combination conduction aphasia. It seems more likely that relative inability to repeat "no ifs, ands, or buts" reflects primarily a deficit in phonological short-term (working) memory. My bedside testing of this idea has consistently revealed digit spans of less than three in patients who exhibit problems repeating this word sequence.

Reproduction Conduction Aphasia

The case that most closely meets the criteria for reproduction conduction aphasia is patient MV of Bub et al. (1987). This patient initially presented with a more traditional conduction aphasia (combination conduction aphasia, in the terminology adopted here) that evolved into an anomic aphasia with otherwise normal spontaneous language, normal phonetic discrimination, and very poor repetition of nonwords with abundant phonemic paraphasias. Repetition of words was not perfect, declining to 67% of low-frequency three-syllable words. It is unclear whether this reflected a minor flaw in pathway 1 (Figure 3.1), which would make her disorder an extreme form of combination conduction aphasia, or the inability of normal bottom-up and top-down processing in pathway 1 to correct all errors generated in pathway 5. The term "reproduction conduction aphasia" seems appropriate, as this patient had little difficulty *producing* words (aside from anomia), and her signal deficit was in *reproducing* phonemic strings (in repetition) that was apparently related to phonological processing per se and could not be tied to some other underlying disorder (e.g., in auditory–verbal short-term memory).

Phonological Aphasia

Three reported cases, one classified as having transcortical motor aphasia, exemplify phonological aphasia. All three had relatively spared repetition, with phonemic paraphasias most frequent during naming and spontaneous language (Kohn & Smith, 1991, 1994; McCarthy

& Warrington, 1984). One patient (Kohn & Smith, 1991) was distinctive in that he resorted to spelling during picture naming, apparently making use of the word representation in the graphemic lexicon in a largely vain attempt to overcome phonological paraphasias in verbal output. Because repetition was not perfect in these cases, these patients could be viewed as having extreme forms of combination conduction aphasia, in which damage to the articulatory hierarchy (Figure 3.1, pathway 1) was relatively severe but damage to the acoustic–articulatory link (pathway 5) was very mild. Classification of this entity as conduction aphasia seems inappropriate given the spared repetition, and classification as transcortical motor aphasia does not seem entirely satisfactory, as the major cause of nonfluency in the case of McCarthy and Warrington (1984) was a mix of phonemic paraphasias and phonetic disintegration. Nor does it resemble any other type of aphasia, most notably Wernicke's (because of relatively good comprehension) or Broca's (because fluency is relatively normal, repetition is spared, phonetic disintegration is not a consistent feature, and grammatical function is relatively preserved). Hence the designation "phonological aphasia." The cases of Burns and Canter (1977), with Wernicke's or conduction aphasia, had better real-word repetition than naming (although polysyllabic word repetition was poor), raising the possibility that these patients had combination conduction aphasia with damage predominantly involving pathway 1. Nonword repetition was not tested.

Combination Conduction Aphasia

Sequences in Conduite D'Approche

Patients with combination conduction aphasia produce significantly more phonologically similar sequences than patients with Broca's or Wernicke's aphasia (Kohn, 1984). Some of these sequences are very long (one reported by Gandour et al., 1994, contained 27 items). The persistent neural network instantiation of the lexical target fails to elicit reliably (i.e., to bring above threshold) the single hierarchical set of sublexical components ultimately determining the correct phonemic sequence. The network damage that causes this failure also permits phonologically similar elements at the various levels in the hierarchy to rise transiently above threshold, leading to incorrect output that phonologically resembles the target. The persisting integrity of the lexical target as lexical working memory provides a template with which to compare feedback, whether transmitted retrogradely through the brain or via auditory self-monitoring. The detection of a discrepancy between template and production spurs another attempt at production.

Word Length Effects

The model predicts that longer words will pose greater problems, because they increase the number of sublexical elements that are simultaneously being processed. This increases the opportunity for these elements to induce errors by interacting with each other and their various associated sublexical elements. Also, because the lesion reduces the reliability of bringing every one of multiple syllables above production threshold, this increases the opportunity for sublexical omissions. Such effects are well documented in patients with combination conduction aphasia (Alajouanine & Lhermitte, 1973; Bub et al., 1987; Caplan, Vanier, & Baker, 1986; Caramazza et al., 1986; Dubois et al., 1973; Friedman & Kohn, 1990; Gandour et al., 1994; Kohn, 1989; Kohn & Smith, 1991, 1995; McCarthy & Warrington, 1984; Pate, Saffran, & Martin, 1987; Valdois et al., 1988; Yamadori & Ikumura, 1975). On the other hand, repetition of long words is less likely to result in verbal paraphasias, because a single phonemic error is less likely to activate other real words, with their associated top-down reinforcement effects; this effect may become evident when there is damage to the acoustic hierarchy that leads to the introduction of a phonemic slip very early in the process of repetition. With a short word, such a slip is likely to activate a host of other short words, increasing the likelihood of a verbal paraphasia (Howard & Franklin, 1988).

Variable Lexical Bias Effects

The model predicts variable lexical bias, depending on locus of lesion. This lexical bias may be mediated directly when repetition occurs via the concept representation, and indirectly, via bottom-up and top-down spread of activation through the articulatory hierarchy, when repetition occurs via the acoustic–articulatory links. Two effects of lesion locus may be expected. First, I have posited that combination conduction aphasia reflects a partial lesion of two pathways: the phonological articulatory hierarchy (Figure 3.1, pathway 1) and the higher-level acoustic–articulatory link (pathway 5). One discrete lesion at the nexus of these pathways could damage both equally, but more commonly, one would expect to see worse damage to one pathway than to the other. To the extent that the phonological articulatory hierarchy (pathway 1) is damaged, lexical bias effects will be reduced and repetition of nonwords spared. To the extent that the acoustic–articulatory link (pathway 5) is damaged, lexical bias effects will be increased and repetition of nonwords will be impaired.

Second, lexical bias effects will vary according to the integrity of upper levels of the phonological articulatory hierarchy (semantic field, articulatory word forms) and the type of word being repeated. The superiority in repeating words over nonwords should be maximal when lexical–semantic representations are essentially intact and are able to provide strong top-down reinforcement of words and correction of phonemic slips (e.g., Caramazza et al., 1986; Strub & Gardner, 1974). However, lexical bias should be less in patients with damaged lexical representations reflected in anomia (e.g., Caplan et al., 1986; Dubois et al., 1973). Because functors (closed-class words) have little meaning and are primarily of grammatical importance, they normally receive little top-down reinforcement from semantic representations. Thus in patients capable of strong lexical–semantic bias (no anomia), the repetition of major lexical items may be superior to that of functors; in patients with anomia, by contrast, major lexical items should have much less advantage over functors, as then neither receives much top-down reinforcement (Caplan et al., 1986). On the other hand, functors should be relatively resistant to phonemic paraphasias because of strong top-down reinforcement from the lexical level that is instantiated in strong connections between word and phoneme levels in the phonological hierarchy acquired through frequent use (see "Frequency and Imageability Effects," below). This has been borne out in practice (Caplan et al., 1986; Kohn, 1989; Lecours, 1982). To summarize, the relative advantage in repetition of functors over major lexical items will reflect the balance of three factors: degree of preservation of representations supporting word frequency effects (favoring functors), degree of preservation of grammar (favoring functors), and naming ability (favoring major lexical items). In the typical case of combination conduction aphasia, the first two factors appear to dominate, and functors are relatively spared.

There is indirect evidence that lexical bias effects may be exerted by sublexical components at the syllabic level. Valdois et al. (1988) found that in a group of patients with conduction aphasia, performance in a repetition task was the same for nonwords as for real words—a surprising result. However, the nonword stimuli in their task differed from real words only in their vowels. Thus there is a high likelihood that the resultant syllables were in their subjects' "syllabic lexicons" and capable, like real words, of providing top-down reinforcement that would inhibit or correct phonemic slips. Other sublexical bias effects can account for the reliability with which phonemic slips obey phonotactic constraints. Unacceptable phonemic sequences provide bottom-up activation of the joint phonemes, syllables, and words that contain them, and these in turn provide top-down influences that induce further phoneme slips and correct the phonotactically unacceptable productions. It is also possible that processes normally involved in phonetic modification that ultimately exert their effect at the articulatory level are serving to eliminate phonotactically unacceptable sequences.

Malapropisms (formal verbal paraphasias) in a sense represent lexical bias run amok. As a lexical item is activated, it activates all of its various sublexical and phonological components. These return activation to the lexical target, but also to phonologically similar targets, regardless of their degree of semantic unrelatedness. This pattern of top-down followed by bottom-up spread of activation can have perverse consequences. Natural noise in the system can lead to selection of an item phonologically similar to the lexical target because its activation level ends up being a little higher—a classic malapropism. In the presence of a lesion of the articulatory hierarchical processor, the downward spread of activation from a lexical target may generate patterns of activity corresponding to a phonemic paraphasic error. This error in turn generates bottom-up spread of activation, enhancing the likelihood that a phonologically similar word will receive maximum activation in lieu of the target (see Blanken, 1990, for empirical evidence of this). This process, the lexicalization of neologisms (described in Dell's model; see above), adds one or more errors to the original phonological slip as it arrives at the new word. Gagnon, Schwartz, Martin, Dell, and Safran. (1995) have confirmed that formal paraphasias on average contain a greater number of phonological deviations from the target than do neologisms. A formal paraphasia loses its semantic relationship to the target, because words with similar meaning do not generally sound alike.

Verbal paraphasias can arise in a completely different way, in which a phonological slip yields a real word by chance without lexical or grammatical influence. For example, given the target "cat," a selection error late in phonological processing can result in "sat." Verbal paraphasias commonly reflect what are referred to as "combination errors," in which phonological, semantic, and grammatical influences are all evident. Combination errors may develop in two ways. First, a phonemic slip that initially eliminates semantic and grammatical resemblance to the target (e.g., "cat" → "sat") is followed by bottom-up and top-down processing that induces a second slip and generates a semantic, grammatical, and phonological associate of the target ("cat" → "sat" → "rat"), "rat" being the ultimate result because it received some direct activation as a semantic associate of "cat," and some bottom-up activation from sublexical elements of "sat." Second, the selection of a concept is associated with the activation of semantically related concept representations. All of these semantically related representations engage articulatory word forms that, through spread of activation down through their sublexical components, ultimately produce bottom-up activation of phonologically related articulatory word forms. In the presence of natural or lesion-induced noise in the system that prevents the engagement of the target word, an alternate that is both semantically and phonologically related and thus receives activation from two sources may be more likely to be selected than one that is only semantically related, only phonologically related, or unrelated (Brédart & Valentine, 1992; Dell & Reich, 1981; Dell et al., 1997; Harley, 1984, 1990; Laine & Martin, 1996; Martin, Weisberg, & Saffran, 1989).

Frequency and Imageability Effects

As the model incorporates PDP principles, those linguistic items represented most strongly and redundantly in neural connectivity will be the most resistant to the degradative effects of lesions or noise. The most immediate result is that high-frequency items will be retained to a greater degree than low-frequency items. This may reflect two factors: (1) Frequency is likely to be reflected in greater strength of bidirectional connections between words and various types of sublexical elements (phonemes included) that build up in the course of word use; and (2) high-frequency items at every level receive greater top-down reinforcement, high-frequency open-class items from the semantic field, high-frequency closed-class items from networks supporting grammar, and high-frequency sublexical elements and phonemes from the large number of words including them (for a review, see Stemberger, 1991).

Normal subjects repeat high-frequency words better than low-frequency words (Watkins & Watkins, 1977). Naming errors in aphasia are more likely with low-frequency targets (Kay & Ellis, 1987). Neologistic errors and phonemic paraphasias in jargon and conduction aphasia are more common with low-frequency than with high-frequency targets (Allport, 1984b; Bub et al., 1987; Martin & Saffran, 1992; McCarthy & Warrington, 1984; Miller & Ellis, 1987; Pate et al., 1987; Strub & Gardner, 1974), as are phonological slips in naturally occurring and experimentally induced slips of the tongue (Dell, 1988; Stemberger, 1984; Stemberger & MacWhinney, 1986). In both aphasic language and slips of the tongue, less common phonemes and phoneme combinations tend to be replaced by more common phonemes and combinations; this reflects in part the fact that high-frequency phonemes are included in more words, which in turn provide top-down reinforcement of these phonemes.

A corollary to the effect of word frequency is the effect of imageability. Highly imageable words are likely to have extensive representations in sensory association cortices (most often visual), which in turn serve as an additional source of top-down reinforcement of these words. Imageability effects on repetition have been reported (Allport, 1984a; Howard & Franklin, 1988; Martin & Saffran, 1992).

Word frequency and imageability effects will be constrained by the same factors that govern lexical bias. Thus frequency and imageability effects in repetition will be maximal when lexical and semantic representations, and the pathways that link them to phonological representations (pathways 1 and 2), are intact and pathways 4 and 5 are damaged. On the other hand, if repetition can occur rapidly and accurately via pathways 4 and 5, then lexical access will have minimal impact (still less if there is damage to upper portions of pathways 1 and 2) because of the delays inherent in bottom-up and top-down activity spread, and frequency, imageability, and lexical bias effects will be minimal. Martin and Saffran (1997) have provided tentative confirmation of these concepts.

Effects of Delay

The model predicts that patients with conduction aphasia will benefit from delay in the repetition of real words when damage to the phonological processor is greater than to lexical–semantic representations, because delay allows the corrupted trace in phonological working memory to die out and lexical–semantic representations to dominate output. It predicts that delay will differentially impair the repetition of nonwords. Both predictions have been borne out (Bub et al., 1987; Gardner & Winner, 1978; Hough & DeMarco, 1995; Strub & Gardner, 1974).

ANATOMY OF PHONOLOGICAL PROCESSING

The data I have reviewed suggest that phonological processing is a hierarchical process. Can this be reconciled with the traditional Wernicke–Geschwind model (Geschwind, 1965;

Wernicke, 1874), in which a center for auditory word images in area 22 is linked (presumably via the arcuate fasciculus) to the area of motor expression in the posterior inferior frontal lobe (Broca's area)? The answer is "Partly." Recent data from functional imaging studies (Démonet et al., 1992; Paulesu, Frith, & Frackowiak, 1993) and from intraoperative electrocortical stimulation studies (Ojemann, 1991) strongly suggest that there *is* a discontinuity in the perisylvian language cortex that supports phonological processing. That is, there is indeed a posterior language region centered on area 22 and extending variably into area 40, and an anterior region centered on Broca's area and extending variably backward into opercular areas 4 and 6. The parietal operculum between the central sulcus and area 40 appears less likely to be implicated directly in language processes of any type in the majority of patients. There is a caveat here, and that is that data are emerging—particularly from Ojemann's electrocortical stimulation studies (Ojemann, 1991; Ojemann, Ojemann, Lettich, & Berger, 1989), but more recently from functional imaging studies (Binder et al., 1995; Cuenod et al., 1995)—that there is substantial individual variability in the location and extent of cortex devoted to language processing in general and to phonological processing in particular.

Although functional imaging and electrocortical stimulation studies provide validation of the basic concept of the two-part Wernicke–Geschwind model, empirical studies of phonological processing clearly indicate that a hierarchical series of interlinked processes is occurring in distributed fashion over two anatomically separated cortical regions, and that it is not simply a question of transmission of word images to a language output zone. This revised conceptualization is actually somewhat reminiscent of that espoused by Kurt Goldstein (1948). The precise division of labor between the posterior and anterior language zones with respect to phonological processing remains to be determined. Furthermore, ischemic damage is widely distributed in any given stroke patient, and multiple components of language function are generally impaired to a variable degree. The region of maximal damage, usually apparent in imaging studies, will tend to define the predominant aphasic characteristics, but damage to other areas, often invisible on imaging studies, may contribute in an important way to the particular attributes of the aphasia; this problem is most evident in nonthalamic subcortical aphasia (Nadeau & Crosson, 1997). Finally, the degree to which other cortices, particularly in the right hemisphere, may compensate for aphasic deficits is quite variable. Conduction aphasia often begins as Wernicke's aphasia. Then, through some combination of recovery of deranged neural function and recruitment of compensatory neural function, possibly involving the right hemisphere (Benson et al., 1973; Brown, 1975; Kinsbourne, 1971), lexical access and comprehension improve to the degree that the major residual deficit is phonological. These unfortunate complexities of the lesion model pose major challenges both to the behavioral neurologist, who attempts to establish clinical-pathological correlations, and to the cognitive neuropsychologist, who is committed to explaining aphasic behavior in terms of a defect in a single functional system.

Disconnection theories of conduction aphasia originated with Carl Wernicke and have been a subject of continual debate ever since (Palumbo, Alexander, & Naeser, 1992). The long white matter links between Wernicke's and Broca's areas (e.g., the arcuate fasciculus) presumably evolved with the physical separation of these two cortices that developed during phylogenesis and ontogenesis. Thus there is no particular reason to think that these long white matter tracts are either functionally more important or fundamentally different from white matter connections *within* Wernicke's and Broca's areas. The model of phonological processing I have discussed consists of a hierarchy of progressively larger and more complex phonological structures built on a base of articulatory representations in Broca's area and opercular areas 4 and 6, a parallel hierarchy built on a base of acoustic representations in the superior temporal gyrus (Howard et al., 1992), and direct links between the two bases. The arcuate fasciculus or another long, anterior–posterior perisylvian white matter pathway could subserve two functions in phonology: (1) direct linkage between the acoustic and articulatory representations (pathways 4 and 5 in Figure 3.1); and (2) linkages within the articulatory hierarchy, presumably connecting distinctive features and motoric representations in Broca's area to phonological sublexical and lexical representations more posteriorly (part of pathway 1 in Figure 3.1). The position within the articulatory hierarchy of this white matter pathway is uncertain and may vary from person to person.

Conduction aphasia, both as traditionally defined and as redefined in this chapter as combination conduction aphasia, is produced by lesions in the supramarginal gyrus, the posterior aspect of Wernicke's area, and the angular gyrus (Benson et al., 1973; Damasio & Damasio, 1980; Naeser & Hayward, 1978; Palumbo et al., 1992). The insula is also commonly involved, but it is unlikely that this phylogenetically ancient structure with predominantly orbito-frontal and limbic connectivity participates in language processes. However, white matter connections from the superior temporal gyrus to the frontal cortex do pass in the extreme capsule, immediately beneath the insula (Damasio & Damasio, 1980). To the extent that conduction aphasia reflects damage to acoustic–articulatory links (Figure 3.1, pathways 4 and 5), it can be viewed as a disconnection syndrome. However, combination conduction aphasia also involves, to varying degrees, damage to pathway 1; as such, it is best viewed as a limited form of Wernicke's aphasia, distinguished by better lexical access and a relatively preserved acoustic hierarchy (pathway 2). This view of conduction aphasia was first espoused by Freud (1891/1953).

Although there is reasonable consistency in the anatomical lesions associated with combination conduction aphasia, in occasional cases cortical lesions are much larger, there is extensive subcortical involvement (consistent with proximal middle cerebral artery occlusion; Nadeau & Crosson, 1997), or aphasia has been caused by intracerebral hemorrhage (Damasio & Damasio, 1980; McCarthy & Warrington, 1984; Palumbo et al., 1992). The functional consequences of this lesion heterogeneity have not been thoroughly explored. However, it is noteworthy that whereas Damasio and Damasio (1980) reported normal digit spans in their six cases with fairly circumscribed lesions, McCarthy and Warrington (1984) reported severely reduced digit spans in their two cases of lobar hemorrhage. This suggests that with larger lesions, there may be substantial destruction of pathway 4 (Figure 3.1), reducing the substrate for phonological working memory. Large posterior ischemic perisylvian lesions raise the possibility of right-hemisphere participation in the recovery process of at least some patients with combination conduction aphasia. Patients with repetition conduction aphasia, who by and large seem to have larger lesions (unfortunately rather poorly documented), provide even more compelling evidence of surrogate right-hemisphere language function. In fact, it may not be too extreme to attribute the entire range of variability in repetition conduction aphasia not to lesion variability (a possibility raised earlier), but to variations in nondominant-hemispheric capacity for phonological function.

REHABILITATION

I have presented a complex model of phonological function and provided evidence that aphasia may result in differential impairment of specific segments of the phonological apparatus. The profile of impairment in any given patient can readily be defined with specific tests (Table 3.4). This chapter has, from the beginning, used a PDP conceptualization to approach the problems of phonological processing. It is therefore to the PDP attributes of the model that I look for implications regarding rehabilitation.

TABLE 3.4. Clinical Tests of the Phonological Apparatus

Pathway	Test
1	Spontaneous language
	Naming to confrontation or definition
2	Auditory lexical decision
4	Phonetic discrimination
	Rhyming judgment
5	Nonword repetition

Although the model presented seems quite complex, and although PDP models are in many ways counterintuitive, the phonological apparatus actually appears to be much simpler when viewed in full PDP terms (Figure 3.3). It consists of a network of connections linking concept representations to articulatory motor representations, a network of connections linking concept representations to acoustic representations, and networks linking acoustic to articulatory representations. I refer to these as "pattern associator networks," because they enable the translation of one pattern of neural representation into another pattern in a different modality. The networks linking acoustic to articulatory representations store the neural knowledge of the relationships between acoustic sequences and articulatory sequences. Implicit in this knowledge of paired sequential relationships is knowledge of acoustic and articulatory aggregations—the clumping mentioned early in the chapter that instantiates joint phonemes, rhymes, syllables, morphemes, and articulatory word forms. Therefore, all sublexical knowledge resides in the acoustic–articulatory network. I have posited a link between concept representations and the hidden units in the middle of the acoustic–articulatory network, in order to explain a phenomenon that has been a major focus in this chapter: Patients with damage to the phonological apparatus make sublexical paraphasic errors, not just in repetition but also in spontaneous language and naming (hence phonological and combination conduction aphasias). Direct links between concept representations and articulatory motor representations do not instantiate sublexical knowledge because concepts are fundamentally unitary, and to the extent that they imply subconcepts, these subconcepts do not correspond to parts of words, but rather to different whole words. If the only link between concept representations and articulatory motor representations were the direct one, affected patients would be anomic or make semantic paraphasic (whole-word) errors, but would never generate sublexical errors during spontaneous language and naming.

I touch on some specific aspects of this more completely PDP-based conceptualization of phonology in what follows. The point to be made here is that the various parts of the phonological apparatus are almost certainly interlinked to a degree not previously suspected. This suggests in turn that phonologically oriented therapy may have a role to play in many types of aphasias, not just in aphasias in which there is evidence of sublexical breakdown of language.

Implications of Hebbian Learning

In PDP models, the information lies in the strengths of connections between units. The concept that this might be true in the brain was first proposed independently by Ramón y Cajal (1923) and Tanzi (1893), but it was really developed by Donald Hebb (1949). Hebb proposed that connection strengths develop to the degree that there is simultaneous acti-

Distributed Concept Representations

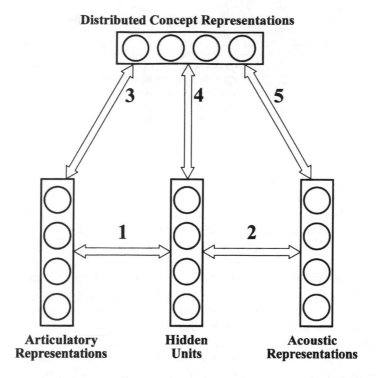

FIGURE 3.3. In this figure, pools of neurons supporting distributed representations are depicted as sets of four circles, and the massive interconnectivity between the pools (probably two-way) as open arrows. The core of the language processor, which supports word and nonword repetition and is located predominantly in dominant perisylvian cortex, consists of the articulatory representations, the acoustic representations, their interposed hidden units, and connecting links 1 and 2. This core supports the knowledge of the relationship between sound sequences and articulatory motor sequences characteristic of the language spoken. This is not an acoustic-element-to-phoneme transcoder; rather, it is a transcoder of acoustic sequences to articulatory sequences. The role of hidden units is further elucidated in Chapter 12 of this volume. Suffice it to say at this point that they are essential to the capability of the network for instantiating sequence knowledge.

Connecting links 3, 4, and 5 represent connections between cortex supporting semantic distributed representations and the core phonological processor. Additional pools of intermediate hidden units are left out for purposes of clarity. Two output links are posited (3 and 4) because patients with combination conduction and phonological aphasias routinely demonstrate sublexical paraphasias (e.g., phonemic paraphasias) in spontaneous language, at the same time that they may exhibit dramatic dissociations between the frequency of sublexical paraphasias in spontaneous language and in repetition. These observations suggest that there must be semantic–articulatory links that are whole-word-based (pathway 3) and that incorporate knowledge of phonological sequences (pathway 4). It should be stressed that pathway 3 does not instantiate sublexical knowledge except at the movement level. This conceptualization parallels that thought to underlie reading, in which there is unequivocal evidence of lexical–semantic and phonological pathways (Plaut et al., 1996). Pathways 1, 3, and 4 and the units they link constitute the basis for the phonological output lexicon.

vation of two connected neurons. Neuroscientific studies of species ranging from primitive mollusks (*Aplysia*) to higher primates suggest that learning in the brain does incorporate some variation of the Hebbian principle.

What implications does the Hebbian principle have for rehabilitation? Rehabilitation in patients with essentially intact concept representations consists predominantly of training one or more pattern associator networks—for example, the pattern associator linking distributed concept representations with articulatory motor representations in patients with anomic, phonological, combination conduction, or Broca's aphasia; the pattern associators linking acoustic and articulatory motor representations in patients with reproduction conduction aphasia (as redefined here); or the pattern associator linking orthographic sequence representations to articulatory motor sequence representations in patients with acquired phonological dyslexia.

To maximize the efficiency of Hebbian learning, the input and desired output patterns need to be approached as directly as possible. Thus an algorithm for treating anomia or alexia that relies primarily on acoustic feedback is less likely to be effective than one that also includes articulatory motor feedback, particularly if the brain links between acoustic and articulatory representations are damaged, as they are in all the perisylvian aphasias (Broca's, Wernicke's, conduction, and global). After all, the major point of the treatment is to facilitate articulatory production. Even normal subjects will tend to hear the phonetic sequence they see being mouthed, even when the actual acoustic stimulus corresponds to a slightly different phonetic sequence—the McGurk effect (McGurk & MacDonald, 1976). At the least, clinicians can provide articulatory motor feedback simply by having patients view their faces as they provide feedback. There is evidence that treatment algorithms employing intensive and explicit means of providing articulatory motor feedback can be highly successful (Conway et al., 1998).

The Hebbian principle also makes signal delay potentially relevant. Focal cerebral activation will be maximal at time of stimulus onset and will remain high only to the extent that working memory is normal in the particular modalities involved. Given the often disseminated damage associated with strokes, working memory may not be normal, and focal activation patterns may decay rapidly with time. This suggests that feedback regarding the correct response should occur either simultaneously with or very shortly after stimulus presentation, or that errorless learning strategies, which facilitate a prompt correct response, should be employed (Brownjohn, 1988; Strand & Morris, 1986; Worley et al., 1992).

Implications of Associative Properties of PDP Networks

The Need for Rich and Converging Inputs

In PDP networks, activation flows freely from one part of a network to another and from network to network, constrained only by the strengths of the network connections. Thus multiple sources of input that converge to establish a given representation increase the probability that the desired representation will be generated and that variously related competing distributed representations will not. The implication of this principle for rehabilitation is that stimuli should be as rich and polymodal as possible. High-quality color graphics or real objects, which enable visual, tactile, and even olfactory input, are likely to be more effective than black-and-white line drawings.

Multiple Parallel Pathways

There is accumulating evidence that many if not all language functions in the brain are subserved by two (perhaps more) parallel pathways. The most clearly explicated process is reading, wherein grapheme-to-phoneme, lexical, and semantic routes have been posited (see Greenwald, Chapter 7, this volume). PDP models incorporating two routes, a grapheme sequence → phoneme sequence route and a grapheme cluster → semantic distributed representation → phoneme cluster route, can adequately account for all the observed behavior (Plaut et al., 1996). There is corresponding evidence of two routes involved in writing (see Rapcsak & Beeson, Chapter 8, this volume).

The mechanisms underlying the syndrome of optic aphasia are controversial, but one major hypothesis is that there are two routes to object naming: one involving a pattern associator network that links visual representations directly to articulatory motor representations (enabling us to learn and remember the name of an utterly meaningless symbol or drawing, for example); and a second route linking visual representations to concept representations, and thence to articulatory motor representations (Shuren & Heilman, 1993). In this conceptualization, optic aphasia occurs because a damaged visual–articulatory route generates incorrect patterns of activation in articulatory motor cortex, which compete with correct patterns of activation generated via the concept route. This renders the patient incapable of output (i.e., anomic) when naming to confrontation, but fluent when speaking spontaneously, in which case there is no competition from the corrupted visual–articulatory route.

Spontaneous language production has not hitherto been recognized as a two-route process. However, as I have noted in the introduction to this section, there is compelling evidence that it is.

I have made this long digression to emphasize the plausibility of pervasive dual-network mechanisms underlying language function, including the most essential language function of all—the capacity for spontaneous output and naming. The importance of the point is that the product of dual networks is likely to be mutually reinforcing; however, when one of the networks is damaged, not only is mutual reinforcement lost, but there is a possibility of interference, as I have posited in regard to optic aphasia. The relevance for treatment is that in the aphasic patient, it may be important to explicitly recognize the existence of dual networks and conduct two different, network-specific rehabilitation strategies. For example, in a patient with conduction aphasia with substantial anomia, rehabilitation of the acoustic–articulatory network could potentially improve anomia by reducing interference (from the links between the semantic and acoustic–articulatory networks) with names more successfully generated via direct, semantic–articulatory motor connections.

"Gatekeeper" Networks

The prototypic gatekeeper network is that which underlies articulatory motor representations. In principle, these can be accessed via the acoustic route (repetition), the orthographic route (reading aloud), or the semantic route (naming to confrontation, naming to definition). The interface between these various sources of input with articulatory motor representations may be different. It is not clear which might provide the best route for rebuilding articulatory motor representations. The optimal route may vary from patient to patient, and it is possible that a two- or three-pronged rehabilitation approach (perhaps mutually reinforcing) would be preferable. The present understanding of neural structure is not an adequate basis for predictions, and ultimately this is an empirical question to be answered in each patient uniquely.

Generalization

The PDP structure of neural networks has strong implications for generalization effects in rehabilitation. Pattern associators that instantiate links between sequences—such as the acoustic–articulatory motor network underlying repetition, or the orthographic–articulatory motor network underlying reading aloud—provide the basis for intrinsic generalization. That is, rehabilitation with any reasonable corpus of words will provide the patient with experience applicable to many if not most other words, because words in any given language share a limited spectrum of acoustic–articulatory sequences. This tends not to be true of pattern associators that instantiate links between concept representations and, for example, articulatory motor representations, for the simple reason that there is no relationship between the meaning of a word and the articulatory motor programs needed for its production. There is still some limited opportunity for generalization from therapies designed to reestablish semantic–articulatory links—to the extent that trained and untrained items share semantic features (Plaut, 1996). To the extent that the lesion is nearer semantic representations and their links to the phonological apparatus (i.e., posterior), this generalization is likely to be maximal. To the extent that the lesion is nearer articulatory motor representations (e.g., some of the patients discussed under "Phonological Aphasia," above), there is likely to be minimal generalization from rehabilitation designed to improve naming and word access in spontaneous language.

Two other major factors favor generalization. First, PDP networks degrade gracefully. This means that there is still a great deal of useful knowledge in a damaged network. Unlike a digital computer, the network has not been rendered completely dysfunctional. Rather, the likelihood that correct responses will reach threshold for production has been reduced, and the probability of errors (generally near-misses) has been increased. To the degree that the substance of rehabilitation shares features with knowledge still latent within the network, there will be generalization to these related concepts and skills.

Second, I have alluded at the beginning of this section to the degree of linkage that exists within the various components of the phonological processor, and I have elaborated on this concept in my discussion of the prevalence of parallel routes in various language processes. Because of the existence of this linkage, there is a substantial probability in any given patient of cross-modal generalization between treatments (e.g., a patient with anomia may benefit from phonologically motivated treatment as well as semantically motivated treatment).

CONCLUSION

I have reviewed the literature on phonological dysfunction in normal subjects and patients with aphasia, and have developed a revised neural model (derived from Dell's PDP model) that explicitly incorporates many of the parameters evident in the language data and provides a logical account for many of the patterns of phonological dysfunction observed. The most fundamental principle of this model is that its function, whether normal or disrupted by natural or lesion-induced noise, is related entirely to the topography of network connections. It is possible that there are important nontopographic factors, yet to be demonstrated—for example, individual variability in the anatomical instantiation of language, and in the relative development of the alternate routes in dual-route processes (Plaut et al., 1996).

The revised neural model presented here appears to have no major shortcomings in accounting for the behavioral data. However, this is in considerable part because I have not attempted to apply the model to problems for which there are not yet satisfactory PDP solutions; nor have I attempted to apply the model to such major parallel processes as parsing, prosody, and phonetic modification. Furthermore, the model as discussed here does not fully incorporate the concept of distributed representations (see Nadeau, Chapter 12, this volume).

I have proposed a new classification of conduction aphasias that is explicitly linked to the revised neural model. It seems to account reasonably well in a general way for most experimental data. However, things are not as tidy as they might seem: The studies I have referenced were motivated by a variety of different models, and questions that might challenge the conceptualization I have proposed were not asked.

The basis for both short-term and long-term auditory–verbal memory is made explicit in this model—short-term memory as a transient pattern of neural activation, long-term memory as the information encoded in connection strengths, both synonymous with the language processor itself. These ideas are rooted in fundamental PDP principles, but their empirical support comes largely from the work of investigators like Martin, Saffran, and their colleagues, who have brought to maturity a line of research initiated years ago by Baddeley and others. I have not even mentioned the role of the frontal lobes and other systems also involved in the transient selective engagement of neural nets that underlies working (short-term) memory; nor have I mentioned the potential role of the hippocampal system in making episodic long-term declarative memory contributions to the performance of short-term memory tasks.

Several major rehabilitation principles have been proposed: (1) Desired input and output patterns must be approached as directly as possible (e.g., semantic and articulatory, not just acoustic, in the treatment of anomia); (2) response delay is likely to reduce response success and hence rehabilitative efficacy; (3) the employment of rich, multimodality (i.e., converging) inputs is likely to enhance efficacy; (4) the prevalence of dual pathways subserving language processes provides both the potential for reduced performance through interference effects, and the opportunity for greater rehabilitation efficacy by targeting both pathways; (5) multimodality approaches may be preferable in rehabilitating gatekeeper networks such as articulatory motor representations; (6) generalization effects are most likely to be seen in the rehabilitation of pattern associator networks instantiating sequence knowledge (e.g., acoustic–articulatory), and are least likely to be seen with rehabilitation of pattern associators linking nonsequential representations (e.g., semantic–articulatory), in which case probability of generalization will probably depend on lesion locus.

NOTE

1. It is not possible to elaborate fully on the term "distributed" here. The reader is referred to Chapter 12 of this volume for a full discussion. Although this limitation somewhat constrains the discussion in this chapter (much like discussing physics without using calculus), it also makes the present model somewhat more transparent, and hence easier to understand. A complete PDP model of phonological processes incorporating distributed representations has not yet been developed.

REFERENCES

Akmajian, A., Demers, R. A., & Harnish, R. M. (1984). *Linguistics: An introduction to language and communication*. Cambridge: MIT Press.

Alajouanine, T., & Lhermitte, F. (1973). The phonemic and semantic components of jargon aphasia. In H. Goodglass & S. Blumstein (Eds.), *Psycholinguistics and aphasia* (pp. 318–329). Baltimore: Johns Hopkins University Press.

Allport, D. A. (1984a). Auditory–verbal short-term memory and conduction aphasia. In H. Bouma & D. G. Bouwhuis (Eds.), *Attention and performance X: Control of language processes* (pp. 313–325). Hillsdale, NJ: Erlbaum.

Allport, D. A. (1984b). Speech production and comprehension: One lexicon or two? In W. Prinz & A. F. Sanders (Eds.), *Cognition and motor processes* (pp. 209–228). Berlin: Springer-Verlag.

Baars, B. J., Motley, M. T., & MacKay, D. G. (1975). Output editing for lexical status in artificially elicited slips of the tongue. *Journal of Verbal Learning and Verbal Behavior, 14,* 382–391.

Barton, M. I. (1971). Recall of generic properties of words in aphasic patients. *Cortex, 7,* 73–82.

Benson, D. F., Sheremata, W. A., Bouchard, R., Segarra, J. M., Price, N., & Geschwind, N. (1973). Conduction aphasia: A clinicopathological study. *Archives of Neurology, 28,* 339–346.

Berndt, R. S., & Mitchum, C. C. (1990). Auditory and lexical information sources in immediate recall: Evidence from a patient with deficit to the phonological short-term store. In G. Vallar & T. Shallice (Eds.), *Neuropsychological impairments of short-term memory* (pp. 115–144). Cambridge, England: Cambridge University Press.

Binder, J. R., Rao, S. M., Hammeke, T. A., Frost, J. A., Bandettini, P. A., Jesmanowicz, A., & Hyde, J. S. (1995). Lateralized human brain language systems demonstrated by task subtraction functional magnetic resonance imaging. *Archives of Neurology, 52,* 593–601.

Blanken, G. (1990). Formal paraphasias: A single case study. *Brain and Language, 38,* 534–554.

Blumstein, S. (1973a). *A phonological investigation of aphasic speech.* The Hague: Mouton.

Blumstein, S. (1973b). Some phonologic implications of aphasic speech. In H. Goodglass & S. Blumstein (Eds.), *Psycholinguistics and Aphasia* (pp. 123–137). Baltimore: Johns Hopkins University Press.

Blumstein, S. (1978). Segment structure and the syllable in aphasia. In A. Bell & J. B. Hooper (Eds.), *Syllables and segments* (pp. 189–200). Amsterdam: North-Holland.

Blumstein, S., Baker, E., & Goodglass, H. (1977). Phonological factors in auditory comprehension in aphasia. *Neuropsychologia, 15,* 19–30.

Brédart, S., & Valentine, T. (1992). From Monroe to Moreau: An analysis of face naming errors. *Cognition, 45,* 187–223.

Brener, R. (1940). An experimental investigation of memory span. *Journal of Experimental Psychology, 26,* 467–482.

Brooks, J. O., & Watkins, M. J. (1990). Further evidence of the intricacy of memory span. *Journal of Experimental Psychology: Learning, Memory, and Cognition, 16,* 1134–1141.

Brown, A. S. (1991). A review of the tip-of-the-tongue experience. *Psychological Bulletin, 109,* 204–223.

Brown, J. W. (1975). The problem of repetition: A study of "conduction" aphasia and the "isolation" syndrome. *Cortex, 11,* 37–52.

Brown, R., & McNeill, D. (1966). The "tip of the tongue" phenomenon. *Journal of Verbal Learning and Verbal Behavior, 5,* 325–337.

Brownjohn, M. D. (1988). Acquisition of Makaton symbols by a young man with severe learning difficulties. *Behavioural Psychotherapy, 16,* 85–94.

Bub, D., Black, S., Howell, J., & Kertesz, A. (1987). Damage to input and output buffers: What's a lexicality effect doing in a place like that? In E. Keller & M. Gopnik (Eds.), *Motor and sensory processes of language* (pp. 83–110). Hillsdale, Erlbaum.

Buckingham, H. W. (1980). On correlating aphasic errors with slips-of-the-tongue. *Applied Psycholinguistics, 1,* 199–220.

Buckingham, H. W. (1987). Phonemic paraphasias and psycholinguistic production models for neologistic jargon. *Aphasiology, 1,* 381–400.

Buckingham, H. W., Avakian-Whitaker, H., & Whitaker, H. A. (1978). Alliteration and assonance in neologistic jargon aphasia. *Cortex, 14,* 365–380.

Buckingham, H. W., & Kertesz, A. (1974). A linguistic analysis of fluent aphasia. *Brain and Language, 1,* 43–62.

Burke, D. M., MacKay, D. G., Worthley, J. S., & Wade, E. (1991). On the tip of the tongue: What causes word finding failures in young and older adults? *Journal of Memory and Language, 30,* 542–579.

Burns, M. S., & Canter, G. J. (1977). Phonemic behavior of aphasic patients with posterior cerebral lesions. *Brain and Language, 4,* 492–507.

Butterworth, B. (1979). Hesitation and the production of verbal paraphasias and neologisms in jargon aphasia. *Brain and Language, 8,* 133–161.

Canter, G. J., Trost, J. E., & Burns, M. S. (1985). Contrasting speech patterns in apraxia of speech and phonemic paraphasia. *Brain and Language*, 24, 204–222.

Caplan, D. (1993). *Language: Structure, processing and disorders*. Cambridge, MA: MIT Press.

Caplan, D., Vanier, M., & Baker, C. (1986). A case study of reproduction conduction aphasia: I. Word production. *Cognitive Neuropsychology*, 3, 99–128.

Caramazza, A., Basili, A. G., Koller, J. J., & Berndt, R. S. (1981). An investigation of repetition and language processing in a case of conduction aphasia. *Brain and Language*, 14, 235–271.

Caramazza, A., Miceli, G., & Villa, G. (1986). The role of the (output) phonological buffer in reading, writing, and repetition. *Cognitive Neuropsychology*, 3, 37–76.

Carpenter, R. L., & Rutherford, D. R. (1973). Acoustic cue discrimination in adult aphasia. *Journal of Speech and Hearing Research*, 16, 534–544.

Cermak, L. S., & Tarlow, S. (1978). Aphasic and amnesic patients' verbal vs. nonverbal retentive capabilities. *Cortex*, 14, 32–40.

Coltheart, M., & Byng, S. (1989). A treatment for surface dyslexia. In X. Seron & G. Deloche (Eds.), *Cognitive approaches in neuropsychological rehabilitation* (pp. 159–174). Hillsdale, NJ: Erlbaum.

Conway, T., Heilman, P., Rothi, L. J. G., Alexander, A. W., Adair, J., Crosson, B., & Heilman, K. M. (1998). Treatment of a case of phonological alexia with agraphia using the Auditory Discrimination in Depth (ADD) program. *Journal of the International Neuropsychological Society*, 4, 608–620.

Coslett, H. B., Roeltgen, D. P., Rothi, L. J. G., & Heilman, K. M. (1987). Transcortical sensory aphasia: Evidence for subtypes. *Brain and Language*, 32, 362–378.

Cuenod, C. A., Bookheimer, S. Y., Hertz-Pannier, L., Zeffiro, T. A., Theodore, W. H., & Le Bihan, D. (1995). Functional MRI during word generation, using conventional equipment: A potential tool for language localization in the clinical environment. *Neurology*, 45, 1821–1827.

Damasio, H., & Damasio, A. R. (1980). The anatomical basis of conduction aphasia. *Brain*, 103, 337–350.

Dell, G. S. (1985). Positive feedback in hierarchical connectionist models: Applications to language production. *Cognitive Science*, 9, 3–23.

Dell, G. S. (1986). A spreading-activation theory of retrieval in sentence production. *Psychological Review*, 93, 283–321.

Dell, G. S. (1988). The retrieval of phonological forms in production: Tests of predictions from a connectionist model. *Journal of Memory and Language*, 27, 124–142.

Dell, G. S. (1990). Effects of frequency and vocabulary type on phonological speech errors. *Language and Cognitive Processes*, 5, 313–349.

Dell, G. S., & Reich, P. A. (1981). Stages in sentence production: An analysis of speech error data. *Journal of Verbal Learning and Verbal Behavior*, 20, 611–629.

Dell, G. S., Schwartz, M. F., Martin, N., Saffran, E. M., & Gagnon, D. A. (1997). Lexical access in normal and aphasic speakers. *Psychological Review*, 104, 801–838.

Démonet, J.-F., Chollet, F., Ramsay, S., Cardebat, D., Nespoulous, J.-L., Wise, R., Rascol, A., & Frackowiak, R. (1992). The anatomy of phonological and semantic processing in normal subjects. *Brain*, 115, 1753–1768.

Dubois, J., Hécaen, H., Angelergues, R., Maufras de Chatelier, A., & Marcie, P. (1973). Neurolinguistic study of conduction aphasia. In H. Goodglass & S. Blumstein (Eds.), *Psycholinguistics and aphasia* (pp. 283–300). Baltimore: Johns Hopkins University Press.

Duhamel, J.-R., & Poncet, M. (1986). Deep dysphasia in a case of phonemic deafness: Role of the right hemisphere in auditory language comprehension. *Neuropsychologia*, 24, 769–779.

Ellis, A. W. (1980). Errors in speech and short-term memory: The effects of phonemic similarity and syllable position. *Journal of Verbal Learning and Verbal Behavior*, 19, 624–634.

Ellis, A. W. (1984). Introduction to Byron Bramwell's (1897) case of word meaning deafness. *Cognitive Neuropsychology*, 1, 245–258.

Ellis, A. W., Miller, D., & Sin, G. (1983). Wernicke's aphasia and normal language processing: A case study in cognitive neuropsychology. *Cognition*, 15, 111–144.

Elman, J. L., & McClelland, J. L. (1988). Cognitive penetration of the mechanisms of perception: Compensation for coarticulation of lexically restored phonemes. *Journal of Memory and Language*, 27, 143–165.

Fay, D., & Cutler, A. (1977). Malapropisms and the structure of the mental lexicon. *Linguistic Inquiry*, 8, 505–520.

Freud, S. (1953). *On aphasia: A critical study* (E. Stengel, Ed. 2nd Trans.). New York: International Universities Press. (Original work published 1891)

Friedman, R. B., & Kohn, S. E. (1990). Impaired activation of the phonological lexicon: Effects upon oral reading. *Brain and Language, 38,* 278–297.

Friedrich, F. J., Glenn, C. G., & Marin, O. S. M. (1984). Interruption of phonological coding in conduction aphasia. *Brain and Language, 22,* 266–291.

Fromkin, V. A. (1971). The non-anomalous nature of anomalous utterances. *Language, 47,* 27–52.

Gagnon, D. A., Schwartz, M. F., Martin, N., Dell, G. S., & Saffran, E. M. (1995). The origins of form-related word and nonword errors in aphasic naming. *Brain and Cognition, 28,* 192.

Gainotti, G., Miceli, G., Silveri, M. C., & Villa, G. (1982). Some anatomo-clinical aspects of phonemic and semantic comprehension disorders in aphasia. *Acta Neurologica Scandinavica, 66,* 652–665.

Gandour, J., Akamanon, C., Dechongkit, S., Khunadorn, F., & Boonklam, R. (1994). Sequences of phonemic approximations in a Thai conduction aphasic. *Brain and Language, 46,* 69–95.

Gardner, H., & Winner, E. (1978). A study of repetition in aphasic patients. *Brain and Language, 6,* 168–178.

Garrett, M. F. (1975). The analysis of sentence production. In G. H. Bower (Eds.), *The psychology of learning and motivation* (Vol. 9, pp. 133–177). New York: Academic Press.

Garrett, M. F. (1976). Syntactic processes in sentence production. In R. J. Wales & E. Walker (Eds.), *New approaches to language mechanisms* (pp. 231–256). Amsterdam: North-Holland.

Geschwind, N. (1965). Disconnexion syndromes in animals and man. *Brain, 88,* 237–294, 585–644.

Goldman-Rakic, P. S. (1990). Cellular and circuit basis of working memory in prefrontal cortex of nonhuman primates. *Progress in Brain Research, 85,* 325–336.

Goldstein, K. (1948). *Language and language disorders.* New York: Grune & Stratton.

Goodglass, H., Kaplan, E., Weintraub, S., & Ackerman, N. (1976). The "tip of the tongue" phenomenon in aphasia. *Cortex, 12,* 145–153.

Goodglass, H., Gleason, J. B., & Hyde, M. R. (1970). Some dimensions of auditory language comprehension in aphasia. *Journal of Speech and Hearing Research, 13,* 595–606.

Green, E. (1969). Phonological and grammatical aspects of jargon in an aphasic patient: A case study. *Language and Speech, 12,* 103–118.

Green, E., & Howes, D. H. (1977). The nature of conduction aphasia: A study of anatomic and clinical features and of underlying mechanisms. In H. Whitaker & H. A. Whitaker (Eds.), *Studies in neurolinguistics* (Vol. 3, pp. 123–156). New York: Academic Press.

Harley, T. A. (1984). A critique of top-down independent levels models of speech production: Evidence from non-plan-internal speech errors. *Cognitive Science, 8,* 191–219.

Harley, T. A. (1990). Phonologic activation of semantic competitors during lexical access in speech production. *Language and Cognitive Processes, 8,* 291–309.

Hebb, D. O. (1949). *The organization of behavior.* New York: Wiley.

Heilman, K. M., Scholes, R., & Watson, R. T. (1976). Defects of immediate memory in Broca's and conduction aphasia. *Brain and Language, 3,* 201–208.

Hoit-Dalgaard, J., Murry, T., & Kopp, H. G. (1983). Voice onset time production and perception in apraxic subjects. *Brain and Language, 20,* 329–339.

Hough, M. S., & DeMarco, S. (1995). Phonemic retrieval in conduction aphasia: Memory trace decay or blocking effect? *Brain and Cognition, 28,* 196.

Howard, D., & Franklin, S. (1987). Three ways for understanding written words, and their use in two contrasting cases of surface dyslexia (together with an odd routine for making 'orthographic' errors in oral word production). In A. Allport, D. Mackay, W. Prinz, & E. Scheerer (Eds.), *Language perception and production: Relationships between listening, speaking, reading and writing* (pp. 340–366). London: Academic Press.

Howard, D., & Franklin, S. (1988). *Missing the meaning?: A cognitive neuropsychological study of the processing of words by an aphasic patient.* Cambridge, MA: MIT Press.

Howard, D., Patterson, K., Wise, R., Brown, W. D., Friston, K., Weiller, C., & Frackowiak, R. (1992). The cortical localization of the lexicons. Positron emission tomography evidence. *Brain, 115,* 1769–1782.

Joanette, Y., Keller, E., & Lecours, A. R. (1980). Sequences of phonemic approximations in aphasia. *Brain and Language, 11,* 30–44.

Katz, R. B., & Goodglass, H. (1990). Deep dysphasia: Analysis of a rare form of repetition disorder. *Brain and Language, 39,* 153–185.

Kay, J., & Ellis, A. W. (1987). A cognitive neuropsychological case study of anomia: Implications for psychologic models of word retrieval. *Brain, 110,* 613–629.

Keller, E. (1978). Parameters for vowel substitutions in Broca's aphasia. *Brain and Language, 5,* 265–285.

Kertesz, A., & Benson, D. F. (1970). Neologistic jargon: A clinicopathological study. *Cortex, 6,* 362–386.

Kinsbourne, M. (1971). The minor cerebral hemisphere as a source of aphasic speech. *Archives of Neurology, 25,* 302–306.

Klatt, D. H. (1989). Review of selected models of speech perception. In W. Marslen-Wilson (Ed.), *Lexical representation and process* (pp. 169–226). Cambridge, MA: MIT Press.

Klich, R. J., Ireland, J. V., & Weidner, W. E. (1979). Articulatory and phonological aspects of consonant substitutions in apraxia of speech. *Cortex, 15,* 451–470.

Kohn, S. E. (1984). The nature of the phonological disorder in conduction aphasia. *Brain and Language, 23,* 97–115.

Kohn, S. E. (1989). The nature of the phonemic string deficit in conduction aphasia. *Aphasiology, 3,* 209–239.

Kohn, S. E., & Friedman, R. B. (1986). Word meaning deafness: A phonological–semantic dissociation. *Cognitive Neuropsychology, 3,* 291–308.

Kohn, S. E., & Smith, K. L. (1990). Between-word speech errors in conduction aphasia. *Cognitive Neuropsychology, 7,* 133–156.

Kohn, S. E., & Smith, K. L. (1991). The relationship between oral spelling and phonological breakdown in a conduction aphasic. *Cortex, 27,* 631–639.

Kohn, S. E., & Smith, K. L. (1993). Lexical–phonological processing of functors: Evidence from fluent aphasia. *Cortex, 29,* 53–64.

Kohn, S. E., & Smith, K. L. (1994). Evolution of impaired access to the phonological lexicon. *Journal of Linguistics, 8,* 267–288.

Kohn, S. E., & Smith, K. L. (1995). Serial effects of phonemic planning during word production. *Aphasiology, 9,* 209–222.

Koriat, A., & Lieblich, I. (1974). What does a person in a "TOT" state know that a person in a "don't know" state doesn't know? *Memory and Cognition, 2,* 647–655.

La Pointe, L. L., & Johns, D. F. (1975). Some phonemic characteristics in apraxia of speech. *Journal of Communication Disorders, 8,* 259–269.

Laine, M., & Martin, N. (1996). Lexical retrieval deficit in picture naming: Implications for word production models. *Brain and Language, 53,* 283–314.

Laubstein, A. S. (1987). Syllable structure: The speech error evidence. *Canadian Journal of Linguistics, 32,* 339–363.

Lecours, A. R. (1982). On neologisms. In J. Mehler, E. C. T. Walker, & M. Garrett (Eds.), *Perspectives on mental representation* (pp. 217–250). Hillsdale, NJ: Erlbaum.

Lecours, A. R., & Lhermitte, F. (1969). Phonemic paraphasias: Linguistic structures and tentative hypotheses. *Cortex, 5,* 193–228.

Levelt, W. J. M. (1989). *Speaking: From intention to articulation.* Cambridge, MA: MIT Press.

Liberman, A. M., Cooper, F. S., Shankweiler, D. P., & Studdert-Kennedy, M. (1967). Perception of the speech code. *Psychological Review, 74,* 431–461.

Liberman, A. M., & Mattingly, I. G. (1985). The motor theory of speech perception revisited. *Cognition, 21,* 1–36.

Luria, A. R. (1974). Language and brain: Towards the basic problems of neurolinguistics. *Brain and Language, 1,* 1–14.

MacKay, D. G. (1970). Spoonerisms: The structure of errors in the serial order of speech. *Neuropsychologia, 8,* 323–350.

MacKay, D. G. (1972). The structure of words and syllables: Evidence from errors in speech. *Cognitive Psychology, 3,* 210–227.

MacNeilage, P. (1982). Speech production mechanisms in aphasia. In S. Grillner, B. Lindblom, J. Lubker, & A. Persson (Eds.), *Speech motor control* (pp. 43–60). Oxford: Pergamon Press.

Martin, A. D., & Rigrodsky, S. (1974). An investigation of phonological impairment in aphasia: Part 1. *Cortex, 10,* 317–346.

Martin, N., & Saffran, E. M. (1992). A computational account of deep dysphasia: Evidence from a single case study. *Brain and Language, 43,* 240–274.

Martin, N., & Saffran, E. M. (1997). Language and auditory–verbal short-term memory impairments: Evidence for common underlying processes. *Cognitive Neuropsychology, 14,* 641–682.

Martin, N., Saffran, E. M., & Dell, G. S. (1996). Recovery in deep dysphasia: Evidence for a relation between auditory–verbal STM capacity and lexical errors in repetition. *Brain and Language, 52,* 83–113.

Martin, N., Weisberg, R. W., & Saffran, E. M. (1989). Variables influencing the occurrence of naming errors: Implications for a model of lexical retrieval. *Journal of Memory and Language, 28*, 462–485.

McCarthy, R., & Warrington, E. K. (1984). A two-route model of speech production: Evidence from aphasia. *Brain, 107*, 463–485.

McClelland, J. L., Rumelhart, D. E., & the PDP Research Group. (Eds.). (1986). *Parallel distributed processing: Explorations in the microstructure of cognition. Vol. 2. Psychological and biological models.* Cambridge, MA: MIT Press.

McGurk, H., & MacDonald, J. (1976). Hearing lips and seeing voices. *Nature, 264*, 746–748.

Miceli, G., Caltagirone, C., Gainotti, C., & Payer-Rigo, P. (1978). Discrimination of voice versus place contrasts in aphasia. *Brain and Language, 6*, 47–51.

Miceli, G., Gainotti, G., Caltagirone, C., & Masullo, C. (1980). Some aspects of phonological impairment in aphasia. *Brain and Language, 11*, 159–169.

Michel, F., & Andreewsky, E. (1983) Deep dysphasia: An analog of deep dyslexia in the auditory modality. *Brain and Language, 18*, 212–223.

Miller, D., & Ellis, A. W. (1987). Speech and writing errors in "neologistic jargonaphasia": A lexical activation hypothesis. In M. Coltheart, G. Sartori, & R. Job (Eds.), *The cognitive neuropsychology of language* (pp. 253–271). Hillsdale, NJ: Erlbaum.

Morton, J. (1980). Two auditory parallels to deep dyslexia. In. M. Coltheart, K. Patterson, & J. Marshall (Eds.), *Deep dyslexia* (pp. 189–196). London: Routledge & Kegan Paul.

Motley, M. T., & Baars, B. J. (1976). Semantic bias effects on the outcomes of verbal slips. *Cognition, 4*, 177–187.

Nadeau, S. E., & Crosson, B. (1997). Subcortical aphasia. *Brain and Language, 58*, 355–402, 436–458.

Naeser, M. A., & Hayward, R. W. (1978). Lesion localization in aphasia with cranial computed tomography and the Boston Diagnostic Aphasia Exam. *Neurology, 28*, 545–551.

Nespoulous, J.-L., Joanette, Y., Béland, R., Caplan, D., & Lecours, A. R. (1984). Phonologic disturbances in aphasia: Is there a "markedness effect" in aphasic phonetic errors? *Advances in Neurology, 42*, 203–214.

Nespoulous, J.-L., Joanette, Y., Ska, B., Caplan, D., & Lecours, A. R. (1987). Production deficits in Broca's and conduction aphasia: Repetition versus reading. In E. Keller & M. Gopnik (Eds.), *Motor and sensory processes of language* (pp. 53–81). Hillsdale, NJ: Erlbaum.

Nooteboom, S. G. (1969). The tongue slips into patterns. In A. G. Sciarone, A. J. van Essen, & A. A. Van Raad (Eds.), *Leyden studies in linguistics and phonetics* (pp. 114–132). The Hague: Mouton.

Ojemann, G., & Mateer, C. (1979). Human language cortex: Localization of memory, syntax, and sequential motor–phoneme identification systems. *Science, 205*, 1401–1403.

Ojemann, G. A. (1991). Cortical organization of language. *Journal of Neuroscience, 11*, 2281–2287.

Ojemann, G. A., Ojemann, J., Lettich, E., & Berger, M. (1989). Cortical language localization in left, dominant hemisphere: An electrical stimulation mapping investigation in 117 patients. *Journal of Neurosurgery, 71*, 316–326.

Palumbo, C. L., Alexander, M. P, & Naeser, M. A. (1992). CT scan lesion sites associated with conduction aphasia. In S. E. Kohn (Ed.), *Conduction aphasia* (pp. 51–75). Hillsdale, NJ: Erlbaum.

Pate, D. S., Saffran, E. M., & Martin, N. (1987). Specifying the nature of the production impairment in a conduction aphasic. *Language and Cognitive Processes, 2*, 43–84.

Paulesu, E., Frith, C. D., & Frackowiak, R. S. J. (1993). The neural correlates of the verbal component of working memory. *Nature, 362*, 342–345.

Plaut, D. C. (1996). Relearning after damage in connectionist networks: Toward a theory of rehabilitation. *Brain and Language, 52*, 25–82.

Plaut, D. C., McClelland, J. L., Seidenberg, M. S., & Patterson, K. (1996). Understanding normal and impaired word reading: Computational principles in quasi-regular domains. *Psychological Review, 103*, 56–115.

Poncet, M., Degos, C., DeLoche, G., & Lecours, A. R. (1972). Phonetic and phonemic transformations in aphasia. *International Journal of Mental Health, 1*, 46–54.

Posner, M. I. (1964). Rate of presentation and order of recall in immediate memory. *British Journal of Psychology, 55*, 303–306.

Ramón y Cajal, S. (1923). *Recuerdos de mi vida*. Madrid: Pueyo.

Rumelhart, D. E., McClelland, J. L., & the PDP Research Group. (Eds.). (1986). *Parallel distributed processing: Explorations in the microstructure of cognition. Vol. 1. Foundations.* Cambridge, MA: MIT Press.

Saffran, E. M., & Marin, O. S. M. (1975). Immediate memory for word lists in a patient with deficient auditory short-term memory. *Brain and Language, 2,* 420–433.

Schwartz, M. F., Saffran, E. M., Bloch, D. E., & Dell, G. S. (1994). Disordered speech production in aphasic and normal speakers. *Brain and Language, 47,* 52–88.

Shallice, T., & Vallar, G. (1990). The impairment of auditory–verbal short-term storage. In G. Vallar & T. Shallice (Eds.), *Neuropsychological impairments of short-term memory* (pp. 11–53). Cambridge, England: Cambridge University Press.

Shallice, T., & Warrington, E. K. (1977). Auditory–verbal short-term memory impairment and conduction aphasia. *Brain and Language, 4,* 479–491.

Shattuck-Hufnagel, S. (1979). Speech errors as evidence for a serial-ordering mechanism in sentence production. In W. E. Cooper & E. C. T. Walker (Eds.), *Sentence processing: Psycholinguistic studies* (pp. 295–341). Hillsdale, NJ: Erlbaum.

Shattuck-Hufnagel, S. (1983). Sublexical units and suprasegmental structure in speech production planning. In P. F. MacNeilage (Eds.), *The production of speech* (pp. 109–136). New York: Springer-Verlag.

Shattuck-Hufnagel, S. (1987). The role of word-onset consonants in speech production planning: New evidence from speech error patterns. In E. Keller & M. Gopnik (Eds.), *Motor and sensory processes of language* (pp. 17–51). Hillsdale, NJ: Erlbaum.

Shewan, C. M. (1980). Phonological processing in Broca's aphasics. *Brain and Language, 10,* 71–88.

Shinn, P., & Blumstein, P. (1983). Phonetic disintegration in aphasia: Acoustic analysis of spectral characteristics for place of articulation. *Brain and Language, 20,* 90–114.

Shuren, J., & Heilman, K. M. (1993). Non-optic aphasia. *Neurology, 43,* 1900–1907.

Stemberger, J. P. (1982). The nature of segments in the lexicon: Evidence from speech errors. *Lingua, 56,* 235–259.

Stemberger, J. P. (1984). Structural errors in normal and agrammatic speech. *Cognitive Neuropsychology, 4,* 281–313.

Stemberger, J. P. (1985). An interactive activation model of language production. In A. W. Ellis (Ed.), *Progress in the psychology of language* (Vol. 1, pp. 143–186). Hillsdale, NJ: Erlbaum.

Stemberger, J. P. (1991). Apparent anti-frequency effects in language production: The addition bias and phonological underspecification. *Journal of Memory and Language, 30,* 161–185.

Stemberger, J. P., & MacWhinney, B. (1986). Frequency and the lexical storage of regularly inflected forms. *Memory and Cognition, 14,* 17–26.

Strand, S. C., & Morris, R. C. (1986). Programmed training of visual discriminations: A comparison of techniques. *Applied Research in Mental Retardation, 7,* 165–181.

Strub, R. L., & Gardner, H. (1974). The repetition defect in conduction aphasia: Mnestic or linguistic? *Brain and Language, 1,* 241–255.

Tallal, P., & Piercy, M. (1975). Developmental aphasia: The perception of brief vowels and extended stop consonants. *Neuropsychologia, 13,* 69–74.

Tanzi, E. (1893). I fatti e le induzioni nell'odierna istologia del sistema nervoso. *Riv Sper Freniatr Med Leg Alienazioni Ment, 19,* 419–472.

Trojano, L., Stanzione, M., & Grossi, D. (1992). Short-term memory and verbal learning with auditory phonological coding defect: A neuropsychological case study. *Brain and Cognition, 18,* 12–33.

Trost, J. E., & Canter, G. J. (1974). Apraxia of speech in patients with Broca's aphasia: A study of phoneme production accuracy and error patterns. *Brain and Language, 1,* 63–79.

Ungerleider, L. G. (1995). Functional brain imaging studies of cortical mechanisms of memory. *Science, 270,* 769–775.

Valdois, S., Joanette, Y., & Nespoulous, J.-L. (1989). Intrinsic organization of sequences of phonemic approximations: A preliminary study. *Aphasiology, 3,* 55–73.

Valdois, S., Joanette, Y., Nespoulous, J.-L., & Poncet, M. (1988). Afferent motor aphasia and conduction aphasia. In H. A. Whitaker (Ed.), *Phonological processes and brain mechanisms* (pp. 59–92). New York: Springer-Verlag.

Vallar, G., & Baddeley, A. D. (1984). Phonological short-term store, phonological processing and sentence comprehension: A neuropsychological case study. *Cognitive Neuropsychology, 1,* 121–141.

Warrington, E. K., Logue, V., & Pratt, R. T. C. (1971). The anatomical localization of selective impairment of auditory verbal short-term memory. *Neuropsychologia, 9,* 377–387.

Warrington, E. K., & Shallice, T. (1969). The selective impairment of auditory verbal short-term memory. *Brain, 92,* 885–896.

Warrington, E. K., & Shallice, T. (1972). Neuropsychological evidence of visual storage in short term memory tasks. *Quarterly Journal of Experimental Psychology, 24,* 30–40.

Watkins, M. J., & Watkins, O. C. (1977). Serial recall and the modality effect: Effects of word frequency. *Journal of Experimental Psychology: Human Learning and Memory, 3,* 712–718.

Wernicke, C. (1874). *Der Aphasische Symptomenkomplex.* Breslau: Cohn & Weigart.

Wickelgren, W. A. (1969). Context-sensitive coding, associative memory, and serial order in (speech) behavior. *Psychological Review, 76,* 1–15.

Worley, M., Holcombe, A., Cybriwsky, C., Doyle, P., Schuster, J. W., Ault J., & Gast, D. L. (1992). Constant time delay with discrete responses: A review of effectiveness and demographic, procedural and methodological parameters. *Research in Developmental Disabilities, 13,* 239–266.

Yamadori, A., & Ikumura, G. (1975). Central (or conduction) aphasia in a Japanese patient. *Cortex, 11,* 73–82.

Yarmey, A. D. (1973). I recognize your face but I can't remember your name: Further evidence on the tip-of-the-tongue phenomenon. *Memory and Cognition, 1,* 287–290.

Zatorre, R. J., Evans, A. C., Meyer, E., & Gjedde, A. (1992). Lateralization of phonetic and pitch discrimination in speech processing. *Science, 256,* 846–849.

4

DISORDERS OF WORD RETRIEVAL IN APHASIA: THEORIES AND POTENTIAL APPLICATIONS

CAROLYN E. WILSHIRE
H. BRANCH COSLETT

An impairment in word retrieval is a common, if not universal, symptom of aphasia. Regardless of diagnostic classification, virtually all aphasic patients have difficulty retrieving words for spoken production, and this is most clearly observed in their generally poor performance on tasks such as picture naming (Benson, 1979; Kohn & Goodglass, 1985). Nevertheless, as most clinicians will report, the nature of the word retrieval problem does not appear to be the same across all individuals, and many of the differences observed are not captured well by the traditional diagnostic categories. Consider the following four examples:

Mr. A makes semantic paraphasias (semantically related word substitutions; e.g., "camel" → "horse") on tasks of picture naming. He often doesn't notice his mistakes. Also, when required to select a picture that matches a word he has just heard, he makes semantic substitutions (such as selecting "horse" for the word "camel"). However, he has no trouble repeating a word if he first hears it spoken.

Like Mr. A, Ms. B makes some semantic paraphasias in naming, but she also produces phonemic paraphasias (phonologically related errors; e.g., "castle" → "caskle," "chimney" → "pinnely") and circumlocutions (semantic descriptions of the item she is seeking; e.g., for "penguin," "It lives where it's cold, eats fish, it's in the water . . ."). In addition, she is keenly aware of the inappropriateness of her errors. However, unlike Mr. A, she has no difficulty on tasks such as word–picture matching. She also repeats words without error.

Mr. C's errors on naming tasks are mainly phonemic paraphasias. Unlike Mr. A. or Ms. B., he makes few semantic paraphasias. Like Ms. B, Mr. C recognizes his own errors and performs well on word–picture matching. However, he also has some problems in repetition, during which he produces errors of a type similar to his naming errors.

Ms. D, a nonfluent aphasic patient, produces short circumlocutions and semantic paraphasias in naming, and she often corrects her own errors. Some of her naming attempts are mildly phonetically distorted but nonetheless recognizable. Ms. D's success on a given item varies from attempt to attempt, and sometimes words she can retrieve in isolation are unavailable to her during running speech. Her verb naming is particularly poor. Ms. D performs well on word–picture matching, however, and she repeats well, given her mild articulatory difficulties.

These four individuals have one problem in common: difficulty retrieving words, which manifests itself clearly in tasks of picture naming. However, each person's problem seems to be somewhat different. These differences may have practical implications; they may be telling us something important about each individual's underlying impairment, and about the way it might best be treated. Therefore, a system that allows us to characterize these differences can be an extremely useful clinical tool. The "cognitive" or "cognitive-neuropsychological" approach to aphasia aims to provide such a system. Its goal is to take a particular aspect of language processing (in this case, spoken-word retrieval), to break it down into its various cognitive components, and to identify which component or components are impaired in a given individual. Ideally, this information can then be used to motivate a particular treatment approach.

In this chapter, we review recent research that has applied the cognitive approach to the analysis and treatment of word retrieval problems in aphasia. The focus is on retrieval of words for spoken production; due to space limitations, we do not deal in any detail with word comprehension deficits, impairments involving other output modalities (e.g., writing), or difficulties that occur only under specific stimulus conditions (e.g., "optic aphasia"; Beauvois & Saillant, 1985; Coslett & Saffran, 1989). We further limit ourselves to those aspects of spoken word retrieval that precede articulatory–motor programming— that is, how a speaker arrives at a sequence of phonemes that appropriately describes the concept he or she had in mind, but not how this phonemic "plan" is subsequently programmed for articulation (for evidence to support the distinction between more abstract, phonemic-level sound planning and motor–articulatory programming, see Blumstein, Cooper, Goodglass, Statlender, & Gottlieb, 1980; Nespoulous, Joanette, Beland, Caplan, & Lecours, 1984). The discussion to follow begins with a review of current theories of word retrieval in normal speakers. It then outlines a number of cognitive accounts of word retrieval impairments in aphasic patients, and offers a new system of classification which identifies four different primary subtypes of impairment. Finally, some recent literature is reviewed in which cognitive models of aphasic patients' word retrieval have been used to guide therapy programs. The coverage of the vast literature on these topics is by no means exhaustive, and is likely to be highly biased by our own theoretical leanings. Nevertheless, we have attempted to offer alternative points of view on the most important issues, and to provide a discussion that gives the reader some appreciation for the various approaches, controversies, and unresolved issues in this area.

MODELS OF NORMAL WORD RETRIEVAL

According to most current models of spoken-word production, the process of translating concepts into strings of phonemes involves two stages. During the first stage, a semantic description of the concept to be expressed is converted into a lexical representation. This lexical representation specifies the identity of the target word, and possibly also its grammatical properties, but does not specify its full phonological form. It is sometimes referred to as a "lemma."[1] During the second stage, this "lemma" is converted into a fully specified phonological description of the word (Butterworth, 1989; Dell, 1986; Garrett, 1975; Kempen & Huijbers, 1983; Levelt, 1989; Schriefers, Meyer, & Levelt, 1990).[2] According to this two-stage model, retrieval failures should take different forms, depending on the stage at which the breakdown occurs. A failure to retrieve the target lemma for a given semantic description may result in selection of another lemma that has a similar semantic description (i.e., a semantic paraphasia, such as "camel" → "horse"). On the other hand, a failure to retrieve a word's phonological description is more likely to result in a response in which some of the phonemes are correctly generated, but others are misselected (i.e., a phonemic paraphasia, such as "chimney" → "pinnely"). This notion is illustrated in Figure 4.1.

In many current models, this two-stage view of word retrieval is phrased in spreading-activation terms: The corresponding units at the various levels of representation (semantic features, lemmas, and phonemes) are seen as being interconnected within a network. When a word must be retrieved, activation is passed down from the semantic to the lemma level—generating activity in the target lemma—and then subsequently from the lemma level to the representations of individual phonemes (see, e.g., Dell, 1986, 1988; Levelt et al., 1999; Roelofs, 1992, 1997; Stemberger, 1985, 1990). A failure to sufficiently activate the target lemma may result in a semantic substitution, because lemmas of semantically related words, which will already have been partly activated by the semantic description, are the most likely to be incorrectly selected if the target lemma itself is unavailable. (Of course, a semantic error may also occur if the semantic representation itself is incomplete or impaired; we discuss this further below.) A failure to sufficiently activate all of the target word's phonemes may result in a phonemic paraphasia: If the activation reaching the phoneme level is weak or noisy, some phonemes may be successfully activated, but others may not become activated enough to be selected out from among their competitors, so the response may contain a mixture of correct and incorrect phonemes (e.g., "chimney" → "pinnely"). This idea is illustrated in Figure 4.2.

Although most models agree that word retrieval involves two stages, they do differ as to how the stages relate to one another. In some models, the stages occur in strict sequence: A lemma is first selected, and once this process is complete, its phonemes are then recov-

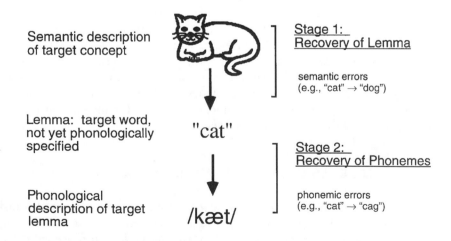

FIGURE 4.1. Illustration of the two-stage model of word retrieval.

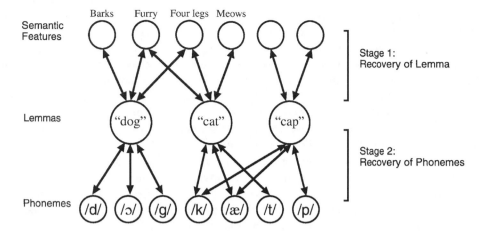

FIGURE 4.2. Illustration of a simplified spreading-activation model of word retrieval.

ered (e.g., Levelt, 1989, 1992; Levelt et al., 1999; Roelofs, 1992, 1997). In others, there is a constant upward and downward flow of information between the lemma and phoneme levels of representation; in these models, phonological recovery can begin even before lemma recovery is complete (e.g., several candidate lemmas may begin to be phonologically processed before a single one is definitively selected at the higher level), and the phoneme recovery process can actually influence events at the former, lemma level (e.g., Dell, 1986, 1988; Stemberger, 1985, 1990). These types of models, often called "interactive" models, make specific predictions about the kinds of errors likely to be observed in cases of breakdown. For example, they predict a higher than chance incidence of form-related word substitutions (purely form-related errors such as "camel" → "candle," as well as "mixed" errors such as "skunk" → "squirrel"). This is because activation can "feed back" from phoneme representations to any lemmas that contain those phonemes; thus any partially active lemma representation that shares phonemes with the target will be boosted (see Figure 4.2). Evidence from both aphasic patients' and normal subjects' performance supports this prediction (Dell & Reich, 1981; Harley, 1984; Martin, Weisberg, & Saffran, 1989; see Rapp & Goldrick, in press, for a review). This same property of interactive models also provides an elegant account for the effects of phoneme cueing: If the target lemma cannot be retrieved, the provision of a first-phoneme cue may help, because the phonemes presented will feed activation back to the lemma level, thereby "boosting" the activation levels of the target lemma. If that lemma is already partially activated, this boost may be sufficient to enable its production.

The question as to whether the word retrieval process is indeed interactive in the ways described above is still the subject of ongoing debate (for a recent discussion, see Rapp & Goldrick, in press). Nevertheless, it does appear that some phenomena are difficult to explain without postulating some degree of interaction between levels. And as we have seen, the notion of interaction provides a useful and elegant way of conceptualizing some common clinical phenomena, such as the phonemic cueing effect.

Another point on which models differ concerns the processes that take place after the fully specified phonological representation of the word has been recovered. According to some, this step is followed by a second, "postlexical" phonological processing stage, in which the recovered phonological information is reorganized into the form it will ultimately take in the speech plan (e.g., Béland, Caplan, & Nespoulous, 1990; Garrett, 1975; Levelt, 1992; Roelofs, 1997; Shattuck-Hufnagel, 1979, 1983, 1987, 1992). In some models, the purpose of this second stage is to "flesh out" the highly abbreviated, underspecified phonological material in the phonological description that has just been retrieved (e.g., Béland et al., 1990). In others, its purpose is to make the phonological changes that are required when a sequence of words must be combined into a phrase (e.g., Roelofs, 1997; Shattuck-Hufnagel, 1979, 1983). Although models of this postlexical phonological stage vary widely, most predict that failures at this level should result in errors in which phonemes within a word or phrase are misordered. For example, between-word phoneme movement errors, which are occasionally produced by normal speakers (e.g., "Guinea kig page"), are generally said to arise at this level. In contrast, errors involving complete omission of many of the phonemes within a word, such as those seen in certain types of aphasia (e.g., "chimney" → "pinnely"), are generally attributed to a problem in phoneme recovery itself.

Nevertheless, it should be borne in mind that not all models commit themselves to the notion of an explicit "postlexical" phonological processing stage. In many, the various operations—and the types of errors—attributed to this level of processing are said to occur during phoneme recovery itself. For example, in interactive models such as Dell's (1986) model, recovery of a given phoneme will be influenced by within-word factors (accessibility of the stored phonological information) and between-word factors (presence of competition from other words in the phrase) simultaneously. So misselection and misordering errors can potentially arise at the same processing level. Therefore, while it is clear that different types of phonological errors are likely to have different underlying causes, it is not yet clear whether this necessitates the postulation of an entirely separate, additional level of processing.

In summary, current models view the process of word retrieval as occurring in two stages: First, a word is located that corresponds to the concept the speaker has in mind; and second, the phonological form of that target word is recovered. Models differ as to whether they view these two stages as completely separate and sequential, or as overlapping and interactive. Finally, some (but not all) models propose that the phonological information recovered about a word undergoes additional processing during a subsequent, postlexical phonological processing stage. In the discussion to follow, we examine how the various word retrieval problems observed in aphasia might be described in terms of these current theoretical formulations.

COGNITIVE MODELS OF WORD RETRIEVAL IN APHASIA

The aim of a cognitive model of word retrieval in aphasia is to identify the specific cognitive processes that are malfunctioning for each particular aphasic individual or type of problem. Ideally, it should be possible to start with a model of how word retrieval takes place in normal speakers, and then to identify which cognitive operations are impaired for a given individual (see Saffran, 1982, and Shallice, 1988, for more detailed discussions of this notion and of its inherent assumptions). The first cognitive-neuropsychological analyses of word retrieval impairments, many of which grew up independently of normal theory, placed a strong emphasis on representations; that is, they aimed to identify what kinds of representation(s) were unavailable to a patient (e.g., whether semantic or phonological representations were inaccessible). More recently, there has been a shift toward greater emphasis on the processes that map between these representations—an approach that is more sympathetic to that taken in the literature on normal word retrieval. Indeed, in recent years the relationship between models of normal and aphasic individuals' performance has grown increasingly tight. We review some examples that illustrate this progression. Note that in the discussion to follow, we make a clear separation between word retrieval impairments in fluent aphasia (which usually result from damage to posterior speech areas) and in nonfluent aphasia (which usually occur after damage affecting anterior speech areas). Descriptions apply to fluent aphasia, unless otherwise stated.

Semantic and Output Anomia

As noted above, many of the earliest cognitive-neuropsychological analyses of word retrieval impairments in aphasia placed strong emphasis on representations. They sought to identify which representations were unavailable to a patient during word retrieval. These early analyses identified two types of representations that may be unavailable due to aphasic impairment: (1) the complete semantic description of the concept required, and (2) the fully phonologically specified representation of the word to be produced (see Gainotti, Silveri, Villa, & Miceli, 1986; Kay & Ellis, 1987). An inability to recover the first of these was termed "semantic anomia" (or alternatively, a "central semantic deficit"), and a problem involving the second was called "output anomia" (or an "impairment accessing the phonological output lexicon"). We consider each of these in turn (see also Nickels, 1997, for further discussion).

Let us consider first the condition of semantic anomia. Howard and Orchard-Lisle (1984) described what is often considered a "classic" case of this disorder. Their globally aphasic patient JCU made frequent semantic paraphasias in naming tasks, and often failed to recognize her own errors as incorrect. She also had difficulty on tasks involving semantic comprehension, such as word–picture matching with semantically related distractors (e.g., being shown a picture of a bike, and responding to the question "Is this a car?"). Furthermore, JCU's naming was facilitated by the provision of first-letter cues (e.g., "starts with 'p'"), but she could also be misled by such a cue if it was inappropriate (e.g., for the target "tiger," the cue "starts with 'l'" could elicit "lion"). The authors argued that JCU suffered from an inability to recover complete semantic descriptions of the relevant concepts.[3] Semantic descriptions were incompletely specified, so that related concepts sometimes became confused with one another. This resulted in semantic paraphasias in picture naming. And since these same semantic descriptions were also said to be called upon in comprehension, this accounted for why similar errors were observed in word–picture matching. The authors attributed the facilitatory effect of first-letter cues to their ability to provide additional information capable of distinguishing semantically similar concepts. For example, if the semantic descriptions of "lion" and "tiger" were equally activated in response to a picture, the provision of a first letter, "l," might help to resolve the situation. However, these letter cues, if incorrect, would favor the inappropriate alternative, and the errors so induced would not be detected. Subsequent studies have described individuals exhibiting features similar to those of patient JCU (e.g., Hillis, Rapp, Romani, & Caramazza, 1990).

The symptom complex exhibited by JCU and others, which is characterized by semantic confusions in both production and comprehension tasks, is often referred to as "semantic anomia" (or, alternatively, a "central semantic deficit" or an "impairment accessing semantic representations"). Such patients may be unaware of their errors, and some (such as JCU) may be susceptible to "miscueing." In addition, affected individuals may exhibit sensitivity to "semantic" variables, such as concreteness/imageability (Breedin, Saffran, & Coslett, 1994; Nickels & Howard, 1994), or semantic category (e.g., living things [Warrington &

Shallice, 1984] or inanimate objects [Warrington & McCarthy, 1983, 1987] may be disproportionately impaired). In terms of models of normal word retrieval, semantic anomia can be thought of as occurring prior to the two hypothesized stages of word retrieval (see above). It is a disorder that affects an important prerequisite of the word retrieval process—that is, the ability to adequately specify the semantic representation of the item to be retrieved.

"Output anomia," on the other hand, refers to a condition that affects only word production. Patient EST, reported by Kay and Ellis (1987), is a case often used to illustrate this kind of disorder. EST was a relatively mildly impaired patient with a diagnosis of anomic aphasia, whose spontaneous speech was fluent, albeit somewhat circumlocutory. Unlike JCU, EST made a number of different types of errors on naming tasks, including phonemic paraphasias (about 25%) and semantic paraphasias (about 20%). He also differed from JCU in that he had much less difficulty with word–picture matching. Also, he could not be "miscued" in naming. The authors argued that EST's good comprehension and resistance to miscueing suggested that his semantic representations were intact. They proposed that his difficulties in naming arose during retrieval of output-specific representations; that is, EST was unable to retrieval the full phonological description for the word to be produced. This pattern of performance—difficulty in retrieving words within the context of well-preserved word comprehension—earned the term "output anomia" (or, alternatively, a "deficit in accessing the phonological output lexicon").

Since Kay and Ellis's (1987) study, a number of other similar cases exhibiting this type of output-specific word retrieval disorder have been documented (Badecker, Miozzo, & Zanuttini, 1995; Franklin, Howard, & Patterson, 1995; Henaff Gonon, Bruckert, & Michel, 1989; patient CSS in Rapp & Goldrick, in press). These subsequent studies have highlighted several other features of the disorder that distinguish it from semantic anomia. Unlike the performance of patients with semantic anomia, in which "semantic" variables appear to have the strongest effects, the performance of patients with output anomia appears to be more sensitive to variables such as frequency and grammatical class.[4] For example, a number of documented cases are disproportionately impaired on lower-frequency targets (e.g., Badecker et al., 1995; Caramazza & Hillis, 1990; Kay & Ellis, 1987; although this may also be true of other types of naming impairment), and some show greater difficulty with nouns than with verbs (e.g., Miozzo, Soardi, & Cappa, 1994; Zingeser & Berndt, 1988).[5] These studies not only highlight the ways in which output anomia differs from semantic anomia, but they also provide important evidence about the kinds of variables that are relevant during the process of recovering output-level lexical representations, and how these differ from those relevant at the semantic level itself (see Kay & Ellis, 1987, and Zingeser & Berndt, 1988, for discussions).

Output anomia, then, can be thought of as a "primary" disorder of word retrieval, unlike semantic anomia, in which the problem is a consequence of a wider deficit in semantic function. In terms of normal models, the impairment is in some part of the two-stage mapping process that takes semantic representations and converts them into fully phonologically specified representations. Which of the two stages is affected is not clear. Many descriptions of this disorder do not relate it directly to normal models. Others use language that emphasizes representation, not process, and it is therefore difficult to map these directly onto current theories. Nevertheless, some offer descriptions that are suggestive of a problem in accessing lemmas from semantic representations. For instance, Ellis and Young, (1998) describe this as an impairment in mapping from "lexico-semantic" representations (which store word meanings) to the "speech output lexicon" (which, in many formulations, consists of lemmas not yet specified as to their phonological form). Below we consider some recent attempts to relate various forms of output anomia more directly to the two-stage view of word retrieval.

Output Anomia: Further Fractionations

We have described output anomia as a "primary" disorder of word retrieval—that is, a disorder involving the word retrieval process itself. Therefore, in a chapter on word retrieval impairments, it is worthy of more detailed examination. As noted above, early cognitive analyses of output anomia did not make strong claims as to how this kind of disorder mapped onto the two stages of word retrieval commonly proposed in normal models. However, more recent evidence suggests that it may be possible to subdivide this disorder according to the precise stage at which the impairment occurs. There is certainly some diversity within the general class of output anomia. In contrast to classic cases like EST, some patients with output anomia produce semantic errors as their primary error type (e.g., patients RGB and HW of Caramazza & Hillis, 1990). These patients' good semantic comprehension would rule out a semantic anomia; nevertheless, their high rate of semantic paraphasias would suggest a deficit arising early in the word retrieval process at the stage before a lemma has been definitively selected. Other patients make relatively few semantic paraphasic errors and show extremely well-preserved grammatical, first-letter, and gender knowledge for the words they cannot retrieve, and in some cases even knowledge of the target's homophones (see, e.g., Badecker et al., 1995; Henaff Gonon et al., 1989). These patients' ability to retrieve information that cannot be directly inferred from a semantic description alone suggests a deficit relatively late in the word retrieval process; the exact lexical item seems to have been located, but its complete phonological description is unavailable.

The existence of this kind of evidence has led to the postulation of models that identify two dissociable forms of output anomia, which correspond to the two stages proposed in models of normal word retrieval. These are (1) a deficit in recovering lemmas from their semantic descriptions, and (2) a deficit in recovering the phonological descriptions of words from their lemmas (e.g., Badecker et al., 1995; Foygel & Dell, in press; Henaff Gonon et al., 1989; Rapp & Goldrick, in press; but see Dell, Schwartz, Martin, Saffran, & Gagnon, 1997, for an alternative view that describes all word retrieval deficits in terms of global impairments involving both these stages of word retrieval).

Deficits in Lemma Recovery

Patients whose primary error type is the semantic paraphasia, and whose comprehension is relatively well preserved, have been hypothesized to have a difficulty recovering lemmas from their semantic representations. Rapp and Goldrick (in press) offer such an account for the performance of one individual who made many semantic paraphasias but had no difficulty with semantic comprehension tasks (patient PW). They account for PW's performance by proposing that his lemma representations were subject to an abnormal degree of fluctuation in their activity levels. Because of this fluctuation (or "noise," as the authors call it), activation reaching the lemma level is not always successful in activating the appropriate target above its related competitors. Foygel and Dell (in press) also suggest a lemma recovery problem as the underlying cause of semantic paraphasias in patients who are prone to such errors in naming. However, unlike Rapp and Goldrick, they describe this problem not in terms of fluctuating activity within the lemmas themselves, but in terms of weakened connections between semantic representations and their corresponding lemmas. According to Foygel and Dell, the activation being received by the lemma representations is insufficient for the target lemma to be reliably selected from its (usually semantically related) competitors.

Although the error type most commonly associated with a lemma recovery deficit is the semantic paraphasia, some authors suggest that other types of errors might also sometimes arise. Miller and Ellis (1987), and subsequently Harley and MacAndrew (1992), have suggested that the more distant phonemic paraphasias and "neologistic" responses of patients with severe Wernicke's aphasia (e.g., "doctor" → "dockumen," "queen" → "robbli") may result from a lemma recovery deficit. They propose that if the target lemma is insufficiently activated, this may have a consequent effect at the phonological level, such that the phonemes of the target word do not become active enough to overcome competition from those of other, coactivated words. This results in neologistic responses with a distant or unidentifiable phonological relationship to the target, perhaps occasionally with a "blend"-like quality (e.g., "penguin" → "pelikwin"). Such an explanation is only possible in a model of naming that allows for considerable overlap in the processes of lemma and phoneme recovery, as in some interactive models (see above). The reason why lemma recovery failures might sometimes result in such phonemic errors, while others lead to whole-word semantic substitutions, is unclear. One suggestion is that the presence of accompanying perceptual-level impairments may inhibit some patients' ability to self-monitor, and therefore to suppress production if no target word has been clearly selected out from among its competitors (see Ellis & Young, 1988). The extent of any accompanying impairment at the phoneme recovery level might also be a relevant factor, as might the speech context (whether word production is constrained, as in picture naming, or free, as in spontaneous speech).

Another type of error that has been associated with lemma retrieval deficits is the form-related word substitution, or formal paraphasia (e.g., "camel" → "candle"). The interactive model of Foygel and Dell (in press) predicts that such errors will accompany semantic paraphasias in patients with a deficit at the lemma recovery level. This is because their model allows for interaction or "feedback" between levels, so that the lemmas of words that have a formal relationship to the target will receive some activation by virtue of the phonemes they share with the target (see discussion above). If the target lemma itself is insufficiently or inconsistently activated, this feedback will sometimes be enough to enable such a word to be selected in place of the target.

In summary, then, current accounts propose the existence of a type of word retrieval impairment that involves the lemma recovery process, and whose primary presenting feature is the production of semantic paraphasias on naming tasks, accompanied by good performance on semantic comprehension tasks. Accounts vary as to the precise conceptualization of the impairment (whether due to "noise" or weakened connections), and in their predictions regarding the occurrence of other types of errors (phonemic paraphasias/neologistic errors and formal paraphasias). Nevertheless, they have in common the notion that the first of the two stages of word retrieval can become selectively impaired in aphasia.

Deficits in the Recovery of Phonological Descriptions

Some recent evidence also supports the existence of a complementary form of output anomia that involves not lemma recovery, but rather the recovery of phonological descriptions. Individuals who show good comprehension, commit few semantic errors, and exhibit partial knowledge of words they cannot fully retrieve have been described as being able to recover the target lemma, but not its phonological description. Some patients argued to have this type of deficit produce many nonresponses/circumlocutions, but are nevertheless able to recall some of the phonological and/or syntactic properties of target words. As noted above, Badecker et al. (1995) offer such an account for an individual who showed good recall of gender information for words he could not produce. Henaff Gonon et al. (1989) offer a similar explanation for a patient with preserved knowledge of gender, first-letter, and homophone information about irretrievable words. Other hypothesized cases may produce substantial numbers of phonemic paraphasias. Rapp and Goldrick (in press) attribute the occurrence of phonemic paraphasias in one patient (CSS) to a deficit in recovering phonological descriptions from their corresponding lemmas. Specifically, they suggest that such errors may occur if there is an abnormal degree of fluctuating activity (or "noise") within the phoneme representations themselves. Foygel and Dell (in press) offer a similar explanation for individuals who produce substantial numbers of phonemic paraphasias. However, they characterize this difficulty not in terms of fluctuating levels of activity, but in terms of weakened connections between lemmas and their corresponding phonemes.

In patients with a pure deficit involving recovery of phonological descriptions, the primary error types are generally predicted to be phonemic paraphasias and failures to respond. Whether form-related real-word substitutions (or formal paraphasias) would also be expected is unclear: Foygel and Dell (in press) suggest that although some such errors may be observed (e.g., "cat" → "cap"), they may resemble real lexical items by coincidence alone, and may be better thought of as "homophonic" phonemic paraphasias. On the other hand, however, there are some models of the phonological recovery process that do seem to predict higher than chance occurrence of formal paraphasias (e.g., Dell, Juliano, & Govindjee, 1993). Also, it is at present unclear why some patients with a purported phoneme recovery deficit seem to produce mainly circumlocutions and target descriptions (such as those described by Badecker, Henaff Gonon, and their colleagues), while others produce a large number of phonemic paraphasias. This may suggest an additional source of variation not accounted for by the two-stage model. Alternatively, it might indicate that the "circumlocutors" could perhaps be better described as having a deficit at the earlier, lemma recovery level.[6] Semantic paraphasias are not predicted to occur as a result of a deficit at this level; the occurrence of such errors would suggest a co-occurring impairment at the lemma recovery or higher levels, or possibly the operation of a conscious strategy to find an alternative when the target is unavailable.

One interesting prediction of Foygel and Dell's (in press) account concerns the performance of these "phoneme recovery deficit" patients on word repetition tasks. These authors proposed that the availability of an auditory target in tasks of repetition enables the speaker to bypass the lemma recovery process (the target lemma being activated directly as a result of hearing the word itself), but not the phoneme recovery process. Consequently, for patients with a deficit involving the lemma recovery process, being able to bypass this impaired stage should lead to improved performance (i.e., better performance on repetition than on free naming). However, those with an impairment at the later, phoneme recovery stage should show little improvement, and should continue to produce similar kinds of errors as in free naming. Foygel and Dell's predictions were largely confirmed. They found that the hypothesized locus of a patient's primary impairment—within their interactive two-stage model of word retrieval—was a good predictor of repetition performance. That is, patients said to have marked impairment at the phoneme recovery level were predicted to, and did, make more errors in repetition than those with little or no impairment at this level.[7] This suggests the possibility that impairments involving the two stages of word retrieval might be further discriminated using an additional task—word repetition.

In summary, the accounts described above all take the view that a second subtype of output anomia exists that involves not the process of recovering lemmas from semantic representations, but rather the process of recovering phonological descriptions for the target lemma representations. A primary presenting feature of this disorder is the production of phonemic paraphasias. Again, accounts vary as to the precise conceptualization of the impairment (whether it is due to "noise" or weakened connections). Also, there are some unresolved issues concerning the status of other error types—for example, whether no responses/target descriptions and formal paraphasias might also be observed with this type of disorder. Nevertheless, these accounts have in common the notion that the second, lemma-to-phoneme stage of word retrieval can also become selectively impaired in aphasia.

Conclusions

Is there sufficient evidence to postulate that the two stages of word retrieval map directly onto two distinct types of deficits in aphasia? The defining features of the two types of disorders are certainly not clear-cut (e.g., as noted above, some accounts predict that phonemic paraphasias might be a feature of both types of disorders). Nevertheless, the distinction appears to be a useful one for capturing two important sources of variation among patients, neither of which appears to be explicable simply in terms of overall severity. These are (1) variation in the relative incidence of different error types in "output" anomics (most notably phonemic and semantic paraphasias), and (2) variation in the extent to which patients exhibit a similar problem in word repetition tasks. Furthermore, the two-stage model accounts for these two diverse features in an elegant and intuitively satisfying way. Therefore, we believe that the distinction is likely to prove useful as a tool for characterizing the differences between patients.

One point about these various cognitive classifications of word retrieval impairments in aphasia is worth emphasizing here. Unlike the traditional aphasia syndromes, where an individual is assigned to only one category, this cognitive approach allows for the possibility that a person may suffer from more than one type of cognitive deficit. For example, an individual with a large lesion may suffer from both a lemma recovery deficit *and* a phoneme recovery deficit, and may therefore exhibit performance that shows features of both. Foygel and Dell's (in press) recent study of patterns in naming errors provides some evidence to support this; these authors found that the error patterns of most patients they studied were best described within their interactive two-stage model in terms of some combination of deficits involving each of the two stages. Indeed, authors such as Dell et al. (1997) take the view that a "global" deficit involving both stages of word retrieval may be the norm rather than the exception, and that a great deal of individual variability may be due to variation in the *nature* of the breakdown, rather than its *locus*. We return to this point later.

Phonemic Paraphasias and "Postlexical" Processing

As noted above, some models of normal speech production propose an additional "postlexical" level of phonological processing, during which retrieved phonological information is reorganized into the form it will ultimately take in the planned utterance. According to many authors, this postlexical process can also become impaired in aphasia, which may lead to the production of phonemic paraphasias—just as is the case for impairments involving phoneme recovery itself (e.g., Caplan, 1992; Caplan, Vanier, & Baker, 1986;

Kohn, 1989; Kohn & Smith, 1990, 1994). This issue is worthy of some consideration here, because it suggests that phonemic paraphasias may have different origins in different individuals, and that not all arise during "word retrieval" per se.

However, this is a difficult question to address. Models with a "postlexical" processing stage vary so widely that it is difficult to establish a universal set of testable predictions as to how breakdowns at this level should differ from those occurring during the phoneme recovery process. Also, some predictions are difficult to test, as they rely on error characteristics that may vary with severity as well as type of lesion. For example, breakdowns arising at the "postlexical" level are generally predicted to be phonologically closer to their targets than those that are "lexical" in origin, but this may be a factor that varies with overall severity as well. And for those characteristics that do not suffer from these problems, results have been unpromising. For example, one characteristic often postulated to discriminate "postlexical" impairments from "phoneme recovery" impairments is a high frequency of phoneme-misordering errors. However, in a recent study of picture naming, these phoneme-misordering errors were found to be relatively rare in all phonologically-impaired aphasic patients (Wilshire, 1998, 2000). Although the issue is far from resolved, it appears that at present there is not yet sufficient evidence to support the existence of an additional "postlexical" origin for certain types of aphasic phonemic errors. So until such evidence comes to light, considerations of economy and parsimony dictate that we should try to explain phonemic errors without recourse to a "postlexical" level of processing.

Word Retrieval Disorders in Nonfluent Aphasia

The above-described models are usually employed to account for word retrieval disorders that occur in fluent aphasia, and that arise as a result of impairment to the posterior language areas (namely, the superior temporal and inferior parietal regions of the left hemisphere). However, patients with nonfluent aphasia also commonly exhibit a word retrieval disorder that is not just simply consequence of a more general articulatory programming deficit (see Kertesz, 1979, Kohn & Goodglass, 1985, and Williams & Canter, 1982, on Broca's aphasia, and Kertesz, 1979, on transcortical motor aphasia). Like patients with fluent aphasia, those with nonfluent aphasia may completely fail to name pictures, or may produce semantic paraphasias; however, they may be more likely than patients with fluent aphasia to correct these errors (e.g., Kohn & Goodglass, 1985). Furthermore, word retrieval in patients with nonfluent aphasia may show considerable sensitivity to context: Williams and Canter (1982) found that patients with Broca's aphasia were poorer at retrieving the names of objects within a complex picture description task than in a standard object naming task—the opposite trend to patients with Wernicke's aphasia. Indeed, some individuals have been found to exhibit such effects even in tasks that do not require the production of actual sentences. For example, in a case reported by Wilshire and McCarthy (1999), manipulations of rate of presentation and degree of semantic relatedness between successive items exerted a powerful influence on picture-naming performance; this effect was not observed for a fluent "output anomic" patient presented for comparison (see also McCarthy & Kartsounis, 1999, for a similar case).

Word retrieval by patients with nonfluent aphasia has been found to exhibit a number of other unique features. First, such patients, if they show a grammatical-class effect, are more likely to have greater difficulty with verbs than with nouns—the reverse of the pattern usually exhibited by patients with fluent aphasia (see, e.g., Berndt, Mitchum, Haendiges, & Sandson, 1997; Miceli et al., 1984; Zingeser & Berndt, 1990). This noun superiority effect may occur even in patients without agrammatism (Caramazza & Hillis, 1991; Daniele, Silveri, Giustolini, Colosimo & Gainotti, 1994). Also, nonfluent aphasic patients are often reported to have disproportionate difficulty with tasks involving multiple-word generation ("verbal fluency"), particularly if the search criterion involves aspects of form (e.g., "Tell me all the words you can think of that begin with 's'"; Benton, 1968; see also Coslett, Bowers, Verfaellie, & Heilman, 1991). Finally, word retrieval may be influenced by different kinds of variables. The patient of Wilshire and McCarthy (1999) referred to above had difficulty mainly in the production domain (there was little accompanying difficulty on semantic comprehension tasks); nevertheless, he was found to be strongly sensitive to "semantic" variables—not only the semantic proximity between successive items, but also target concreteness/imageability. By contrast, in fluent aphasia sensitivity to semantic variables is generally accompanied by more general disturbances in semantic function, such as those seen in the disorder of semantic anomia (see discussion above).

Cognitive models of word retrieval in normal and aphasic individuals generally have little to say about the underlying deficit in these nonfluent cases. The "mental lexicon"—that is, the storehouse or network of information about words and their phonological descriptions—is generally proposed to be located in the posterior language areas (Benson, 1979; Coughlan & Warrington, 1978; Damasio, Gradowski, Tranel, Hichwa, & Damasio, 1996; Hécaen & Angelergues, 1964). So why do we see word retrieval impairments at all in nonfluent aphasia? One possibility consistent with much existing evidence is that the anterior speech areas have a special role in generating syntactic "frames"—that is, descriptions specifying which grammatical type must be selected for each "slot" in the utterance (e.g., Caplan, 1985; Schwartz, 1987). In many models, these frames directly activate lexical items. As each "slot" is ready to be filled, the relevant frame activates all the words that can legally appear at that position. Therefore, an inability to generate such frames may place an individual at a distinct disadvantage when retrieving words, particularly when their selection is strongly syntactically determined—for example, function words, and perhaps also verbs (see also Zingeser & Berndt, 1990, for a discussion).

Another explanation that has been offered for word retrieval disorders in nonfluent aphasia is that the anterior speech areas have an important function in initiating and/or controlling activity in the (posterior) lexical network (Wilshire & McCarthy, 1999). Consequently, damage to anterior speech areas may affect a person's ability to initiate the word retrieval process, and/or his or her ability to prevent highly activated, unintended words from interfering with the selection of the target. This may result in performance that is highly variable from trial to trial. It would also explain why tasks involving multiple-word generation ("verbal fluency") may be particularly difficult for these patients. This kind of task, especially when it is based on form properties of words (e.g., words that start with "s"), requires highly "strategic" search of the lexicon. Such an account might also explain why retrieval of words in sentences is often more difficult than isolated word retrieval. In connected speech, many representations may be concurrently active at the time a given word must be selected, so there may be a greater need for lexical "control" to ensure appropriate selection of the right word at the right time.

Although these "syntactic" and "control" accounts of word retrieval in nonfluent aphasia are quite different, they may not necessarily be in direct competition. It is still possible that each account describes a separate and distinguishable subtype of word retrieval impairment in nonfluent aphasia. However, at present we can only speculate on such possibilities; there is simply not enough yet known about this topic to address these kinds of issues directly. What *is* clear, however, is that the various accounts offered for word retrieval disorders in nonfluent aphasia differ markedly from those put forward to explain such disorders in fluent aphasia. They do not focus on the particular stage of word retrieval at which the problem occurs, but instead emphasize qualitative differences in the way word retrieval tasks place. Indeed, some authors go so far as to suggest that word retrieval disorders in nonfluent aphasia might not be isolable to a single stage of word retrieval in quite the same way as those in fluent aphasia (Wilshire & McCarthy, 1999). If this is indeed the case, this might explain why patients with nonfluent aphasia often produce such a range of different types of errors, and why their performance is often influenced by a number of apparently unrelated variables. It might also explain why some variables that strongly influence performance in patients with fluent aphasia may have only weak or imperceptible effects in those with nonfluent aphasia (e.g., frequency effects may be weak or absent; McCarthy & Kartsounis, 1999; Warrington & Cipolotti, 1996; Zingeser & Berndt, 1990). Nevertheless, we need to find out much more about word retrieval disorders in nonfluent aphasia before we can draw any firm conclusions regarding the cognitive underpinnings of these disorders.

Toward a System of Classification for Word Retrieval Impairments

As the discussion above illustrates, there are still many disagreements as to the cognitive impairments responsible for different word retrieval disorders in aphasia, and many questions remain unresolved. Nevertheless, we attempt to draw some tentative conclusions about the state of the literature, in the form of a four-way classification of word retrieval impairments. The conclusions are necessarily very personal and subjective, but we think that the system may nonetheless prove useful for the purposes of identifying and classifying different types of word retrieval difficulties.

The classifications below are based on performance on the following types of tasks: picture naming, word repetition, and word–picture matching (note that the patient names/ initials in parentheses refer back to the hypothetical case descriptions given in the introduction to this chapter). It is important to emphasize here that the categories describe the features of relatively "pure" deficits of the kind in question. It is of course possible—perhaps even probable—that a given patient may have more than one type of deficit, and may therefore exhibit features corresponding to more than one of the types described. Also, it should be borne in mind that this scheme provides merely an outline of the word retrieval process and how it might break down in aphasia. And, as the sections on "other possible features" illustrate, many details of the various processing stages or components, and how they behave after language breakdown, are still unknown or are subjects of disagreement. Many of these outstanding questions may begin to be resolved in the new decade, as theoretical models of word retrieval become more sophisticated, and as more becomes known about the patterns of impairment observed in aphasia.

Pure Semantic Anomia (Mr. A)

Defining Features. The production of semantic paraphasias in naming tasks, accompanied by significant (although not necessarily equivalent) rates of semantic substitutions in word–picture matching tasks. In naming, semantic paraphasias are the primary error type, once failures to respond have been eliminated. Some of these errors appear to go undetected and are not corrected by the patient. Repetition is intact.

Other Possible Features. The individual may show imageability effects or may exhibit disproportionate difficulty with one or more semantic categories. He or she may be susceptible to "miscueing."

Cognitive Deficit. An inability to recover a complete semantic description of the concept to be expressed.

Aphasia Diagnosis of Sufferers. Patients with this deficit might present with Wernicke's aphasia or anomic aphasia, depending upon severity of impairment.

Primary Impairment in Lemma Retrieval (Ms. B)

Defining Features. The production of circumlocutions and semantic paraphasias in naming tasks, accompanied by relatively well-preserved performance on word–picture matching tasks. Errors are frequently detected by the patient, and circumlocutions may include detailed semantic descriptions of the item sought. The effect of word frequency is strong. Repetition is intact.

Other Possible Features. According to some authors, more distant phonemic paraphasias or neologisms may also occur in some individuals and/or under some circumstances. By some accounts, formal paraphasias may also be expected. Some patients may exhibit greater difficulty with noun than with verb retrieval.

Cognitive Deficit. Good preservation of semantic representations concerning a target item, but inability to reliably recover the lemma corresponding to a given semantic description.

Aphasia Diagnosis of Sufferers. Patients with this deficit may present with anomic aphasia. Wernicke's aphasia may be diagnosed in cases where there are accompanying deficits in input phonological processing.

Primary Impairment in Phoneme Retrieval (Mr. C)

Defining Features. The production of phonemic paraphasias in naming tasks, accompanied by preserved to near-preserved performance on word–picture matching tasks. Errors on naming tasks may also include failures to respond and circumlocutions, but semantic paraphasias should be relatively rare. Errors are frequently detected by the patient. Repetition elicits some phonemic paraphasias of the same type observed in naming (although not necessarily as many).

Other Possible Features. According to some authors, certain cases may produce mainly lexically specific descriptions of the target word rather than outright phonemic paraphasias (e.g., information about first letter, gender, homophones). By some accounts, formal paraphasias may also occur.

Cognitive Deficit. Good preservation of semantic representations, intact ability to recover lemmas, but inability to reliably recover the phonological description corresponding to the target lemma.

Aphasia Diagnosis of Sufferers. Patients may present with anomic aphasia or conduction aphasia. Wernickie's aphasia may be diagnosed in cases where there are accompanying deficits in input phonological processing.

Word Retrieval Deficits in Nonfluent Aphasia (Ms. D)

Defining Features. A nonfluent aphasic presentation, accompanied by the production of semantic substitutions and other error types on picture naming. Errors may be frequently self-corrected. Performance on a given word is likely to vary between sessions or between different situational contexts. Word generation tasks involving form-based criteria (e.g., all words starting with "l") are likely to be particularly difficult. Frequency effects, often strong in other patient groups, may be weak or absent.

Other Possible Features. Performance on word–picture matching may be preserved for mildly impaired patients, but may be impaired for more severe cases. Verb retrieval may be more impaired than noun retrieval. Agrammatism may or may not be present. Some individuals may repeat without error, but for others, accompanying articulatory–motor impairments may be responsible for some distortion of targets.

Cognitive Deficit. Unclear, but likely to be different from those in the previous three categories. There may be impairment in one or more lexical "control" processes, or difficulty generating syntactic frames to guide the word retrieval process.

Aphasia Diagnosis of Sufferers. Patients may present with Broca's aphasia or transcortical motor aphasia.

COGNITIVE APPROACHES TO THE TREATMENT OF WORD RETRIEVAL DISORDERS

The cognitive approach to the analysis of word retrieval impairments in aphasia can certainly provide us with valuable insights into the nature of a person's language difficulties. Nevertheless, it is of little practical use unless those insights can somehow be used to the benefit of the person concerned. The question we consider in this final section is whether the cognitive approach provides practical information that can be used to guide a course of treatment for impaired individuals. The idea that cognitive theory might have such applications has gained so much ground over the last decade that it has earned its own name—as the "cognitive" or "cognitive-neuropsychological" approach to therapy (see, e.g., Coltheart, Bates, & Castles, 1994; Howard & Hatfield, 1987; Lesser, 1989; Mitchum & Berndt, 1995; Seron, van der Linden, & de Partz, 1991). Below we describe this cognitive approach to therapy and some recent efforts to apply it to the treatment of word retrieval disorders. We discuss the current usefulness of the approach, its potential difficulties and limitations, and its prospects for the future.

Just what is the cognitive approach to therapy? Generally speaking, it is an approach in which a clinician makes use of cognitive models of language impairment in choosing or designing a therapy program for a given patient. More specifically, it involves describing the patient's language impairment in terms of existing cognitive models (using the kinds of approaches described above), and then using this information to select a treatment for that impairment—perhaps from the clinician's existing repertoire, or perhaps even an entirely new technique. The idea that choice of therapy can be grounded in a cognitive theory of aphasia is intuitively appealing. It can provide the therapist with a possible explanation as to *why* a particular therapy might result in improving a person's language performance. Also, it provides a framework that has the potential to explain some of the variability seen in patient responses to treatment—why a given treatment works for one patient and not another.

An Illustration

To illustrate this approach as it applies to word retrieval disorders, let us consider the hypothetical case of Mr. J, who has a profile consistent with semantic anomia, and who presents with severe naming difficulties. According to a "traditional" approach, Mr. J's naming difficulties might be treated with a generally applicable type of naming therapy, such as a cueing hierarchy (e.g., Linebaugh, 1983) or a "deblocking" strategy (e.g., Helm-Estabrooks, Emery, & Albert, 1987). According to the cognitive approach, however, the underlying cognitive impairment would first be identified—in this case, it would probably be an inability to retrieve complete semantic descriptions of the words. Then a therapy would be chosen that is capable of directly addressing this problem. For Mr. J, the treatment of choice would be one focusing on restitution of the (impaired) semantic representations. An example of such a treatment is Hillis's (1991, 1998) "feature-contrasting" technique, in which the therapist points out the precise semantic features that distinguish commonly confused words (e.g., if the patient misnames a picture of a cherry as a "lemon," a picture of the interfering item "lemon" is presented, and the differences between this and a cherry are pointed out—e.g., yellow vs. red, sour vs. sweet).

There are several points to note about this approach to therapy. First, it requires that a detailed pretreatment evaluation be conducted for each individual, so that his or her complete cognitive profile can be drawn up before a course of treatment is decided upon. A consequence of this is that treatment of any particular language function—say, word retrieval—may not necessarily be the same for all affected patients. Another practical consequence is that therapy time must be allowed for this initial detailed diagnostic procedure. Second, the cognitive approach emphasizes "restitution of function"; that is, it has a strong focus on improving the functioning of damaged cognitive component, rather than merely encouraging strategies that compensate for those impairments. Therefore, it assumes that the damaged component has some potential for recovery. Therefore, its use may be best suited to less severely impaired individuals. Third, the approach deals with individual cognitive components/processing stages separately; therapy is aimed at ameliorating the functioning of one particular stage or component at a time. Again, this suggests that the approach may be best suited to more moderately impaired individuals with relatively circumscribed deficits, for whom it is practical to isolate and treat individual cognitive problems.

Recent Applications

Although the idea of "cognitive therapy" is still relatively new, there have been a number of recent documented efforts to apply it to the treatment of word retrieval difficulties, with some promising results (see also Nickels & Best, 1996a, for a review). Most such efforts have adopted a simple model of word retrieval impairment, which distinguishes only two subtypes—semantic anomia and output anomia (see discussion above). That is, these studies differentiate word retrieval problems arising from inadequate semantic descriptions (semantic anomia) from those arising somewhere during the conversion of those descriptions into phonologically specified words (output anomia), but they do not further subdivide the latter into two separate stages. Generally speaking, the approach taken in these studies is to identify whether a particular individual's problem involves the recovery of semantic representations (semantic anomia), of output phonological descriptions (output anomia), or of both. A therapy task is then chosen that focuses on retraining the particular component(s) thought to be impaired. That is, patients with semantic anomia are treated with tasks hypothesized to restore semantic representations, whereas patients with output anomia are treated with tasks hypothesized to retrain access to the phonological descriptions of words.

Treatments for Semantic Anomia

One task commonly used to treat semantic anomia is word–picture matching, usually featuring distractors that are semantically related to the target. Targets may be spoken or written words, and the task may or may not require a patient to actually produce the word (see, e.g., Davis & Pring, 1991; Hillis & Caramazza, 1994; Howard, Patterson, Franklin, Orchard-Lisle, & Morton, 1985; LeDorze & Pitts, 1995; Marshall, Pound, White-Thomson, & Pring, 1990; Nettleton & Lesser, 1991; Nickels & Best, 1996b). The rationale here is that these tasks force the patient to focus on the semantic features that distinguish related items, thereby encouraging him or her to "relearn" the complete semantic description. Other tasks used to treat semantic anomia include (1) the "feature-contrasting" technique of Hillis (1991, 1998) described earlier, in which the distinguishing features between two confused items are explicitly pointed out; and (2) the use of questions that require access to detailed semantic knowledge about the target word (e.g., "Does a cow eat grass?", Is a bear a tree or an animal?"; Howard et al., 1985; Nettleton & Lesser, 1991). Again, the argument is that these tasks force the patient to focus on the precise semantic features of the items being treated. Many studies adopting one or more of these techniques have demonstrated significant and long-lasting improvements in naming performance for the trained items (see especially Marshall et al., 1990; see also Davis & Pring, 1991; Hillis, 1991; Hillis & Caramazza, 1994; Howard et al., 1985; Nickels & Best, 1996b). In addition, some studies have shown some generalization of the therapy to other, untreated words—particularly semantically related items that were used as distractors in the treatment tasks themselves (e.g., Hillis, 1991; Howard et al., 1985).

An example of successful application of a "semantic" therapy to a patient with semantic anomia is that of Marshall et al. (1990). These authors report data from patient IS, whose semantic comprehension was impaired, and who produced substantial numbers of semantic paraphasias in naming (she also produced some phonemic paraphasias, suggesting a possible accompanying output anomia, which was not the focus of the study). IS was given therapy based on the semantic matching paradigm: She was presented with four semantically related written words, together with (1) a picture or (2) a spoken definition, and was asked to select the written word that corresponded to the picture/definition. She was given feedback on errors. After a relatively small amount of therapy (just 5 hours' treatment spread over 2 weeks), IS showed significant improvement in her naming of the treated items, which persisted at least 1 month after therapy. Her performance also improved on semantic comprehension tasks that featured the items used in treatment.

Hillis (1991, 1998) also reports successful treatment of a patient with semantic anomia; in this case, the "feature-contrasting" technique described earlier was used. Hillis reports data from patient HG, who produced semantic paraphasias across a range of tasks and modalities, including spoken and written naming and word–picture matching (again, there were also some accompanying difficulties at the phonological/output level). In this case, HG was asked to write the names of pictures; if a semantic paraphasia was produced, a picture depicting the substituted, semantically related word was presented and its contrasting semantic features were pointed out, as described earlier. This treatment resulted in improved written naming for the treated items, and there was also significant generalization to untreated but semantically related items. Furthermore, performance on other word-processing tasks, such as spoken naming and word–picture matching, also improved.

Treatments for Output Anomia

Therapeutic tasks used to treat output anomia have tended to emphasize actual production of the phonological form of the word itself, and/or conscious reflection on the word's phonological properties. For example, the patient may be trained to name pictures with the help of phonological cues, such as the initial phoneme, the initial syllable, or a rhyming word (Greenwald, Raymer, Richardson, & Rothi, 1995; LeDorze & Pitts, 1995; Howard et al., 1985; Miceli, Amitrano, Capasso, & Caramazza, 1996; Raymer, Thomson, Jacobs, & LeGrand, 1993; Nettleton & Lesser, 1991). Or the person may be asked to repeat or read aloud the test words, either in isolation or in view of the corresponding picture, and sometimes also with the help of phonemic cues (e.g., Davis & Pring, 1991; Greenwald et al., 1995; Hillis & Caramazza, 1994; Miceli et al., 1996; Nettleton & Lesser, 1991). Alternatively, the patient may be asked to perform various operations that involve attending to a word's phonological form, such as judging whether two words rhyme (Howard et al., 1985; Nettleton & Lesser, 1991) or identifying the number of syllables and/or initial phoneme of a word (LeDorze & Pitts, 1995; Robson, Marshall, Pring, & Chiat, 1998). Again, several studies using one or more of these techniques have documented improvement in naming performance as a result of treatment (e.g., Hillis & Caramazza, 1994; Miceli et al., 1996; Nettleton & Lesser, 1991; Robson et al., 1998), although these improvements have usually been limited to the treated items themselves (but see Robson et al., 1998, for an example of successful generalization).

An example of successful application of "phonological" therapy to the treatment of output anomia is that of Robson et al. (1998). Their patient, GF, was severely impaired on naming tasks and produced omissions, semantic paraphasias, and some phonemic paraphasias. However, her performance on semantic comprehension tasks was well preserved, and her error awareness was excellent. The therapeutic protocol chosen for GF was aimed at encouraging her to reflect on each word's phonological form, particularly its initial phoneme and number of syllables. The rationale here was that this training might enable GF to "self-cue" during naming (she was found to be responsive to externally presented phonemic cues). One task trained GF to judge the number of syllables in a spoken word presented with a picture. Later she had to respond to the picture presented alone. A second task required GF to identify the target word's first sound. Subsequently she was encouraged to access this phonological information and use it as a self-cue. As a result of this treatment, naming performance for the treated words improved significantly, and there was also some generalization to untreated words.[8]

Evaluation

Although studies have generally achieved some measure of success using "cognitively motivated" therapies for word retrieval disorders, a question arises as to whether these therapies do in fact produce better outcomes than more traditional forms of therapy. That is, would comparable rates of improvement be obtained if more traditional techniques were used, which were aimed at ameliorating word retrieval deficits in general? Hillis (1998) suggests this may be the care, at least for patients with multiple impairments. She has demonstrated that for a patient with impairments at both the "semantic" and "output" levels (patient HG, described above), cognitively motivated therapy focusing on just one of these levels was no more beneficial than the use of a more traditional "cueing hierarchy" designed to treat all types of naming problems (she used a hierarchy that incorporated both semantic and phonemic cues). Perhaps this is not surprising, since Hillis's "traditional" therapy may have included elements that acted upon both (impaired) cognitive components at the same time.

However, when we consider patients with more circumscribed cognitive impairments, the picture is somewhat more promising. Hillis and Caramazza (1994, Study 3) provide strong support for the use of cognitively motivated treatment by demonstrating a "double dissociation" between the effects of different types of treatment for different types of cognitive impairments. Two patients, one with semantic anomia (JJ) and the other with output anomia (HW), were each treated with two forms of therapy—one aimed at strengthening semantic representations (written-word-to-picture matching), and the other aimed at facilitating phonological word form retrieval (reading aloud with phonemic cueing). The patient with semantic anomia (JJ) showed improvement with the semantic treatment but not the phonological treatment, whereas the patient with output anomia (HW) exhibited the converse pattern, showing significant improvement with the phonological treatment but not the semantic treatment. This suggests that if a more complete design is used, which incorporates contrasting patient types and treatments, it is possible to demonstrate advantages for cognitively motivated treatments. Nevertheless, the fact that such advantages only seem to emerge for designs incorporating relatively "pure" cases of impairment illustrates the very real possibility that the cognitive approach may not be well suited to more severe cases with multiple cognitive impairments.

Whatever the strengths and weaknesses of existing efforts at cognitive therapy, it is important to bear in mind that the cognitive approach is only as good as the theoretical model(s) on which it is based. We have noted earlier that most existing studies adopt a very simple model, which distinguishes only two types of word retrieval impairments—a "semantic" deficit and an "output" deficit. We have already shown above that this simple bipartite model fails to capture some important sources of variability in patient performance. Although the four-way classification system we have advanced might improve the situation somewhat, it still has relatively little to say about what actually takes place within the various stages or levels of processing, and even less to say about how their function may improve with behavioral interventions (see Hillis, 1998, and Hillis & Caramazza, 1994, for excellent discussions of these issues). Choice of actual treatment tasks is similarly limited by our current understanding. Most studies have identified tasks as semantic or phonological largely on the basis of intuition, and have not attempted to describe in detail precisely how each task is accomplished. Therefore, it is difficult to be certain whether a task is really operating at the targeted level of processing. For example, a "phonological" task such as naming pictures to a phoneme cue clearly involves some degree of phonological activity; however, it may also involve semantic stimulation and, perhaps even more importantly, reinforcement of associations between semantic representations and phonological forms (see Nickels & Best, 1996a, for a discussion of these kinds of issues). As our understanding increases about the processes that take place during word retrieval, the various types of impairments that can occur, and the ways in which individual tasks may facilitate recovery of these impairments, it is likely that the cognitive approach will have a good deal more to contribute. Some of the outstanding questions and issues regarding cognitive therapy—for example, when and why we sometimes see generalization to untreated items, and how we can encourage this—may then begin to be answered.

Conclusion

A number of (valid) criticisms have been raised about the cognitive approach—that it may be too time-consuming, that it is unsuitable for many patients, and that models of the impairments and treatment tasks are not sufficiently well developed to offer much guidance. Given these criticisms, it is probably too early to offer up "cognitive therapy" for word retrieval disorders as a new alternative to traditional therapies. Nevertheless, we should not underestimate the potential of this approach to influence therapeutic practices in more subtle ways. As therapists become more and more familiar with cognitive models of word retrieval impairment in aphasia, this is likely to influence the way they think about such impairment and the way they approach treatment. And as models of word retrieval disorders and treatments develop, the cognitive approach may have a more substantive contribution to make: It may eventually lead to the design of more formal systems that aim to match therapy with cognitive impairments, and possibly even to the formulation of entirely new treatment paradigms.

FINAL REMARKS

As we have seen in the discussion above, cognitive psychology and cognitive neuropsychology offer ways of characterizing word retrieval disorders in aphasia that have possible practical applications, and may even be useful in therapy. Evidence gathered from studies in this tradition strongly supports the notion that not all word retrieval disorders are the same. Such studies have identified at least two different cognitive deficits that can give rise to word retrieval difficulties—an inability to access semantic representations (semantic anomia) and an inability to access a word for output (output anomia). More recent research also suggests that deficits of the second kind—those involving access to words for output—may be further subdivided according to whether the deficit involves an inability to locate words that meet the desired meaning specifications (lemma recovery) or an inability to access the phonemes of the located word (phoneme recovery). Furthermore, it may be possible to draw a cognitive distinction between word retrieval disorders occurring within the general syndrome of fluent aphasia and those arising in nonfluent aphasia; indeed, some cognitive accounts for the latter type of disorders have already been advanced. Finally, recent treatment studies suggest that these kinds of cognitive characterizations of word retrieval disorders may be useful in guiding therapy for certain types of patients.

Nevertheless, one point we have raised during our discussion is that most of our understanding of the cognitive underpinnings of word retrieval disorders is still at a very general level. Many studies make claims about the broad architecture of the word retrieval process and the level of processing impaired in certain types of retrieval disorders, but relatively few have anything to say about what precisely goes on within these levels of processing and how this changes as a result of brain damage. This kind of information is very much needed. First, it may help us to understand some of the variation we see among patients that cannot be captured in terms of the broad loci of their deficits. Dell et al. (1997) argue the strongest version of this view by suggesting that a large proportion of patient-to-patient variation in word retrieval performance may be due to differences in the *way* processing at the relevant stages breaks down, rather than at *which* stages processing breaks down. Second, information about the internal workings of the various stages of word retrieval—and about how their function can be altered through behavioral intervention—is essential if we are to understand the way in which therapeutic tasks work to ameliorate a particular deficit, and what precise tasks might be best suited for a particular purpose.

Recent studies are definitely moving in this direction. We have seen that authors such as Dell et al. (1997), Foygel and Dell (in press), and Rapp and Goldrick (in press) offer descriptions of word retrieval that not only incorporate stages, but also offer suggestions as to *how* processing at these stages breaks down in the various aphasic conditions. Also, while theories about word retrieval in aphasia have not yet confronted issues of recovery and relearning, some progress has been made in this direction in related areas. For example, Plaut (1996) advances a model of word reading that includes the capacity to relearn after breakdown, and that behaves in some interesting and potentially informative ways (e.g., relearning occurs faster with exposure to typical examples of a category than it does with exposure to atypical examples). Within the next decade, it is very likely that we will see more progress in this direction in the field of spoken-word retrieval.

ACKNOWLEDGMENTS

Much of the work on this chapter was completed while the first author was a Research Fellow at the Center for Cognitive Neuroscience, Department of Neurology, Temple University, Philadelphia, Pennsylvania. Her work was supported by NIH grant no. Ro1 DC00191. The second author wishes to cite NIH grant no. Ro1 DC02754 for support of this project.

NOTES

1. Here we use the term "lemma" to refer to a lexical representation not yet fully specified as to its phonological form. We remain neutral as to whether this representation is used only in spoken-word retrieval, or whether it is also retrieved in written naming (for discussions, see Caramazza, 1997; Rapp & Goldrick, in press).

2. Some models also propose an intervening stage of morphological representation, at which a word is represented in terms of its stem and bound morphemes (Levelt, Roelofs, & Meyer, 1999). However, in the present chapter we limit our consideration to monomorphemic words, and take the liberty of glossing over these (important) issues of morphological composition and decomposition.

3. Some authors argue that this deficit need only affect "verbal semantics" (or knowledge of word meanings); nonverbal conceptual knowledge about the real world (e.g., what a toothbrush is used for) may be preserved (see Howard & Orchard-Lisle, 1987; Nickels & Howard, 1994).

4. Some studies also report imageability effects (e.g., Franklin et al., 1995), but these effects may be attributable to input/maintenance processes (tasks such as repetition are heavily used) or to the confounding effects of frequency.

5. A number of individuals exhibit the reverse pattern of performance (e.g., Miceli, Silveri, Villa, & Caramazza, 1984; Zingeser & Berndt, 1990). However, most such individuals have been nonfluent aphasic patients. Such cases are discussed in a separate section below.

6. The ability to recover grammatical gender and homophone information about words does seem to suggest successful recovery of the appropriate lemma. But it is also possible that the lemma may have been only partially activated—enough to permit access to some of the more coarse-grained properties of the word, but not enough to initiate a sufficiently strong activation pattern at the phonological level of representation.

7. The predictions were not perfect: The "phoneme recovery" patients were generally better at repetition than would be predicted on the basis of the authors' model of the repetition task. This suggests that the spoken stimulus not only supports lemma recovery, but may also partially support phoneme recovery—perhaps by priming the target phonemes at the output level.

8. Surprisingly, while GF's naming performance improved, her ability to provide the phonological "self-cues" she was trained to generate did not. Nevertheless, it is possible that this training indirectly improved her naming, by encouraging her to generate her own internal phonological representations for each word.

REFERENCES

Badecker, W., Miozzo, M., & Zanuttini, R. (1995). The two-stage model of lexical retrieval: Evidence from a case of anomia with selective preservation of grammatical gender. *Cognition*, *34*, 205–243.

Beauvois, M.-F., & Saillant, B. (1985). Optic aphasia for colour and colour agnosia: A distinction between visual and visuo-verbal impairments in the processing of colours. *Cognitive Neuropsychology*, *2*, 1–48.

Béland, R., Caplan, D., & Nespoulous, J.-L. (1990). The role of abstract phonological representations in word production: Evidence from phonemic paraphasias. *Journal of Neurolinguistics*, *5*, 125–164.

Benson, D. F. (1979). Neurologic correlates of anomia. In H. Whitaker & H. A. Whitaker (Eds.), *Studies in neurolinguistics* (Vol. 4). New York: Academic Press.

Benton, A. L. (1968). Differential behavioral effects in frontal lobe disease. *Neuropsychologia*, *6*, 53–60.

Berndt, R. S., Mitchum, C. C., Haendiges, A. N., & Sandson, J. (1997). Verb retrieval in aphasia: 1. Characterizing single word impairments. *Brain and Language*, *56*, 68–106.

Blumstein, S. E., Cooper, N. E., Goodglass, H., Statlender, S., & Gottlieb, J. (1980). Production deficits in aphasia: A voice-onset time analysis. *Brain and Language*, *9*, 153–170.

Breedin, S. D., Saffran, E. M., & Coslett, H. B. (1994). Reversal of the concreteness effect in a patient with semantic dementia. *Cognitive Neuropsychology*, *11*, 617–660.

Butterworth, B. (1989). Lexical access in speech production. In W. Marslen-Wilson (Ed.), *Lexical representation and process*. Cambridge, MA: MIT Press.

Caplan, D. (1985). Syntactic and semantic structure in Agrammatism. In M. L. Kean (Ed.), *Agrammatism*. Orlando, FL: Academic Press.

Caplan, D. (1992). *Language: Structure, processing and disorders*. Cambridge, MA: MIT Press.

Caplan, D., Vanier, M., & Baker, C. (1986). A case study of reproduction conduction aphasia: I. Word production. *Cognitive Neuropsychology*, *3*, 99–128.

Caramazza, A. (1997). How many levels of processing are there in lexical access? *Cognitive Neuropsychology*, *14*, 177–208.

Caramazza, A., & Hillis, A. E. (1990). Where do semantic errors come from? *Cortex*, *26*, 95–122.

Caramazza, A., & Hillis, A. E. (1991). Lexical organization of nouns and verbs in the brain. *Nature*, *349*, 788–790.

Coltheart, M., Bates, A., & Castles, A. (1994). Cognitive neuropsychology and rehabilitation. In M. J. Riddoch & G. W. Humphreys (Eds.), *Cognitive neuropsychology and cognitive rehabilitation*. Hillsdale, NJ: Erlbaum.

Coslett, H. B., Bowers, D., Verfaellie, M., & Heilman, K. M. (1991). Frontal verbal amnesia. *Archives of Neurology*, *48*, 949–955.

Coslett, H. B., & Saffran, E. M. (1989). Preserved object recognition and reading comprehension in optic aphasia. *Brain*, *112*, 1091–1110.

Coughlan, A. D., & Warrington, E. K. (1978). Word comprehension and word retrieval in patients with localized cerebral lesions. *Brain*, *100*, 163–185.

Damasio, H., Gradowski, T. J., Tranel, D., Hichwa, R. D., & Damasio, A. R. (1996). A neural basis for lexical retrieval. *Nature*, *380*, 499–505.

Daniele, A., Silveri, M. C., Giustolini, L., Colosimo, C., & Gainotti, G. (1994). Evidence for a possible neuroanatomical basis for lexical processing of nouns and verbs. *Neuropsychologia*, *32*, 1325–1341.

Davis, A., & Pring, T. (1991). Therapy for word finding deficits: More on the effects of semantic and phonological approaches to treatment with dysphasic patients. *Neuropsychological Rehabilitation*, *1*, 135–145.

Dell, G. S. (1986). A spreading-activation theory of retrieval in sentence production. *Psychological Review*, *93*, 283–321.

Dell, G. S. (1988). The retrieval of phonological forms in production: Test of predictions from a connectionist model. *Journal of Memory and Language, 27,* 124–142.

Dell, G. S., Juliano, C., & Govindjee, A. (1993). Structure and content in language production: A theory of frame constraints in phonological speech errors. *Cognitive Neuroscience, 17,* 149–195.

Dell, G. S., & Reich, P. A. (1981). Stages in sentence production: An analysis of speech error data. *Journal of Verbal Learning and Verbal Behaviour, 20,* 611–629.

Dell, G. S., Schwartz, M. F., Martin, N., Saffran, E. M., & Gagnon, D. A. (1997). Lexical access in aphasic and nonaphasic speakers. *Psychological Review, 104,* 801–838.

Ellis, A. W., & Young, A. W. (1988). *Human cognitive neuropsychology.* Hillsdale NJ: Erlbaum.

Foygel, D., & Dell, G. S. (in press). Models of impaired lexical access in speech production. *Journal of Memory and Language.*

Franklin, S. E., Howard, D., & Patterson, K. E. (1995). Abstract word anomia. *Cognitive Neuropsychology, 12,* 549–566.

Gainotti, G., Silveri, M. C., Villa, G., & Miceli, G. (1986). Anomia with and without comprehension disorders. *Brain and Language, 29,* 18–33.

Garrett, M. F. (1975). The analysis of sentence production. In G. Bower (Ed.), *The psychology of learning and motivation* (Vol. 9). New York: Academic Press.

Greenwald, M. L., Raymer, A. M., Richardson, M. E., & Rothi, L. J. G. (1995). Contrasting treatments for severe impairments of picture naming. *Neuropsychological Rehabilitation, 5,* 17–49.

Harley, T. A. (1984). A critique of top-down independent levels models of speech production: Evidence from non-phrase-internal errors. *Cognitive Science, 8,* 191–219.

Harley, T. A., & MacAndrew, S. B. G. (1992). Modelling paraphasias in normal and aphasic speech. In *Proceedings of the Fourteenth Annual Conference of the Cognitive Science Society, Bloomington, IN.* Hillsdale, NJ: Erlbaum.

Hécaen, H., & Angelergues, R. (1964). Localization of symptoms in aphasia. In A. V. S. De Rueck & M. O'Connor (Eds.), *Disorders of language.* London: Churchill.

Helm-Estabrooks, N., Emery, P., & Albert, M. L. (1987). Treatment of Aphasic Perseveration (TAP) program. *Archives of Neurology, 44,* 1253–1255.

Henaff Gonon, M., Bruckert, R., & Michel, F. (1989). Lexicalization in an anomic patient. *Neuropsychologia, 27,* 391–407.

Hillis, A. E. (1991). The effects of separate treatments for distinct impairments within the naming process. In T. Prescott (Ed.), *Clinical aphasiology* (Vol. 19). Austin, TX: Pro-Ed.

Hillis, A. E. (1998). Effects of separate treatments for distinct impairments within the naming process. *Journal of the International Neuropsychological Society, 4,* 648–660.

Hillis, A. E., & Caramazza, A. (1994). Theories of lexical processing and rehabilitation of lexical deficits. In M. J. Riddoch & G. W. Humphreys (Eds.), *Cognitive neuropsychology and cognitive rehabilitation.* Hillsdale, NJ: Erlbaum.

Hillis, A. E., Rapp, B., Romani, C., & Caramazza, A. (1990). Selective impairments of semantics in lexical processing. *Cognitive Neuropsychology, 7,* 191–243.

Howard, D., & Hatfield, F. M. (1987). *Aphasia therapy: Historical and contemporary issues.* Hillsdale, NJ: Erlbaum.

Howard, D., & Orchard-Lisle, V. (1984). On the origin of semantic errors in naming: Evidence from the case of a global aphasic. *Cognitive Neuropsychology, 1,* 163–190.

Howard, D., Patterson, K. E., Franklin, S., Orchard-Lisle, V., & Morton, J. (1985). The treatment of word retrieval deficits in aphasia: A comparison of two therapy methods. *Brain, 108,* 817–829.

Kay, J., & Ellis, A. (1987). A cognitive neuropsychological case study of anomia. *Brain, 110,* 613–629.

Kempen, G., & Huijbers, P. (1983). The lexicalization process in sentence production and naming: Indirect selection of words. *Cognition, 14,* 184–209.

Kertesz, A. (1979). *Aphasia and associated disorders: Taxonomy, localization and recovery.* New York: Grune & Stratton.

Kohn, S. E. (1989). The nature of the phonemic string deficit in conduction aphasia. *Aphasiology, 3,* 209–239.

Kohn, S. E., & Goodglass, H. (1985). Picture naming in aphasia. *Brain and Language, 24,* 266–283.

Kohn, S. E., & Smith, K. L. (1990). Between-word speech errors in conduction aphasia. *Cognitive Neuropsychology, 7,* 133–156.

Kohn, S. E., & Smith, K. L. (1994). Distinctions between two phonological output deficits. *Applied Psycholinguistics, 15,* 75–95.

LeDorze, G., & Pitts, C. (1995). A case study evaluation of the effect of different techniques for the treatment of anomia. *Neuropsychological Rehabilitation, 5,* 17–49.

Lesser, R. (1989). Some issues in the neuropsychological rehabilitation of anomia. In X. Seron & G. Deloche (Eds.), *Cognitive approaches in neuropsychological rehabilitation.* Hillsdale, NJ: Erlbaum.

Levelt, W. J. M. (1989). *Speaking: From intention to articulation.* Cambridge, MA: MIT Press.

Levelt, W. J. M. (1992). Accessing words in speech production: Stages, processes and representations. *Cognition, 42,* 1–22.

Levelt, W. J. M., Roelofs, A., & Meyer, A. S. (1999). A theory of lexical access in speech production. *Behavioral and Brain Sciences, 22,* 1–75.

Linebaugh, C. (1983). Treatment of anomic aphasia. In C. Perkins (Ed.), *Current therapies for communication disorders: Language handicaps in adults.* New York: Thieme–Stratton.

Marshall, J., Pound, C., White-Thomson, M., & Pring, T. (1990). The use of picture/word matching tasks to assist word retrieval in aphasic patients. *Aphasiology, 4,* 167–184.

McCarthy, R. A., & Kartsounis, L. D. (1999). *Wobbly words: Refractory anomia with preserved semantics.* Manuscript in preparation.

Martin, N., Weisberg, R. N., & Saffran, E. M. (1989). Variables influencing the occurrence of naming errors: Implications for models of lexical retrieval. *Journal of Memory and Language, 28,* 462–485.

Miceli, G., Amitrano, A., Capasso, R., & Caramazza, A. (1996). The remediation of anomia resulting from output lexical damage: Analysis of two cases. *Brain and Language, 52,* 150–174.

Miceli, G., Silveri, M. C., Villa, G., & Caramazza, A. (1984). On the basis for the agrammatics' difficulty in producing main verbs. *Cortex, 20,* 207–220.

Miller, D., & Ellis, A. (1987). Speech and writing errors in "neologistic jargonaphasia": A lexical activation hypothesis. In M. Coltheart, G. Sartori, & K. Job (Eds.), *The cognitive neuropsychology of language.* Hillsdale, NJ: Erlbaum.

Miozzo, A., Soardi, M., & Cappa, S. F. (1994). Pure anomia with spared action naming due to a left temporal lesion. *Neuropsychologia, 32,* 1101–1109.

Mitchum, C. C., & Berndt, R.S. (1995). The cognitive neuropsychological approach to the treatment of language disorders. *Neuropsychological Rehabilitation, 5,* 1–16.

Nespoulous, J.-L., Joanette, Y., Beland, R., Caplan, D., & Lecours, A. R. (1984). Phonological disturbance in aphasia: Is there a "markedness effect" in aphasic phonemic errors? In F. C. Rose (Ed.), *Advances in neurology: Vol. 42. Progress in aphasiology.* London: Raven Press.

Nettleton, J., & Lesser, R. (1991). Therapy for naming difficulties in aphasia: Application of a cognitive neuropsychological model. *Journal of Neurolinguistics, 6,* 139–157.

Nickels, L. (1997). *Spoken word production and its breakdown in aphasia.* Hove, England: Psychology Press.

Nickels, L., & Best, W. (1996a). Therapy for naming disorders: Part I. Specifics, surprises and suggestions. *Aphasiology, 10,* 21–47.

Nickels, L., & Best, W. (1996b). Therapy for naming disorders: Part II. Principles, puzzles and progress. *Aphasiology, 10,* 109–136.

Nickels, L., & Howard, D. (1984). A frequent occurrence?: Factors affecting the production of semantic errors in aphasic naming. *Cognitive Neuropsychology, 11,* 289–320.

Plaut, D. (1996). Relearning after damage in connectionist networks: Toward a theory of rehabilitation. *Brain and Language, 52,* 25–82.

Rapp, B., & Goldrick, M. (in press). Discreteness and interactivity in spoken word production. *Psychological Review.*

Raymer, A. M., Thomson, C. K., Jacobs, B., & LeGrand, H. R. (1993). Phonological treatment of naming deficits in aphasia: Model-based generalization analysis. *Aphasiology, 7,* 27–53.

Robson, J., Marshall, J., Pring, T., & Chiat, S. (1998). Phonological naming therapy in jargon aphasia: Positive but paradoxical effects. *Journal of the International Neuropsychological Society, 4,* 675–686.

Roelofs, A. (1992). A spreading activation model of lemma retrieval in speaking. *Cognition, 42,* 107–142.

Roelofs, A. (1997). The WEAVER model of word-form encoding in speech production. *Cognition, 64,* 249–284.

Saffran, E. M. (1982). Neuropsychological approaches to the study of language. *British Journal of Psychology, 73,* 317–337.

Schriefers, H., Meyer, A. S., & Levelt, W. J. M. (1990). Exploring the time course of lexical access in language production: Picture–word interference studies. *Journal of Memory and Language, 29*, 86–102.

Schwartz, M. F. (1987). Patterns of speech production deficit within and across aphasic syndromes: Application of a psycholinguistic model. In M. Coltheart, G. Sartori, & K. Job (Eds.), *The cognitive neuropsychology of language*. Hillsdale, NJ: Erlbaum.

Seron, X., van der Linden, M., & de Partz, M.-P. (1991). In defence of cognitive approaches to neuropsychological therapy. *Neuropsychological Rehabilitation, 1*, 303–318.

Shallice, T. (1988). *From neuropsychology to mental structure*. Cambridge, England: Cambridge University Press.

Shattuck-Hufnagel, S. (1979). Speech errors as evidence for a serial ordering mechanism in sentence production. In W. E. Cooper & E. C. T. Walker (Eds.), *Sentence processing: Psycholinguistic studies presented to Merrill Garrett*. Hillsdale, NJ: Erlbaum.

Shattuck-Hufnagel, S. (1983). Sublexical units and suprasegmental structure in speech production planning. In P. F. MacNeilage (Ed.), *The production of speech*. New York: Springer-Verlag.

Shattuck-Hufnagel, S. (1987). The role of word onset consonants in speech production planning: New evidence from speech error patterns. In E. Keller & M. Gopnik (Eds.), *Motor and sensory processes of language*. Hillsdale, NJ: Erlbaum.

Shattuck-Hufnagel, S. (1992). The role of word structure in segmental serial ordering. *Cognition, 42*, 213–259.

Stemberger, J. P. (1985). An interactive activation model of language production. In A. Ellis (Ed.), *Progress in the psychology of language*. Hillsdale, NJ: Erlbaum.

Stemberger, J. P. (1990). Wordshape errors in language production. *Cognition, 35*, 123–157.

Warrington, E. K., & Cipolotti, L. (1996). Word comprehension: The distinction between refractory and storage impairments. *Brain, 119*, 611–625.

Warrington, E. K., & McCarthy, R. A. (1983). Category specific access dysphasia. *Brain, 106*, 859–878.

Warrington, E. K., & McCarthy, R. A. (1987). Categories of knowledge: Further fractionation and an attempted integration. *Brain, 110*, 1273–1296.

Warrington, E. K., & Shallice, T. (1984). Category specific semantic impairments. *Brain, 107*, 829–854.

Williams, S. E., & Canter, G. (1982). The influence of situational context on naming performance in aphasic syndromes. *Brain and Language, 17*, 92–106.

Wilshire, C. E. (1998). Three "abnormal" features of aphasic phonological errors. *Brain and Language, 65*, 219–222.

Wilshire, C. E. (2000). *Where do aphasic phonological errors come from? Evidence from phoneme movement errors in picture naming*. Manuscript submitted for publication.

Wilshire, C. E., & McCarthy, R. A. (1999). *Evidence for a context-sensitive word retrieval disorder in a case of nonfluent aphasia*. Manuscript submitted for publication.

Zingeser, L. B., & Berndt, R. S. (1988). Grammatical class and context effects in a case of pure anomia: Implications for models of language production. *Cognitive Neuropsychology, 5*, 473–516.

Zingeser, L. B., & Berndt, R. S. (1990). Retrieval of nouns and verbs in agrammatism and anomia. *Brain and Language, 39*, 14–32.

5

THE SEMANTIC SYSTEM

ANASTASIA M. RAYMER
LESLIE J. GONZALEZ ROTHI

The "semantic system" is the store of knowledge regarding concepts (Caplan, 1993). It is the mechanism of language processing through which people apply meaning to their sensory and productive experiences of spoken and written words, viewed objects, and gestures. As such, the ideas we discuss in this chapter devoted to the semantic system and impairments of semantic processing are closely related to those reviewed by Wilshire and Coslett in Chapter 4 of this book, as lexical and semantic mechanisms are typically active and highly interactive in the course of word processing (Hodges, Patterson, & Tyler, 1994). Although there is a large cognitive-psychological literature on semantic function, we focus our review on studies in cognitive neuropsychology that have provided evidence of the structure and function of the semantic system, using studies of individuals with brain impairment.

A HISTORICAL PERSPECTIVE

Wernicke (1874) was the first to develop a model of "centers" involved in spoken language, to localize these centers in circumscribed brain regions, and to predict divergent patterns of language breakdown associated with lesions of these language centers or their connections. Subsequently, Lichtheim (1885) expanded upon Wernicke's model, adding centers for reading, writing, and concepts. Lichtheim's "concept system," through which we derive word meanings, is akin to the "semantic system," the term used in modern accounts of language processing. Unlike the centers for spoken and written language, which are presumably localized in specific brain regions, Lichtheim proposed that concepts are distributed throughout the brain. On the basis of his expanded model, Lichtheim predicted additional aphasia syndromes, in association with dysfunction in and among these centers, including transcortical aphasias. He used the term "transcortical sensory aphasia," for example, to refer to the dissociation of the central language mechanisms from the concept system, leading to retained ability to repeat, but impairment in comprehending language.

Lissauer (1890/1988) implied that semantic memory may be "modality-specified." He proposed that meaning is derived through an association process in which there is "activation of memories laid down through different sensory modalities" (p. 182).

According to Freud (1891/1953), one of the problems with the original connectionist model was its incompleteness in accounting for behaviors noted in brain damage. Also, he viewed the centers proposed by Wernicke and Lichtheim as oversimplified in their description of how complex cognitive processes such as speaking and reading are accomplished. Freud's objection to the incompleteness and simplification of early connectionist models is relevant to the state of affairs in cognitive neuropsychology today. The nature of the concept system, or the semantic system as we refer to it now, is a case in point. As in the work of Lichtheim (1885) and Lissauer (1890/1988), much discussion centers on whether the semantic system is unitary and is accessed through all modalities of processing, or whether it is a more complex, multicomponent system.

In this chapter we provide an overview of more modern cognitive-neuropsychological conceptions of semantic processing. Citing studies of individuals with acquired brain damage, as well as brain activation studies in healthy individuals, we review the neuroanatomy that supports the semantic system's functioning. Finally, a portion of our discussion is focused on issues related to clinical practice with individuals whose aphasia includes disturbances of semantic processing.

MODERN PERSPECTIVES ON THE SEMANTIC SYSTEM

Today, using evidence accumulated in studies of normal and brain-impaired individuals, models of cognitive mechanisms involved in semantic processing are considerably more explicit than the originally proposed Wernicke–Lichtheim model. For example, a model of components involved in semantic processing, shown in Figure 5.1 includes modality-specific input and mode-specific output lexicons storing memory representations for familiar spoken and written words and gestures, as well as recognition systems for processing familiar viewed objects (Rothi, Raymer, Maher, Greenwald, & Morris, 1991). These mode- and modality-specific input and output mechanisms are thought to be activated in a cascading fashion (Humphreys, Riddoch, & Quinlan, 1988) and are interconnected by way of a semantic system through which meanings for words, gestures, or objects are derived (Caramazza, Hillis, Rapp, & Romani, 1990; Riddoch, Humphreys, Coltheart, & Funnell, 1988).

Much debate in recent years has focused on this semantic system and how it is structured. Researchers have promoted two general theories, which we review briefly: unitary semantics (Caramazza et al., 1990; Hillis, Rapp, & Caramazza, 1995; Humphreys & Riddoch, 1988; Lambon Ralph, Patterson, & Hodges, 1997; Rapp, Hillis, & Caramazza, 1993; Seymour, 1973, 1978) and modality-specific semantics (Beauvois & Saillant, 1985; Farah & McClelland, 1991; Paivio, 1971, 1986; Shallice, 1988; Warrington & McCarthy, 1994).

Unitary Semantics

One proposal regarding the structure of the semantic mechanism is that a single, unitary semantic system is responsible for providing meaning for a stimulus, regardless of the modality of stimulus input or the ultimate mode of response (as represented in Figure 5.1). A single semantic representation specifies information such as perceptual properties, functions, and other associated knowledge relevant to the meaning of a given referent (Caramazza et al., 1990; Rapp et al., 1993; Hillis et al., 1995). This same semantic representation is activated to achieve meaning for all modalities of input, including spoken and written words, as well as viewed objects and gestures.

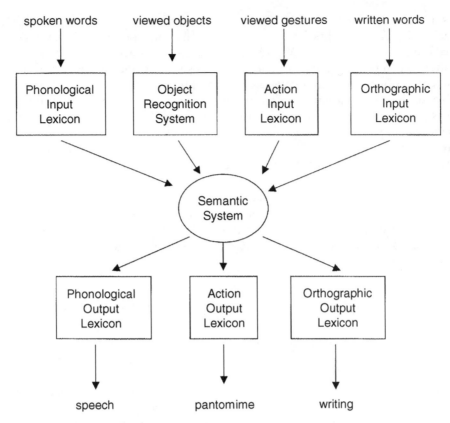

FIGURE 5.1. Model of input, output, and semantic mechanisms involved in lexical–object–gesture processing.

Neuropsychological evidence has been cited in support of a unitary semantic system. Caramazza, Berndt, and Brownell (1982) demonstrated a relationship between failure to classify objects and impaired labeling of objects in a subgroup of their subjects with aphasia. That is, some individuals with aphasia who had difficulty classifying objects tended also to have difficulty naming objects. They attributed this pattern of impairments to dysfunction in a single semantic system.

Other evidence for unitary semantics comes from the performance of individuals with brain damage who demonstrate quantitatively and qualitatively similar semantic impairment in multiple lexical tasks. For example, Hillis, Rapp, Romani, and Caramazza (1990) described the performance of an individual with aphasia who produced the same proportion of semantic errors in all lexical tasks: oral picture naming, oral word reading, written picture naming, writing to dictation, and word comprehension. The authors proposed that this pattern of co-occurrence of deficits was related to impairment of a unitary semantic mechanism that all tasks engaged.

More recently, Caramazza and Shelton (1998) have elaborated on the organization of the unimodal semantic representations to account for dissociations in semantic categories of processing often observed in brain-damaged individuals. Specifically, patients may have impairments in naming and recognition limited to specific semantic categories, such as living and nonliving things (Bunn, Tyler, & Moss, 1998; Warrington & McCarthy, 1983), fruits and vegetables (Farah & Wallace, 1992; Hart, Berndt, & Caramazza, 1985), and animals (Caramazza & Shelton, 1998; Ferreira, Giusiano, & Poncet, 1997; Hart & Gordon, 1992; Hillis & Caramazza, 1991). Caramazza and Shelton (1998) attributed category specificity in lexical–semantic impairments to texturing of the semantic representations across categories of objects. The semantic properties for an object are "highly intercorrelated" (p. 8) and are shared across members of a category of objects. Categories for natural objects such as plants or animals are particularly intercorrelated. Therefore, it is not unreasonable that localized brain damage could affect certain critical sets of semantic representations for a natural category and lead to category-specific semantic impairments. Thus, even though this theory posits a unitary semantic system, the system envisaged is heterogeneous in its structure across categories.

Modality-Specific Semantics

A contrasting view of the structure of the semantic system was suggested by Paivio (1971, 1986), who proposed a theory of cognition incorporating two semantic subsystems: an "imagery" system, which subserves meaning concerning items and events that are viewed (hereafter referred to as "visual semantics"); and a system devoted to meaning that is specifically relevant to language (hereafter referred to as "verbal semantics"). Others have elaborated upon this idea and proposed that the semantic system may include subsystems specialized for information relevant to each sensory modality and/or output mode (as in Figure 5.2) (Allport, 1985; Saffran, 1997; Shallice, 1988). Neuropsychological evidence presented in support of specialized subsystems of semantic knowledge comes from a number of sources, including optic aphasia and category-specific aphasias.

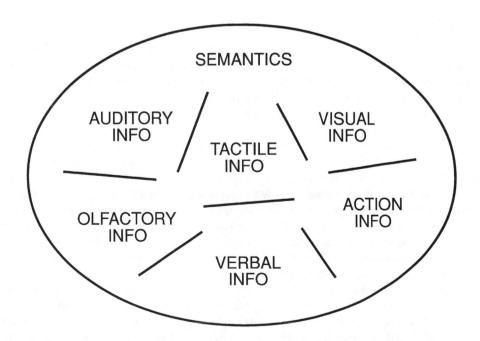

FIGURE 5.2. Model of semantics incorporating regionalized subsystems of knowledge.

Optic Aphasia

Individuals with optic aphasia have difficulty naming viewed pictures and objects. They can name the same items if they are defined verbally or have a characteristic sound; this argues against a general multimodality anomia, and indicates that semantic and phonological lexical retrieval mechanisms remain functional when activated through alternative input modalities. Moreover, these individuals can demonstrate recognition of a viewed object that they cannot name, by either providing an appropriate gesture or describing the object's use; this argues against impairment of visual object input processing (visual agnosia) as the basis for the modality-specific naming failure.

To account for the dissociations observed in optic aphasia, researchers have advocated a number of interpretations, a review of which is beyond the scope of this chapter (but see Farah, 1990; Iorio, Falanga, Fragassi, & Grossi, 1992). One particular interpretation of optic aphasia (Beauvois & Saillant, 1985; Ferreira, Giusiano, Ceccaldi, & Poncet, 1997) refers to a lexical model incorporating modality-specific semantic systems for visual and verbal semantics. Beauvois and Saillant (1985) suggested that optic aphasia results from an impairment in the interactions of the two specialized subsystems of semantics. Individuals with optic aphasia can provide gestures for viewed items, because visual semantic information is sufficient to activate action output systems for gesture. These individuals cannot name viewed items, however, because both visual and verbal semantic systems must be activated in order for visual information to gain access to the phonological output lexicon for picture naming.

The situation is further complicated by reports of other modality-specific aphasias, such as those specific to auditory input (Denes & Semenza, 1975) and tactile input (Beauvois, Saillant, Meininger, & Lhermitte, 1978; Rapcsak, Rothi, & Heilman, 1987). Taking this line of reasoning to its full extent, one may propose a complex structure for the semantic system, with subsystems specified for all modalities of input.

Category-Specific Aphasia

As noted earlier, researchers have described other individuals with aphasia whose naming and word comprehension disabilities are fractionated along semantic category lines. That is, patients display selective preservation or selective impairment of language processing for specific semantic categories (e.g., living and nonliving things, fruits and vegetables, and animals). Caramazza and his colleagues have interpreted such dissociations as evidence that knowledge is represented in a unitary semantic system characterized by some heterogeneity in the structure of the semantic representations across categories (Caramazza, Hillis, Leek, & Miozzo, 1994; Caramazza & Shelton, 1998). However, others have proposed alternative accounts for these selective category deficits.

Warrington and her colleagues (Warrington & McCarthy, 1983, 1994; Warrington & Shallice, 1984) have explained category-specific deficits in relation to the type of semantic information that is a defining attribute for particular semantic categories. For example, function information (verbal semantics) is important for characterizing categories of nonliving things, such as tools and kitchen items. In contrast, sensory feature information (visual semantics) is important for distinguishing categories of living things, such as animals.

Warrington and McCarthy (1987) further elaborated their proposal when they observed another individual, patient YOT, who experienced more difficulty comprehending names of small manipulable objects than names of large objects. All of these items, small and large, were nonliving items, which depend upon function information for semantic interpretation. The patient's differential performance on these categories could not be explained by their theory. Therefore, in addition to verbal and visual semantics, Warrington and McCarthy considered the influence of motor information on the specification of the semantics of certain categories of objects (e.g., small manipulable objects)—an idea consistent with Allport's (1985) notion of an action-oriented semantic domain. In their model of action processing, Rothi, Ochipa, and Heilman (1991, 1997) refer to this form of information as "action semantics."

Ochipa, Rothi, and Heilman (1989) reported the case of a left-handed man who, following a right-hemisphere stroke, demonstrated impaired knowledge of action semantics: He could not use tools correctly, name the function of tools, or point to tools described by function. However, he apparently had preserved knowledge of verbal semantics as he was able to name these same tools and point correctly to the tools when named. A contrasting pattern of preserved miming with impaired semantic knowledge was noted in an individual with progressive language deterioration described by Schwartz, Marin, and Saffran (1979).

In general, these unusual category-specific dissociations, observed among a variety of individuals, suggest that the semantic system may be fractionated in terms of both sensory input modality and output mode, as depicted in Figure 5.2. This is consistent with proposals that the semantic system is a complex network of subsystems of semantic knowledge (Allport, 1985; Saffran, 1997).

One implication of this interpretation that category-specific aphasias are a byproduct of the mode or modality of critical semantic information for that impaired category is that many semantic categories are presumably regionalized in the brain in less than transparent ways. For example, "ball" and "screwdriver," which are from distinct semantic categories, should be represented (at least in part) in similar cerebral regions, by virtue of the fact that actions constitute a critical feature of the meaning of each of these words. However, the more closely associated words "ball" and "net" should be less closely localized, as motor information is not a critical attribute of the meaning of a net.

Shallice (1988) has suggested that the semantic system is composed of modality- and mode-specific subsystems, which may not be discrete modules per se, but which represent a distributed semantic network in which regions are specialized for different modalities and modes of information. Meaning for a word, gesture, or object should be derived through the activation of subsets of semantic information distributed throughout the semantic subsystems that become linked over time through repeated experience (Saffran, 1997). Although Caramazza and Shelton (1998) hold to a unitary view of the semantic system, they propose that there exist specialized domains of semantic knowledge for animate–inanimate categories, which reflect critical neural adaptations in the representation of human knowledge.

As we proceed in this chapter, we acknowledge the disparate opinions that continue to exist regarding the structure of the semantic system. We are not clear what the actual ramifications of the two main views of semantic processing—unitary semantics versus modality-specific semantics—are for our daily clinical interactions with brain-impaired patients. Clinical research has begun to explore some of the direct clinical implications of semantic system theories. We advocate the position that structure and texture in semantic processing influence the semantic impairments we observe in our brain-injured patients, and thus have direct implications for the management of these impairments.

SEMANTIC IMPAIRMENTS

Individuals with aphasia due to acquired brain damage from stroke, Alzheimer's disease, and other brain disorders may develop language impairments that reflect dysfunction in various aspects of semantic processing. Because of the complex structure of the semantic system, impairment may be fairly selective, as is evident in the previous discussion of modality- and category-specific aphasias. However, patients often present with more generalized semantic system impairment, which ultimately affects processing in all semantic subsystems and domains across all tasks requiring semantic processing. Semantic impairment leads to reduced ability to retrieve words (anomia) and to comprehend words, either spoken or written, and may affect performance in quantitatively and qualitatively similar ways across different lexical–semantic tasks (e.g., Hillis et al., 1990; Howard & Orchard-Lisle, 1984). Impairments of semantic processing often underlie the language deficits seen in certain traditional syndromes of aphasia (including transcortical sensory aphasia and anomic aphasia), as well as the impaired language of Alzheimer's disease. Observations in these types of individuals also provide information on the neurological substrate of semantic processing.

Transcortical Sensory Aphasia

Individuals with transcortical sensory aphasia (hereafter referred to as TCSA) demonstrate impairments of auditory comprehension and retrieval of words, whereas repetition is remarkably spared. The specific mechanism of the language impairment varies across patients and represents dysfunction of the semantic system itself, or disconnection of the semantic system from other language-processing mechanisms. Spared repetition in TCSA presumably relates to the availability of alternative nonsemantic, sublexical, or lexical–phonological means to repeat words that remain functional in these individuals (Coslett, Roeltgen, Rothi, & Heilman, 1987; Kremin, 1987; Martin & Saffran, 1990). In one study examining the sentence repetition abilities of patients with TCSA (Berthier et al., 1991), patients demonstrated that whereas most of them were able to correct syntactic irregularities during repetition, they had great difficulty detecting semantic anomalies in the sentences. These patients were also able to repeat nonwords well. These findings suggest that patients with TCSA have access to both phonological and syntactic knowledge, but have particular difficulty using semantic knowledge to perform language tasks.

TCSA is observed in individuals with vascular lesions in the left temporo-parieto-occipital region (Kertesz, Sheppard, & MacKenzie, 1982) or with lesions of the left thalamus (Crosson, 1992; McFarling, Rothi, & Heilman, 1982). In addition, as patients with Alzheimer's disease experience decline in their language abilities, they often go through a phase in which they exhibit what can be characterized as TCSA (Cummings, Benson, Hill, & Reed, 1985).

Anomic Aphasia

Another aphasia syndrome that may relate to an impairment of the semantic system is anomic aphasia (Raymer, Foundas, et al., 1997). In anomic aphasia, individuals demonstrate selective difficulty in word retrieval, with adequate auditory comprehension and repetition of the same words (Benson & Ardila, 1996). For example, we and our colleagues (Raymer, Foundas, et al., 1997) observed a gentleman, HH, who had a cross-modality anomia (word retrieval difficulties in speaking and writing the names of viewed pictures and spoken definitions) and relatively preserved lexical comprehension following a lesion in the left inferior temporo-occipital region (Brodmann's area 37). In addition, we have described two other individuals with a similar pattern of acute cross-modality anomia in the context of preserved lexical comprehension, in conjunction with circumscribed lesions of the left thalamus (Raymer, Moberg, Crosson, Nadeau, & Rothi, 1997). Because the impairments were cross-modal (speaking and writing) output deficits that spanned modalities of input (viewed pictures and verbal descriptions), we attributed the anomia in all three individuals to failure in the lexical retrieval process at the point in which semantic representations activate subsequent lexical (phonological and orthographic) output representations.

In contrast, Hart and Gordon (1990) described three individuals with lesions of left posterior temporal and inferior parietal cortex (areas 21, 22, 39), with difficulties in word comprehension in contrast to preserved oral naming skills. They attributed the selective word comprehension impairment to dysfunction of an input stage in semantic processing.

The anomic aphasia and selective comprehension disturbances described in these six cases (Hart & Gordon, 1990; Raymer, Foundas, et al., 1997; Raymer, Moberg, et al., 1997) suggest that semantic processing can be fractionated along an additional dimension. Whereas modality-specific and category-specific impairments suggest "horizontal" dysfunction of semantic processing among mode- and modality-specific subsystems, input and output semantic impairments indicate a "vertical" fractionation in semantic processing.

Hillis and Caramazza (1995b) articulated a similar view in their review of the lexical–semantic impairments represented by three different patients who produced semantic errors in naming. Semantic errors in each patient arose at different stages in the semantic process: impaired semantic access by way of object processing, impaired semantic representations themselves, and impaired output from semantics to subsequent lexical–phonological representations. These types of selective impairments of semantic processing are probably less common, as neurological damage typically exceeds the biological substrates of semantic processing, also affecting performance in other language domains (e.g., phonology, syntax, morphology).

Language Impairment in Dementia

In initial stages of cognitive deterioration, individuals with Alzheimer's disease (hereafter referred to as AD) often demonstrate impairments of memory and language (Cummings et al., 1985; Huff et al., 1987). The language difficulty is typically characterized by impairments in word retrieval similar to those seen in anomic aphasia. However, as deterioration progresses and both auditory and reading comprehension are affected, the language impairment is more characteristic of the pattern seen in TCSA (Cummings et al., 1985; Hier, Hagenlocker, & Shindler, 1985). Individuals with AD are impaired in picture naming, and tend to produce semantically related or unrelated words (Bayles & Tomoeda, 1983; Bowles, Obler, & Albert, 1987). They are often unable to comprehend words, including the names of objects for which they are anomic (Chertkow, Bub, & Seidenberg, 1989). An extensive literature examining the basis for language impairment in individuals with AD has attributed these deficits to semantic system dysfunction (Daum, Riesch, Sartori, & Birbaumer, 1996; Martin, 1992).

In recent years, researchers have described a number of individuals with progressive aphasias in the absence of deterioration in other cognitive domains. Rogers and Alarcon (1999) noted that a portion of these individuals eventually develop the full symptomatology of dementia. However, others develop no symptoms other than the progressive deterioration of language abilities. One-third of the progressive aphasias are classified as fluent aphasias, at least a portion of which represent selective deterioration of semantic knowledge (Hodges & Patterson, 1996; Hodges, Patterson, Oxbury, & Funnell, 1992; Hodges et al., 1994; Kertesz, Davidson, & McCabe, 1998). The individuals with semantic dementia show increasing impairments of word retrieval, auditory and reading comprehension, and nonverbal semantic processing (e.g., matching associated pictures), in the presence of retained abilities with phonology and syntax.

Whereas the ongoing semantic deterioration in individuals with AD and selective semantic dementia typically affects processing across semantic domains, careful analysis of performance in individual subjects may demonstrate selective domains of spared and impaired semantic processing. Recent systematic investigations have revealed that certain semantic categories may be preferentially affected in individuals with progressive language impairments. Of particular interest is the living–nonliving distinction, described earlier.

Montanes, Goldblum, and Boller (1995) studied the naming performance of a group of patients with AD and determined that living items were more difficult to name than nonliving items if the pictures were presented as black-and-white line drawings. The category effect diminished when naming colored pictures, suggesting the importance of color in accessing semantic knowledge for the category of living items. In contrast, Silveri and et al. (1997) reported one patient with progressive semantic dementia who had the reverse category dysfunction when other linguistic factors were controlled for: impaired naming of nonliving items as compared to living items.

Lambon Ralph and colleagues (1997) evaluated decline in semantic processing across various semantic categories in a group of patients with AD. With advancing disease, the patients described fewer sensory characteristics when providing definitions for objects in natural categories (e.g., animals), whereas they provided less associative information for objects in artifact categories (e.g., household objects). These findings lend additional support to the view that category-specific impairments relate to deterioration of subsystems of semantic processing.

NEUROANATOMY OF SEMANTICS

Evidence from Acquired Lesions

Although our discussion of semantic system impairments has provided us with interesting evidence regarding the functional structure of the semantic system, we also have many important clues as to the neural instantiation of semantic knowledge. AD, with its predilection for more posterior temporo-occipital association cortices bilaterally (Engel, Cummings, Villanueva-Meyer, & Mena, 1993), is known for its effects on semantic aspects of language processing. Individuals with more selective degenerative impairment of semantic processing, termed "semantic dementia," have been noted to have abnormalities particularly affecting the left temporal lobe (Hodges et al., 1992; Kertesz et al., 1998).

Lesion locations in individuals with semantic impairments due to acute vascular events also implicate left-hemisphere posterolateral cortical regions in semantic processing. Kertesz and his colleagues (Kertesz, Harlock, & Coates, 1979; Kertesz et al., 1982) noted the involvement of the left parieto-temporo-occipital junction in individuals with TCSA, a syndrome associated with semantic impairments. This localization is characteristic of many individuals with selective impairments of input and output to semantic processing (Figure 5.3).

Hart and Gordon (1990) noted that the left posterior temporal and inferior parietal cortex (areas 21, 22, 39) was critical for input to semantic processing in their subjects with selective comprehension impairments and retained picture naming. We (Raymer, Foundas, et al., 1997) provided evidence that the left inferior temporal cortex (area 37) played a

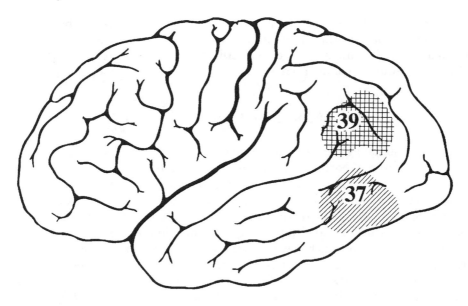

FIGURE 5.3. Lateral view of posterior left-hemisphere cortex, highlighting two cortical regions that appear to play a critical role in semantic processing.

crucial role in semantic output processing in our subject HH with an acute cross-modal anomia. This finding was supported in a subsequent report describing two additional patients with lesions affecting area 37 (Foundas, Daniels, & Vasterling, 1998).

Finally, left thalamic structures seem to be implicated in this complex semantic network, as implied by the observation of TCSA in many individuals with vascular lesions of the left thalamus (Crosson, 1992). We (Raymer, Moberg, et al. (1997), based on our observations of cross-modal anomia in two subjects with left thalamic infarcts, have proposed that thalamic input is especially involved in engaging portions of cortex in the process of semantic activation of lexical output representations.

There is also evidence bearing on the neural instantiation of modality-specific semantic subsystems. For example, impairments for the category of living items in individuals with viral encephalitis and damage to anterior and medial temporal regions (Warrington & Shallice, 1984) suggest that these regions are particularly important for the mediation of visual semantic information.

A recent study investigated lesion locations associated with word retrieval impairments for three different semantic categories often affected by category-specific impairments (names of persons, animals, and tools) (Damasio, Grabowski, Tranel, Hichwa, & Damasio, 1996). Distinct left-hemisphere lesions were associated with impairment in each category: Impairment for persons was linked with temporal pole lesions; impairment for animals was associated with lesions in anterior inferotemporal cortex; and impairment for tools was linked with lesions in lateral tempo-parieto-occipital and posterolateral inferotemporal cortex. In another recent study, we and our colleagues (Crosson, Moberg, Boone, Rothi, & Raymer, 1997) described a patient with a selective word retrieval impairment for the category of medical terminology associated with a left thalamic lesion. Although it was not clear whether the level of impairment was related to semantic or lexical retrieval stages of processing, the thalamus clearly had an important role to play for this selective semantic category. Findings from these lesion studies indicate not only that there are distinct domains of semantic knowledge (as suggested in the earlier discussion), but that discrete brain regions are involved in representation and processing in these semantic domains. Additional studies of patients with circumscribed brain lesions are necessary before the neural architecture of semantic domains of knowledge can be further elaborated.

Neuroimaging Studies of Semantic Processing

Additional corroborating evidence for the anatomy of semantic processing comes from the burgeoning literature reporting neuroimaging investigations in unimpaired individuals performing tasks requiring semantic processing. Several studies have now provided evidence across a variety of lexical–semantic tasks to suggest a neural substrate for semantic processing. Studies consistently report activation in left posterior temporo-parietal regions (including area 39) and inferior temporal regions (including area 37), as well as in left inferior frontal cortex, all of which may be associated with semantic processing (Buchel, Price, & Friston, 1998; Cappa, Perani, Schnur, Tettamanti, & Fazio, 1998; Demonet et al., 1992; Grabowski, Damasio, & Damasio, 1998; Smith et al., 1996; Vandenberghe, Price, Wise, Josephs, & Frackowiak, 1996). For example, Vandenberghe et al. (1996) used positron emission tomography (PET) to examine regions of activation in tasks in which subjects made semantic judgments for words and pictures. They identified a common region of activation in left posterior regions (parieto-temporal junction, fusiform–inferior temporal junction, middle temporal gyrus), as well as in left inferior frontal cortex (Brodmann's area 47). Cappa et al. (1998) evaluated activation across four tasks requiring subjects to make visual semantic and associative semantic decisions for words. They proposed that lexical–semantic processing occurs in left prefrontal and temporo-parietal cortex.

Neuroimaging findings that left inferior frontal regions are involved in semantic processing deviate from our knowledge of the neural substrates of semantic processing proposed on the basis of lesion studies. One possible reason for this discrepancy is that it can be difficult to dissociate lexical from semantic stages of processing in some neuroimaging paradigms. For example, Grabowski et al. (1998) reported activation of the left inferior frontal gyrus when naming three different categories of pictures, whereas the left middle frontal gyrus was active only for the category of famous faces. They proposed that the left frontal gyrus plays a role in word retrieval. However, although they attempted to use a control task that subtracted the influences of speech processes from the experimental naming tasks, it is not clear that lexical stages of processing were truly removed from their contrast, leaving only semantic processes active.

Other neuroimaging investigations have not identified left inferior frontal activation associated with semantic processing (Martin, Wiggs, Ungerleider, & Haxby, 1996; Williamson et al., 1995; Wise et al., 1991). Zelkowicz, Herbster, Nebes, Mintun, and Becker (1998) proposed that the left frontal activation seen during picture naming in their study appeared to be related to phonological and not semantic processing demands of the tasks, as the same left frontal region was active in the production of nonsense syllables when subjects were looking at nonsense objects. Thompson-Schill, D'Esposito, Aguirre, and Farah (1997) proposed an alternative explanation on the basis of a study using semantic processing tasks, in which they manipulated the level of semantic processing demands (high and low). Left inferior frontal activation was only observed in high-demand conditions across tasks. Therefore, they proposed that the left frontal cortex is active only when a task demands selection from among close alternatives, suggesting a general role in selecting responses from memory. This argument is similar to that proposed by Grabowski et al. (1998) for the activation of the left middle frontal gyrus during naming in a more difficult category (famous faces), suggesting a role in more effortful mental search operations. Regardless of the interpretation, the left inferior and posterior temporal regions are consistently implicated as a substrate for semantic processing, whereas left inferior frontal activation may relate to other cognitive demands in the course of lexical processing.

Neuroimaging studies have also begun to provide evidence for the neural basis of semantic subsystems of knowledge. Martin, Haxby, Lalonde, Wiggs, and Ungerleider (1995) reported a PET experiment in which subjects viewed line drawings and written words, and silently generated either the color or the action corresponding to each item. In the color task the investigators observed increased activation in the ventral temporal region, and in the action task they observed increased activation in the middle temporal gyrus. In a subsequent investigation (Martin et al., 1996), subjects viewed a series of pictures from the same semantic category—either animals (living things) or tools (nonliving items)—and silently named each picture. Both categories of pictures resulted in bilateral activation of ventral temporal and inferior frontal regions. However, animals elicited preferential activation of the left medial occipital lobe, and tools resulted in activation of the left premotor and left middle temporal regions.

Other studies have subsequently confirmed left premotor cortex activation for tool naming as well as for action naming (Grabowski et al., 1998; Grafton, Fadiga, Arbib, & Rizzolatti, 1997), suggesting an important role of this region in semantic processing for tools and actions. Cappa et al. (1998) reported that semantic processing for the category of animals, as contrasted with the category of tools, was associated with increased activation in right middle frontal and fusiform gyri. Martin (1996) proposed that although the left temporal region is critically involved in the storage of semantic knowledge about objects in general, brain activation studies suggest that domains of semantic knowledge are distributed throughout the brain in association areas adjacent to the primary sensory and motor cortices with which they are affiliated, in keeping with the fractionated view of the semantic system that we have described earlier.

As lesion studies have suggested a modality-specific account for the category effects seen in some brain-damaged patients, we might expect some overlap in regions of activation for certain semantic categories and types of semantic knowledge (e.g., animals and visual knowledge, tools and associative knowledge). Cappa et al. (1998) considered this possibility in their PET investigation, in which they evaluated regions of brain activation as subjects made semantic decisions about a visual or an associative characteristic of words from the categories of animals and tools. Rather than demonstrating regions of overlap, results revealed distinct regions of activation over right and left frontal, parietal, and temporal cortices for the two object categories and the two types of semantic information. Their study provides further evidence that a complex network of brain regions underlies semantic processing for different categories and types of semantic knowledge.

APPLICATION OF THEORY TO PRACTICE

Prognosis for Recovery from Semantic Impairments

Semantic impairments have been reported in individuals with a variety of neurological disorders. In general, the etiology of the brain disorder and the size and extent of brain lesion in each case will have the greatest influence on the prognosis for recovery from semantic impairment (Rothi, 1997). For example, semantic impairments associated with degenerative dementias, whether these are AD or more selective types of cortical atrophy, are unlikely to improve and are apt to become worse over time.

Recovery from semantic impairments related to acute neurological disorders is reported to be more favorable. Many individuals with acute onset of selective semantic impairment leading to TCSA or anomic aphasia demonstrate good recovery of language skills; their impairment often evolves to a less severe form (e.g., anomic aphasia) or even to full language recovery (Kertesz, 1979). In addition, semantic language impairments associated with left thalamic lesions typically resolve substantially (Crosson, 1992).

Recently, several groups of investigators have described more detailed analyses of language recovery in individuals with impairments in some aspect of semantic processing. For example, an analysis of recovery of word retrieval abilities in HH, the patient described earlier with a discrete lesion in the left temporo-occipital junction (area 37), demonstrated substantial recovery of lexical–semantic function (Raymer, Maher, Foundas, Rothi, & Heilman, in press). Specifically, HH showed improvement across word retrieval tasks systematically manipulating oral and written output modes and visual and phonological input modalities. The number of semantic errors lessened over time across tasks. We have proposed that this parallel pattern of improvement across phonological and orthographic output modes provides further support for our original proposal of impairment arising at a common late stage in semantic processing.

Laiacona, Capitani, and Barbarotto (1997) reported the recovery of language abilities for two patients, LF and EA. LF, who initially had a milder deficit, exhibited category-specific impairment for living things. EA initially exhibited impairment in both living and nonliving domains, but it was worse in the former. Thirteen months later, LF had improved to normal levels of function. Two years later, EA demonstrated significant improvement only for the nonliving category; performance with living items remained severely impaired.

The mechanism for the fairly good prognosis for recovery of semantic processing in individuals with acute semantic impairment is unclear. One likely contributing factor is the role the right hemisphere may play in semantic processing. In the extensive literature exploring the contribution of the right hemisphere to language processing, researchers have reported that whereas the right hemisphere seems to have limited abilities related to grammatical and phonological aspects of language, it is capable of a fair degree of language comprehension related to semantic processing (Bogen, 1993). However, an intact right hemisphere did not allow for substantial recovery for the category of living items in patient EA (Laiacona et al., 1997). Although based on limited observations, these findings suggest that the right hemisphere may have less potential for enhancing processing for selective semantic categories.

Assessment of Semantic Functioning

As we commence our discussion of assessment of semantic processing, we are at a crossroads. We have described two competing theories as to the structure of the semantic system, each with different implications for the techniques to use in the assessment of semantic impairments. Because of the practicality of this difference, we must make a choice, while aware that the two theories of the structure of the semantic system remain controversial. We elect to assume a more unitary view of the semantic system, with some attention to category specificity in the representation of semantic knowledge. That is, we assume that the semantic system is the unitary system of meaning recruited by the lexical system, interacting with all input modalities and output modes of representation. Impairment of this critical system will be demonstrated in a variety of lexical–semantic tasks that require semantic processing for successful completion (e.g., picture naming, word–picture matching). Tasks such as oral word reading, writing words to dictation, and word repetition, which can be accomplished via alternative sublexical or lexical (and nonsemantic) processes, may not be affected if these processes remain functional. A semantic system impairment will be characterized by the consistency of impairment across input modalities and/or output modes, and a qualitatively similar error pattern may be evident across lexical–semantic tasks (Hillis, 1998; Hillis et al., 1990; Rothi, Raymer, et al., 1991).

Standardized aphasia batteries such as the Boston Diagnostic Aphasia Examination (Goodglass & Kaplan, 1983) or the Western Aphasia Battery (Kertesz, 1982) may be useful in detecting language impairments related to semantic processing, as subjects will show impaired performance on comprehension and naming subtests. However, the purpose of these types of batteries is to identify the aphasia syndrome that best characterizes an individual's language performance. These analyses may overlook important distinctions in language impairments, which in turn may have important consequences for management.

The Florida Semantics Battery

We (Raymer, Rothi, & Greenwald, 1995) contrasted the performance of two individuals, HH and SS, with different left posterior cortical lesions, in whom standardized aphasia testing indicated a pattern consistent with anomic aphasia in both cases. (See also Raymer, Foundas, et al., 1997, for a complete description of HH's performance, and Raymer, Greenwald, Richardson, Rothi, & Heilman, 1997, for a description of SS's performance). Both individuals were administered the Florida Semantics Battery (Table 5.1) (Raymer et al., 1990), a battery of lexical–semantic tasks developed to characterize language impairments with respect to the cognitive-neuropsychological model of lexical processing (Figure 5.1). This battery incorporates the same basic corpus of stimuli across tasks, but the modality of stimulus input and mode of response output are systematically varied across tasks. The stimuli are 120 nouns from 10 different semantic categories (e.g., transportation, fruits, clothing, tools) classified as high-, middle-, or low-frequency in the English language.

In contrast to their similar performance on standardized aphasia assessment, SS and HH exhibited significant differences in their lexical–semantic impairments on the Florida Semantic Battery (Raymer et al., 1995). Both individuals demonstrated multimodality naming failure that was attributed to impairment in semantic activation of subsequent stages

---

TABLE 5.1. Subtests of the Florida Semantics Battery

Oral naming of pictures
Written naming of pictures
Oral naming to spoken definitions
Reading words aloud
Writing words to dictation
Cross-modal matching
   Auditory word-to-picture matching
   Written word-to-picture matching
Associative matching
   Match spoken word to associated spoken word
   Match picture to associated picture
Category sorting
   Sort pictures into semantic categories
   Sort written words into semantic categories

---

of lexical processing. However, SS had an additional visual-modality-specific impairment in naming viewed objects, or optic aphasia, allowing him to name correctly only 15% of viewed pictures. Additional testing of visual object processing suggested that this modality-specific impairment arose from impaired activation of the semantic system by the object recognition system (Raymer, Greenwald, et al., 1997). The results of the cognitive-neuropsychological assessment, in which we varied input modalities and output modes while using the same items, and evaluated patterns of errors across tasks, ultimately had important consequences for the way we treated SS's naming impairment (Greenwald, Raymer, Richardson, & Rothi, 1995).

Other assessment tools are now available that are useful in evaluating semantic performance from a cognitive-neuropsychological perspective. Subtests of the Psycholinguistic Assessments of Language Processing in Aphasia (PALPA)(Kay, Lesser, & Coltheart, 1992), similar to those listed in Table 5.1, may be sensitive to impairments of semantic processing. The Pyramids and Palm Trees Test (Howard & Patterson, 1992) is a useful visual nonverbal semantic task requiring subjects to select from three drawings the two that are most closely associated.

At times it can be difficult to detect semantic impairment in tasks evaluating the comprehension of single words. For example, in word–picture matching tasks, individuals may accomplish the task on the basis of only superficial semantic information if a target picture (e.g., apple) and the distractor pictures (e.g., chair, hammer, dress) are unrelated (Raymer & Berndt, 1996). For this reason it is useful to evaluate comprehension performance in the context of related semantic distractors as well (e.g., orange, banana, grapes), which will require subjects to activate more specific semantic information to derive the correct answer. This modification may allow the examiner to identify subtle semantic system impairments that otherwise might be overlooked.

In the Florida Semantics Battery, we have also included a semantic associates subtest patterned after Pyramids and Palm Trees (Howard & Patterson, 1992). We require subjects to match a target to a semantically related item from three choices (e.g., target = carrot, associate = rabbit, distractors = squirrel, cake). We contrast modalities of presentation, requiring matching of viewed objects to viewed objects, spoken object names to spoken object names, viewed objects to spoken object names, and spoken object names to viewed objects. We have found this subtest to be sensitive to more subtle impairments in semantic activation (e.g., Raymer, Greenwald, et al., 1997).

Few published tests are available that assist the clinician in detecting semantic impairments or retained abilities restricted to individual semantic categories (e.g., animals, fruits, tools, furniture). We have incorporated semantic category distinctions into our Florida Semantics Battery (Raymer et al., 1990), as we test 10 items from 12 different semantic categories. We suspect that although reports of category-specific impairments in the literature are fairly limited, these interesting impairments may occur more often than is thought. These differences are not presently detected only because of limitations in current test methods. However, if clinicians ask their patients, they may be helpful in identifying specific categories of objects that seem especially difficult for them. One of our past patients complained of inordinate difficulty he was experiencing with medical terms during his extended hospitalization. Careful, controlled examination substantiated his complaint (Crosson et al., 1997).

Clinicians may find it useful to develop informal sets of stimuli that include items from a variety of semantic categories stressing different types of semantic content. Visual information is purportedly important in the representation of living categories, such as animals, fruits, and vegetables; auditory information is relevant to the categories of musical instruments and animals; and motor information is relevant to the categories of garage tools, kitchen implements, and office implements. Results of such testing may allow clinicians to streamline their efforts in intervention to focus on each individual's difficulties with words in specific semantic categories.

Semantic Errors

The pattern of errors produced as an individual attempts to perform lexical tasks such as picture naming or word comprehension can render clues regarding the functional basis for the individual's language impairment. For example, for the target picture of an apple, semantic naming errors might include the production of inappropriate superordinate ("fruit"), coordinate ("orange"), or associated ("pie") word responses. In comprehension tasks, subjects may select semantically related distractors rather than unrelated or phonologically related distractors for a given target.

As we might expect, individuals with semantic system impairment often produce semantically based errors in both lexical comprehension and production tasks (Hillis, 1998; Howard & Orchard-Lisle, 1984). Hillis et al. (1990) reported that their subject, KE, who had a selective impairment of lexical–semantic processing, produced a similar number of semantic errors in all lexical tasks (oral and written picture naming, oral word reading, writing to dictation, and word–picture matching). Semantic errors constituted the predominant type of error observed in the individuals with anomia related to semantic output disturbances as described earlier (Raymer, Foundas, et al., 1997; Raymer, Greenwald, et al., 1997). The conclusion here is that if naming errors emanate from semantic impairment, and if the lexical–semantic system is a unitary semantic system, errors should be evident each time the deficient system is required in lexical processing, regardless of the input or output domains.

Picture-naming errors in individuals with AD are also often semantically related to the target (Bayles & Tomoeda, 1983; Bowles et al., 1987). However, individuals with AD may also produce large portions of off-target, semantically empty naming responses (e.g., for hammer, "that thing for making things"), indicating significant deterioration in semantic processing (Williamson, Adair, Raymer, & Heilman, 1998). Likewise, in word comprehension tasks, semantically related distractors induce greater difficulty than unrelated distractors in mild stages of the disease; however, as the disease progresses and semantic dysfunction increases, individuals with AD may be equally impaired with either semantic or unrelated distractors (Raymer & Berndt, 1996, Case 4).

It is important to note, however, that the production of semantic errors does not necessarily signal an impairment at the level of semantic processing (Hillis & Caramazza, 1995b). Caramazza and Hillis (1990) described two subjects, RGB and HW, who produced large numbers of semantic errors in tasks of oral picture naming and oral word reading, but none in written picture naming, writing to dictation, and word comprehension tasks. They interpreted this mode-specific output impairment as a disturbance of the phonological output lexicon. In contrast, patients with optic aphasia often produce a large number of semantic errors in picture-naming tasks, but perform much better when naming to tactile input or spoken description (Hillis & Caramazza, 1995a; Raymer, Greenwald, et al., 1997). Researchers have attributed the visual-modality-specific occurrence of semantic errors in picture naming to a failure in accessing the complete semantic representation from visual input. These observations underscore the need to analyze error patterns across all lexical tasks, in order to develop more accurate hypotheses regarding the functional basis for lexical impairment in each individual.

Overall, the implication of the cognitive-neuropsychological approach for assessment of semantic dysfunction is that clinicians must include additional tasks, some of which challenge our patients to tap into their semantic reserves (e.g., semantic associates tasks, naming to spoken definitions). We must be careful diagnosticians to evaluate consistency of performance and patterns of errors across tasks, which will allow us to develop more accurate hypotheses about the nature of lexical and semantic impairments we observe. This can be a difficult process, as many patients will demonstrate impairments that implicate multiple levels of processing in the lexical–semantic system. However, this endeavor should be worthwhile, as the information we gain in assessment will be valuable in guiding efforts toward intervention (Raymer et al., 1995).

Management of Semantic Impairments

The directions clinicians take in the management of disorders of semantic function will depend in large part on the etiology of the neurological processes underlying semantic dysfunction. Semantic impairments stemming from degenerative diseases will often be managed more cautiously than those related to acute conditions in which recovery may be anticipated.

Degenerative Semantic Dysfunction

Interventions for patients with degenerative etiologies of semantic dysfunction may include more conservative approaches (Bayles, 1993). For example, a clinician may provide family counseling to describe the nature of the degenerative disease process and how it affects language abilities related to the semantics or meanings of words before it affects the grammar and sound structure of words. The clinician may assist in structuring the language environment to optimize current levels of semantic processing in communication and to prepare caregivers for further semantic decline. For example, Bayles (1993) has suggested that clinicians instruct caregivers to talk about concrete, familiar concepts, to use redundancy in their communication, and to avoid the use of abstract and figurative language.

In contrast, there are clinicians who pursue a more direct intervention approach for patients with degenerative conditions causing semantic dysfunction; they may institute treatments in attempts to maintain current levels or even to improve performance in lexical–semantic tasks. For example, McNeil, Small, Masterson, and Fossett (1995) reported that a combination of behavioral and pharmacological (*d*-amphetamine) treatment improved word retrieval abilities in a patient who had lexical–semantic impairment in association with a primary progressive aphasia. We do not know how long those benefits were maintained once treatment was discontinued, however.

Acute Semantic Dysfunction

For individuals with acute neurological disorders (e.g., stroke) leading to semantic dysfunction, clinicians may anticipate neurological improvement and may choose to provide direct intervention for semantic impairments. Specific decisions regarding the type of intervention strategy to apply will relate to the chronicity of the semantic impairment (Rothi, 1995). Both "restitutive" strategies (which encourage restoration of semantic system function) and "substitutive" strategies (which attempt to circumvent the effects of semantic dysfunction) will be appropriate in early stages of recovery, whereas substitutive strategies will receive emphasis at more chronic stages. Treatments for semantic impairments specifically associated with the syndrome of TCSA have received little attention in the aphasia literature (Rothi, 1997). However, several studies have reported treatment approaches useful for overcoming impairments of word retrieval and auditory comprehension related to semantic dysfunction across a number of aphasia syndromes.

Restitutive forms of semantic treatment have been used with success for some subjects whose word retrieval impairments are related to semantic dysfunction. For example, some researchers have used a treatment strategy in which clinicians provide subjects with repeated exposure to semantically weighted comprehension tasks. Subjects perform word–picture matching tasks using semantic distractors (e.g., pointing to an apple from among pictures of an apple, banana, orange, and grapes), and answer yes–no questions about semantic details of pictures (e.g., "Does this grow on a tree?"). The assumption is that these types of tasks may influence changes at the level of the semantic system that will also be reflected in improved word retrieval abilities, as semantic processing is necessary for accurate word retrieval. Following this type of semantic treatment, patients have demonstrated improvement in naming pictures (Davis & Pring, 1991; Marshall, Pound, White-Thomson, & Pring, 1990; Nickels & Best, 1996; Pring, White-Thomson, Pound, Marshall, & Davis, 1990). Drew and Thompson (1999) reported, however, that a word–picture matching semantic treatment was only effective for their subjects if the actual target word was spoken in the course of treatment.

Grayson, Hilton, and Franklin (1997) implemented a similar type of treatment, incorporating exposure to four different semantic processing tasks, to improve auditory comprehension in their patient with jargon aphasia. They asked their subject to point to named objects, to categorize objects, and to match semantic associates as they systematically increased the number and relatedness of semantic distractors and provided gestural and verbal cues. Their patient demonstrated improvement in standardized tasks requiring semantic processing (auditory word–picture matching, written word–picture matching), but not on tasks tapping phonological processing (minimal pairs discrimination) and syntactic processing (sentence–picture matching). They did not report whether or not the patient improved in word retrieval.

Other clinicians have used a different type of semantic treatment, which emphasizes relearning distinctive semantic characteristics for pictures subjects are unable to name (Hillis, 1991, 1998; Ochipa, Maher, & Raymer, 1998). This approach is useful for individuals who tend to misname pictures as semantically related items (e.g., for a picture of an apple, the response is "orange"). In these studies, when a subject misnamed a picture, a clinician provided the subject with contrasting semantic information that differentiated the target picture from the close semantic coordinate (e.g., an apple grows on trees, is red, and tastes good in pie). Hillis (1998) reported that when her subject with traumatic brain injury received this type of semantic treatment, she demonstrated improvement in writing names of pictures for trained words and semantically related untrained words, as well as using these same words in other semantic processing tasks (spoken naming, repetition, writing to dictation, picture verification tasks). Hillis also noted that her patient used trained words in daily activities.

More recently, researchers have described a semantic treatment involving semantic feature analysis (Boyle, 1997; Boyle & Coelho, 1995; Coelho, McHugh, & Boyle, 2000; Lowell, Beeson, & Holland, 1995). Clinicians train subjects to proceed through a feature matrix that reviews different pieces of semantic information relevant to a pictured object. The information may include the category, function, properties, location, and any associations for that object. So for a picture of an apple, a subject would say that it is a fruit, it can be eaten, it is red and has a core with seeds, it is found on a tree, and it is associated with pies. Following semantic feature treatment, subjects have demonstrated improvements in naming untrained pictures and have shown generalized improvements in untrained pictures.

Whereas all of these treatment studies have focused on improving semantic processing abilities in general, Behrmann and Lieberthal (1989) applied a category-specific approach to treatment in one patient, CH. CH had significant comprehension impairments for verbal and written material, but he performed better on items in the category of animals and especially poorly on items in the categories of body parts and furniture. The investigators applied a treatment protocol in which CH was introduced to superordinate and specific details for items in the categories of body parts, furniture, and transportation. CH then performed visual and verbal matching tasks applying the trained semantic information. Following therapy, CH improved his ability to categorize trained items in the three semantic categories. He also showed improvement in classifying untrained items in one of three trained categories (body parts) and one of three untrained semantic categories (foods). However, negligible improvement was seen in general semantic testing following completion of treatment.

Overall, studies have shown that a number of semantic treatments that are restitutive in nature may generate improvement in semantic processing for trained words and pictures, with some generalization possible to untrained semantically related exemplars. In addition to restitutive treatments, subjects may benefit from treatments that focus on use of substitutive strategies to circumvent or overcome semantic dysfunction. Substitutive treatments can take one of two forms: (1) a "vicariative" strategy, in which a different mode of cognitive processing is paired with verbal behavior, in an attempt to encourage other parts of the brain not usually supporting language functions to become involved in the verbal process; or (2) a "compensatory" strategy, in which other brain regions support the process of communication, such that communication is accomplished in a fundamentally different manner than it was previously. Information about the complexity of semantic representations in terms of modality- and mode-specific regions of knowledge may be influential in this regard. Clinicians may encourage patients to use retained aspects of semantic knowledge either to activate or to circumvent unavailable semantic information.

For example, given our knowledge of action semantics, one potential substitutive strategy is the use of gestural communication, such as AmerInd gestures (Skelly, 1979). In a vicariative use of gesture, some researchers have reported pairing gesture with verbal output in treatment, and later curtailing the use of gesture once verbal abilities have improved (e.g., Hoodin & Thompson, 1983). Alternatively, gestural use may be continued as a compensatory strategy to circumvent instances of word retrieval failure across time. No studies have directly investigated the use of a gestural strategy in patients with semantic system dysfunction to determine whether gesture is a viable modality for facilitating semantic system recovery.

Other substitutive strategies may be useful to circumvent semantically based word retrieval impairments. A clinician may encourage a subject to circumlocute and provide as much semantic information as possible from remaining semantic knowledge, as a strategy that allows the listener to decode the intent of a subject's semantically depleted message. Or the subject may use drawing as a means to convey the content of an intended message (Lyon & Helm-Estabrooks, 1987). Like the use of gesture, these compensatory strategies may provide sufficient activation in the semantic system that the actual target word can ultimately be retrieved in a vicariative manner. Alternatively, the strategies may provide a long-term means to compensate for word retrieval abilities related to semantic impairment.

CONCLUSIONS

Issues related to the semantic system's functioning and its neurological instantiation are complex and continue to evolve. However, we have accumulated a substantial body of information that has practical implications for our clinical endeavors. Already we have seen how advances in semantic theory have led to modifications in assessment procedures and elaboration of treatments for use in patients with semantic dysfunction. Additional research is necessary to evaluate the effectiveness of semantic treatments across patients with different sources of semantic dysfunction. In time patients will surely benefit as clinicians continue to apply principles derived from basic semantic theory in clinical practice.

REFERENCES

Allport, D. A. (1985). Distributed memory, modular subsystems and dysphasia. In S. Newman & R. Epstein (Eds.), *Current perspectives in dysphasia* (pp. 32–60). Edinburgh: Churchill Livingstone.

Bayles, K. A. (1993). Management of neurogenic communication disorders associated with dementia. In R. A. Chapey (Ed.), *Language intervention strategies in adult aphasia* (pp. 535–545). Baltimore: Williams & Wilkins.

Bayles, K. A., & Tomoeda, C. K. (1983). Confrontation naming impairment in dementia. *Brain and Language, 19,* 98–114.

Beauvois, M.-F., & Saillant, B. (1985). Optic aphasia for colours and colour agnosia: A distinction between visual and visuo-verbal impairments in the processing of colours. *Cognitive Neuropsychology, 2,* 1–48.

Beauvois, M.-F., Saillant, B., Meininger, V., & Lhermitte, F. (1978). Bilateral tactile aphasia: A tacto-verbal dysfunction. *Brain, 101,* 381–401.

Behrmann, M., & Lieberthal, T. (1989). Category-specific treatment of a lexical–semantic deficit: A single case study of global aphasia. *British Journal of Disorders of Communication, 24,* 281–299.

Benson, D. F., & Ardila, A. (1996). *Aphasia: A clinical perspective.* New York: Oxford University Press.

Berthier, M. L., Starkstein, S. E., Leiguarda, R., Ruiz, A., Mayberg, H. S., Wagner, H., Price, T. R., & Robinson, R. G. (1991). Transcortical aphasia: Importance of the nonspeech dominant hemisphere in language repetition. *Brain, 114,* 1409–1427.

Bogen, J. E. (1993). The callosal syndromes. In K. M. Heilman & E. Valenstein (Eds.), *Clinical neuropsychology* (3rd ed., pp. 337–407). New York: Oxford University Press.

Bowles, N. L., Obler, L. K., & Albert, M. L. (1987). Naming errors in healthy aging and dementia of the Alzheimer type. *Cortex, 3,* 519–524.

Boyle, M. (1997, November). *Semantic feature analysis treatment for dysnomia in two aphasia syndromes.* Poster presented at the annual meeting of the American Speech–Language–Hearing Association, Boston.

Boyle, M., & Coelho, C. A. (1995). Application of semantic feature analysis as a treatment for aphasic dysnomia. *American Journal of Speech–Language Pathology, 4,* 94–98.

Buchel, C., Price, C., & Friston, K. (1998). A multimodal language region in the ventral visual pathway. *Nature, 394,* 274–277.

Bunn, E. M., Tyler, L. K., & Moss, H. E. (1998). Category-specific semantic deficits: The role of familiarity and property type reexamined. *Neuropsychology, 12,* 367–379.

Caplan, D. (1987). *Neurolinguistics and linguistic aphasiology.* New York: Cambridge University Press.

Caplan, D. (1993). *Language: Structure, processing, and disorders.* Cambridge, MA: MIT Press.

Cappa, S. F., Perani, D., Schnur, T., Tettamanti, M., & Fazio, F. (1998). The effects of semantic category and knowledge type on lexical–semantic access: A PET study. *Neuroimage, 8,* 350–359.

Caramazza, A., Berndt, R. S., & Brownell, H. (1982). The semantic deficit hypothesis: Perceptual parsing and object classification by aphasic patients. *Brain and Language, 15,* 161–189.

Caramazza, A., & Hillis, A. E. (1990). Where do semantic errors come from? *Cortex, 26,* 95–122.

Caramazza, A., Hillis, A. E., Leek, E. C., & Miozzo, M. (1994). The organization of lexical knowledge in the brain: Evidence from category- and modality-specific deficits. In L. Hirschfeld & S. Gelman (Eds.), *Mapping the mind: Domain specificity in cognition and culture* (pp. 68–84). New York: Cambridge University Press.

Caramazza, A., Hillis, A. E., Rapp, B., & Romani, C. (1990). The multiple semantics hypothesis: Multiple confusions? *Cognitive Neuropsychology, 7,* 161–189.

Caramazza, A., & Shelton, J. R. (1998). Domain-specific knowledge systems in the brain: The animate–inanimate distinction. *Journal of Cognitive Neuroscience, 10,* 1–34.

Chertkow, H., Bub, D., & Seidenberg, M. (1989). Priming and semantic memory loss in Alzheimer's disease. *Brain and Language, 36,* 420–446.

Coelho, C. A., McHugh, R. E., & Boyle, M. (2000). Semantic feature analysis as a treatment for aphasic dysnomia: A replication. *Aphasiology, 14,* 133–142.

Coslett, H. B., Roeltgen, D. P., Rothi, L. J. G., & Heilman, K. M. (1987). Transcortical sensory aphasia: Evidence for subtypes. *Brain and Language, 32,* 362–378.

Crosson, B. (1992). *Subcortical functions in language and memory.* New York: Guilford Press.

Crosson, B., Moberg, P. J., Boone, J. R., Rothi, L. J. G., & Raymer, A. M. (1997). Category-specific naming deficit for medical terms after dominant thalamic/capsular hemorrhage. *Brain and Language, 60,* 407–442.

Cummings, J. L., Benson, D. F., Hill, M. A., & Reed, A. (1985). Aphasia in dementia of the Alzheimer's type. *Neurology, 35,* 394–397.

Damasio, H., Grabowski, T. J., Tranel, D., Hichwa, R. D., & Damasio, A. R. (1996). A neural basis for lexical retrieval. *Nature, 380,* 499–505.

Daum, I., Riesch, G., Sartori, G., & Birbaumer, N. (1996). Semantic memory impairment in Alzheimer's disease. *Journal of Clinical and Experimental Neuropsychology, 18,* 648–665.

Davis, A., & Pring, T. (1991). Therapy for word-finding deficits: More on the effects of semantic and phonological approaches to treatment with dysphasic patients. *Neuropsychological Rehabilitation, 1,* 135–145.

Demonet, J. F., Chollet, F., Ramsay, S., Cardebat, D., Nespoulous, J. L., Wise, R., & Frackowiak, R. S. J. (1992). The anatomy of phonological and semantic processing in normal subjects. *Brain, 115,* 1753–1768.

Denes, G., & Semenza, C. (1975). Auditory modality-specific anomia: Evidence from a case of pure word deafness. *Cortex, 11,* 401–411.

Drew, R. L., & Thompson, C. K. (1999, June). Model-based semantic treatment for naming deficits in aphasia. *Journal of Speech, Language, and Hearing Research, 42,* 972–989.

Engel, P., Cummings, J. L., Villanueva-Meyer, J., & Mena, I. (1993). Single photon emission computed tomography in dementia: Relationship of perfusion to cognitive deficits. *Journal of General Psychiatric Neurology, 6,* 144–151.

Farah, M. (1990). *Visual agnosia.* Cambridge, MA: MIT Press.

Farah, M., & McClelland, J. L. (1991). A computational model of semantic memory impairment: Modality specificity and emergent category specificity. *Journal of Experimental Psychology: General, 120,* 339–357.

Farah, M. J., & Wallace, M. A. (1992). Semantically-bounded anomia: Implications for the neural implementation of naming. *Neuropsychologia, 30,* 609–621.

Ferreira, C. T., Giusiano, B., Ceccaldi, M., & Poncet, M. (1997). Optic aphasia: Evidence of the contribution of different neural systems to object and action naming. *Cortex, 33,* 499–513.

Ferreira, C. T., Giusiano, B., & Poncet, M. (1997). Category-specific anomia: Implication of different neural networks in naming. *NeuroReport, 8,* 1595–1602.

Foundas, A. L., Daniels, S. K., & Vasterling, J. J. (1998). Anomia: Case Studies with lesion localization. *Neurocase, 4,* 35–43.

Freud, S. (1953). *On aphasia: A critical study* (E. Stengel, Ed. and Trans.). New York: International Universities Press. (Original work published 1891)

Goodglass, H., & Kaplan, E. (1983). *The assessment of aphasia and related disorders.* Philadelphia: Lea & Febiger.

Grabowski, T. J., Damasio, H., & Damasio, A. R. (1998). Premotor and prefrontal correlates of category-related lexical retrieval. *Neuroimage, 7,* 232–243.

Grafton, S. T., Fadiga, L., Arbib, M. A., & Rizzolatti, G. (1997). Premotor cortex activation during observation and naming of familiar tools. *Neuroimage, 6,* 231–236.

Grayson, E., Hilton, R., & Franklin, S. (1997). Early intervention in a case of jargon aphasia: Efficacy of language comprehension therapy. *European Journal of Disorders of Communication*, *32*, 257–276.

Greenwald, M. L., Raymer, A. M., Richardson, M. E., & Rothi, L. J. G. (1995). Contrasting treatments for severe impairments of picture naming. *Neuropsychological Rehabilitation*, *5*, 17–49.

Hart, J., Berndt, R. S., & Caramazza, A. (1985). Category-specific naming deficit following cerebral infarction. *Nature*, *316*, 439–440.

Hart, J., & Gordon, B. (1990). Delineation of single-word semantic comprehension deficits in aphasia, with anatomical correlation. *Annals of Neurology*, *27*, 226–231.

Hart, J., & Gordon, B. (1992). Neural subsystems for object knowledge. *Nature*, *359*, 60–64.

Hier, D. B., Hagenlocker, K., & Shindler, A. G. (1985). Language disintegration in dementia: Effects of etiology and severity. *Brain and Language*, *25*, 117–133.

Hillis, A. E. (1991). The effects of separate treatments for distinct impairments within the naming process. In T. Prescott (Ed.), *Clinical aphasiology* (Vol. 19, pp. 255–265). San Diego, CA: College Hill Press.

Hillis, A. E. (1998). Treatment of naming disorders: New issues regarding old therapies. *Journal of the International Neuropsychological Society*, *4*, 648–660.

Hillis, A. E., & Caramazza, A. (1991). Category-specific naming and comprehension impairment: A double dissociation. *Brain*, *114*, 2081–2094.

Hillis, A. E., & Caramazza, A. (1995a). Cognitive and neural mechanisms underlying visual and semantic processing: Implications from "optic aphasia." *Journal of Cognitive Neuroscience*, *7*, 457–478.

Hillis, A. E., & Caramazza, A. (1995b). The compositionality of lexical semantic representations: Clues from semantic errors in object naming. *Memory*, *3*, 333–358.

Hillis, A. E., Rapp, B., & Caramazza, A. (1995). Constraining claims about theories of semantic memory: More on unitary versus multiple semantics. *Cognitive Neuropsychology*, *12*, 175–186.

Hillis, A. E., Rapp, B., Romani, C., & Caramazza, A. (1990). Selective impairment of semantics in lexical processing. *Cognitive Neuropsychology*, *7*, 191–243.

Hodges, J. R., & Patterson, K. (1996). Nonfluent progressive aphasia and semantic dementia: A comparative neuropsychological study. *Journal of the International Neuropsychological Society*, *2*, 511–524.

Hodges, J. R., Patterson, K., Oxbury, S., & Funnell, E. (1992). Semantic dementia: Progressive fluent aphasia with temporal lobe atrophy. *Brain*, *115*, 1783–1806.

Hodges, J. R., Patterson, K., & Tyler, L. K. (1994). Loss of semantic memory: Implications for the modularity of mind. *Cognitive Neuropsychology*, *11*, 505–542.

Hoodin, R. B., & Thompson, C. K. (1983). Facilitation of verbal labeling in adult aphasia by gestural, verbal or verbal plus gestural training. In R. H. Brookshire (Ed.), *Clinical Aphasiology Conference proceedings* (pp. 62–64). Minneapolis, MN: BRK.

Howard, D., & Orchard-Lisle, V. (1984). On the origin of semantic errors in naming: Evidence from the case of a global aphasic. *Cognitive Neuropsychology*, *1*, 163–190.

Howard, D., & Patterson, K. (1992). *Pyramids and Palm Trees Test*. Bury St. Edmunds, England: Thames Valley.

Huff, F. J., Becker, J. T., Belle, S. H., Nebes, R. D., Holland, A. L., & Boller, F. (1987). Cognitive deficits and clinical diagnosis of Alzheimer's disease. *Neurology*, *37*, 1119–1124.

Humphreys, G. W., & Riddoch, M. J. (1988). On the case for multiple semantic systems: A reply to Shallice. *Cognitive Neuropsychology*, *5*, 143–150.

Humphreys, G. W., Riddoch, M. J., & Quinlan, P. T. (1988). Cascade processes in picture identification. *Cognitive Neuropsychology*, *5*, 67–103.

Iorio, L., Falanga, A., Fragassi, N. A., & Grossi, D. (1992). Visual associative agnosia and optic aphasia: A single case study and a review of the syndromes. *Cortex*, *28*, 23–37.

Kay, J., Lesser, R., & Coltheart, M. (1992). *Psycholinguistic Assessments of Language Processing in Aphasia (PALPA)*. Hillsdale, NJ: Erlbaum.

Kertesz, A. (1979). *Aphasia and associated disorders: Taxonomy, localization, and recovery*. New York: Grune & Stratton.

Kertesz, A. (1982). *The Western Aphasia Battery*. New York: Grune & Stratton.

Kertesz, A., Davidson, W., & McCabe, P. (1998). Primary progressive semantic aphasia: A case study. *Journal of the International Neuropsychological Society*, *4*, 388–398.

Kertesz, A., Harlock, W., & Coates, R. (1979). Computer tomographic localization, lesion size, and prognosis in aphasia and nonverbal impairment. *Brain and Language, 8,* 34–50.

Kertesz, A., Sheppard, A., & MacKenzie, R. (1982). Localization in transcortical sensory aphasia. *Archives of Neurology, 39,* 475–478.

Kremin, H. (1987). Is there more than ah-oh-oh?: Alternative strategies for writing and repeating lexically. In M. Coltheart, R. Job, & G. Sartori (Eds.), *The cognitive neuropsychology of language* (pp. 295–335). Hillsdale, NJ: Erlbaum.

Laiacona, M., Capitani, E., & Barbarotto, R. (1997). Semantic category dissociations: A longitudinal study of two cases. *Cortex, 33,* 441–461.

Lambon Ralph, M. A., Patterson, K., & Hodges, J. R. (1997). The relationship between naming and semantic knowledge for different categories in dementia of Alzheimer's type. *Neuropsychologia, 35,* 1251–1260.

Lichtheim, L. (1885). On aphasia. *Brain, 7,* 433–484.

Lissauer, H. (1988). Ein fall von seelenblindheit nebst einem beitrag zur theorie derselben [A case of visual agnosia with a contribution to theory]. *Cognitive Neuropsychology, 5,* 157–192. (Original work published 1890)

Lowell, S., Beeson, P. M., & Holland, A. L. (1995). The efficacy of a semantic cueing procedure on naming performance of adults with aphasia. *American Journal of Speech–Language Pathology, 4,* 109–114.

Lyon, J., & Helm-Estabrooks, N. (1987). Drawing: Its communicative significance for expressively restricted aphasic adults. *Topics in Language Disorders, 8,* 61–71.

Marshall, J., Pound, C., White-Thomson, M., & Pring, T. (1990). The use of picture/word matching tasks to assist word retrieval in aphasic patients. *Aphasiology, 4,* 167–184.

Martin, A. (1992). Degraded knowledge representations in patients with Alzheimer's disease: Implications for models of semantic and repetition priming. In L. R. Squire & N. Butters (Eds.), *Neuropsychology of memory* (2nd ed., pp. 220–232). New York: Guilford Press.

Martin, A. (1996). *Semantic memory and the brain.* Seminar presented at the European meeting of the International Neuropsychological Society, Veldhoven, The Netherlands.

Martin, A., Haxby, J. V., Lalonde, F. M., Wiggs, C. L., & Ungerleider, L. G. (1995). Discrete cortical regions associated with knowledge of color and knowledge of action. *Science, 270,* 102–105.

Martin, A., Wiggs, C. L., Ungerleider, L. G., & Haxby, J. V. (1996). Neural correlates of category-specific knowledge. *Nature, 379,* 649–652.

Martin, N., & Saffran, E. M. (1990). Repetition and verbal STM in transcortical sensory aphasia. *Brain and Language, 39,* 362–378.

McFarling, D., Rothi, L. J. G., & Heilman, K. M. (1982). Transcortical aphasia from ischaemic infarcts of the thalamus: A report of two cases. *Journal of Neurology, Neurosurgery and Psychiatry, 45,* 107–112.

McNeil, M. R., Small, S. L., Masterson, R. J., & Fossett, T. R. D. (1995). Behavioral and pharmacological treatment of lexical–semantic deficits in a single patient with primary progressive aphasia. *American Journal of Speech–Language Pathology, 4,* 76–87.

Montanes, P., Goldblum, M. C., & Boller, F. (1995). The naming impairment of living and nonliving items in Alzheimer's disease. *Journal of the International Neuropsychological Society, 1,* 39–48.

Nickels, L., & Best, W. (1996). Therapy for naming disorders: Part II: Specifics, surprises, and suggestions. *Aphasiology, 10,* 109–136.

Ochipa, C., Maher, L. M., & Raymer, A. M. (1998). One approach to the treatment of anomia. *ASHA Special Interest Division 2: Neurophysiology and Neurogenic Speech and Language Disorders, 15,* 18–23.

Ochipa, C., Rothi, L. J. G., & Heilman, K. M. (1989). Ideational apraxia: A deficit in tool selection and use. *Annals of Neurology, 25,* 190–193.

Paivio, A. (1971). *Imagery and verbal processes.* New York: Holt, Rinehart & Winston.

Paivio, A. (1986). Mental comparisons involving abstract attributes. *Memory and Cognition, 2,* 199–208.

Pring, T., White-Thomson, M., Pound, C., Marshall, J., & Davis, A. (1990). Picture/word matching tasks and work retrieval: Some follow-up data and second thoughts. *Aphasiology, 4,* 479–483.

Rapcsak, S. Z., Rothi, L. J. G., & Heilman, K. M. (1987). Phonological alexia with optic and tactile anomia: A neuropsychological and anatomical study. *Brain and Language, 31,* 109–121.

Rapp, B. C., Hillis, A. E., & Caramazza, A. (1993). The role of representations in cognitive theory: More on multiple semantics and the agnosias. *Cognitive Neuropsychology, 10*, 235–249.

Raymer, A. M., & Berndt, R. S. (1996). Reading lexically without semantics: Evidence from patients with probable Alzheimer's disease. *Journal of the International Neuropsychological Society, 2*, 340–349.

Raymer, A. M., Foundas, A. L., Maher, L. M., Greenwald, M. L., Morris, M., Rothi, L. J. G., & Heilman, K. M. (1997). Cognitive neuropsychological analysis and neuroanatomical correlates in a case of acute anomia. *Brain and Language, 58*, 137–156.

Raymer, A. M., Greenwald, M. L., Richardson, M. E., Rothi, L. J. G., & Heilman, K. M. (1997). The right hemisphere and optic aphasia/optic apraxia. *Neurocase, 3*, 173–183.

Raymer, A. M., Maher, L. M., Foundas, A. L., Rothi, L. J. G., & Heilman, K. M. (in press). Analysis of lexical recovery in an individual with acute anomia. *Aphasiology.*

Raymer, A. M., Maher, L. M., Greenwald, M. L., Morris, M., Rothi, L. J. G., & Heilman, K. M. (1990). *The Florida Semantics Battery: Experimental edition.* Gainesville: University of Florida, Department of Neurology.

Raymer, A. M., Moberg, P., Crosson, B., Nadeau, S. E., & Rothi, L. J. G. (1997). Lexical–semantic deficits in two patients with dominant thalamic infarction. *Neuropsychologia, 35*, 211–219.

Raymer, A. M., Rothi, L. J. G., & Greenwald, M. L. (1995). The role of cognitive models in language rehabilitation. *NeuroRehabilitation, 5*, 183–193.

Riddoch, M. J., Humphreys, G. W., Coltheart, M., & Funnell, E. (1988). Semantic systems or system?: Neuropsychological evidence re-examined. *Cognitive Neuropsychology, 5*, 3–25.

Rogers, M. A., & Alarcon, N. B. (1999, October). Characteristics and management of primary progressive aphasia. *ASHA SID2: Neurophysiology and Neurogenic Speech and Language Disorders, 9*(4), 12–26.

Rothi, L. J. G. (1995). Behavioral compensation in the case of treatment of acquired language disorders resulting from brain damage. In R. A. Dixon & L. Backman (Eds.), *Psychological compensation: Managing losses and promoting gains* (pp. 219–230). Hillsdale, NJ: Erlbaum.

Rothi, L. J. G. (1997). Transcortical motor, sensory, and mixed aphasias. In L. L. LaPointe (Ed.), *Aphasia and related neurogenic language disorders* (2nd ed., pp. 91–111). New York: Thieme.

Rothi, L. J. G., Ochipa, C., & Heilman, K. M. (1991). A cognitive neuropsychological model of limb praxis. *Cognitive Neuropsychology, 8*, 443–458.

Rothi, L. J. G., Ochipa, C., & Heilman, K. M. (1997). A cognitive neuropsychological model of limb praxis and apraxia. In L. J. G. Rothi & K. M. Heilman (Eds.), *Apraxia: The neuropsychology of action* (pp. 29–49). Hove, England: Psychology Press.

Rothi, L. J. G., Raymer, A. M., Maher, L. M., Greenwald, M. L., & Morris, M. (1991). Assessment of naming failures in neurological communication disorders. *Clinics in Communication Disorders, 1*, 7–20.

Saffran, E. M. (1997). Aphasia: Cognitive neuropsychological aspects. In T. E. Feinberg & M. J. Farah (Eds.), *Behavioral neurology and neuropsychology* (pp. 151–165). New York: McGraw-Hill.

Schwartz, M. F., Marin, O. S. M., & Saffran, E. M. (1979). Dissociation of language function in dementia: A case study. *Brain and Language, 7*, 277–306.

Seymour, P. H. K. (1973). A model for reading, naming and comparison. *British Journal of Psychology, 64*, 35–49.

Seymour, P. H. K. (1978). *Human visual cognition.* New York: St. Martin's Press.

Shallice, T. (1988). *From neuropsychology to mental structure.* Cambridge, England: Cambridge University Press.

Silveri, M. C., Gainotti, G., Perani, D., Cappelletti, J. Y., Carbone, G., & Fazio, F. (1997). Naming deficit for non-living items: Neuropsychological and PET study. *Neuropsychologia, 35*, 359–367.

Skelly, M. (1979). *Amer-Ind gestural code based on universal American Indian hand talk.* New York: Elsevier.

Smith, C. D., Anderson, A. H., Chen, Q., Blonder, L. X., Kirsch, J. E., & Avison, M. J. (1996). Cortical activation in confrontation naming. *NeuroReport, 7*, 781–785.

Thompson-Schill, S. L., D'Esposito, M., Aguirre, G. K., & Farah, M. J. (1997). Role of left inferior prefrontal cortex in retrieval of semantic knowledge: A reevaluation. *Proceedings of the National Academy of Sciences USA, 94*, 14792–14797.

Vandenberghe, R., Price, C., Wise, R., Josephs, O., & Frackowiak, R. S. J. (1996). Functional anatomy of a common semantic system for words and pictures. *Nature, 383*, 254–256.

Warrington, E. K., & McCarthy, R. A. (1983). Category-specific access dysphasia. *Brain, 100*, 1273–1296.

Warrington, E. K., & McCarthy, R. A. (1987). Categories of knowledge: Further fractionation and an attempted integration. *Brain, 110*, 1273–1296.

Warrington, E. K., & McCarthy, R. A. (1994). Multiple meaning systems in the brain: A case for visual semantics. *Neuropsychologia, 32*, 1465–1473.

Warrington, E. K., & Shallice, T. (1984). Category-specific semantic impairments. *Brain, 107*, 829–853.

Wernicke, C. (1874). *Der Aphasische Symptomenkomplex.* Breslau: Cohn & Weigart.

Williamson, D. J. G., Adair, J. C., Raymer, A. M., & Heilman, K. M. (1998). Object and action naming in Alzheimer's disease. *Cortex, 34*, 601–610.

Williamson, D. J. G., Crosson, B., Rothi, L. J. G., Shurla, S., Heilman, K. M., & Nadeau, S. E. (1995). Regional cerebral blood flow during the generation of language. *Journal of the International Neuropsychological Society, 1*, 37.

Wise, R., Chollet, F., Hadar, U., Friston, K., Hoffner, E., & Frackowiak, R. (1991). Distribution of cortical neural networks involved in word comprehension and word retrieval. *Brain, 114*, 1803–1817.

Zelkowicz, B. J., Herbster, A. M., Nebes, R. D., Mintun, M. A., & Becker, J. T. (1998). Examination of regional cerebral blood flow during object naming tasks. *Journal of the International Neuropsychological Society, 4*, 160–166.

6

GRAMMAR AND AGRAMMATISM

ANJAN CHATTERJEE
LYNN MAHER

Humans string words together to form sentences. Sentences convey information about states and events, and thus form the vehicles by which humans express thoughts and communicate with each other. The ability to convey and comprehend sentence-level information relies on knowledge of grammar, or how words relate to one another. "Agrammatism" is the aphasic disorder in which this knowledge, or its application, is disrupted by brain damage. Agrammatism frequently accompanies Broca's aphasia, but disturbances of grammar may also be seen in other aphasic patients. In this chapter we review the clinical features of agrammatism, its theoretical and neurological underpinnings, and potential treatment strategies. Because clinicians may be unfamiliar with linguistic terms often used to describe sentence-level disorders, we have included a short glossary at the end of the chapter.

CLINICAL DESCRIPTION

Most patients with agrammatism are dysfluent. Sequencing words together seems to require effort. Their spontaneous speech is often "telegraphic"; that is, they communicate with nouns and simple phrases, such as "Dog eat" rather than "The dog is eating." Their utterances often lack elaboration. They generally comprehend simple statements, but often have difficulty comprehending grammatically complex sentences. The hallmark of English agrammatical speech is the omission of function words and parts of words (Goodglass, 1993). Agrammatical patients are more likely to omit function words like prepositions, articles, and conjunctions than nouns. Function words, or "functors," are "closed-class words." "Closed-class" means that there are only a finite number of functors in any language; by contrast, the number of "open-class words," which are nouns, verbs, adjectives, and adverbs, is unlimited. Agrammatical patients also omit bound grammatical morphemes in their speech. Bound grammatical morphemes are parts of words that cannot stand by themselves and that modify the meaning of open-class words. For example, the grammatical morpheme "ed," which modifies the tense of a verb (as in "walked"), may be omitted by a patient with agrammatism.

Although patients with agrammatism use open-class words preferentially, their use of verbs may deviate from normal. They tend to use nouns rather than verbs to describe actions. They also tend to omit auxiliary verbs in spontaneous speech. Auxiliary verbs modify the main verb. In the phrase "might have to run," "might" and "have" are auxiliary verbs modifying the main verb "to run." The omission of bound and free-standing grammatical morphemes and auxiliary verbs contributes to the general clinical impression of simplified, telegraphic speech.

Agrammatical patients vary widely in the details of their language impairment. Production and comprehension may be differentially affected. Agrammatical patients fall into two general groups: Some patients have difficulties with the relationship of words to each other (syntactic deficits), whereas others have deficits in processing grammatical morphemes (Goodglass, 1993). Syntactic and morphological symptoms often coexist in the same patient but may be dissociated.

In summary, the speech output of patients with agrammatism often appears effortful. The structure of their sentences and phrases is simplified. Their language is characterized by the omission of grammatical words and grammatical morphemes. They comprehend simple utterances, but may not understand sentences that are grammatically complex. This description does not mean that they form a unified, homogeneous group. Nor does it imply that there is a discrete "grammar center" in the brain, damage to which produces agrammatism. In this chapter we use a model of normal sentence production to guide the analysis of agrammatical symptoms. By identifying the steps involved in transforming a thought into a sentence, one can begin to recognize points of disruption that produce sentence-level deficits.

A MODEL OF NORMAL SENTENCE PRODUCTION

Models of sentence production dating back to the early part of the century have been concerned with the stages involved in transcoding prelinguistic thought into verbal form (for a review, see Kolk, Van Grunsven, & Keyser, 1985). Garrett's (1980, 1984) recent model of normal sentence production has the virtue of being derived empirically and is detailed enough to provide a framework for the analysis of agrammatical speech (Figure 6.1). This model posits a sequence of independent processes operating at different levels of linguistic representation. The hypothesized processes and representations are derived from observations of speech errors made by normal speakers. Word substitutions and movement or exchange errors are of particular interest. These errors are not necessarily the same errors that are made by agrammatical patients. Rather, the errors made by normal subjects help to uncover different levels and operations of sentence processing. These levels and operations can then be used as a framework to interpret agrammatical symptoms.

Word substitution errors expose processes underlying lexical selection. These substitutions are usually meaning-based or sound-based, and only rarely a combination of both. An example of a meaning-based error might be "finger" for "toe." An example of a sound based error might be "mushroom" for "mustache." Garrett suggests that the existence of these two types of word substitution errors implies that the selection of the meaning and the form of words occurs independently and at distinct points in sentence construction.

Movement errors, such as word and sound exchanges, allow inferences about the processing of phrases (see also Nadeau, Chapter 3, this volume). Exchange errors involve words or parts of words. These exchanges have specific effects on their morphological and phonological environments. Garrett offers the following examples:

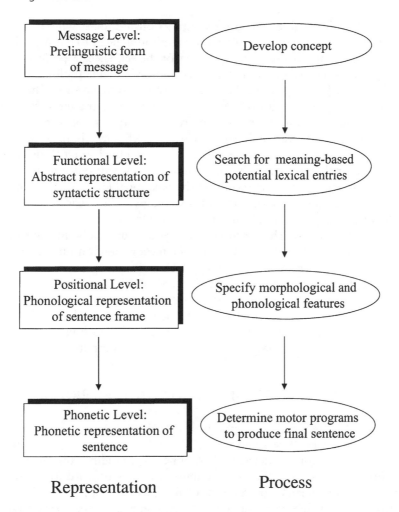

FIGURE 6.1. Illustration of Garrett's (1980, 1984) model of sentence production, indicating levels of representation and processes that are proposed to occur at each level.

1. We'll sit around the *song* and sing *fires*" ("fire and sing songs").
2. "*an an*gwage *l*acquisition device" ("a language acquisition device"; "a" is replaced by "an").
3. "Even the best team lost*s*" ("Even the best team*s* lost"; the phoneme /z/ changes to /s/).

Several generalizations follow from these observations. Word exchanges take place predominantly between phrases, often with several intervening words. Word exchanges only occur between words of corresponding grammatical categories. By contrast, sound exchanges occur within phrases, usually only span a word or two, and are not constrained by grammatical category. Exchange errors may produce local morphological alterations as in the second example above, and local phonological alterations as in the third example. From these kinds of data Garrett postulates that sentences are constructed through different levels of representations. A message level contains the pre-linguistic form of the message to be conveyed. A functional level contains a multi-phrase level, which establishes the meaning relationship between words but not their phonological form. A positional level organizes the segments and phonological features of the sentence. A phonetic level specifies the final sounds to be produced prior to their motor implementation.

The model has little to say about the structure of the message level. The data used to derive the model do not shed light on this level. The message triggers a meaning-based search from the lexicon (the mental store of words) for entries to be inserted at the functional level. The functional level establishes "who does what to whom"—that is, the thematic roles of the message to be conveyed. This level is quite abstract. It does not specify the order of words or the phrasal environments in which words will finally be produced.

The functional level triggers operations at the positional level. At this level a sentence frame is planned. A second search through the lexicon gives the entries selected in the previous level their phonological form. After the sentence frame is constructed, grammatical morphemes are then inserted. These processes occur automatically, giving rise to a phonetic level of processing, which then determines the motor programs involved in articulating or writing the final sentence.

The positional and functional levels of Garrett's model are more closely related to language processes relevant to agrammatism. The positional level describes morphological and phonological features of the final sentence, and the functional level describes abstract features of sentence syntactic structure and the meaning relationships among words. Disruption at either of these levels may result in agrammatical output.

MORPHOLOGIC ERRORS IN AGRAMMATICAL PRODUCTION

Agrammatical patients frequently omit grammatical morphemes in their sentences. Grammatical morphemes may be "free-standing" or "bound." Free-standing grammatical morphemes, such as prepositions, articles, and conjunctions, modify other words or specify the relationship between words. Bound morphemes are parts of words (typically affixes in English) that modify the meaning of the root forms of words (e.g., the "ed" in "walked"). Deficits at this level of sentence production implicate representations or processes operating at Garrett's positional level (Caramazza & Hillis, 1989).

Bradley, Garrett, and Zurif (1980) have emphasized the distinction between open- and closed-class words, arguing that these classes of words have different computational roles in sentences. Closed-class words (which are also free-standing grammatical morphemes) determine phrasal construction, whereas open-class words primarily refer to objects and events. Bradley et al. argue that these computational differences must imply separate retrieval mechanisms for these different kinds of words. The word retrieval mechanisms for closed-class words are postulated to be selectively disrupted in agrammatism. The consequences of these selective retrieval deficits are evident in the spontaneous speech, repetition, oral reading, and writing of agrammatical patients (Nespoulous et al., 1988).

Kean (1977, 1978) has offered a formal phonological account for agrammatical morphological errors. She argues that the pattern of agrammatical omissions may be related to the stress applied to words or word segments. In the word "definiteness," the presence of the bound morpheme "ness" does not influence the phonological stress pattern of the root word. By contrast, in "definitive," "ive" crucially alters the stress pattern. Kean argues that patients with agrammatism selectively omit bound morphemes that do not alter stress patterns, such as possessive, tense, or plural markers. Similarly, functors, which do not alter the stress pattern of words in a sentence, are omitted from their speech.

Goodglass, Fodor, and Schulhoff (1967) have proposed a psychological notion of "saliency," arguing that less salient words or parts of words are more likely to be omitted by agrammatical patients. This notion of saliency incorporates informativeness, intonational and amplitudinal stress, phonological prominence, and affective quality; however, saliency is claimed to account for only a subset of agrammatical symptoms. Goodglass and Berko (1960) reported that all grammatical morphemes are not equally vulnerable to omission. In sentence completion tasks, they found that agrammatical subjects performed best with plurals; did worst with possessives; and achieved intermediate scores with inflectional morphemes reflecting tense, comparatives, and superlatives.

The pattern of agrammatical morphological errors may be idiosyncratic to individual patients. Miceli, Silveri, Romani, and Caramazza (1989), in a study of 20 agrammatical subjects, found little consistency in the frequency of omission errors involving five types of free-standing grammatical morphemes: prepositions, definite articles, indefinite articles, clitics, and auxiliary verbs. Although they found a general correlation between the frequencies of errors in free-standing and bound morphemes, individual patients often deviated from this pattern. These observations led the authors to suggest that free-standing and bound grammatical morphemes are produced by separate mechanisms. Miceli and Caramazza (1988) also reported a dissociation within bound morphology in an Italian agrammatical patient. He was severely impaired in producing inflectional (i.e., grammatical) morphemes, but only mildly impaired with derivational (i.e., nongrammatical) morphemes.

SYNTACTIC DEFICITS IN AGRAMMATICAL PRODUCTION

Saffran, Schwartz, and Marin (1980) first drew attention to the "word order problem" in agrammatism. Agrammatical patients have problems with mapping thematic roles, or the conceptual knowledge of who does what to whom, onto linguistic form. These kinds of thematic role deficits may occur independently of morphological deficits and reflect deficits within Garrett's functional level (Caramazza & Miceli, 1991; Maher, Chatterjee, Gonzalez-Rothi, & Heilman, 1995; Martin & Blossom-Stach, 1986). Agrammatical patients often use lexical–semantic knowledge to guide their productions. They are more likely to produce accurate sentences when only one of the potential agents is animate, as in "The boy kicks the rock," than when both potential agents are animate, as in "The boy kisses the girl." Presumably production of the former sentence is guided by real-world knowledge that a rock cannot kick a boy. However, with the latter—a reversible sentence, without such semantic constraints—these patients often misorder their words. "Word order error" does not imply that these patients produce words randomly; they do not produce sentences with noun–noun–verb or verb–noun–noun sequences. Rather, the placement of nouns around the verb is misordered. These deficits are usually uncovered via picture description tasks, but may also be observed in the spontaneous speech of agrammatical patients (Byng & Black, 1989).

Thematic role assignment deficits in agrammatical patients may relate to deficits in the processing of the verbs that constrain the sentence structure. In support of this hypothesis, patients with Broca's aphasia have greater difficulty retrieving verbs than nouns (Damasio & Tranel, 1993; McCarthy & Warrington, 1985; Miceli, Silveri, Villa, & Caramazza, 1984). Although verbs in English are morphologically more complex than nouns, this difference probably does not explain the disproportionate difficulties agrammatical patients experience with verbs. Chinese patients with Broca's aphasia show deficits in naming actions similar to those observed in English-speaking patients, even though Chinese verbs are not conjugated and are no more complex morphologically than Chinese nouns (Bates, Chen, Tzeng, Li, & Opie, 1991). The effect of verb retrieval deficits on sentence frames is not straightforward. For example, Zingeser and Berndt (1990) report that syntactic frames help some aphasic patients to retrieve verbs, but impede their retrieval of others. The specific semantic, lexical, and syntactic properties of verbs and their influence on sentence production are complex and remain an active area of investigation (Bates, Chen, et al., 1991; Kegl, 1995; Kohn & Lorch, 1989; Miceli, Silveri, Nocentini, & Caramazza, 1988; Shapiro & Levine, 1990; Zingeser & Berndt, 1990).

MESSAGE-LEVEL CONSIDERATIONS IN AGRAMMATISM

Little is known about the structure of the message level and its influences on sentence production. This lack of knowledge stems in part from the fact that Garrett's model was derived from normal speech errors, and these data do not address the message level (although see Levelt, 1989, for some thoughts on this level).

We have suggested that patients with functional-level deficits may provide insight into the structure of the message level. We reported a patient with a thematic-role-mapping deficit who consistently used a temporal or spatial strategy rather than linguistic rules to map thematic roles onto grammatical categories (Chatterjee, Maher, Gonzalez-Rothi, & Heilman, 1995; Maher et al., 1995). Specifically, participants on the left were consistently considered to be agents or doers of actions, and those on the right were considered to be patients or recipients of actions. Normal subjects also demonstrated subtle spatial biases in how they conceptualized these thematic roles (Chatterjee, Maher, & Heilman, 1995; Chatterjee, Southwood, & Basilico, 1999). These observations suggest that the message level may in part have a spatial structure, rather than the propositional structure of more "downstream" sentence representations.

One explanation for agrammatical production implicates a message-level strategic decision. According to this view, agrammatical patients limit their output to the bare essentials required to convey their message, because speaking is effortful. Under restricted conditions, agrammatical speakers may produce grammatical morphemes that they usually omit in spontaneous speech (Kolk et al., 1985). This observation suggests that they have not lost lexical or phonological representations of grammatical morphemes. Selecting among possible grammatical morphemes to convey the message in a sentential form requires considerable, nearly simultaneous, on-line processing. Capacity limitations of on-line sentence processing brought on by brain damage may encourage adaptations and result in telegraphic speech. Kolk and coworkers suggest that this adaptive strategy involves a message-level prelinguistic decision to formulate sentences and communication that minimize the demands of production (Heeschen & Kolk, 1988; Kolk et al., 1985). By contrast, Berndt (1991) suggests that the lack of sentence elaboration may reflect conceptual impoverishment at the message level, rather than a strategic decision per se.

COMPREHENSION IN AGRAMMATISM

In general, agrammatical patients have been considered to have difficulties in production but relatively preserved comprehension. The insights of investigators in the early part of the century (cited in Goodglass, 1976) implicating coexisting comprehension deficits in these patients were unappreciated until recently. Zurif, Caramazza, and Myerson (1972) compared agrammatical and normal subjects' perception of the relationship between content and function words. Patients were shown cards with all possible sets of three words from each sentence. As the cards were presented, they were asked to choose the two words most closely related to each other, based on their use in the original sentence. Subjects' selections were analyzed via hierarchical cluster analysis, yielding phrase structure trees that graphically displayed perceived strengths of relationships between words. For example, in the sentence "The man was hurt," normal subjects linked "the" to "man" and "was" to "hurt," whereas the aphasic subjects linked "man" to "hurt." In general, normal subjects linked elements within noun phrases to each other and elements within verb phrases to each other. For example, articles and demonstratives were linked to their respective nouns. The copula ("to be" and its conjugations), when used as an auxiliary verb in the passive tense, was linked to the past participle, and when used as a main verb, it was linked to the predicate adjective. By contrast, agrammatical subjects tended to ignore articles, pronouns, copulas, and similar grammatical words. Their perceived clusters violated sentence constituent boundaries, suggesting that even when the agrammatical subjects were not required to produce language, they were insensitive to the structure of sentences.

Subsequently, agrammatical patients' comprehension difficulties were demonstrated more directly, using sentences in which meaning could only be extracted by syntactic processing. Heilman and Scholes (1976) reported that patients had difficulties interpreting sentences with dative constructions, such as "He showed her the baby pictures" and "He showed her baby the pictures." Caramazza and Zurif (1976) reported that patients had difficulties with sentences containing relative embedded clauses. In "The dog that the cat was chasing was brown," they had difficulty recognizing whether the dog or the cat was brown.

Several hypotheses to explain asyntactic comprehension have been postulated. The analysis of asyntactic comprehension is not guided by a general framework along the lines of Garrett's (1980, 1984) model of sentence production. However, there may be processes common to comprehension and production deficits. Grammatical morphemes are selected and inserted at the positional level of sentence production. A selective deficit in processing grammatical morphemes would make it difficult to comprehend sentences in which such processing is necessary to extract meaning. Damage or insufficient access to the store of grammatical morphemes could produce sentence-level deficits in both production and comprehension (Bradley et al., 1980).

An alternative hypothesis, which also focuses on difficulties with grammatical morphemes, implicates deficits in short-term memory or phonological working memory. Words encountered early in a sentence must be held in a short-term memory store for subsequent analysis (Kolk & Van Grunsven, 1985; Vallar & Baddeley, 1984). Words with little intrinsic semantic content, such as functors, must be retained in a phonological form. A phonological storage deficit should result in a selective lack of retention of grammatical words and produce asyntactic comprehension. Kolk and Van Grunsven (1985) argue that variability across patients and across sentence type within patients are better explained by such memory deficits than by a primary linguistic deficit.

Central syntactic deficits in sentence comprehension are analogous to production deficits at the functional level. Saffran et al. (1980) have reported that thematic-role-mapping deficits also occur in comprehension. Patients may successfully use lexical–semantic strategies in deciphering nonreversible sentences (e.g., "The boy kicked the stone"), but make role reversal errors in reversible sentences, in which such strategies are futile. Because such patients perform quite well on grammaticality judgment tasks, Saffran and Schwartz

(1994) posit a deficit in access to grammatical knowledge, rather than loss of grammatical knowledge itself, to account for their comprehension deficits.

Caplan and Grodzinsky offer linguistically motivated interpretations of asyntactic comprehension. These theories stem from general theories of transformational grammar and do not map directly onto Garrett's levels of sentence processing. Both views start from the premise that sentences have a hierarchical structure, and that a deeper ("D-structure") representation is translated into a surface ("S-structure") form. Caplan argues that patients are deficient in their ability to appreciate the hierarchical structure underlying surface forms of sentences. Consequently, they use nonlinguistic linear strategies to guide their interpretations of word strings. With linear ordering, they assign the thematic role of agent to the first noun that they encounter, and assume that the next noun is the recipient of an action (Caplan, 1983; Caplan & Futter, 1986). Grodzinsky (1986) proposes a more restricted deficit, framed by Chomsky's (1981) theory of government and binding. His trace deletion hypothesis, with subsequent modifications (Grodzinsky, Wexler, Chien, Marakovitz, & Solomon, 1993; Hickok, Zurif, & Canseco-Gonzalez, 1993), proposes that patients with agrammatism have greater syntactic knowledge than postulated by Caplan. The reasoning is as follows. An active and a passive sentence may have an identical deep structure, but transformations are performed on the deep structure to produce the passive surface structure. Constituent noun phrases are moved from their original positions in the deep structure, but leave an abstract trace of their original position in the surface structure. The moved noun phrase is grammatically bound to the trace of its original position. Thus a passive sentence such as "The boy was hit by the girl," has the underlying structure $\{_S\{_{NP}e\}$ was $\{_{VP}$ hit $\{_{NP}$ the boy$\}$ $\{_{PP}$ by the girl$\}\}\}$. This structure is transformed into the S-structure $\{_S\{_{NP}$ The boy$\}_i$ was $\{_{VP}$ hit t_i $\{_{PP}$ by the girl$\}\}\}$.[1] "The girl" derives its thematic role from the preposition "by" that directly governs it. However, the thematic role for "the boy" is assigned to its trace (t_i) position, which is grammatically bound to its moved location. Grodzinsky hypothesizes that patients with asyntactic comprehension are unable to appreciate the grammatical link between the moved constituent and its underlying trace. They delete the trace in the S-structure of sentences and are unable to recover the deeper structure required to comprehend the meaning of the sentences (Grodzinsky, 1989).

Agrammatical patients also have difficulties understanding sentences with "wh" words (e.g., "who," "what," "where," "which"). These difficulties are also explained via transformational grammar. The question "What did the man buy?" has a deep structure "The man bought a car." "A car" from the deep structure is replaced by the "wh" word and moved to the beginning of the sentence, leaving a trace at the original location. Again, agrammatical patients have difficulties with these sentences, since they do not appreciate the movement of constituents and their relationships to trace locations (Thompson & Shapiro, 1995).

Although each of these hypotheses potentially accounts for asyntactic comprehension in specific patients, it is unlikely that a single explanation will account for all instances of asyntactic deficits. Patients with asyntactic comprehension in the absence of a deficit in phonological or working memory have been reported (Chatterjee, Maher, Rothi, et al., 1995; Martin & Blossom-Stach, 1986; Martin, Wetzel, Blossom-Stach, & Feher, 1989). Patients with reduced working memory spans and near-normal comprehension of syntactically complex sentences have also been reported (Goodglass, Gleason, & Hyde, 1970; Martin, 1987; Martin & Feher, 1990). The thematic-role-mapping hypothesis predicts similar deficits with simple active and simple passive sentences. Yet many patients perform better on active than on passive sentences (Caplan & Futter, 1986; Caramazza & Miceli, 1991; Schwartz, Linebarger, Saffran, & Pate, 1987). Caplan's and Grodzinsky's hypotheses predict normal performance on simple active sentences. However, some patients perform poorly on active as well as passive sentences (Badecker, Nathan, & Caramazza, 1991; Chatterjee, Maher, Gonzalez-Rothi, et al., 1995; Jones, 1984). Preliminary data even suggest that patients with conceptual message-level deficits may be more likely to perform poorly on active sentences (Chatterjee, Southwood, Calhoun, & Thompson, 1999).

Patients with morphological deficits and asyntactic comprehension are still capable of making accurate grammaticality judgments. They are sensitive to the subcategorization requirements of lexical items, have a functor vocabulary, and can handle discontinuous syntactic dependencies across clauses (Linebarger, Schwartz, & Saffran, 1983). The ability to make grammaticality judgments suggests that these patients do not have complete loss of morphological knowledge or syntactic knowledge. These data argue for the preservation of grammatical knowledge while implicating application or processing of this knowledge. However, other studies raise doubts about the integrity of such knowledge. Grossman and Haberman (1982) report that patients with nonfluent aphasia often fail to detect violations of case marking and number agreement in syntactically complex or passive frames. A further distinction has been drawn between on-line and off-line grammaticality judgment tasks, which may relate to working memory deficits. The idea is that on-line sensitivity to grammaticality relies more on automatic processes, whereas off-line judgments rely on controlled processes. Several studies have demonstrated on-line deficits of grammaticality judgment in patients with nonfluent aphasia who may nevertheless be capable of normal off-line judgments (Baum, 1988; Tyler, 1985).

The situation is then similar to that of agrammatical production. There does not seem to be a critical deficit that explains all forms of asyntactic comprehension. Rather, any one of several facilities necessary to comprehend sentences that cannot be decoded by simply applying lexical–semantic knowledge may be selectively impaired, resulting in asyntactic comprehension.

PARALLELISM IN AGRAMMATICAL PRODUCTION AND ASYNTACTIC COMPREHENSION

It is clear that asyntactic comprehension and agrammatical production may dissociate from each other (Berndt, 1991). The short-lived enthusiasm for the hypothesis that a single central grammar center, encapsulated functionally and localized in the brain, could be disrupted selectively has given way to the sense that agrammatism ought not to be considered a coherent syndrome (Badecker & Caramazza, 1985). Patients with agrammatical production and preserved syntactic comprehension (Caramazza & Hillis, 1989; Kolk et al., 1985; Miceli, Mazzucchi, Menn, & Goodglass, 1983; Nespoulous et al., 1988), as well as patients with grammatical production but asyntactic comprehension, have been reported (Vallar & Baddeley, 1984; Vallar, Basso, & Bottini, 1990). Yet, as pointed out by Berndt (1991), it may be premature to abandon the possibility of a critical juncture at which sentence production and comprehension converge. Damage at this juncture may then be accompanied by parallel production and comprehension deficits. We have suggested that sentence representation levels most closely aligned to the message level may be such a convergence point. We are unaware of any patients reported in whom there is a dissociation between comprehension and production of thematic role assignment. Our patient who used a temporal–spatial strategy to make thematic role assignments did so in both production and comprehension (Chatterjee, Maher, Rothi, et al., 1995).

AGRAMMATISM AND PARAGRAMMATISM

As mentioned before, while patients classified clinically as having Broca's aphasia are often agrammatical, disturbances of grammar may be seen in other types of aphasia (Berndt, 1991). Patients with fluent aphasia also make errors with grammatical morphemes (in addition to errors with major lexical items). Whereas agrammatical errors consist of omissions, paragrammatical errors consist of substitutions (Grodzinsky, 1984). Heeschen argues that patients with agrammatical and patients with paragrammatical aphasia share a common morphological–syntactic deficit, but apply different adaptive strategies to deal with their deficit. The choice of strategy is determined by deficits of fluency and not by a primary linguistic difference (Heeschen, 1985). Kolk et al. (1985) have similarly emphasized adaptive mechanisms in interpreting these aphasic patients' behavior. By contrast, Goodglass, Christiansen, and Gallagher (1993) describe systematic differences (as well as similarities) in morphological errors made by agrammatical and paragrammatical patients. Agrammatical patients performed more poorly than fluent aphasic patients on the use of auxiliaries, verb inflections, and passive word order.

Studies of aphasia in other languages have raised questions about whether omission errors in English agrammatism are actually lexical substitution errors. For example, omitting the "ed" past tense morpheme for the verb "walk" still results in a word. It remains unclear whether an agrammatical patient who utters "walk" inappropriately is omitting a necessary bound morpheme or substituting a different word form. In languages in which the word stem cannot be free-standing, patients do not omit bound morphemes to produce nonword stems (Menn, O'Connor, Obler, & Holland, 1995). These observations suggest, by analogy, that agrammatism in English may also be paragrammatism. That is, agrammatical patients are actually making substitution errors.

THE NEUROLOGY OF AGRAMMATISM

Study of the neurology of agrammatism lags behind that of functional deficits in sentence processing. Investigators with sophisticated theoretical approaches to language deficits sometimes minimize the role of biological variables (Caramazza, 1992). Biologically oriented investigators have historically focused on language behaviors (fluency, repetition, etc.) and not language structure. Their investigations often rely on traditional clinical classifications and not on deficits of language components. They also tend to avoid the technical and theoretical complexities of agrammatism, which are usually shrouded in psycholinguistic terminology.

Bouillaud, in the mid-19th century, emphasized the role of the frontal lobes in speech production (see Benton, 1991). Broca subsequently demonstrated that these processes were lateralized to the left frontal lobe. He emphasized the role of the third frontal convolution, the area that now bears his name (again, see Benton, 1991). With the advent of modern neuroimaging, Mohr et al. (1978) and Tonkonogy and Goodglass (1981) convincingly demonstrated that lesions confined to Broca's area do not produce long-lasting Broca's aphasia. Rather, the responsible lesions are considerably larger, usually also involving the operculum.

Luria (1974) argued that the basic approach of ascribing a specific functional component of language to a specific brain location is untenable. In his view, the goals of neurolinguistics are to single out basic components underlying the processes of language behavior, to identify the factors involved in their realization, and then to study which parts of the brain provide these factors. According to this view, these factors need not be confined to linguistic operations; they are utilized when needed, regardless of the cognitive domain. Luria drew a broad distinction between anterior and posterior regions of the brain. He argued that the frontal lobes are involved in programming, regulating, and controlling human actions in accordance with conscious goals and motivations. With respect to language, these properties of frontal cortices are necessary in the synthesis of successive elements into a single, continuous, coherent series. Damage to these structures should make it difficult to produce fluent propositional language. By contrast, posterior cortices are involved in operations requiring the simultaneous synthesis of stimuli into more abstract signals. Cognitive operations dependent on the use of such synthesized codes should break down with posterior damage (Luria, 1958, 1977).

In the spirit of Luria's approach to neurolinguistics, Nadeau (1988) analyzed two patients with large left frontal lesions. These patients evidenced central syntactic deficits and relatively preserved morphological abilities. Nadeau contrasted them with a patient reported by Kolk et al. (1985), whose primary deficit was morphological and whose lesion was located posteriorly. Nadeau has argued that frontal cortices plan behavior, particularly in novel situations, in a variety of cognitive contexts. Accordingly, frontal systems mediate the selection of word order and functors to tailor linguistic output to the subtleties of the intended message. Such planning of sentences allows variety and shifts in emphasis through changes in word order, use of passive constructions, embedded sentences, direct–indirect object constructions, cleft subjects and objects, and so on. Nadeau suggests that postcentral cortices, in contrast to frontal cortices, operate on associative principles formed during language ontogenesis. In effect, these cortices mediate a vast memory store of morphological and phonological associations, which are inserted as dictated by sentential elements in each word's neighborhood, the word's position, and its phonological prominence. This conceptualization modifies the traditional role of the arcuate fasciculus, the white matter connections between postcentral and frontal language cortex. Geschwind (1965) postulated that the arcuate fasciculus is the conduit by which language data processed posteriorly are then delivered to frontal cortices to be prepared for output. According to Nadeau (1988), the arcuate fasciculus may serve, at least in part, to mediate access to morphologial structures to be inserted into the final sentence, whose frame is determined by frontal cortices. In support of this hypothesis, he cites a case of agrammatism reported by Miceli et al. (1983). This patient had a lesion sparing Broca's area, but involving the posterior portions of the pars opercularis, precentral gyrus, and posterior and superior aspects of the insula extending into the deep white matter. The patient evolved to having a syntactic deficit with relatively preserved morphology. Nadeau suggested that this patient was agrammatical because damage to the arcuate fasciculus prevented the frontal lobes from exerting their influence on posterior regions. Further work will need to be done to confirm the accuracy of this functional–hypothesis regarding sentence production.

Sentence-level comprehension deficits have been observed with lesions to the left perisylvian cortices. Selnes, Knopman, Niccum, Rubens, and Larson (1983) related lesion location and volume in 39 patients with left middle cerebral artery strokes to auditory comprehension deficits and subsequent recovery. They found that lesions of the posterior superior temporal and infrasylvian supramarginal gyrus were most predictive of severe deficits and poor outcomes as indexed by the Token Test. Patients with initially preserved auditory comprehension had lesions that spared these regions. Most patients with initially severe deficits but subsequent recovery also had lesions that spared these regions. Lesion volume was only predictive for very large and very small lesions. Subsequent reports have confirmed that posterior lesions are associated with more persistent syntactic comprehension deficits (Tramo, Baynes, & Volpe, 1988).

Caplan, Hildebrandt, and Makris (1996) published a systematic study of asyntactic comprehension in 60 stroke patients, 46 with left-hemisphere strokes and 14 with right-hemisphere strokes. Patients enacted thematic roles in 12 examples of 25 sentence types designed to test a wide variety of syntactic operations. Both right- and left-brain-damaged patients performed worse than normal control subjects, and left-brain-damaged patients performed more poorly than right-brain-damaged patients. The finding that right-brain-damaged patients performed poorly on syntactically complex sentences, independent of sentence length, was surprising. The authors suggest that perhaps the right hemisphere contributes some general working memory capacity needed to comprehend syntactically complex sentences in ways not yet understood. Neuroradiological data from 18 of the left-brain-damaged subjects showed that asyntactic comprehension was associated with lesions to all parts of the perisylvian association cortex, and that severity of deficit did not correlate with size of lesion.

TREATMENT OF AGRAMMATISM

Treatments of aphasic patients with agrammatism have been designed to produce general effects, or have been targeted to specific deficits of sentence processing. The general interventions include metalinguistic approaches and pharmacological interventions. These interventions are not necessarily designed specifically to treat agrammatical patients, but may have beneficial effects nevertheless. The targeted interventions are motivated by theoretical frameworks along the lines we have discussed, and are directed specifically at patients with deficits of grammar.

General Interventions

Melodic Intonation Therapy

Melodic intonation therapy (MIT) is the only therapy for aphasia that has been endorsed by the American Academy of Neurology's (1994) Therapeutics and Technology Assessments Subcommittee. MIT is a hierarchically structured program based on the idea that intonation and melodic patterns of language are mediated by the right hemisphere, and that these speech attributes can be used to improve deficits associated with left-hemisphere damage. At the first two levels of the treatment, multisyllabic words and short, high-probability phrases are musically intoned in a prescribed, graduated manner. The third level incorporates longer and phonologically more complex sentences. This treatment is only appropriate in patients with Broca's aphasia and its variants. Patients with bilateral lesions, significant comprehension deficits, or relatively preserved repetition are unlikely to benefit. Reports of efficacy of treatment vary. When improvements occur, they are most likely to be observed in language fluency.

Pharmacotherapy in Aphasia

Pharmacological treatments of aphasia focus on manipulating catecholamine systems. Some studies have been motivated by the observation in experimental animal stroke models that recovery improves with augmentation of noradrenergic systems (Feeney, 1998a, 1998b). These treatments are not targeted at aphasic symptoms specifically, but instead are expected to improve recovery of function in general. It appears that *d*-amphetamine accelerates the growth of axonal sprouts in areas surrounding a stroke and in homologous areas of the contralateral hemisphere during the early stages of recovery after stroke (Stroemer, Kent, & Hulsebosch, 1998). Walker-Bateson et al. (1992) reported improvements in aphasic patients who were given *d*-amphetamine an hour before traditional speech therapy. These patients improved over 10 sessions beyond expectations based on the Porch Index of Communicative Ability norms (Porch, 1967). Importantly, this treatment strategy paired the use of *d*-amphetamine with a behavioral intervention. Future treatment studies of such pairings (Small, 1994), perhaps with more targeted interventions, may hold promise.

Other treatments have been motivated by the potential adjuvant effects of dopamine on frontal lobe function. Albert, Bachman, Morgan, and Helm-Estabrook (1988) reported that fluency improved in a patient with transcortical motor aphasia with the administration of the dopamine agonist bromocriptine. Others have reported similar results, but improvement is not observed consistently across aphasic subjects (Gupta, Mlcoch, Scolaro, & Moritz, 1995; MacLennan, Nicholas, Morley, & Brookshire, 1991). Whether a select group of patients are likely to improve with dopaminergic augmentation is not known.

Targeted Treatments of Agrammatism

Current views of sentence production and the nature of agrammatism have led to the development of new, theoretically motivated approaches to remediation. If sentence processing can be impaired at different levels and can result in a variety of deficits, then no one treatment will be effective in all individuals with agrammatism. To develop a targeted treatment, the levels of sentence processing involved and the components damaged need to be identified. Implicit in this view is the expectation that treatments targeted to specific deficits will be more effective than general therapies (Mitchum, Haendiges, & Berndt, 1995; Schwartz, Fink, & Saffran, 1995). However, specifically targeted interventions will be unlikely to generalize to deficits at other levels of sentence processing or to nontargeted component deficits within the same level (Thompson, 1998; Thompson, Shapiro, Tait, Jacobs, & Schneider, 1996). Lack of treatment generalization also serves as a test of the hypothesis that components of sentence processing are organized modularly.

Despite the difficulty of designing treatment studies for a disorder as complex as agrammatism, several recent individual-case and small-group studies suggest that effective intervention for specific deficits is possible. We discuss interventions in the context of Garrett's (1980, 1984) model of sentence production, recognizing that the authors of these studies do not necessarily tie their approach to features of this model (although see (Mitchum et al., 1995, and Schwartz et al., 1995, for direct applications of the model). Treatment at one level may have effects on specific aspects of other levels, and treatment efficacy at one level may be affected by deficits at other levels.

Treatment of the Positional Level

Based on the neurolinguistic studies of agrammatism by Goodglass and his colleagues (Gleason, Goodglass, Green, Ackerman, & Hyde, 1975; Goodglass & Berko, 1960), Helm-Estabrooks, Fitzpatrick, and Barresi (1981) developed a remediation approach to stimulate the retrieval of morphemes in sentence production. The Helm Elicited Language Program for Syntax Stimulation (HELPSS) incorporates a hierarchy of sentence difficulty and presents sentences in a story completion format. The approach is one of stimulation and direct correction, based on the theory that the morphological–syntactic failure is one of retrieval and can be improved by practicing sentences with the same word order and morphology but different major lexical items. Because the focus of the intervention is on the phonological realization of grammatical morphemes within the sentence frame, the HELPSS appears to target positional-level representations. However, verb retrieval is probably stimulated simultaneously in this approach.

Helm-Estabrooks et al. (1981) demonstrated the effectiveness of the HELPSS with an individual with chronic Broca's aphasia. The subject improved on standard aphasia tests following HELPSS treatment. In a follow-up study (Helm-Estabrooks & Ramsberger, 1986), six patients improved on expressive measures, but not on receptive syntactic measures. These findings were partially replicated by Doyle, Goldstein, and Bourgeois (1987), but generalization to untrained stimuli was not consistent. Three of the four patients improved on trained sentences following treatment, but the treatment effect was not maintained consistently across subjects and sentence types. Only one subject had any training on complex sentences (passives). Deficits in thematic role mapping and word order were not addressed. Therefore, it is not clear whether HELPSS treatment affected argument structure deficits, although the lack of improvement in syntactic comprehension suggests that it did not.

Mitchum and Berndt (1994) studied the effects of treating verb morphology on sentence construction. They used triads of picture sequences to focus on past-, present-, and future-tense inflectional morphology, and cued their subjects to include tense markers when needed. Their subjects improved in verb use and used tense morphology more accurately in picture description, as well as on less constrained sentence production tasks. This improvement was limited to the trained tense morphology and resulted in inappropriate transfer to untrained forms, yielding anomalous constructions (e.g., "The bike is riding the girl"). This treatment, which targeted the positional level, improved verb retrieval. The authors suggested that increased availability of grammatical morphemes may have freed up limited resources, which in turn facilitated verb retrieval. Alternatively, the grammatical morphology may have served as a form of syntactic priming, enhancing verb retrieval. Perhaps interventions at later stages of sentence construction may also "stimulate" earlier levels, in particular verb retrieval. Interestingly, thematic role assignment and syntactic comprehension did not improve as a result of this intervention.

Haendiges, Berndt, and Mitchum (1996) were successful at improving the comprehension of thematic roles by drawing attention to passive morphology, which is realized at the positional level. Comprehension improved only after active and passive constructions were explicitly compared and related to an action picture. Treatment effects were maintained when the subject was presented with the complete sentence frame, but not when presented with a truncated form (e.g., "The man was splashed by the woman," but not "The man was splashed"). This suggested that the subject was able to recognize the correct thematic roles based on the presence of passive morphology at the positional level. Berndt and Mitchum (1998) also described a patient who improved in passive sentence comprehension only after receiving explicit instruction in the differences between passive and active sentence forms. This improvement also generalized to untreated passive sentences, but not to truncated forms. An item analysis revealed that some verbs were more difficult to process, based on the number of possible arguments implied by the verb (i.e., the complexity of the predicate–argument structure). This finding is consistent with the report (Thompson, Lange, Schneider, & Shapiro, 1997) that ease of verb processing and the number of possible verb arguments influence treatment.

Thompson and her colleagues have described another approach that targets the positional level, and to some extent the functional level, of sentence production. They have reported a number of treatment studies designed to improve complex sentence production that involve noncanonical sentence construction (Thompson, Shapiro, & Roberts, 1993; Thompson & Shapiro, 1995; Thompson, 1998; Thompson, Shapiro, Ballard, et al., 1997). The intervention is based on Chomskian linguistic theory of movement (the "move alpha" rule) from the underlying canonical "D-structure" to the noncanonical "S-structure" of complex sentences (e.g., passives or "wh" interrogatives). The treatment approach involves first identifying the verbs and the verb argument structure for simple active sentences, moving the target sentence constituents to form the "wh" question, and finally producing the surface "wh" question form. This intervention resulted in two patterns of performance: One group was able to acquire the complex form with good generalization to other types of sentences requiring the same type of movement (either argument movement or adjunctive movement). The other group required additional training to select the correct "wh" specifier for the position. For both groups, generalization to untreated sentences occurred only for surface structures that used the same type of movement rule. Treatment for movement of the argument noun phrase (e.g., "who" questions) only generalized to other argument movement sentences (e.g., "what" questions), but not to adjunctive movement sentences (e.g., "when" questions).

Treatment of the Functional Level

Functional-level treatments focus on verb retrieval and on mapping of thematic roles. Retrieving the verb is critical to establishing the argument structure of the sentence; therefore, improving verb retrieval might be expected to improve sentence production. The results of this strategy have been mixed (Berndt, Haendiges, Mitchum, & Sandson, 1997; Fink, Martin, Schwartz, Saffran, & Myers, 1993; Loverso, Prescott, & Selinger, 1986; Mitchum & Berndt, 1994).

Mitchum and Berndt (1994) used rapid serial naming of pictured verbs to improve verb naming. Unfortunately, the improvement in naming verbs did not influence verb retrieval in sentence production. Verb retrieval alone may not be sufficient to establish an adequate functional-level sentence representation.

Fink et al. (1993) described two verb retrieval treatment approaches. The first, "direct training," involved two components: phonemic cueing and modeling to facilitate access to verbs, followed by generation of the noun phrases associated with the verb to produce a sentence. The second approach consisted of verb priming through sentence repetition. Gains in verb retrieval for treated verbs were observed in the direct training approach and were maintained in follow-up testing. This approach resulted in reduced omissions of untreated verbs and an increase in acceptable verb substitutions for the targets. The verb-priming approach also resulted in greater verb use, although this improvement was not long-lasting. Both procedures demonstrated that the sentence production of agrammatical individuals who demonstrate verb retrieval impairments can be manipulated to increase the production of verbs in sentences.

Loverso and his colleagues (Loverso et al., 1986; Loverso & Milione, 1992; Prescott, Selinger, & Loverso, 1982) used a verb-cueing treatment for sentence production. In this treatment, the subjects were provided with the written and auditory form of the verb. Through a hierarchy of "wh" cues, they selected the noun phrase (or phrases) to structure around the verb in both spoken and written form. The patients' spoken and written verb production improved. This improvement generalized somewhat to untreated verbs, and was maintained 1 month after treatment. This treatment may have helped develop accurate argument structures rather than verb retrieval per se. However, these results are consistent with the finding that some individuals with verb impairments can benefit from being provided with the verb (Berndt et al., 1997).

Deficits in thematic role assignment involving semantically reversible sentences have led to several remediation approaches commonly referred to as "mapping therapy" (Byng, 1988; Jones, 1986; Mitchum et al., 1995; Schwartz, Saffran, Fink, & Myers, 1994). These treatment are likely to influence both comprehension and production, if as we suggest, this mapping procedure is critical to both. Byng (1988) used written sentences to explicitly train interpretation of thematic roles in the sentence. Spatial and color-coded diagrams were used with the written sentences to guide sentence interpretation and verify responses. The predicate argument structure was limited to locative preposition constructions. This study was completed as a 2-week home program, after which remarkable improvement was observed in both written and auditory sentence comprehension. This improvement occurred for both trained and untrained prepositions, and also generalized to verbs. As might be predicted, morphology, which is not assigned at the functional level of sentence processing, did not improve.

Jones's (1986) mapping therapy also used written input. The patient was first trained to identify the verb in the sentence, and then trained to answer questions to identify the logical roles in the sentence, and to underline each of these in a different specified color. This treatment also resulted in a significant improvement in syntactic comprehension and production, with some functional carryover outside the clinic.

Following earlier reports, several replications of mapping therapy have reported varying degrees of effectiveness (Byng, Nickels, & Black, 1994; Haendiges et al., 1996; Schwartz et al., 1995). Many of the follow-up studies have included a wider range of agrammatical individuals, who have additional deficits besides those in thematic role assignment. At present it is premature to predict which patients will benefit the most from mapping treatment. This has led Schwartz et al. (1995) to propose that several components of a skill may need to be targeted simultaneously (e.g., verb retrieval, argument structure, and thematic role assignment).

Nonlinguistic strategies may also help patients with functional level deficits. Since aphasic subjects are usually able to recognize pictures, icons can be used to augment their ability to communicate (Weinrich, 1991). These approaches do not target the patients' linguistic abilities per se. Rather, patients learn a vocabulary of different icons representing nouns and verbs, and they are trained to select them to communicate their intent. This system is also available as a computer-based program and appears to help patients with severe communication deficits (Steele, Weinrich, Wertz, Kleczewska, & Carlson, 1989; Weinrich, 1991).

Treatment of the Message Level

Although no treatment studies focus explicitly on message-level deficits, results of interventions at subsequent levels of sentence production provide some useful information about the message level (Byng et al., 1994; Schwartz et al., 1994). Byng et al. (1994) attempted to treat deficits in comprehension and production of thematic roles (Byng, 1988; Jones, 1986) in three individuals with a wide range of grammatical impairment. This treatment involved three phases. In the first phase, only pictures depicting irreversible sentences were used. To describe the pictures, the subjects were provided with written verb and noun phrases, which were color-coded based on syntactic roles. The subjects' task initially was to match written sentence constituents to the correct position in the sentence frame, using color coding of the constituents as cues, and to check the results of performance. This phase emphasized that events can be structured linguistically, and required that patients develop a conceptual representation of an event from a picture depicting the roles of the participants. Phase 2 of the treatment involved the explicit verbal description of the picture without the written sentence constituents, and Phase 3 was a generalization phase using Promoting Aphasics Communication Activities (PACE; Davis & Wilcox, 1981). PACE attempts to improve communication by placing patients in more natural settings in which they communicate with other people, rather than the restricted setting of patient and therapist.

One subject in this study benefited the most from the first phase of the treatment. Post hoc testing revealed that this subject had considerable difficulty "conceptualizing" the event occurring in the picture—arguably a message-level deficit. She benefited from the phase of treatment that drew attention to the idea that an action was occurring in the picture and that the animate noun in the picture was the agent of that action. However, she continued to have difficulty describing events when the agent for the action pictured varied with the verb selected (e.g., for a picture of a man reading a book to a woman, if the verb is "read," the man is the actor; however, if the verb is "listen," then the woman is the actor).

Like the other proposed levels of sentence processing, the message level probably involves multiple components, each of which may require remediation. Since our knowledge of the message level is limited, it is unclear how often deficits at this level occur in conjunction with "downstream" linguistic deficits, or how often they mimic these deficits. Message-level deficits are likely to influence both production and comprehension. Subjects with conceptual deficits may not do as well as subjects with primarily linguistic deficits if the treatment is targeted at linguistic variables (Schwartz et al., 1994; Thompson, Lange, et al., 1997). Neither the identification nor the treatment of such conceptual deficits has received much attention.

General Observations from Treatment Studies

Treatment studies have led to a better understanding of variables that can affect treatment outcome. General therapies such as MIT and pharmacological interventions have the advantage that they can be used widely. When effective, they appear to improve fluency associated with agrammatism, but do not alter the grammatical deficits per se. Theoretically motivated targeted treatments are labor-intensive, and by their very nature, they are restricted to individually designed treatments based on patients' deficits. As such, broad claims about their efficacy cannot be made at this time. However, some principles seem to emerge from the studies to date. "Deeper" message-level deficits and deficits in the mapping of the message onto the functional level are likely to influence both production and comprehension. Treatment for these deficits, if effective, is likely to benefit both production and comprehension. "Deeper" or "upstream" deficits may also impede treatments targeted at "downstream" levels. For example, individuals unable to conceptualize events do not benefit as much from mapping therapy (Byng et al., 1994). Treatment of one component within a level may be impeded by concomitant deficits within the same level. For example, aphasic patients who make frequent reversal errors may benefit more from mapping therapy than those who also have difficulty with verb comprehension and parsing (Crerar, Ellis, & Dean, 1996). Subjects with more severe, wider-ranging deficits, through demonstrating some gains, do not improve as much as individuals with "purer" forms of agrammatism (Haendiges et al., 1996; Schwartz et al., 1994). Finally, "upstream" treatment may not improve "downstream" deficits. For example, individuals who have a morphological impairment rather than a syntactic deficit are unlikely to benefit from mapping therapy (Schwartz et al., 1995). By contrast, interventions at the positional level may have restricted effects "upstream," particularly since some of these training procedures may also involve verb processing simultaneously.

In summary, much work remains to be done in the treatment of agrammatism. Treatments with careful selection of patients based on theoretical models, and targeted interventions of component deficits (perhaps paired with pharmacological therapies anticipated to improve recovery and learning), offer the most promise for these complex patients.

AFTERWORD

Disorders of sentence processing are by their nature complex, and continue to be actively investigated. Disagreements about appropriate experimental methodology, statistical rigor, interpretation of results, and criteria for patient selection are as yet unresolved (Caplan, 1995; Mauner, 1995). Questions about the fundamental nature of specific grammatical deficits remain contentious (Kean, 1995). This chapter, by necessity, can only provide an overview. Full-length books have been devoted to agrammatism (Caplan & Hildebrandt, 1988; Kean, 1985; Menn & Obler, 1990), and two recent issues of *Brain and Language* (Volume 45, No. 3, Grodzinsky, 1993, and Volume 50, Nos. 1–3, Fromkin, 1995) have also been devoted to disorders of grammar. In particular, four topics not covered in this chapter deserve further discussion.

1. Recent modifications of Garrett's model give greater significance to other cognitive variables and lexical properties that might constrain syntax (Bock, 1982; Bock & Loebell, 1990; Dell, 1986). How such models will extend our understanding of message-level deficits or guide the analysis of verb-processing deficits in sentence production remains to be seen.

2. Most of the empirical work cited in this chapter involves off-line investigations. A striking feature of normal communication is the fluidity with which sentences are produced and comprehended on-line. Several studies have investigated on-line features of agrammatism (Friederici, 1995; Kolk, 1995; Shapiro, Gordon, Hack, & Killackey, 1993; Swinney & Zurif, 1995), incorporating important temporal factors in sentence processing.

3. We have only mentioned in passing the very interesting work being done in cross-linguistic investigations of agrammatism (Bates, Wulfeck, & MacWhinney, 1991; Menn et al., 1995; Menn & Obler, 1990). This approach has the potential to help distinguish symptoms that are language-specific from those that may represent more fundamental deficits reflecting universal principles of language structure and its neural organization.

4. In reviewing the neurology of agrammatism, we have not discussed functional neuroimaging. Methods of analyses of sentence-level stimuli are still being determined. This approach, if motivated theoretically, may begin to provide additional information on the "network" characteristics of different components of sentence processing (Just, Carpenter, Keller, Eddy, & Thulborn, 1996).

GLOSSARY

agent. The person or animate being that causes an action. This is a semantic, not a syntactic notion.
argument structure. "Who did what to whom" in a sentence. The semantic relationship between things or events in a sentence.
aspect. A grammatical category that marks temporal features of an activity denoted by a verb.
auxiliary verb. A functor verb that modifies the main verb. It may help to express tense, mood, or aspect.

bound grammatical morpheme. A grammatical morpheme that is attached to or modifies the form of some other word or word stem. Examples of bound morphemes in English are plural and past-tense endings.

case. A grammatical category that indicates how noun phrases in a sentence relate to each other. Cases typically correspond to subject, direct object, indirect object, and prepositional objects.

clitic. A word-like form that cannot stand on its own, but must be attached to a preceding or following word. Pronouns, copulas, and auxiliary verbs often have clitic forms. In English, many clitics are contracted forms, such as "I*'ve* arrived," "He*'s* gone."

closed-class words. Functors, or grammatical words like prepositions, conjunctions, and articles. "Closed-class" refers to the limited number of such words in any language.

constituent. A morphological or syntactic unit that is part of a larger unit. For example, clauses are constituents of sentences.

copula. A verb form, typically of the verb "to be" in English, that links a subject noun phrase with another noun phrase, an adjective phrase, or a clause by indicating equivalence or a description (e.g., "The man is 6 feet tall").

dative. A sentence incorporating both direct and indirect objects (e.g., "He gave *John* the picture").

derivational morpheme. An affix that creates a new word from an existing one (e.g., "crea*tive*," "sister*hood*").

function word, functor. A free-standing grammatical word that is defined in terms of its grammatical or syntactic function (e.g., "the," "of," "in").

governed. A word whose case is determined by another word is "governed"' by that word.

inflectional morpheme. A bound grammatical affix indicating tense, number, person, or case (e.g., "walk*ed*," "tree*s*").

lexicon. A set of words known to a speaker, with their associated morphological, phonological, semantic, and syntactic properties.

morpheme. The smallest meaningful component of a word. A morpheme may be a whole word ("the," "peach"), an affix ("walk*ing*"), or part of a compound word ("*hydro*static").

open-class words. Words that refer to objects and events, such as nouns, verbs, adjectives and adverbs. "Open-class" refers to the fact that they are unlimited in number.

patient. A thematic role for the recipient of an action. Jill is the patient in the sentence "Jack pushes Jill."

predicate. The verb phrase of the sentence, which provides information about the subject.

relative clause. A clause that cannot stand alone and modifies a noun or noun phrase (e.g., "The cow *that jumped over the moon . . .*").

subcategorization frames. The frame established by a verb that indicates whether it may or must be used with a direct object, an indirect object, or other sentence constituents.

surface structure. The phrase structure of a sentence after transformations have been carried out on its deep structure.

syntax. The organization of words into grammatical phrases, clauses, and sentences.

tense. The time at which an action or state of affairs indicated by a verb took place.

thematic role. The role of a noun phrase in a sentence, such as agent or patient.

trace. A silent, implicit element in a sentence, corresponding to the deep-structure position of a moved phrase. In "Jack was pushed [trace] by Jill," "Jack" has been moved, leaving the trace after the verb.

ACKNOWLEDGMENT

We thank Drs. Helen Southwood, Britt Anderson, and Mark Mennemeier for their helpful comments on this chapter.

NOTE

1. In this technical notation, S refers to sentence, NP to noun phrase, PP to prepositional phrase, VP to verb phrase, t_i to trace index, and e to the empty slot.

REFERENCES

Albert, M. L., Bachman, D. L., Morgan, A., & Helm-Estabrook, N. (1988). Pharmacotherapy for aphasia. *Neurology, 38,* 877–879.

American Association of Neurology. (1994). Melodic intonation therapy: Report of the Therapeutics and Technology Assessments Subcommittee. *Neurology, 44,* 566–568.

Badecker, W., & Caramazza, A. (1985). On consideration of method and theory governing the use of clinical categories in neurolinguistics and cognitive neuropsychology: The case against agrammatism. *Cognition, 20,* 97–126.

Badecker, W., Nathan, P., & Caramazza, A. (1991). Varieties of sentence comprehension deficits: A case study. *Cortex, 27,* 311–321.

Bates, E., Chen, S., Tzeng, O., Li, P., & Opie, M. (1991). The noun–verb problem in Chinese aphasia. *Brain and Language, 41,* 203–233.

Bates, E., Wulfeck, B., & MacWhinney, B. (1991). Cross-linguistic research in aphasia: An overview. *Brain and Language, 41,* 123–148.

Baum, S. (1988). Syntactic processing in agrammatism: Evidence from lexical decision and grammaticality judgment tasks. *Aphasiology, 2*(2), 117–135.

Benton, A. (1991). Aphasia: Historical perspectives. In M. T. Sarno (Ed.), *Acquired aphasia* (pp. 1–26). New York: Academic Press.

Berndt, R. S. (1991). Sentence processing in aphasia. In M. T. Sarno (Ed.), *Acquired aphasia* (pp. 223–269). New York: Academic Press.

Berndt, R. S., Haendiges, A. N., Mitchum, C. C., & Sandson, J. (1997). Verb retrieval in aphasia: 2. Relationship to sentence processing. *Brain and Language, 56,* 107–137.

Berndt, R. S., & Mitchum, C. C. (1998). An experimental treatment of sentence comprehension. In N. Helm-Estabrook & A. Holland (Eds.), *Approaches to the treatment of aphasia* (pp. 91–111). San Diego: Singular Publishing.

Bock, J. (1982). Toward a cognitive psychology of syntax: Information processing contributions to sentence formulation. *Psychological Review, 89*(1), 1–47.

Bock, K., & Loebell, H. (1990). Framing sentences. *Cognition, 35,* 1–39.

Bradley, D. C., Garrett, M. F., & Zurif, E. B. (1980). Syntactic deficits in Broca's aphasia. In D. Caplan (Ed.), *Biological studies of mental processing* (pp. 269–286). Cambridge, MA: MIT Press.

Byng, S. (1988). Sentence processing deficits: Theory and therapy. *Cognitive Neuropsychology, 5*(6), 629–676.

Byng, S., & Black, M. (1989). Some aspects of sentence production in aphasia. *Aphasiology, 3*(3), 241–263.

Byng, S., Nickels, L., & Black, M. (1994). Replicating therapy for mapping deficits in agrammatism: Remapping the deficit? *Aphasiology, 8,* 315–341.

Caplan, D. (1983). A note on the "word-order problem" in agrammatism. *Brain and Language, 20,* 155–165.

Caplan, D. (1995). Issues arising in contemporary studies of disorders of syntactic processing in sentence comprehension in agrammatic patients. *Brain and Language, 50,* 325–338.

Caplan, D., & Futter, C. (1986). Assignment of thematic roles by an agrammatic aphasic patient. *Brain and Language, 27,* 117–134.

Caplan, D., & Hildebrandt, N. (1988). *Disorders of syntactic comprehension.* Cambridge, MA: MIT Press.

Caplan, D., Hildebrandt, N., & Makris, N. (1996). Location of lesions in stroke patients with deficits in syntactic processing in sentence comprehension. *Brain, 119,* 933–949.

Caramazza, A. (1992). Is cognitive neuropsychology possible? *Journal of Cognitive Neuroscience, 4,* 80–95.

Caramazza, A., & Hillis, A. E. (1989). The disruption of sentence production: Some dissociations. *Brain and Language, 36,* 625–650.

Caramazza, A., & Miceli, G. (1991). Selective impairment of thematic role assignment in sentence processing. *Brain and Language, 41*, 402–436.

Caramazza, A., & Zurif, E. (1976). Dissociation of algorithmic and heuristic processes in language comprehension: Evidence from aphasia. *Brain and Language, 3*, 572–582.

Chatterjee, A., Maher, L. M., & Heilman, K. M. (1995). Spatial characteristics of thematic role representation. *Neuropsychologia, 33*, 643–648.

Chatterjee, A., Maher, L. M., Gonzalez-Rothi, G., & Heilman, K. M. (1995). Asyntactic thematic role assignment: The use of a temporal–spatial strategy. *Brain and Language, 49*, 125–139.

Chatterjee, A., Southwood, M. H., & Basilico, D. (1999). Verbs, events and spatial representations. *Neuropsychologia, 37*, 395–402.

Chatterjee, A., Southwood, M. H., Calhoun, J., & Thompson, K. A. (1999) Conceptual and linguistic knowledge of thematic roles in aphasia [Abstract]. *Neurology, 52*, A458.

Chomsky, N. (1981). *Lectures on government and binding.* Dordrecht, The Netherlands: Foris.

Crerar, M. A., Ellis, A. W., & Dean, E. C. (1996). Remediation of sentence processing deficits in aphasia using a computer-based microworld. *Brain and Language, 52*, 229–275.

Damasio, A. R., & Tranel, D. (1993). Nouns and verbs are retrieved with differently distributed neural systems. *Proceedings of the National Academy of Sciences USA, 90*, 4957–4960.

Davis, G. A., & Wilcox, M. J. (1981). Incorporating parameters of natural conversation in aphasia treatment. In R. Chapey (Eds.), *Language intervention strategies in adult aphasia* (pp. 169–193). Baltimore: Williams & Wilkins.

Dell, G. S. (1986). A spreading-activation theory of retrieval in sentence production. *Psychological Review, 93*, 283–321.

Doyle, P. J., Goldstein, H., & Bourgeois, M. S. (1987). Experimental analysis of syntax training in Broca's aphasia: A generalization and social validation study. *Journal of Speech and Hearing Disorders, 52*, 143–155.

Feeney, D. M. (1998a). Mechanisms of noradrenergic modulation of physical therapy: Effects on functional recovery after cortical injury. In L.B. Goldstein (Ed.), *Restorative neurology: Advances in pharmacotherapy for recovery after stroke* (pp. 35–48). Armonk, NY: Futura.

Feeney, D. M. (1998b). Rehabilitation pharmacology: Noradrenergic enhancement of physical therapy. In M. D. Ginsberg & J. Bogousslavsky (Eds.), *Cerebrovascular disease; Pathophysiology, diagnosis and management* (Vol. 1, pp. 620–636).Oxford: Blackwell.

Fink, R. B., Martin, N., Schwartz, M. F., Saffran, E. M., & Myers, J. C. (1993). Facilitation of verb retrieval skills in aphasia: A comparison of two approaches. *Clinical Aphasiology, 21*, 263–275.

Friederici, A. D. (1995). The time course of syntactic activation during language processing: A model based on neuropsychological and neurophysiological data. *Brain and Language, 50*, 259–281.

Fromkin, V. A. (Ed.). (1995). Introduction. *Brain and Language, 50*, 1–3.

Garrett, M. F. (1980). Levels of processing in sentence production. In B. Butterworth (Ed.), *Language production* (pp. 177–220). New York: Academic Press.

Garrett, M. F. (1984). The organization of processing structure for language production: Application to aphasic speech. In D. Caplan, A. R. Lecours, & A. Smith (Eds.), *Biological perspectives on language* (pp. 172–193). Cambridge, MA: MIT Press.

Geschwind, N. (1965). Disconnexion syndromes in animals and man. *Brain, 88*, 237–294, 585–644.

Gleason, J. B., Goodglass, H., Green, E., Ackerman, N., & Hyde, M. (1975). The retrieval of syntax in Broca's aphasia. *Brain and Language, 24*, 451–471.

Goodglass, H. (1976). Agrammatism. In H. Whitaker & H. A. Whitaker (Eds.), *Studies in neurolinguistics* (pp. 237–260). New York: Academic Press.

Goodglass, H. (1993). *Understanding aphasia.* New York: Academic Press.

Goodglass, H., & Berko, J. (1960). Agrammatism and inflectional morphology in English. *Journal of Speech and Hearing Research, 3*, 267–267.

Goodglass, H., Christiansen, J. A., & Gallagher, R. (1993). Comparison of morphology and syntax in free narrative and structured tests: Fluent vs. nonfluent aphasics. *Cortex, 29*, 377–407.

Goodglass, H., Fodor, I. G., & Schulhoff, C. (1967). Prosodic factors in grammar: Evidence from aphasia. *Journal of Speech and Hearing Research, 10*, 5–20.

Goodglass, H., Gleason, J. B., & Hyde, M. R. (1970). Some dimensions of auditory language comprehension in aphasia. *Journal of Speech and Hearing Research, 13*, 596–606.

Grodzinsky, Y. (1984). The syntactic characterization of agrammatism. *Cognition, 16*, 99–120.

Grodzinsky, Y. (1986). Language deficits and the theory of syntax. *Brain and Language, 27*, 135–159.

Grodzinsky, Y. (1989). Agrammatic comprehension of relative clauses. *Brain and Language*, 37, 480–499.

Grodzinsky, Y. (1993). Introduction. *Brain and Language*, 45(3), 229–305.

Grodzinsky, Y., Wexler, K., Chien, Y.-C., Marakovitz, S., & Solomon, J. (1993). The breakdown of binding relations. *Brain and Language*, 45, 396–422.

Grossman, M., & Haberman, S. (1982). Aphasic's selective deficits in appreciating grammatical agreements. *Brain and Language*, 16, 109–120.

Gupta, S. R., Mlcoch, A. G., Scolaro, C., & Moritz, T. (1995). Bromocriptine treatment of nonfluent aphasia. *Neurology*, 45, 2170–2173.

Haendiges, A. N., Berndt, R. S., & Mitchum, C. C. (1996). Assessing the elements contributing to a mapping deficit: A targeted treatment study. *Brain and Language*, 52, 276–302.

Heeschen, C. (1985). Agrammatism versus paragrammatism: A fictitious opposition. In M. L. Kean (Ed.), *Agrammatism* (pp. 207–248). New York: Academic Press.

Heeschen, C., & Kolk, H. (1988). Agrammatism and paragrammatism. *Aphasiology*, 2, 299–302.

Heilman, K. M., & Scholes, R. J. (1976). The nature of comprehension errors in Broca's conduction and Wernicke's aphasics. *Cortex*, 12(3), 257–302.

Helm-Estabrooks, N., Fitzpatrick, P. M., & Barresi, B. (1981). Response of an agrammatic patient to a syntax stimulation program for aphasia. *Journal of Speech and Hearing Disorders*, 46, 422–427.

Helm-Estabrooks, N., & Ramsberger, G. (1986). Treatment of agrammatism in long-term Broca's aphasia. *British Journal of Disorders of Communication*, 21, 39–48.

Hickok, G., Zurif, E., & Canseco-Gonzalez, E. (1993). Structural description of agrammatic comprehension. *Brain and Language*, 45, 371–395.

Jones, E. V. (1984). Word order processing in aphasia: Effects of verb semantics. *Advances in Neurology*, 42, 159–181.

Jones, E. V. (1986). Building the foundations for sentence production in a nonfluent aphasic. *British Journal of Disorders of Communication*, 21, 63–82.

Just, M. A., Carpenter, P. A., Keller, T. A., Eddy, W. F., & Thulborn, K. R. (1996). Brain activation modulated by sentence comprehension. *Science*, 274, 114–116.

Kean, M. L. (1977). The linguistic interpretation of aphasic syndromes: Agrammatism in Broca's aphasia, an example. *Cognition*, 5, 9–46.

Kean, M.-L. (1978). *The linguistic interpretation of aphasic syndromes*. Montgomery, VT: Bradford Books.

Kean, M. L. (Ed.). (1985). *Agrammatism*. New York: Academic Press.

Kean, M.-L. (1995). The elusive character of agrammatism. *Brain and Language*, 50, 369–384.

Kegl, J. (1995). Levels of representation and units of access relevant to agrammatism. *Brain and Language*, 50, 151–200.

Kohn, S. E., & Lorch, M. P. (1989). Verb finding in aphasia. *Cortex*, 25, 57–69.

Kolk, H. (1995). A time-based approach to agrammatic production. *Brain and Language*, 50, 282–303.

Kolk, H. H., & Van Grunsven, M. J. F. (1985). Agrammatism as a variable phenomenon. *Cognitive Neuropsychology*, 2, 347–384.

Kolk, H. H., Van Grunsven, M. J. F., & Keyser, A. (1985). On parallellism between production and comprehension in agrammatism. In M.-L. Kean (Ed.), *Agrammatism* (pp. 165–206). New York: Academic Press.

Levelt, W. (1989). *Speaking: From intention to articulation*. Cambridge, MA: MIT Press.

Linebarger, M. C., Schwartz, M. F., & Saffran, E. M. (1983). Sensitivity to grammatical structure in so-called agrammatic aphasics. *Cognition*, 13, 361–392.

Loverso, F. L., & Milione, J. (1992). Training and generalization of expressive syntax in nonfluent aphasia. *Clinics in Communication Disorders*, 2, 43–53.

Loverso, F. L., Prescott, T., & Selinger, M. (1986). Cueing verbs: A treatment strategy for aphasic adults. *Journal of Rehabilitation Research*, 25, 47–60.

Luria, A. R. (1958). Brain disorders and language analysis. *Language and Speech*, 1, 14–34.

Luria, A. R. (1974). Language and brain: Towards the basic problems of neurolinguistics. *Brain and Language*, 1, 1–14.

Luria, A. R. (1977). *Neuropsychological studies in aphasia*. Amsterdam: Swets & Zeitlinger.

MacLennan, D. L., Nicholas, L. E., Morley, G. K., & Brookshire, R. H. (1991). The effects of bromocriptine on speech and language function in a man with transcortical motor aphasia. *Clinical Aphasiology*, 21, 145–155.

Maher, L., Chatterjee, A., Rothi, L. J. G., & Heilman, K. (1995). Agrammatic sentence production: The use of a temporal–spatial strategy. *Brain and Language, 49,* 105–124.

Martin, R. (1987). Articulatory and phonological deficits in short-term memory and their relation to syntactic processing. *Brain and Language, 32,* 159–192.

Martin, R., & Blossom-Stach, C. (1986). Evidence of syntactic deficits in a fluent aphasic. *Brain and Language, 28,* 196–234.

Martin, R., & Feher, E. (1990). The consequences of reduced memory span for the comprehension of semantic versus syntactic information. *Brain and Language, 38,* 1–20.

Martin, R., Wetzel, W. F., Blossom-Stach, C., & Feher, E. (1989). Syntactic loss versus processing deficit: An assessment of two theories of agrammatism and syntactic comprehension deficits. *Cognition, 32,* 157–191.

Mauner, G. (1995). Examining the empirical and linguistic bases of current theories of agrammatism. *Brain and Language, 50,* 339–368.

McCarthy, R., & Warrington, E. K. (1985). Category-specificity in an agrammatic patient: The relative impairment of verb retrieval and comprehension. *Neuropsychologia, 23,* 709–727.

Menn, L., & Obler, L. K. (1990). *Agrammatic aphasia: A cross-language narrative sourcebook.* Amsterdam: Benjamines.

Menn, L., O'Connor, M., Obler, L. K., & Holland, A. (1995). *Non-fluent aphasia in a multilingual world.* Amsterdam: Benjamines.

Miceli, G., & Caramazza, A. (1988). Dissociation of inflectional and derivational morphology. *Brain and Language, 35,* 24–65.

Miceli, G., Mazzucchi, A., Menn, L., & Goodglass, H. (1983). Contrasting cases of Italian agrammatic aphasia without comprehension disorder. *Brain and Language, 19,* 65–97.

Miceli, G., Silveri, C., Nocentini, U., & Caramazza, A. (1988). Pattern of dissociation in comprehension and production of noun and verbs. *Aphasiology, 2,* 351–358.

Miceli, G., Silveri, M., Romani, C., & Caramazza, A. (1989). Variation in the pattern of omissions and substitutions of grammatical morphemes in the spontaneous speech of so-called agrammatic patients. *Brain and Language, 36,* 447–492.

Miceli, G., Silveri, M. C., Villa, G., & Caramazza, A. (1984). On the basis for the agrammatics difficulty in producing main verbs. *Cortex, 20,* 207–220.

Mitchum, C. C., & Berndt, R. S. (1994). Verb retrieval and sentence construction: Effects of targeted intervention. In M. J. Riddoch & G. W. Humphreys (Eds.), *Cognitive neuropsychology and cognitive rehabilitation* (pp. 317–348). Hillsdale, NJ: Erlbaum.

Mitchum, C. C., Haendiges, A. N., & Berndt, R. S. (1995). Treatment of thematic mapping in sentence comprehension: Implications for normal processing. *Cognitive Neuropsychology, 12,* 503–547.

Mohr, J. P., Pessin, M. S., Finkelstein, S., Funkenstein, H. H., Duncan, G. W., & Davis, K. R. (1978). Broca's aphasia: Pathologic and clinical aspects. *Neurology, 28,* 311–324.

Nadeau, S. E. (1988). Impaired grammar with normal fluency and phonology. *Brain, 111,* 1111–1137.

Nespoulous, J.-L., Dordain, M., Perron, C., Ska, B., Bub, D., Caplan, D., Mehler, J., & Lecours, A. (1988). Agrammatism in sentence production without comprehension deficits: Reduced availability of syntactic structures and/or of grammatical morphemes? A case study. *Brain and Language, 33,* 273–295.

Porch, B. E. (1967). *Porch Index of Communicative Ability: I: Theory and development.* Palo Alto, CA: Consulting Psychologists Press.

Prescott, T. E., Selinger, M., & Loverso, F. L. (1982). An analysis of learning, generalization and maintenance of verbs by an aphasic patient. In R. H. Brookshire (Ed.), *Clinical Aphasiology Conference proceedings* (Vol. 12, pp. 178–182). Minneapolis, MN: BRK.

Saffran, E. M., & Schwartz, M. F. (1994). Impairments of sentence comprehension. *Philosophical Transactions of the Royal Society of London, Series B, 346,* 47–53.

Saffran, E. M., Schwartz, M. F., & Marin, O. S. M. (1980). The word order problem in agrammatism: II. Production. *Brain and Language, 10,* 263–280.

Schwartz, M. F., Fink, R. B., & Saffran, E. M. (1995). The modular treatment of agrammatism. *Neuropsychological Rehabilitation, 5,* 93–127.

Schwartz, M. F., Linebarger, M., Saffran, E., & Pate, D. (1987). Syntactic transparency and sentence interpretation in aphasia. *Linguistic and Cognitive Processes, 2,* 85–113.

Schwartz, M. F., Saffran, E., Fink, R., & Myers, J. (1994). Mapping therapy: A treatment program for agrammatism. *Aphasiology, 8,* 19–54.

Selnes, O. A., Knopman, D. S., Niccum, N., Rubens, A. B., & Larson, D. (1983). Computed tomographic scan correlates of auditory comprehension deficits in aphasia: A prospective recovery study. *Annals of Neurology, 13,* 558–566.

Shapiro, L. P., Gordon, B., Hack, N., & Killackey, J. (1993). Verb–argument structure processing in complex sentences in Broca's and Wernicke's aphasia. *Brain and Language, 45,* 423–447.

Shapiro, L. P., & Levine, B. A. (1990). Verb processing during sentence comprehension in aphasia. *Brain and Language, 38,* 21–47.

Small, S. L. (1994). Pharmacotherapy of aphasia: A critical review. *Stroke, 25,* 1282–1289.

Steele, R., Weinrich, M., Wertz, R. T., Kleczewska, M. K., & Carlson, G. S. (1989). Computer-based visual communication in aphasia. *Neuropsychologia, 27,* 409–426.

Stroemer, R. P., Kent, T. A., & Hulsebosch, C. Z. (1998). Enhanced neocortical sprouting, synaptogenesis, and behavioral recovery with D-amphetamine therapy after neocortical infarction in rats. *Stroke, 29,* 2381–2395.

Swinney, D., & Zurif, E. (1995). Syntactic processing in aphasia. *Brain and Language, 50,* 225–239.

Thompson, C. K. (1998). Treating sentence production in agrammatic aphasia. In N. Helm-Estabrooks & A. Holland (Eds.), *Approaches to the treatment of aphasia* (pp. 113–151). San Diego, CA: Singular Press.

Thompson, C. K., Lange, K., Schneider, S., & Shapiro, L. (1997). Agrammatic and non-brain-damaged subjects' verb argument production in constrained elicitation conditions. *Aphasiology, 11,* 473–490.

Thompson, C. K., & Shapiro, L. P. (1995). Training sentence production in agrammatism: Implications for normal and disordered language. *Brain and Language, 50,* 201–224.

Thompson, C. K., Shapiro, L. P., Ballard, K. J., Jacobs, B. J., Schneider, S. S., & Tait, M. E. (1997). Training and generalized production of wh- and NP- movement structures in agrammatic aphasia. *Journal of Speech, Language, and Hearing Research, 40,* 228–244.

Thompson, C. K., Shapiro, L., & Roberts, M. (1993). Treatment of sentence production deficits in aphasia: A linguistic-specific approach to wh- interrogative training and generalization. *Aphasiology, 7,* 111–133.

Thompson, C. K., Shapiro, L. P., Tait, M. E., Jacobs, B. J., & Schneider, S. L. (1996). Training *Wh-* question production in agrammatic aphasia: Analysis of argument and adjunct movement. *Brain and Language, 52,* 175–228.

Tonkonogy, J., & Goodglass, H. (1981). Language function, foot of the third frontal gyrus, and rolandic operculum. *Archives of Neurology, 38,* 486–490.

Tramo, M. J., Baynes, K., & Volpe, B. T. (1988). Impaired syntactic comprehension and production in Broca's aphasia: CT lesion localization and recovery patterns. *Neurology, 38,* 95–98.

Tyler, L. (1985). Real time comprehension processes in agrammatism: A case study. *Brain and Language, 26,* 259–275.

Vallar, G., & Baddeley, A. (1984). Phonological short term store: Phonological processing and sentence comprehension. *Cognitive Neuropsychology, 1,* 121–141.

Vallar, G., Basso, A., & Bottini, G. (1990). Phonological processing and sentence comprehension. In G. Vallar & T. Shallice (Eds.), *Neurological impairments of short term memory* (pp. 448–476). New York: Cambridge University Press.

Walker-Batson, D., Unwin, H., Curtis, S., Allen, E., Wood, M., Smith, P., Devous, M. D., Reynolds, S., & Greenlee, R. G. (1992). Use of amphetamine in the treatment of aphasia. *Restorative Neurology and Neuroscience, 4,* 47–50.

Weinrich, M. (1991). Computerized visual communication as an alternative communication system and therapeutic tool. *Journal of Neurolinguistics, 6,* 159–176.

Zingeser, L. B., & Berndt, R. S. (1990). Retrieval of nouns and verbs in agrammatism and anomia. *Brain and Language, 39,* 14–32.

Zurif, E. B., Caramazza, A., & Myerson, R. (1972). Grammatical judgments of agrammatic aphasics. *Neuropsychologia, 10,* 405–417.

PART III

Behavioral Disorders Associated with Aphasia

7

THE ACQUIRED DYSLEXIAS

MARGARET L. GREENWALD

A brief clinical assessment of reading is included in virtually all contemporary mental status examinations and aphasia test batteries. Acquired dyslexia (i.e., alexia) in previously literate adults is a common outcome of dementing illness and of ischemic infarctions due to occlusive cerebrovascular disease, but may also result from intracerebral hemorrhage, intracranial neoplasm, arteriovenous malformation, multiple sclerosis, and migraine. Historically, clinical classifications of acquired dyslexia have been closely tied to neuroanatomical theories, and reading was generally viewed as inextricably bound to the spoken language system. More recently, a psycholinguistic focus on critical variables of test stimuli and error analysis has led to more precise differentiation of behavioral subtypes of reading impairment across patients, and to better appreciation of the ways in which written and spoken language systems can be dissociated. Progress in defining behavioral indices of acquired dyslexia in the context of theories of normal cognition has enabled the development of computational models used in computer simulations of both normal and impaired reading behavior. The various contemporary approaches to reading research are rapidly expanding our understanding of how reading is normally accomplished, and the many ways in which reading can be disrupted by neurological disease or injury.

This chapter includes a review of the clinical subtypes of acquired dyslexia, the cognitive and neurological deficits that are thought to underlie them, and current approaches to the diagnosis of acquired dyslexia. It does not include a discussion of developmental dyslexia, or more than a passing consideration of current debates in reading research; for these, the reader is referred to other sources. Lastly, this chapter includes an examination of the clinical utility of detailed diagnosis in motivating distinct approaches to reading treatment, and the ways in which treatment outcome may inform theories of acquired dyslexia.

THEORIES OF NORMAL AND IMPAIRED READING

Neurological Syndromes

Traditional neurological classifications of acquired reading disorders reflected basic distinctions in the language abilities of neurologically impaired patients and the neuroanatomical disruptions thought to underlie these patterns of behavior. Clinicians observed that reading breakdown could be dissociated from breakdown of writing ability (thus alexia with or without agraphia; Dejerine, 1891, 1892), and noted that in some patients acquired dyslexia was accompanied by general impairment of the language system (i.e., "aphasic alexia") or of the visual system (i.e., "agnosic alexia") (e.g., Misch & Frankl, 1929). The various labels that have accumulated for clinical syndromes of acquired dyslexia may be unduly confusing to new students of these disorders. Generally, patients demonstrating "pure alexia" or "primary alexia" without agraphia have been distinguished from patients with both alexia and agraphia associated with more general language impairment, to which the reading disorder has been thought to be "secondary" (Table 7.1). Alexia with agraphia occurring in the absence of more general aphasic disturbance has sometimes been called "parietal alexia" (e.g., Hermann & Poetzl, 1926; Quensel, 1931). When alexia with agraphia is accompanied by substantial aphasia, the features of the reading disorder are often similar to those of the general language disorder (e.g., Benson, 1977), but this is not always the case (e.g., Kremin, 1993). ("Literal alexia," or the inability to read individual letters, was earlier included as a type of alexia [Hinshelwood, 1900; Benson, Brown, & Tomlinson, 1971], but may be better characterized as a form of anomia [e.g., Friedman & Albert, 1985].)

These clinical terms used to describe acquired reading disorders reflect important early progress in our understanding of the neuroanatomical and behavioral bases of acquired dyslexia. However, the extent to which observed dissociations among reading, writing, and other language functions could define theories of dyslexia was limited by the available assessment measures. Psycholinguistic analyses led to increasingly detailed behavioral descriptions of reading deficits. Neuroanatomical analyses progressed to include a variety of neuroimaging and brain activation techniques, as described below.

Psycholinguistic Syndromes

Psycholinguistic classifications of acquired dyslexia represent an approach in which the behavioral patterns of reading impairment are defined as they relate to cognitive and linguistic theories of normal language. Reading performance has been found to be critically dependent upon variables of reading stimuli, such as spelling regularity, imageability, word frequency and novelty, word length, and grammatical class. "Regular" words (e.g., "stamp," "flip") consist of common print-to-sound associations in English, while "irregu-

TABLE 7.1. Traditional Neurological Classifications of Alexia, Reflecting the Distinction between Alexia with and Alexia without Other Language Deficits

Alexia without agraphia	vs.	Alexia with agraphia[a]
Pure alexia[b]		
Pure word blindness	vs.	Parietal alexia–agraphia[c]
Subcortical alexia	vs.	Cortical alexia[d]
Agnosic alexia	vs.	Aphasic alexia[e]
Agnosic alexia	vs.	Visual asymbolia[f]
Visual alexia	vs.	Aphasic alexia[g]
Primary alexia	vs.	Secondary alexia[h]

[a,b]Dejerine (1891, 1892); [c]Hermann and Poetzl (1926); [d]Wernicke (1874), Kleist (1934); [e]Misch and Frankl (1929); Alajouanine, Lhermitte, and Ribaucourt-Ducarne (1960); [f]Brain (1961); [g]Luria (1966); [h]Goldstein (1948).

lar" (i.e., "exception") words contain uncommon print-to-sound associations (e.g., "shoe", "yacht") (Berndt, Reggia, & Mitchum, 1987). "High-image" or concrete words (e.g., "apple") represent concepts that can be easily imagined and that can be experienced through the senses, in contrast to "low-image" or abstract words (e.g., "although") (Kroll & Merves, 1986). "High-frequency" words occur often in language usage, while "low-frequency" words are used relatively infrequently (for the English language, see norms compiled by Francis & Kucera, 1982). Novel words or "nonwords" (e.g., "flig") can be pronounced, but they are neither comprehended nor recognized as familiar words (i.e., they have no semantic or lexical associations).

Various theoretical models of reading have been proposed to account for the performance of normal readers and the patterns of reading breakdown observed in acquired dyslexia (e.g., Morton & Patterson, 1980; Bub, Black, Howell, & Kertesz, 1987; Coltheart, 1985; Funnell, 1983; Patterson & Shewell, 1987; Patterson & Hodges, 1992). Figure 7.1 is a simplified schematic of many of the cognitive processes thought to be involved in normal reading.

Observed dissociations in the types of words that dyslexic patients were able to read led some researchers to propose a dual-route theory of normal single-word reading (e.g., Marshall & Newcombe, 1973; Coltheart, 1978; Allport & Funnell, 1981). According to this view, one route for reading a real word requires activation of its corresponding word form within an orthographic "lexicon" of previously recognized written words, and then activation of the semantic representation of the word; this "lexical–semantic route" was postulated to account for normal whole-word reading of all real words, whether regularly or exceptionally spelled. For oral reading, subsequent activation of the phonological form of the word (i.e., stored pronunciation) allows translation into spoken output. Dual-route theory also

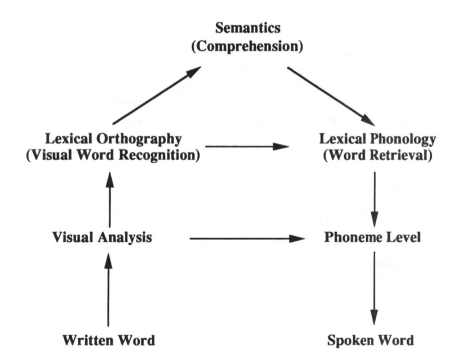

FIGURE 7.1. A simplified schematic of many of the cognitive processes involved in normal reading. Arrows are one-way for simplification only.

includes a "nonlexical route" to oral reading (often referred to as the "sublexical route"), whereby written words are analyzed visually and then converted to sound directly via print-to-sound translation that does not involve lexical or semantic activation (see Shallice & McCarthy, 1985, and Patterson & Hodges, 1992, for alternative views). The nonlexical route was postulated to account for normal reading of novel words or nonwords (which have no meaning or stored pronunciations) and of regularly spelled words, which can be pronounced correctly by piecemeal recoding of constituent letters into their commonly associated sounds. Words with exceptional spellings cannot be translated correctly via this nonlexical route. To account for some patients' ability to read aloud exception words that they do not appear to understand, dual-route theory was often amended to include a third "lexical–nonsemantic route" (e.g., Schwartz, Saffran, & Marin, 1980; but for an alternative view, see Hillis & Caramazza, 1991). One way to describe these reading "routes" and how they relate to one another is in terms of the cognitive subprocesses that are involved in each (see Table 7.2); these subprocesses are included in Figure 7.1 and are described further below.

Dyslexic patients were reported for whom one of these reading routes appeared to be impaired relative to the others, and who produced particular classes of errors. The types of reading errors patients produce can be linked to general areas of impairment within the normal reading process. In a "visual error" (e.g., reading "wheat" as "weather"), the error response is related to the target orthographically, in that at least 50% of the letters of the target word are reproduced in the error response (Coltheart, 1980). These substitutions are thought to reflect disruption to visual analysis or to orthographic lexical access (i.e., word recognition); they are often termed "orthographic errors" when they contain many of the target word letters but are unlike the target words in a strictly visual sense (Friedman, Ween, & Albert, 1993). A "semantic error" is related in meaning to the target word, either as a synonym, as an opposite, or as a semantic associate (e.g., reading "bread" as "butter"), superordinate (e.g., reading "dog" as "animal"), or subordinate (e.g., reading "tool" as "hammer"). Semantic errors may reflect impairment to semantic access, to semantic memory itself, or to semantic egress to phonology, or they may indicate disrupted activation of phonological word forms (Caramazza & Hillis, 1990b). A "phonological error" contains at least 50% of the same phonemes (i.e., sounds) as the target word in the same relative order (e.g., reading "pit"/ [/pIt/] as /pIk/), and is thought to reflect impairment to phonological word forms or their maintenance in short-term memory. A "derivational error" is related morphologically to the target word (e.g., reading "worker" as "working"; Patterson, 1980).

In some instances, reading errors can contain elements of more than one error category. An error may be related to its target word semantically, orthographically, and phonologically (e.g., reading "cart" as "car"). A "visual–phonological error" contains, in the same relative order, at least 50% of the orthographic units and also 50% of the phonological units from the target word. Finally, in a two-stage error (e.g., a "visual-then-semantic error"), the

TABLE 7.2. Components of Normal Reading Involved in the Central Reading "Routes"

Route	Pathway of activation (Figure 7.1)
Lexical–semantic	Visual analysis → lexical orthography → semantics → lexical phonology → phoneme level → spoken word
Lexical–nonsemantic	Visual analysis → lexical orthography → lexical phonology → phoneme level → spoken word
Nonlexical	Visual analysis → sublexical translation → phoneme level → spoken word

error response seems to reflect two errors occurring sequentially. For example, reading "thread" as "movie" may reflect two errors—first a visual error (reading "thread" as "theater") and then a semantic error (reading "theater" as "movie").

Psycholinguistic analyses of dyslexic error responses for subclasses of reading stimuli led to cognitive descriptions of general symptom complexes of acquired dyslexia. Table 7.3 includes a brief description of some of the characteristics of the acquired dyslexias.

TABLE 7.3. Traditional Subtypes of Acquired Dyslexia: Primary Features and Hypothesized Cognitive Deficits

Dyslexia subtype	Primary features/hypothesized cognitive deficits
Deep	*Primary features*: Poor nonword reading/worse than word reading. Word-reading performance: Commonly visual errors/many semantic errors; high-image > low-image words; high-frequency > low-frequency words; content > function words; regularly spelled = irregularly spelled words. *Hypothesized cognitive deficits*: All reading routes impaired, particularly nonlexical route; reliance on faulty lexical–semantic reading route.
Phonological	*Primary features*: Poor nonword reading/worse than word reading. Word-reading performance: Visual/derivational errors; only infrequent semantic errors. Sometimes content > function words; word reading less impaired overall than in deep dyslexia. *Hypothesized cognitive deficits*: All reading routes impaired, particularly nonlexical route; reliance on faulty lexical–semantic reading route.
Surface	*Primary features*: Fairly intact nonword reading/poor word reading, with regularly spelled > irregularly spelled words. Errors are often attempts to "regularize" the pronunciations of irregular words. *Hypothesized cognitive deficits*: Impaired lexical reading routes; reliance on relatively intact nonlexical reading route.
Neglect	*Primary features*: Impaired reading of all words/nonwords; visual errors with positional bias toward retention of letters on the left or right sides. *Hypothesized cognitive deficits*: Visual inattention to either left or right side of the written stimulus.
Attentional	*Primary features*: Impaired text reading, but preserved single-word reading. "Migration errors" are typical. Difficulty reading single letters within a word. *Hypothesized cognitive deficit*: Impaired ability to narrow visual attentional focus.
Letter-by-letter	*Primary features*: All word types are read one letter at a time. Reading latency increases as word length increases. Typical strategy observed in patients with pure alexia. *Hypothesized cognitive deficits*: Impairments to visual letter perception, to letter activation, and/or to letter position encoding have all been suggested.

Note. See text for hypothesized neuroanatomical correlates and further behavioral details.

"Deep dyslexia" (Coltheart, 1980; Coltheart, Patterson, & Marshall, 1980) refers to a pattern of acquired reading impairment in which the nonlexical reading route is impaired relative to the other routes, as evidenced by poor ability to read nonwords. However, the lexical reading systems are also impaired in deep dyslexia, as reflected in visual errors and many semantic errors (e.g., reading "clock" as "time") in word reading. Derivational errors and two-stage visual-then-semantic errors are common. Deep dyslexic patients read concrete/high-image words better than abstract/low-image words, nouns and adjectives better than verbs, and verbs better than function words (e.g., pronouns, conjunctions, articles, prepositions). The frequent occurrence of semantic errors in word reading is viewed as the cardinal feature of deep dyslexia.

"Phonological dyslexia" is similar to deep dyslexia in that the nonlexical reading route is impaired relative to lexical reading, yielding poor reading of nonwords (e.g., Beauvois & Dérouesné, 1979). Errors in nonword reading are often substitutions of visually similar real words. In word reading, errors are typically visual and derivational, and (in contrast to deep dyslexia) are only infrequently semantic in nature. A part-of-speech effect (i.e., nouns are read better than function words) may or may not be present (e.g., Patterson, 1982; Funnell, 1983).

"Surface dyslexia" refers to a relatively selective disturbance to lexical reading characterized by a regularity effect in word reading, such that exceptionally spelled words are poorly read as compared to regular words matched for length and word frequency (e.g., Marshall & Newcombe, 1973; Patterson, Marshall, & Coltheart, 1985). Pronunciation of nonwords and regularly spelled words is relatively intact, reflecting preserved function of the nonlexical reading system. Attempts to read exception words reflect dependence upon grapheme-to-phoneme translation, resulting in "regularizations" of exceptional print-to-sound translations (e.g., reading "yacht" as "yachet"). When these errors result in real-word substitutions, the target word is comprehended as it is pronounced (e.g., reading "shoe" as "show . . . like a movie.").

The dyslexia subtypes described above are sometimes referred to as the "central dyslexias," because impairment involves stages of reading that are central to language function (i.e., semantic, orthographic, and phonological representations). Several subtypes of "peripheral dyslexia" have also been described, defined by impairment of visual or visual–attentional processes that are thought to operate prior to activation of central reading systems during reading. "Neglect dyslexia" describes impaired reading of all word types, characterized by visual errors with a positional bias toward retention of letters on the left (e.g., reading "whisk" as "wheel") or the right sides (e.g., reading "mend" as "hand"). This error pattern has usually been interpreted as reflecting hemispatial visual inattention of the side of word targets that is contralateral to the patient's lesion site (e.g., Ellis, Flude, & Young, 1987; Warrington, 1991; Caramazza & Hillis, 1990a; Hillis & Caramazza, 1990), just as in hemispatial neglect (Jeannerod, 1987). However, right- and left-neglect dyslexia may not represent equivalent deficits, and there is evidence that a positional bias for errors to occur on the right sides of words need not reflect visual inattention (Greenwald & Berndt, 1999). The term "positional dyslexia" (borrowed from Katz & Sevush, 1989) has been suggested to describe those cases in which a positional bias is consistent across visual errors even when the task does not require processing in the "neglected" hemispace, as in reading words in vertical orientation (Ellis, Young, & Flude, 1993).

"Attentional dyslexia" refers to a reading disorder in which text reading is disrupted but single-word reading is preserved (e.g., Shallice & Warrington, 1977; Saffran & Coslett, 1996). This pattern of deficits has been interpreted as reflecting a visual attentional deficit that prevents narrowing of the attentional "spotlight" to focus on a single item in a multiple-item display (e.g., Shallice, 1988). Even though these patients read single words well, they have difficulty identifying letters within those same single words, and difficulty reading single words that are flanked by unrelated letters. A typical feature of this disorder is the production of "migration errors," in which target word letters retain their correct letter position within the word, but "migrate" to the wrong word in the presented string of words (e.g., reading "pan mill" as "man pill").

"Letter-by-letter reading" (sometimes called "spelling dyslexia") refers to the reading strategy adopted by many patients with pure alexia. In pure alexia (Dejerine, 1891, 1892), described above, reading of all word types is impaired, while spelling and other language functions are spared (but see Behrmann, Nelson, & Sekuler, 1998 for an alternative view). Many patients with pure alexia are observed to read in a striking letter-by-letter fashion, and their response time increases predictably with word length. This effortful strategy generally allows such patients to read aloud to the extent that letter naming ability remains intact (Patterson & Kay, 1982). However, letter-by-letter readers may develop undue reliance on this strategy and may be unaware of their own retained ability to comprehend many written words in normal whole-word fashion (Howard, 1991; Shallice & Saffran, 1986; Coslett & Saffran, 1989; Bub & Arguin, 1995).

The psycholinguistic syndromes described here offer a useful shorthand for characterizing the behavioral features of acquired dyslexia; however, these overall patterns of reading performance may reflect different underlying cognitive deficits in various dyslexic patients. Increasingly detailed behavioral assessment of dyslexia within and across individual patients has further defined these differences, contributing to more specific theoretical models of the cognitive subsystems involved in normal reading.

Beyond the Syndromes

Neurological disease or injury can disrupt one or more of multiple elements in the complex process by which visually presented strings of letters are converted to orthographic, semantic, and phonological codes for normal reading (see Figure 7.1). Lexical reading requires activation of orthographic knowledge (for recognition of real words), the semantic system (for comprehension), and phonological knowledge (for pronunciation). "Orthographic lexical activation" (i.e., visual word recognition) refers to the process by which written words are recognized and known to be familiar. Normal visual word recognition requires intact knowledge of words that have been previously encountered (often termed a "lexicon"), as well as intact processes for accessing this knowledge. Lexical activation is influenced by word frequency, in that high-frequency words are generally more easily recognized than low-frequency words. Recognition of written words as familiar, however, does not require comprehension of their meaning.

"Semantic activation" refers to the process by which the lexical knowledge in turn is associated with its corresponding meaning in semantic memory, allowing for written word comprehension. Semantic activation is generally easier for highly imageable or concrete words than for poorly imageable or abstract words. It is widely believed that the semantic knowledge activated from print can also be activated by spoken words, environmental sounds, viewed gestures, and other input modalities (see Shallice, 1988, for an alternative view).

"Phonological lexical activation" refers to the process by which knowledge of the phonological form of words is retrieved. Lexical activation is thought to be more difficult for low-frequency words than for high-frequency words (e.g., Caramazza, 1997; Dell, Schwartz, Martin, Saffran, & Gagnon, 1997). During oral word reading, phonological lexical activation can occur via the semantic system (i.e., the lexical–semantic route) or possibly directly via the orthographic lexicon (i.e., the lexical–nonsemantic route).

Oral reading of letter strings (words or nonwords) that contain regular correspondences from print to sound can be read via a nonlexical (i.e., sublexical) reading route, as described above. Both lexical and nonlexical reading require the following elements of visual analysis.

"Visual perception" of the written word is thought to involve computation of visual intensity changes across the visual field, the two-dimensional geometry of the visual image cast upon the retina, and subsequently the spatial locations of visible surfaces from the viewer's position (e.g., Marr, 1980, 1982). Reading can be disrupted at these early perceptual stages, or as the visual percept becomes increasingly elaborated prior to letter recognition and word recognition. Disorders of visual–spatial attention may also affect these perceptual and recognition processes (e.g., Hillis & Caramazza, 1995).

"Abstract letter identification" is made possible when the output from visual feature analysis is sent to a system for abstract letter recognition (Coltheart, 1981; Johnston & McClelland, 1980). This form of the letter, called a "grapheme," is abstract in the sense that one grapheme may be associated with many physical letter presentations (e.g., the grapheme for "G" would be activated for the visually presented upper-case or lower-case "g," and would be identifiable across different fonts and handwriting styles).

"Encoding of abstract letter position" is a required element of reading, as has long been suggested (Seymour, 1979). Greenwald and Berndt (1999) have recently presented evidence that graphemic order information can be selectively impaired by brain damage, disrupting both lexical and nonlexical reading (Greenwald & Berndt, 1999).

Following these elements of visual analysis and positional encoding, nonlexical reading is often thought to involve three separable stages for piecemeal translation of print to sound (e.g., Coltheart, 1985; Newcombe & Marshall, 1984; Shallice, 1988).

"Graphemic parsing" describes the segmentation of the input string of graphemes into units that correspond to individual sounds (i.e., "phonemes"). Whereas there is sometimes a one-to-one correspondence between the letters in a word and their corresponding sounds (e.g., "hot"), many English words contain multiple-letter segments that correspond to one sound (e.g., "ch" or "sh").

"Grapheme-to-phoneme conversion" refers to translation of graphemic segments into their corresponding sounds. This assignment of phonological representations to graphemic units is thought to follow graphemic parsing of letter strings, and can also allow "sounding out" of isolated letters. There is debate as to the size of the graphemic units that may best support functional reading (e.g., Kay & Bishop, 1987).

"Blending" refers to the assembling of a whole-word-like unit from the phonological units assigned during grapheme-to-phoneme conversion. Dérouesné and Beauvois (1985) have referred to this as the "phonemic stage" in nonlexical reading. Blending of phonological units is required prior to spoken output during oral reading.

Both lexical and nonlexical reading are thought to require activation of a "phoneme level," at which individual distinctive speech sounds are represented. In lexical reading this phoneme level should be activated after phonological lexical access, whereas in nonlexical reading it should be activated in the process of grapheme-to-phoneme conversion. In either case, these individual phonemes are thought to be maintained in short-term memory (i.e., the "phonemic buffer") during speech output.

One or more of these subcomponents of normal reading, or their input or output processes, can be impaired within and across patients with acquired dyslexia. For this reason, it is not enough to describe impairment to an overall "route" of reading, as in describing the syndromes of deep dyslexia and surface dyslexia. The same general pattern of impaired reading performance may be evident in a group of patients who each have a different locus of deficit within a particular reading route.

For example, the pattern of deep dyslexia may result from three different types of disorders (e.g., Shallice & Warrington, 1980): (1) impairment to the semantic system (and reliance on these deficient semantic components); (2) impaired access to the semantic system; or (3) impaired output from the semantic system. Semantic errors in reading may result from any one of these types of disorders. Recent evidence (Greenwald & Berndt, 1999) also suggests that semantic errors in reading may result from impaired orthographic lexical access, in that weak lexical activation may offer degraded input to the semantic system, resulting in semantic substitutions.

The impaired nonlexical reading observed in deep dyslexia and in phonological dyslexia may result from impairment to graphemic parsing, grapheme-to-phoneme conversion, or blending. In some patients, nonlexical reading impairment appears to be associated with reduction in short-term verbal memory (Berndt, 1992).

The impaired lexical reading evident in surface dyslexia may result from disruption to one or more of the lexical–semantic systems described above. Visual errors, often noted in phonological or deep dyslexia, may reflect impairment to one or more of the elements of visual analysis or subsequent orthographic lexical access.

Pure alexia may reflect different deficits across patients. Letter activation (i.e., the encoding of abstract letter identities from print) appears to be abnormal in some (possibly all) patients with pure alexia, though this prelexical deficit may differ in severity from patient to patient (e.g., Behrmann, Plaut, & Nelson, 1998; Behrmann & Shallice, 1995). It is also possible that the pattern of pure alexia may arise from impaired encoding of abstract letter order from print (Greenwald & Berndt, 1999).

Differential diagnosis of functional sources of reading deficit requires interpretation of patient performance across a variety of tasks of language, attention, and memory. Current techniques for assessing these subcomponents of normal reading are outlined later in this chapter.

The degree of independence and interaction among the normal reading subprocesses described here is a matter of debate (e.g., Henderson, 1985; Shallice & McCarthy, 1985; Ellis & Young, 1988; Behrmann, Plaut, & Nelson, 1998), though most current theoretical models of reading assume at least some degree of interactive activation. Variations of computational descriptions (e.g., parallel-distributed-processing models) include highly interactive systems of orthography, phonology, and semantics; these have been influential in recent years in attempts to specify the cognitive mechanisms underlying normal reading and the deficit patterns observed in acquired dyslexia (e.g., Seidenberg & McClelland, 1989; Plaut, McClelland, Seidenberg, & Patterson, 1996). In contrast to dual-route models, connectionist models of reading include distributed word representations that are encoded as patterns of activation computed over time and varying according to the availability of contextual information (Seidenberg, 1997). For recent discussion of neural modeling of cognitive disorders, see Reggia, Ruppin, and Berndt (1996).

Detailed interpretation of the deficit patterns of individual dyslexic patients within the context of theoretical models of normal reading offers a way to test the strength and generality of these models. Fine-grained descriptions of dyslexic error patterns are also likely to contribute to attempts to elucidate the neuroanatomical basis of the dyslexias.

NEUROANATOMICAL CORRELATES OF READING

The left-hemisphere perisylvian region is thought to support much of normal language function, and a wide variety of studies have examined how visual information for reading contacts these language centers during written-word comprehension and oral reading. These have included studies of the syndromes of acquired dyslexia, as well as attempts to isolate the subcomponents of reading described above. For example, in a study of regional cerebral blood flow in normal readers using positron emission tomography (PET), Howard et al. (1992) reported evidence for localization of a lexicon for written-word recognition in the posterior portion of the left middle temporal gyrus. However, the task of correlating particular brain regions with specific aspects of reading is a difficult one. The same general syndrome of dyslexia may arise in patients whose brain lesions vary in both size and specific location. Similarly, in functional neuroimaging studies, variations in experimental design may influence brain activity during reading, which may make it premature to associate specific reading processing functions with individual anatomical areas (Price et al., 1994). However, there is general agreement about some aspects of acquired dyslexia and associated areas of brain dysfunction.

Pure alexia (i.e., alexia without agraphia) is commonly associated with left-hemisphere lesions in the distribution of the posterior cerebral artery (Foix & Hillemand, 1925). Dejerine (1891, 1892) proposed that pure alexia results from disconnection of the calcarine region from the angular gyrus (thought to support word retrieval), with central damage in the white matter of the lingual lobule. Quensel (1931) stressed that damage to the splenium of the corpus callosum in pure alexia prevents visual stimuli from the intact right hemisphere from reaching the angular gyrus in the left hemisphere. Binder and Mohr (1992) examined the reading performance of a group of patients with infarction of the dominant posterior cerebral artery territory, and found that patients retained normal reading ability when their lesions were in the medial and ventral occipital lobe, sparing dorsal white matter pathways and the ventral temporal lobe. In their sample, global and permanent alexia was found only in patients with additional damage to the splenium, forceps major, or white matter above the occipital horn of the lateral ventricle. They observed that patients who read via a letter-by-letter strategy (i.e., spelling dyslexia) had large lesions affecting the ventral temporal lobe, which may participate in later stages of visual processing. In other reports, however, pure alexia has been observed following damage to the left occipital cortex without damage to the splenium (e.g., Behrmann, Black, & Bub, 1990; Behrmann & McLeod, 1995).

Some patients with pure alexia who rely on the letter-by-letter reading strategy nevertheless do appear to retain some residual whole-word reading ability of which they are unaware (e.g., Coslett & Saffran, 1989). Saffran and Coslett (1998) propose that this residual ability reflects covert reading with the right hemisphere, whereas letter-by-letter reading reflects operation of the left hemisphere, using information passed from the right hemisphere. However, it is not yet clear how much reading ability the right hemisphere is able to support, and whether or not graphemic processing may be a property of the left hemisphere (e.g., Miozzo & Caramazza, 1998).

Alexia with agraphia can be observed with or without substantial aphasia. When alexia and agraphia are observed without a substantial language disturbance, the associated brain lesion is often thought to be in the left hemisphere affecting the angular gyrus (e.g., Dejerine,

1892). When alexia is accompanied by Broca's aphasia, it has often been noted that the alexia resembles the aphasia (e.g., a concreteness effect—better reading of concrete/highly imageable words, as in deep dyslexia) and is associated with lesions of the dominant frontal lobe. Alexia accompanied by Wernicke's aphasia has often been noted to share features of the aphasia (e.g., no part-of-speech effect) and to be associated with lesions of the dominant posterior temporal lobe (e.g., Benson, 1977). However, as Kremin (1993) points out, some patients with nonfluent aphasias (e.g., Broca's aphasia) can read function words (e.g., Caramazza, Berndt, & Hart, 1981; Kremin, 1984) or even nonwords (e.g., Goldberg & Benjamins, 1982; Ross, 1983; Kremin, 1985), whereas some patients with fluent aphasia present with deep dyslexia (e.g., de Partz, 1986; Caramazza & Hillis, 1990b).

Thus deep dyslexia has often been associated with damage to left frontal association cortex and Broca's area. The relatively preserved whole-word reading of deep dyslexia, characterized by semantic errors, a concreteness effect, and a part-of-speech effect, has been postulated to involve the operation of an alternative reading system in the right hemisphere (e.g., Coltheart, 1980; Saffran, Bogyo, Schwartz, & Marin, 1980).

The neuroanatomical bases of phonological dyslexia, in which nonword reading is impaired, appears to vary across patients for whom both behavioral and neuroanatomical data are available, although stroke in the left middle cerebral artery distribution has been commonly reported. The angular and supramarginal gyri and the superior temporal lobe are often affected (Friedman et al., 1993). Surface dyslexia, in which nonword reading is relatively spared, is often associated with lesions in the left-hemisphere temporo-parietal cortex and frequently affects the superior temporal gyrus, although lesion site varies across patients with this general pattern of reading disorder. When Rumsey et al. (1997) used PET to examine regional cerebral blood flow in normal readers presented with real words and nonwords, results were consistent with activation of the left superior temporal gyrus during both reading tasks. Activation was greater during nonword reading than during real-word pronunciation.

The possibility that damage to the left frontal operculum may be involved in phonological dyslexia has been a topic of recent neuroimaging investigations of word reading (e.g., Fiez & Petersen, 1998). Sparing of left frontal cortex may be observed with surface dyslexia. However, the role of the left frontal area in the processing of visual words is a matter of dispute. Based upon electroencephalographic recordings of the time course of brain activation during reading in normal subjects, Posner and Pavese (1998) have proposed that frontal cortical areas are most important for the classification of input, whereas posterior areas serve mainly to integrate a single word into the context arising from a sentence.

There is some evidence that portions of the fusiform gyrus may be sensitive to relatively subtle differences in written-word stimuli. By recording cortical surface event-related potentials directly from the inferior temporal and occipital lobes in a group of normal readers, Nobre, Allison, and McCarthy (1994) observed that the anterior fusiform gyrus was sensitive to word–nonword differences and the semantic context in which words were presented, whereas the posterior fusiform gyrus was not. In a PET study of six normal readers, Price, Moore, and Frackowiak (1996) noted that word processing in the lingual gyrus is distinct from that in the posterior fusiform gyrus, with presentation rate and exposure duration of written stimuli yielding differential effects on brain activity across these regions.

Continued attempts to examine the neuroanatomical bases of reading and its disorders may contribute to a better understanding of both *where* and *how* normal reading processes are carried out. Rigorous experimental design across studies will be required for adequate assessment of reading in both normal and impaired subjects.

ASSESSMENT

Acquired dyslexia is often easily identified via screening tests of reading, such as subtests of the Western Aphasia Battery (Kertesz, 1982) or the Boston Diagnostic Aphasia Examination (Goodglass & Kaplan, 1983). However, the type and severity of reading disorder cannot be specified without more detailed testing of reading performance across tasks in which stimuli are controlled for factors known to influence reading performance (e.g., spelling regularity, word frequency, imageability, length). One commercially available assessment tool that allows measurement of more specific aspects of single-word reading is the Psycholinguistic Assessments of Language Processing in Aphasia (PALPA; Kay, Lesser, & Coltheart, 1992). Sentence and text reading are evaluated by a variety of tests, including, for example, the PALPA, the Schonell Test of Oral Word Reading (Schonell, 1961), and the Gray Oral Reading Tests—3 (Wiederholt & Bryant, 1992). Both single-word reading and sentence reading should be evaluated in a dyslexic patient, because attentional and contextual factors may differentially affect performance across these reading conditions. The assessment of reading is most informative when conducted in the context of a general language examination in which lexical and semantic processing can be compared across a variety of input modes and output modalities. The source of reading impairment may also be elucidated by further evaluation of related cognitive functions, such as memory and visual–spatial attention.

Oral reading and reading comprehension tasks provide critical information about phonological and semantic processing during attempts to read. Reading comprehension tasks require access to semantic meaning from print (as well as to syntactic processes in sentence reading). Oral reading tasks involve access to phonological systems, either in tasks that also normally include reading comprehension (i.e., real-word and sentence reading) or in nonlexical tasks (e.g., grapheme-to-phoneme conversion). In both oral and silent reading, specific patterns of reading breakdown, such as those described earlier in this chapter, can only be identified when accuracy of reading is compared across stimulus types (e.g., words vs. nonwords), and following inspection of the types of errors produced.

Selected methods often used to assess subcomponents of normal reading are listed in Table 7.4. Many of the reading tasks described here are included in the PALPA (Kay et al., 1992), and relevant stimuli are also found in experimental measures such as the Battery of Adult Reading Function (Rothi, Coslett, & Heilman, 1984), the Maryland Reading Battery (e.g., Berndt, Haendiges, Mitchum, & Wayland, 1996) and the Johns Hopkins University Dyslexia Battery (Goodman & Caramazza, 1986).

Assessment of visual analysis should address the possibility for impairment at several levels of visual elaboration of the written word. Early visual-perceptual processes can be tested with a task of physical matching of visual stimuli. For example, the patient may be asked to select two identical shapes from an array of three nonsense shapes, or to match two letters of the same case and font.

Activation of abstract letter identities (i.e., graphemes) can be assessed with a task of letter matching across case and/or font (e.g., matching "G" to one of three choices: "g," "c," or "e"), wherein physical similarity cannot determine the correct match. A second task that is commonly used to assess recognition of graphemes from print is the letter decision task. Here the patient is presented with a single real letter or a single nonsense letter, and is asked to respond "yes" or "no" to indicate whether the presented letter is a real letter in English. Of these two tasks, matching letters across case and font may be more sensitive to disruption to abstract letter recognition, in that it imposes a larger visual load and requires that the correct match be selected from a group of real letters. In contrast, it

TABLE 7.4. Examples of Common Tasks Used to Test Elements of Reading Function

Component of reading	Task examples
Early visual perception	Physical matching of shapes/letters
Abstract letter identification	Matching letters across case and font
	Letter decision (real/nonreal letters)
Encoding of abstract letter order	Discriminating word pairs with high degree of letter overlap
Visual word recognition	Visual lexical decision
Semantic processing	Category sorting
	Cross-modality matching
	Verification of cross-modality match
	Matching semantic associates
	Synonym judgments
	Definitions
	Comparisons across inputs/outputs
Lexical-phonological retrieval	Word rhyme judgments
	Comparisons across inputs
Grapheme parsing	Orthographic segmentation
Grapheme-to-phoneme conversion	Letter sounding
Blending	Phoneme blending
	Syllable blending

is possible that less specific knowledge of graphemes may support good performance in the letter decision task, which requires a gross distinction between real and nonreal letter shapes.

Various tasks of visual–spatial attention relevant to reading are described in reports of patients with neglect dyslexia or attentional dyslexia; these have not been listed in Table 7.4. Patients with right-hemisphere lesions who exhibit visual inattention to the left sides of written words also demonstrate hemispatial visual neglect to the left sides of objects or other nonlanguage visual stimuli (e.g., Ellis et al., 1987; Riddoch, Humphreys, Cleton, & Fery, 1990). However, patients with left-hemisphere lesions, whose error pattern in single-word reading includes a tendency to make errors on the rightmost sides of written words, may or may not demonstrate a frank spatial neglect of right hemispace in other tasks (e.g., Greenwald & Berndt, 1999; Hillis & Caramazza, 1990; Buxbaum & Coslett, 1996).

In the absence of apparent visual neglect, a bias toward right-sided errors in word reading may have an ordinal basis rather than a spatial one, reflecting impaired knowledge of abstract letter positions that are encoded in ordinal format (Greenwald & Berndt, 1999). On this account, an ordinal code normally mediates between serial (phonological) and spatial (visual) codes during reading. In patients with intact auditory processing, one way to differentiate an ordinal graphemic disorder from visual–spatial neglect is to compare performance on two types of tasks involving matching of written and auditory words: a task with distractor words that are strongly biased spatially (e.g., "stock" as a distractor for "storm"), and a task with distractors that contain all of the target words' letters but in a different order (e.g., "spots" as a distractor for "stop"). A patient who is neglecting the right sides of written words will have relatively more difficulty rejecting the spatially related distractors, because doing so will require attention to the right sides of the target and distractor words. In contrast, a patient with a deficit in encoding the order of graphemes in written words will have more difficulty rejecting distractors that share all the target words' letters but in the wrong order.

Lexical access from the written word (i.e., visual word recognition) is typically assessed via tasks of visual lexical decision. These tasks involve presenting patients with a written word or nonword and asking them to report whether the stimulus is a real word or not (e.g., Waters & Seidenberg, 1985). Equal numbers of real words and nonwords should be administered. Accuracy can be analyzed along several dimensions: words versus nonwords, high-frequency versus low-frequency words, high-image versus low-image words, regularly spelled versus exception words, and "legal" nonwords versus nonwords that are "illegal" (i.e., do not follow the rules of English orthography). Reaction times (for correct responses only) can also be compared across these classes of stimuli. Better performance in rejecting illegal nonwords compared to legal nonwords is typical, even in patients with impaired lexical access, and high-frequency words are typically accessed more easily than low-frequency words. In the event that the patient performs very poorly in visual lexical decision, the lexical decision task should also be given in other modalities (e.g., auditory lexical decision), in an attempt to determine whether or not the patient understands the task directions.

Impaired semantic processing can result from degraded input to semantics from a primary deficit at the prelexical and/or lexical levels, as described above; from a specific deficit in semantic access; or from disruption to the semantic system itself. If visual lexical decision is intact (even for low-frequency and abstract words), impaired single-word comprehension may reflect either impaired semantic access or impaired semantics. These two sources can be differentiated by comparison of single-word comprehension across input modalities. Whereas disruption to the semantic system itself is thought to affect single-word comprehension across input modalities and output modes, semantic access impairment can be modality-specific (e.g., affecting visual stimuli but not auditory input).

Severely impaired comprehension of written words can be apparent even when only gross semantic distinctions are required. One way of measuring the amount of semantic specificity that the patient is able to obtain from the written word alone is to ask the patient to sort single written words into two piles based upon their meaning. In this sorting task, semantic categories representing varying levels of stimulus difficulty can be presented. For example, relatively less semantic information is required to sort words into "distant" categories (e.g., vehicles vs. clothes) than to sort them into "close" categories (e.g., office items vs. kitchen items) or items "within category" (e.g., summer clothes vs. winter clothes). If the patient is unable to perform this sorting task, the examiner may choose to identify the two target semantic categories or to begin the task, to see whether this assists the patient in sorting the remainder of written words.

Cross-modality matching is often used to assess comprehension of single words. For example, a single written word may be matched to one of several presented pictures. The types of errors produced in these matching tasks can be clues as to the underlying source of comprehension impairment, when the distractors included in the task are properly controlled. If a patient often selects distractors that are semantically related to the target, for example, this suggests some degree of semantic activation from the written word, albeit not sufficient to specify the correct target. A tendency to select pictures visually related to the target picture may indicate a disruption to visual processing of pictures. Selections of pictures that represent written words visually related to the target word (e.g., for "shell," selecting a picture of a shelf) may reflect impaired lexical access from print.

Matching written words to pictures or to spoken words may be easier than sorting written words into semantic categories, if the patient has relatively intact ability to comprehend pictures or spoken words. That is, even when impaired comprehension of the written word *alone* is demonstrated in category sorting, the additional picture or auditory stimuli provided in the matching task may boost the semantic system enough that degraded input from print can activate the correct target. Thus, in some cases, the semantic category task with "close" or "within-category" distractors may be more sensitive as a measure of semantic impairment. The utility of the cross-modality matching task for detecting impairments to semantics or to semantic access from print can be increased by presenting a greater number of choices for each item, or a greater number of distractors that are semantically related to the target.

Verification of correct or incorrect cross-modality matches can be difficult for some patients who nevertheless perform well in the forced-choice cross-modality matching tasks just described. In the verification task, the patient is presented with two items (e.g., a written word and a picture) and asked to respond "yes" or "no" to indicate whether the two items match. In contrast to the cross-modality matching tasks, in which the correct match is available and the patient is required to "guess" a match, the verification task does not always include a correct match and therefore is particularly difficult for patients who are uncertain of the meaning of written words. Although these patients may be able to sort written words into categories (at least distant categories) and to match written words to their corresponding pictures, they may not be aware that their responses are correct and may believe that they are responding incorrectly. The verification task is particularly sensitive as a measure of this uncertainty; poor performance appears to indicate that semantic knowledge is not activated strongly enough to support awareness of that knowledge.

One matching task that is often sensitive to higher-order semantic impairments requires the ability to detect associated semantic concepts. A task involving matching of semantic associates can be used to measure semantic activation within a particular input modality. For example, a single picture can be matched to a choice of two or three pictures, one of which is related semantically to the first picture (e.g., for a picture of soup, pictures of a spoon and a knife); or a written word can be matched to a choice of written words. Additional methods often used for assessing higher-order semantic knowledge include having a patient judge whether two words are synonyms or not, and having the patient provide definitions of single words.

Access to lexical-phonological representations from the written word can be assessed by asking the patient to decide whether two written words rhyme with one another. The written stimuli should be controlled so that correct rhyme judgments cannot be made on the basis of spelling similarity (e.g., "trade–grade," "fever–never," "moose–juice"). Possible disruption to lexical phonology itself can be assessed by comparing oral naming performance across a variety of stimuli (e.g., pictures, written words, viewed objects, tactile objects, orally spelled words, environmental sounds, auditory definitions). If oral naming is inordinately impaired for written words as compared to other types of input, this suggests a deficit earlier in the oral reading process than within lexical phonology itself.

Nonlexical reading ability can be assessed with various tasks of grapheme parsing, grapheme-to-phoneme conversion, and blending (e.g., Berndt, 1992). Graphemic parsing can be evaluated by having the patient attempt to segment printed letter strings into smaller units. For example, the patient may be asked to circle words embedded in nonword strings, to segment real-word stems from inflections, or to indicate syllable boundaries in written words. Grapheme-to-phoneme associations are typically assessed by asking the patient to pronounce the sound that is most frequently associated with a printed letter or letter combination (e.g., "s" or "sh"). The blending component can be tested in tasks requiring the patient to blend separate aurally presented elements into a whole (e.g., blending syllables, phonemes, or the initial phoneme with the remaining "body" of a word). Even though the presented elements may be separated by 2 seconds or more during aural presentation, the patient may recognize that some presented elements form a familiar word when combined; this lexical knowledge may assist performance. For this reason, the ability to blend segments of nonword stimuli should also be tested.

Auditory–verbal short-term memory (i.e., working memory) is often assessed by digit span forward, in which the patient is asked to repeat strings of digits. Additional repetition tasks are used to assess output requiring articulatory rehearsal; other tasks that do not require spoken output can be used to address the possibility of impaired input to the phonological store (e.g., matching judgment tasks).

TREATMENT

Detailed evaluation of acquired dyslexia allows more specific identification of the functional source(s) of reading deficits in individual patients than is possible with more general reading measures. As the complexity of normal reading is gradually elucidated through progress in diagnostic techniques, there is hope that the equally complex effects of reading intervention can be specified across a wide variety of dyslexic patients. Specifying the source of deficit is a necessary step in designing individualized treatments for presumed impairments to various subcomponents of the normal reading system. The functional outcome of innovative treatments, as well as the efficacy of more traditional treatment approaches, can then be interpreted with detailed consideration of differences in cognitive abilities across patients, and of the personal, social, and environmental factors that are critical to treatment success. Sample treatments for acquired dyslexia are described here.

Pure alexia, often characterized by letter-by-letter reading, has been treated via both "restitutive" and "substitutive" approaches. Restitutive treatments, according to Rothi (1992, 1995), are designed to restore an impaired ability by facilitating the same functional processes that supported the ability premorbidly, in the same manner. These treatment approaches are aimed at maximizing recovery based on the reconstructive processes that are assumed to occur in the nervous system, particularly in the early months of recovery. With substitutive treatments, on the other hand, there is no attempt to restore the original system; rather, other systems or processes are recruited as permanent supports of the damaged system, or compensatory strategies for completing the task are trained.

One restitutive approach to the treatment of pure alexia is to attempt to discourage letter-by-letter reading through speeded presentation of written words, with the goal of encouraging reliance on the residual whole-word reading ability that many patients with pure alexia retain. This approach has met with variable success (e.g., Rothi & Moss, 1992; Rothi, Greenwald, Maher, & Ochipa, 1998). One patient studied by Rothi and Moss (1992) completed a 2-week program of twice-daily treatment sessions in which he was presented with single written words at speeded presentation rates in a semantic category decision task. As a result of this treatment (in which words were presented too rapidly to allow letter-by-letter reading), the patient demonstrated improved comprehension of rapidly presented written words, and did so at shorter exposure durations. The success of this restitutive whole-word reading approach may depend upon time elapsed since brain damage; the amount of residual reading ability available to the individual patient; or such related factors as the intensity of the treatment schedule, fatigue, and memory ability.

A second restitutive treatment approach to pure alexia, reported by Behrmann and McLeod (1995), addressed the characteristically slower reading of long words (i.e., the word length effect) in one patient with pure alexia. These authors attempted to convert the patient from a pathological, sequential approach to letter strings to a normal approach, in which the first and last letters of the string are apprehended together. They hypothesized that if the patient could learn to report the last letters of the string as quickly as the first (from speeded stimulus presentation), then the effect of word length on single-word reading would be minimal, as with normal readers. After nine treatment sessions, the patient continued to read longer words more slowly than short words, but treatment did result in significantly improved identification of the final letter of letter strings.

Letter-by-letter reading is generally viewed as a compensatory strategy spontaneously employed by many patients with pure alexia, but one that is particularly laborious and prone to error in those patients with poor ability to name letters from print (e.g., Patterson & Kay, 1982). Substitutive treatment approaches for pure alexia include kinesthetic facilitation of letter naming, in efforts to maximize compensatory letter-by-letter reading in patients with poor letter-naming ability. After practice in copying Japanese characters while reading them aloud, one patient reported by Kashiwagi and Kashiwagi (1989) demonstrated improved oral reading of familiar symbols that had been copied, even after the copying practice was discontinued and only oral reading practice continued. This improvement in oral reading did not extend to unfamiliar symbols that had not been copied. In an attempt to improve visual identification and oral naming of written letters in one patient with pure alexia, Lott, Friedman, and Linebaugh (1994) trained the patient to trace letters onto the palm of his hand during oral letter naming, thus incorporating both tactile and kinesthetic cues into treatment. This approach resulted in improved reading of trained words and, importantly, generalization of training to untrained words. Maher, Clayton, Barrett, Schober-Peterson, and Rothi (1998) recently observed a striking dissociation in reading ability across input modalities in another patient with pure alexia, who was unable to read from print alone but was able to read aloud with 100% accuracy when she used her finger to pretend to copy the letters in words and sentences. After 4 weeks of intervention aimed at maximizing the patient's use of this motor cross-cueing strategy, the patient was able to read while copying from print at double the pretreatment speed. Kinesthetic cues were also used to aid letter naming in a patient who had no reading ability and a profound cross-modality anomia, including letter anomia in visual, tactile, and motor/kinesthetic input modalities (Greenwald & Rothi, 1998). Detailed assessment of this patient's language suggested an excellent prognosis for letter-by-letter reading, by virtue of a remarkable sparing of the ability to pronounce orally spelled words. Daily letter-naming treatment over the course of 6 weeks led to significantly improved oral naming of printed letters, and to slow but successful letter-by-letter reading.

One treatment method aimed at increasing reading speed in pure alexia is the "multiple oral rereading" (MOR) technique (Moyer, 1979). This approach involves giving the patient repetitive practice in reading the same short text passage. Toumainen and Laine (1991) reported that this technique led to improved text-reading for some patients; interestingly, reading performance on lists of single words did not improve. Beeson and Insalaco (1998) also reported increased text-reading speed in two aphasic patients with acquired dyslexia, after a treatment protocol that incorporated use of the MOR technique followed by additional training in reading phase-formatted text. For these patients, the effect of treatment on text-reading speed did generalize to untrained text.

Surface dyslexia (i.e., impairment to lexical reading, with relative sparing of nonlexical phonological reading) has been the target of several reading treatment studies. Byng and Coltheart (1986) reported an attempt to train lexical whole-word reading in one patient with surface dyslexia who had an underlying impairment at the level of visual word recognition. The treatment was designed to facilitate reading of irregularly spelled words by presentation of each word with a picture as a mnemonic aid. Posttreatment assessment was consistent with improved reading of both trained and untrained word sets, with greater improvement noted for the trained set. During subsequent treatment of the same patient, generalization of the training to untrained words was again observed. Weekes and Coltheart (1996), using the treatment method of Byng and Coltheart (1986), attempted to train lexical reading in another patient with surface dyslexia. Again, lexical training using this technique resulted in significantly improved reading of trained words, as well as significant generalization of training to the reading of untrained words.

Friedman and Robinson (1991) designed a different treatment to facilitate lexical whole-word reading in their patient with surface dyslexia. Rather than incorporating a mnemonic or other intermediate aid to learning, they focused on direct training of a set of words with ambiguous pronunciations of specific letter clusters. Across seven treatment sessions (accompanied by home practice) in a 13-week period, the patient's oral reading of trained words steadily improved; reading performance given untrained words fluctuated but did not significantly improve.

Scott and Byng (1989) addressed a severe impairment in comprehension of written homophones in another patient with surface dyslexia, whose reading performance was consistent with partial disconnection of the visual word recognition system from the semantic system. The treatment protocol involved computer presentation of a reading task requiring comprehension of homophones in sentence context. After 10 weeks of training, significant improvement in homophone comprehension was observed for both trained and untrained homophones.

In an attempt to increase reading speed in a patient with surface dyslexia whose reading rate was extremely slow, Moss, Rothi, and Fennell (1991) employed the speeded presentation method described earlier for the treatment of pure alexia (Rothi & Moss, 1992). With the overall goal of enhancing lexical reading, these authors asked their patient to name the semantic category of target words presented at a speed too rapid to allow reading aloud. Ten treatment sessions using this technique resulted in a dramatic decrease in processing time in all reading tasks, including a maintenance of accuracy in reading irregular words at decreasing presentation rates.

Treatment approaches for deep dyslexia (i.e., poor nonlexical reading and many semantic errors in word reading) have emphasized retraining the ability to translate graphemes into phonemes. For example, de Partz (1986) attempted to train grapheme-to-phoneme conversion in one patient with deep dyslexia by using the patient's lexical reading ability to facilitate grapheme sounding. First, the patient was trained to associate each written letter target with a code word that began with that letter; second, each letter was associated with the first sound of the code word; finally, reading of short words and nonwords was attempted. After 9 months of intensive treatment, the patient demonstrated a dramatic increase in overall reading accuracy, and qualitative changes in error production (e.g., only one semantic error, and errors predominantly reflecting misapplication of grapheme-to-phoneme conversion rules). Additional sessions focused on training contextual graphemic conversion rules, after which the patient was able to read correctly but slowly. Although this patient was entered into reading treatment only 3 months after injury (far earlier than is typical in experimental treatments), and therefore spontaneous recovery may have contributed to improved reading, overall performance indicated that at least part of the change was a result of the treatment (e.g., comprehension of semantic categories that were not treated did not improve, whereas comprehension of trained categories did improve).

Nickels (1992) replicated the therapy approach of de Partz (1986) with a patient 16 months after injury. During a 10-week treatment program in which grapheme-to-phoneme correspondences were trained, this patient with deep dyslexia successfully mastered the task of producing the sound associated with a target letter. Oral word reading also improved; surprisingly, however, this change could not be attributed to improved operation of the nonlexical reading system, because the patient was unable to learn to blend phonemes into syllabic units. Rather, the patient seemed to use his knowledge of letter–sound correspondences to generate the first sound of a written word, and from this phonemic cue (if he knew the meaning of the word) he was able to pronounce the whole word. The treatment program thereafter focused on maximizing efficient use of this "autocue" strategy, which proved successful in facilitating both oral word reading and oral naming in conversation.

Mitchum and Berndt (1991) and Berndt and Mitchum (1994) described a treatment designed to facilitate first auditory analysis (see Lindamood & Lindamood, 1975) and then grapheme-to-phoneme conversion in an aphasic patient with deep dyslexia. Grapheme sounding was trained over 11 sessions in which individual letters were associated with pictures of objects beginning with each target sound. The patient was then asked to blend each target letter with a word "body" to make a real word (e.g., "j" + "eep" = "jeep"). Although grapheme-sounding improved significantly in this patient, she was unable to blend sounds sufficiently to form real words or nonwords. Interestingly, improved grapheme-sounding ability appeared to reduce this patient's production of semantic errors in word reading.

The treatment of phonological dyslexia has typically focused on training the conversion of graphemes into phonemes. This nonlexical reading component, as well as the ability to blend phonemes, is often thought to be tied to phonological awareness; that is, the ability to detect or manipulate the constituent sounds in words (Torgesen, Morgan, & Davis, 1992). Over a 2-month period, one patient with mild acquired phonological dyslexia was provided intensive reading treatment in which phonological awareness was specifically targeted for intervention, with the prediction that improved phonological awareness would lead directly to improved nonlexical reading (Conway et al., 1998). For this patient, the Auditory Discrimination in Depth program (Lindamood & Lindamood, 1975), which includes training in motor–articulatory awareness during phoneme production, enabled significant improvement in phonological awareness and in oral reading of words and nonwords. Moreover, the pattern of this patient's reading improvement during sequential stages of the treatment program provided evidence that treatment gains were a specific response to the treatment.

The possibility that general brain activation during reading treatment may lead to nonspecific effects of treatment on cognitive function is an important consideration affecting treatment design and interpretation, as is the possible role of spontaneous recovery of reading function. In a study of dyslexia evolution in one patient with pure alexia, Behrmann et al. (1990) reported a spontaneous decrease in reading latency from the acute onset of pure alexia to 1 year after onset. Klein, Behrmann, and Doctor (1994) reported improved reading performance (i.e., spontaneous evolution from deep dyslexia to phonological dyslexia) in a patient tested at 6 and 18 months after onset. In experimental treatments, issues of treatment specificity are typically addressed by including systematic measures of treatment responses to trained and untrained stimuli and across trained and untrained tasks. These methodological constraints can also partially address the issue of spontaneous recovery of reading function, in that they allow recovery of reading and other language functions to be evaluated in detail. However, though most experimental reading studies are delayed until at least 1 year after injury, the effect of spontaneous recovery on specific aspects of reading function (e.g., evolution of error type) even after that time is in need of further study. Also, while delaying treatment until after the early stages of spontaneous recovery reduces the probability that treatment effects may be influenced by spontaneous recovery, some types of restitutive treatments (Rothi, 1992, 1995) may be most beneficial during these early stages. There is therefore a great need for further investigations of reading recovery in both treated and untreated dyslexic patients, at both early and late stages after injury. Nevertheless, it cannot be denied that acquired dyslexia is responsive to appropriate forms of treatment (e.g., Weekes & Coltheart, 1996). Future studies can focus on the specificity of the effects observed to date.

Treatment for acquired dyslexia may yield benefits beyond those expected in reading performance. Katz and Wertz (1997) compared the effects of a computerized reading treatment with the effects of nonspecific computer stimulation or no treatment at all in a group of 55 aphasic patients with acquired dyslexia who were randomly assigned to one of the three experimental conditions. Although individual differences in dyslexia subtypes were not the focus of this study and thus were not reported, these authors reported that those patients who received reading treatment demonstrated significant improvement in overall language function, whereas patients assigned to the other two conditions did not. Interestingly, these results suggest that reading treatment may have the potential not only to improve reading specifically, but also to facilitate recovery in other areas of language function.

Finally, the results of methodologically rigorous treatment studies for acquired dyslexia can have theoretical as well as clinical implications. Just as theoretical models of normal reading provide a framework within which dyslexia can be interpreted, so clinical observations of reading breakdown force a constant modification of reading theory. Hypotheses about the underlying source of impairment in individual dyslexic patients can be tested in reading intervention studies, which represent one more way to advance our understanding of the complex process of reading and its disorders.

REFERENCES

Alajouanine, T., Lhermitte, F., & Ribaucourt-Ducarne, B. (1960). Les alexies agnosiques et aphasiques. In T. Alajouanine (Ed.), *Les grandes activités du lobe occipital* (pp. 235–265). Paris: Masson.

Allport, D. A., & Funnell, E. (1981). Components of the mental lexicon. *Philosophical Transactions of the Royal Society of London, Series B, 295,* 397–410.

Beauvois, M. F., & Dérouesné, J. (1979). Phonological alexia: Three dissociations. *Journal of Neurology, Neurosurgery and Psychiatry, 42,* 1115–1124.

Beeson, P. M., & Insalaco, D. (1998). Acquired alexia: Lessons from successful treatment. *Journal of the International Neuropsychological Society, 4*(6), 621–635.

Behrmann, M., Black, S .E., & Bub, D. (1990). The evolution of letter-by-letter reading. *Brain and Language, 39,* 405–427.

Behrmann, M., & McLeod, J. (1995). Rehabilitation for pure alexia: Efficacy of therapy and implications for models of normal word recognition. In R. S. Berndt & C. C. Mitchum (Eds.), *Cognitive neuropsychological approaches to the treatment of language disorders* (pp. 149–180). Hillsdale, NJ: Erlbaum.

Behrmann, M., Nelson, J., & Sekuler, E. B. (1998). Visual complexity in letter-by-letter reading: "Pure" alexia is not pure. *Neuropsychologia, 63*(11), 1115–1132.

Behrmann, M., Plaut, D., & Nelson, J. (1998). A meta-analysis and new data supporting an interactive account of postlexical effects in letter-by-letter reading. *Cognitive Neuropsychology, 15,* 7–51.

Behrmann, M., & Shallice, T. (1995). Pure alexia: A nonspatial visual disorder affecting letter activation. *Cognitive Neuropsychology, 12,* 409–454.

Benson, D. F. (1977). The third alexia. *Archives of Neurology, 34,* 327–331.

Benson, D. F., Brown, J., & Tomlinson, E. B. (1971). Varieties of alexia. *Neurology, 21,* 951–957.

Berndt, R. S. (1992). Using data from treatment studies to elaborate cognitive models: Non-lexical reading, an example. In J. Cooper (Ed.), *Aphasia treatment: Current approaches and research opportunities* (NIH Publication No. 93-3424, Vol. 2, pp. 47–64). Bethesda, MD: National Institutes of Health.

Berndt, R. S., Haendiges, A. N., Mitchum, C. C., & Wayland, S. C. (1996). An investigation of non-lexical reading impairments. *Cognitive Neuropsychology, 13*, 763–801.

Berndt, R. S., Reggia, J. A., & Mitchum, C. C. (1987). Empirically derived probabilities for grapheme-to-phoneme correspondences in English. *Behavior Research Methods, Instruments, and Computers, 19*, 1–9.

Binder, J. R., & Mohr, J. P. (1992). The topography of callosal reading pathways. *Brain, 115*, 1807–1826.

Brain, R. (1961). *Speech disorders*. London: Butterworths.

Bub, D. N., & Arguin, M. (1995). Visual word activation in pure alexia. *Brain and Language, 49*, 77–103.

Bub, D. N., Black, S. E., Howell, J., & Kertesz, A. (1987). Speech output processes and reading. In M. Coltheart, G. Sartori, & R. Job (Eds.), *The cognitive neuropsychology of language* (pp. 79–110). Hillsdale, NJ: Erlbaum.

Buxbaum, L. J., & Coslett, H. B. (1996). Deep dyslexic phenomena in a letter-by-letter reader. *Brain and Language, 54*, 136–167.

Byng, S., & Coltheart, M. (1986). Aphasia therapy research: Methodological requirements and illustrative results. In E. Hjelmquist & L. B. Nilsson (Eds.), *Communication and handicap* (pp. 191–213). Amsterdam: North-Holland.

Caramazza, A. (1997). How many levels of processing are there in lexical access? *Cognitive Neuropsychology, 14*, 177–208.

Caramazza, A., Berndt, R. S., & Hart, J. (1981). Agrammatic reading. In F. J. Pirozzolo & M. C. Wittrock (Eds.), *Neuropsychological and cognitive processes in reading* (pp. 297–317). New York: Academic Press.

Caramazza, A., & Hillis, A. E. (1990a). Levels of representation, co-ordinate frames, and unilateral neglect. *Cognitive Neuropsychology, 7*, 391–445.

Caramazza, A., & Hillis, A. E. (1990b). Where do semantic errors come from? *Cortex, 26*, 95–122.

Coltheart, M. (1978). Lexical access in simple reading tasks. In G. Underwood (Ed.), *Strategies of information processing* (pp. 151–216). London: Academic Press.

Coltheart, M. (1980). Deep dyslexia: A right hemisphere hypothesis. In M. Coltheart, K. E. Patterson, & J. C. Marshall (Eds.), *Deep dyslexia* (pp. 326–380). London: Routledge & Kegan Paul.

Coltheart, M. (1981). Disorders of reading and their implications for models of normal reading. *Visible Language, 15*, 245–286.

Coltheart, M. (1985). Cognitive neuropsychology and the study of reading. In M. I. Posner & O. S. M. Marin (Eds.), *Attention and performance XI* (pp. 3–37). Hillsdale, NJ: Erlbaum.

Coltheart, M., Patterson, K., & Marshall, J. C. (Eds.). (1980). *Deep dyslexia*. London: Routledge & Kegan Paul.

Conway, T. W., Heilman, P., Rothi, L. J. G., Alexander, A. W., Adair, J., Crosson, B. A., & Heilman, K. M. (1998). Treatment of a case of phonological alexia with agraphia using the Auditory Discrimination in Depth (ADD) program. *Journal of the International Neuropsychological Society, 4*(6), 608–620.

Coslett, H. B., & Saffran, E. M. (1989). Evidence for preserved reading in pure alexia. *Brain, 112*, 327–359.

Dejerine, J. (1891). Sur un cas de cécité verbal avec agraphie, suivi d'autopsie. *Mémoires de la Societe de Biologie, 3*, 197–201.

Dejerine, J. (1892). Contribution a l'étude anatomo-pathologique et clinique des differentes variétés de cécité verbale. *Mémoires de la Société de Biologie, 4*, 61–90.

Dell, G. S., Schwartz, M. F., Martin, N., Saffran, E. M., & Gagnon, D. A. (1997). Lexical access in aphasic and nonaphasic speakers. *Psychological Review, 104*, 801–838.

de Partz, M. (1986). Reeducation of a deep dyslexic patient: Rationale of the method and results. *Cognitive Neuropsychology, 3*, 149–177.

Dérouesné, J., & Beauvois, M. F. (1985). The "phonemic" stage in the non-lexical reading process: Evidence from a case of phonological alexia. In K. E. Patterson, J. C. Marshall, & M. Coltheart (Eds.), *Surface dyslexia: Neuropsychological and cognitive studies of phonological reading* (pp. 339–457). Hillsdale, NJ: Erlbaum.

Ellis, A. W., Flude, B. M., & Young, A. W. (1987). "Neglect dyslexia" and the early visual processing of letters in words and nonwords. *Cognitive Neuropsychology, 4*, 439–464.

Ellis, A. W., & Young, A. W. (1988). *Human cognitive neuropsychology*. Hillsdale, NJ: Erlbaum.

Ellis, A. W., Young, A. W., & Flude, B. M. (1993). Neglect and visual language. In I. H. Robertson & J. C. Marshall (Eds.), *Unilateral neglect: Clinical and experimental studies* (pp. 233–255). Hillsdale, NJ: Erlbaum.

Fiez, J. A., & Petersen, S. E. (1998). Neuroimaging studies of word reading. *Proceedings of the National Academy of Sciences USA, 95,* 914–921.

Foix, C., & Hillemand, P. (1925). Role vraisemblable du splenium dans la pathologie de l'alexie pure par lesion de la cérébrale posterieure. *Bulletin et Memoires de la Société de Médecins de Hopitaux de Paris, 49,* 393–395.

Francis, W. N., & Kucera, H. (1982). *Frequency analysis of English usage: Lexicon and grammar.* Boston: Houghton Mifflin.

Friedman, R. B., & Albert, M. L. (1985). Alexia. In K. M. Heilman & E. Valenstein (Eds.), *Clinical neuropsychology* (2nd ed., pp. 49–73). New York: Oxford University Press.

Friedman, R. B., & Robinson, S. R. (1991). Whole-word training therapy in a stable surface alexic patient: It works. *Aphasiology, 5,* 521–528.

Friedman, R. B., Ween, J. E., & Albert, M. L. (1993). Alexia. In K. M. Heilman & E. Valenstein (Eds.), *Clinical neuropsychology* (3rd ed., pp. 37–62). New York: Oxford University Press.

Funnell, E. (1983). Phonological processes in reading: New evidence from acquired dysgraphia. *British Journal of Psychology, 74,* 159–180.

Goldberg, T., & Benjamins, D. (1982). The possible existence of phonemic reading in the presence of Broca's aphasia: A case report. *Neuropsychologia, 20,* 547–558.

Goldstein, K. (1948). *Language and language disturbances.* New York: Grune & Stratton.

Goodglass, H., & Kaplan, E. (1983). *The assessment of aphasia and related disorders* (2nd ed.). Philadelphia: Lea & Febiger.

Goodman, R., & Caramazza, A. (1986). *The Johns Hopkins University Dyslexia Battery.* Unpublished manuscript, Johns Hopkins University.

Greenwald, M. L., & Berndt, R. S. (1999). Impaired encoding of abstract letter order: Severe alexia in a mildly aphasic patient. *Cognitive Neuropsychology, 16*(6), 513–556.

Greenwald, M. L., & Rothi, L. J. G. (1998). Lexical access via letter naming in a profoundly alexic and anomic patient: A treatment study. *Journal of the International Neuropsychological Society, 4*(6), 595–607.

Henderson, L. (1985). The psychology of morphemes. In A. W. Ellis (Ed.), *Progress in the psychology of language* (Vol. 1, pp. 15–72). Hillsdale, NJ: Erlbaum.

Hermann, G., & Poetzl, O. (1926). *Uber die Agraphie und ihre Lokaldiagnostischen Beziehungen.* Berlin: Karger.

Hillis, A. E., & Caramazza, A. (1990). The effects of attentional deficits on reading and spelling. In A. Caramazza (Ed.), *Cognitive neuropsychology and neurolinguistics* (pp. 211–275). Hillsdale, NJ: Erlbaum.

Hillis, A. E., & Caramazza, A. (1991). Mechanisms for accessing lexical representations for output: Evidence from a category-specific semantic deficit. *Brain and Language, 40,* 106–144.

Hillis, A. E., & Caramazza, A. (1995). Spatially specific deficits in processing graphemic representations in reading and writing. *Brain and Language, 48,* 263–308.

Hinshelwood, J. (1900). *Letter, word, and mind-blindness.* London: H. K. Lewis.

Howard, D. (1991). Letter-by-letter readers: Evidence for parallel processing. In D. Besner & G. W. Humphreys (Eds.), *Basic processes in reading: Visual word recognition* (pp. 34–76). Hillsdale, NJ: Erlbaum.

Howard, D., Patterson, K., Wise, R., Brown, D., Friston, K., Weiller, C., & Frackowiak, R. (1992). The cortical localization of the lexicon. *Brain, 115,* 1769–1782.

Jeannerod, M. (Ed.). (1987). *Neuropsychological and physiological aspects of spatial neglect.* New York: Elsevier.

Johnston, J., & McClelland, J. L. (1980). Experimental tests of a hierarchical model of word identification. *Journal of Verbal Learning and Verbal Behavior, 19,* 503–524.

Kashiwagi, T., & Kashiwagi, A. (1989). Recovery process of a Japanese alexic without agraphia. *Aphasiology, 3,* 75–91.

Katz, R. B., & Sevush, S. (1989). Positional dyslexia. *Brain and Language, 37,* 266–289.

Katz, R. C., & Wertz, R. T. (1997). The efficacy of computer-provided reading treatment for chronic aphasic adults. *Journal of Speech, Language, and Hearing Research, 40,* 493–507.

Kay, J., & Bishop, D. (1987). Anatomical differences between nose, palm, and foot, or the body in question: Further dissection of the processes of sub-lexical spelling–sound translation. In M. Coltheart (Ed.), *The psychology of reading* (pp. 449–469). Hillsdale, NJ: Erlbaum.

Kay, J., Lesser, R., & Coltheart, M. (1992). *Psycholinguistic Assessments of Language Processing in Aphasia (PALPA)*. Hillsdale, NJ: Erlbaum.

Kertesz, A. (1982). *The Western Aphasia Battery*. New York: Grune & Stratton.

Klein, D., Behrmann, M., & Doctor, E. (1994). The evolution of deep dyslexia: Evidence for the spontaneous recovery of the semantic reading route. *Cognitive Neuropsychology, 11*(5), 579–611.

Kleist, K. (1934). *Gehirnpathologie*. Leipzig: Barth.

Kremin, H. (1984). Comments on pathological reading behavior due to lesions of the left hemisphere. In R. N. Malatesha & H. A. Whitaker (Eds.), *Dyslexia: A global issue* (pp. 273–310). The Hague: Martinus Nijhoff.

Kremin, H. (1985). Routes and strategies: Data on acquired surface dyslexia and surface dysgraphia. In K. E. Patterson, J. C. Marshall, & M. Coltheart (Eds.), *Surface dyslexia: Neuropsychological and cognitive studies of phonological reading* (pp. 105–137). Hillsdale, NJ: Erlbaum.

Kremin, H. (1993). Reading and writing: Cognitive therapies of written language. In M. Paradis (Ed.), *Foundations of aphasia rehabilitation* (pp. 293–318). Oxford: Pergamon Press.

Kroll, J. F., & Merves, J. S. (1986). Lexical access for concrete and abstract words. *Journal of Experimental Psychology: Learning, Memory, and Cognition, 12,* 92–104.

Lindamood, C. H., & Lindamood, P. C. (1975). *Auditory discrimination in depth*. Austin, TX: Pro-Ed.

Lott, S. N., Friedman, R. B., & Linebaugh, C. W. (1994). Rationale and efficacy of a tactile–kinaesthetic treatment for alexia. *Aphasiology, 8,* 181–195.

Luria, A. R. (1966). *Higher cortical functions in man* (B. Haigh, Trans.). New York: Basic Books.

Maher, L. M., Clayton, M. C., Barrett, A. M., Schober-Peterson, D., & Rothi, L. J. G. (1998). Rehabilitation of a case of pure alexia: Exploiting residual abilities. *Journal of the International Neuropsychological Society, 4*(6), 636–647.

Marr, D. (1980). Visual information processing: The structure and creation of visual representations. *Philosophical Transactions of the Royal Society of London, Series B, 290,* 199–218.

Marr, D. (1982). *Vision*. San Francisco: Freeman.

Marshall, J. C., & Newcombe, F. (1973). Patterns of paralexia: A psycholinguistic approach. *Journal of Psycholinguistic Research, 2,* 175–199.

Miozzo, M., & Caramazza, A. (1998). Varieties of pure alexia: The case of failure to access graphemic representations. *Cognitive Neuropsychology, 15*(1–2), 203–238.

Misch, W., & Frankl, K. (1929). Beitrag zur alexielehre. *Monatschrift für Psychiatrie und Neurologie, 71,* 1–47.

Mitchum, C. C., & Berndt, R. S. (1991). Diagnosis and treatment of the non-lexical route in acquired dyslexia: An illustration of the cognitive neuropsychological approach. *Journal of Neurolinguistics, 6*(2), 103–137.

Morton, J., & Patterson, K. E. (1980). A new attempt at interpretation, or an attempt at a new interpretation. In M. Coltheart, K. E. Patterson, & J. C. Marshall (Eds.), *Deep dyslexia* (pp. 91–118). London: Routledge & Kegan Paul.

Moss, S., Rothi, L. J. G., & Fennell, E. B. (1991). Treating a case of surface dyslexia after closed head injury. *Journal of Clinical Neuropsychology, 6,* 35–47.

Moyer, S. (1979). Rehabilitation of alexia: A case study. *Cortex, 15,* 139–144.

Newcombe, F., & Marshall, J. (1984). Varieties of acquired dyslexia: A linguistic approach. *Seminars in Neurology, 4,* 181–195.

Nickels, L. (1992). The autocue?: Self-generated phonemic cues in the treatment of disorders of reading and naming. *Cognitive Neuropsychology, 9,* 155–182.

Nobre, A. C., Allison, T., & McCarthy, G. (1994). Word recognition in the human inferior temporal lobe. *Nature, 372,* 260–263.

Patterson, K. E. (1980). Derivational errors. In M. Coltheart, K. E. Patterson, & J. C. Marshall (Eds.), *Deep dyslexia* (pp. 286–306). London: Routledge & Kegan Paul.

Patterson, K. E. (1982). The relation between reading and phonological coding: Further neuropsychological observations. In A. W. Ellis (Ed.), *Normality and pathology in cognitive functions* (pp. 77–111). London: Academic Press.

Patterson, K. E., & Hodges, J. R. (1992). Deterioration of word meaning: Implications for reading. *Neuropsychologia, 30*(12), 1025–1040.

Patterson, K. E., & Kay, J. (1982). Letter-by-letter reading: Psychological descriptions of a neurological syndrome. *Quarterly Journal of Experimental Psychology, 34A,* 411–441.

Patterson, K. E., Marshall, J. C., & Coltheart, M. (Eds.). (1985). *Surface dyslexia: Neuropsychological and cognitive studies of phonological reading*. Hillsdale, NJ: Erlbaum.
Patterson, K. E., & Shewell, C. (1987). Speak and spell: Dissociations and word-class effects. In M. Coltheart, G. Sartori, & R. Job (Eds.), *The cognitive neuropsychology of language*. Hillsdale, NJ: Erlbaum.
Plaut, D. C., McClelland, J. L., Seidenberg, M. S., & Patterson, K. (1996). Understanding normal and impaired reading: Computational principles in quasi-regular domains. *Psychological Review*, *103*, 56–115.
Posner, M., & Pavese, A. (1998). Anatomy of word and sentence meaning. *Proceedings of the National Academy of Sciences USA*, *95*, 899–905.
Price, C. J., Moore, C. J., & Frackowiak, R. S. J. (1996). The effect of varying stimulus rate and duration on brain activity during reading. *Neuroimage*, *3*, 40–52.
Price, C. J., Wise, R. J. S., Watson, J. D. G., Patterson, K., Howard, D., & Frackowiak, R. S. J. (1994). Brain activity during reading: The effects of exposure duration and task. *Brain*, *117*, 1255–1269.
Quensel, F. (1931). Die alexie. In *Kurzes Handbuch der Ophtalmologie*. Berlin: Springer.
Reggia, J. A., Ruppin, E., & Berndt, R. S. (Eds.). (1996). *Progress in neural processing: Vol. 6. Neural modeling of brain and cognitive disorders*. London: World Scientific.
Riddoch, J., Humphreys, G., Cleton, P., & Fery, P. (1990). Interaction of attentional and lexical processes in neglect dyslexia. *Cognitive Neuropsychology*, *7*, 479–517.
Ross, P. (1983). Phonological processing during silent reading in aphasic patients. *Brain and Language*, *19*, 191–203.
Rothi, L. J. G. (1992). Theory and clinical intervention: One clinician's view. In J. Cooper (Ed.), *Aphasia treatment: Current approaches and research opportunities* (NIH Publication No. 93-3424, Vol. 2, pp. 91–98). Bethesda, MD: National Institutes of Health.
Rothi, L. J. G. (1995). Behavioral compensation in the case of treatment of acquired language disorders resulting from brain damage. In R. A. Dixon & L. Backman (Eds.), *Psychological compensation: Managing losses and promoting gains* (pp. 219–230). Hillsdale, NJ: Erlbaum.
Rothi, L. J. G., Coslett, H. B., & Heilman, K. M. (1984). *Battery of Adult Reading Function*. Unpublished manuscript.
Rothi, L. J. G., Greenwald, M. L., Maher, L. M., & Ochipa, C. (1998). Alexia without agraphia: Lessons from a treatment failure. In N. Helm-Estabrooks & A. Holland (Eds.), *Approaches to the treatment of aphasia* (pp. 179–201). San Diego, CA: Singular Press.
Rothi, L. J. G., & Moss, S. (1992). Alexia without agraphia: Potential for model assisted therapy. *Clinics in Communication Disorders*, *2*(1), 11–18.
Rumsey, J. M., Horwitz, B., Donohue, B. C., Nace, K., Maisog, J. M., & Andreason, P. (1997). Phonological and orthographic components of word recognition: A PET-rCBF study. *Brain*, *120*, 739–759.
Saffran, E. M., Bogyo, L. C., Schwartz, M. F., & Marin, O. S. M. (1980). Does deep dyslexia reflect right hemisphere reading? In M. Coltheart, K. Patterson, & J. C. Marshall (Eds.), *Deep dyslexia* (pp. 381–406). London: Routledge & Kegan Paul.
Saffran, E. M., & Coslett, H. B. (1996). "Attentional dyslexia" in Alzheimer's disease: A case study. *Cognitive Neuropsychology*, *13*(2), 205–228.
Saffran, E. M., & Coslett, H. B. (1998). Implicit vs. letter-by-letter reading in pure alexia: A tale of two systems. *Cognitive Neuropsychology*, *15*(1–2), 141–165.
Schonell, F.J. (1961). *The psychology and teaching of reading*. New York: Philosophical Library.
Schwartz, M. F., Saffran, E. M., & Marin, O. S. M. (1980). Fractionating the reading process in dementia: Evidence for word-specific print-to-sound associations. In M. Coltheart, K. E. Patterson, & J. C. Marshall (Eds.), *Deep dyslexia* (pp. 259–269). London: Routledge & Kegan Paul.
Scott, C., & Byng, S. (1989). Computer assisted remediation of a homophone comprehension disorder in surface dyslexia. *Aphasiology*, *3*, 301–320.
Seidenberg, M. (1997). Language acquisition and use: Learning and applying probabilistic constraints. *Science*, *275*, 1599–1603.
Seidenberg, M., & McClelland, J. L. (1989). A distributed developmental model of word recognition and naming. *Psychological Review*, *96*, 523–568.
Seymour, P. (1979). *Human visual cognition*. New York: St. Martin's Press.
Shallice, T. (1988). Specialisation within the semantic system. *Cognitive Neuropsychology*, *5*(1), 133–142.

Shallice, T., & McCarthy, R. (1985). Phonological reading: From patterns of impairment to possible procedures. In K. E. Patterson, J. C. Marshall, & M. Coltheart (Eds.), *Surface dyslexia: Neuropsychological and cognitive studies of phonological reading* (pp. 361–397). Hillsdale, NJ: Erlbaum.

Shallice, T., & Saffran, E. M. (1986). Lexical processing in the absence of explicit word identification: Evidence from a letter-by-letter reader. *Cognitive Neuropsychology*, *3*, 429–458.

Shallice, T., & Warrington, E. K. (1977). The possible role of selective attention in acquired dyslexia. *Neuropsychologia*, *15*, 31–41.

Shallice, T., & Warrington, E. K. (1980). Single and multiple component central dyslexic syndromes. In M. Coltheart, K. E. Patterson, & J. C. Marshall (Eds.), *Deep dyslexia* (pp. 119–145). London: Routledge & Kegan Paul.

Torgesen, J. K., Morgan, S., & Davis, C. (1992). The effects of two types of phonological awareness training on word learning in kindergarten children. *Journal of Educational Psychology*, *84*, 364–370.

Toumainen, J., & Laine, M. (1991). Multiple oral rereading technique in rehabilitation of pure alexia. *Aphasiology*, *5*, 401–409.

Warrington, E. K. (1991). Right neglect dyslexia: A single case study. *Cognitive Neuropsychology*, *8*, 193–212.

Waters, G. S., & Seidenberg, M. S. (1985). Spelling–sound effects in reading: Time course and decision criteria. *Memory and Cognition*, *13*, 557–572.

Weekes, B., & Coltheart, M. (1996). Surface dyslexia and surface dysgraphia: Treatment studies and their theoretical implications. *Cognitive Neuropsychology*, *13*(2), 277–315.

Wiederholt, J. L., & Bryant, B. P. (1992). *Gray Oral Reading Tests—3*. Austin, TX: Pro-Ed.

Wernicke, C. (1874). *Der Aphasische Ssymptomenkomplex*. Breslau: Cohn & Weigert.

8

AGRAPHIA

STEVEN Z. RAPCSAK
PELAGIE M. BEESON

"Agraphia" is the collective term used for various acquired disorders of writing caused by neurological damage. From a neuropsychological perspective, the writing process has two major functional components: linguistic and motor. The linguistic component is responsible for selecting the appropriate words for written output and for providing information about their correct spelling. In addition to retrieving the orthographic forms of familiar words from lexical memory, linguistic procedures can be used to assemble plausible spellings for unfamiliar words and pronounceable nonwords (e.g., "sprud"). Abstract orthographic (graphemic) representations generated by linguistic spelling systems are not specific to any particular modality of output, since they can be externalized in writing, oral spelling, typing, or spelling with anagram letters. Therefore, we must also postulate an independent set of procedures in writing that convert graphemic information into movements of the pen.

In the neuropsychological literature, agraphia is often discussed in relation to disorders of spoken language. This is a logical approach to take, considering that both in human history and in individual development, writing is a relatively late accomplishment that is superimposed on already established oral language skills. In fact, writing may be defined as a system of communication that utilizes conventional graphic signs to represent various-sized elements of spoken language (i.e., words, syllables, or phonemes) (Gelb, 1963; Ellis & Young, 1988). The close relationship between speech and writing is also evident in pathology, since aphasia and agraphia frequently coexist following damage to the language-dominant hemisphere. Given this common clinical observation, it is perhaps not surprising that a number of investigators have maintained that writing obligatorily involves phonological mediation (Wernicke, 1874, 1886; Grashey, 1885; Déjerine, 1914; Geschwind, 1969; Luria, 1947/1970).

One version of the phonological theory of writing dispenses with the notion of word-specific orthographic representations altogether and posits that written spelling involves segmenting spoken words into their constituent sounds, following which each sound is converted into the appropriate letter (i.e., "phoneme–grapheme conversion") (Grashey, 1885; Wernicke, 1886; Luria, 1947/1970). This view, however, is called into question by the finding that patients who completely fail at the task of converting phonemes into the corresponding graphemes can nevertheless write familiar words with a high degree of accuracy (Shallice, 1981; Bub & Kertesz, 1982a).

Another version of the phonological theory of writing accepts the existence of stored orthographic representations for known words, but maintains that these representations can only be activated indirectly via the phonological forms of the words (Wernicke, 1874; Déjerine, 1914; Geschwind, 1969). The problem with this position is that there are patients who can write words correctly despite severe phonological production deficits (Lhermitte & Dérouesné, 1974; Caramazza, Berndt, & Basili, 1983; Ellis, Miller, & Sin, 1983; Rapp & Caramazza, 1997a), and that even the complete loss of phonological ability is apparently not inconsistent with preserved writing (Levine, Calvanio, & Popovics, 1982). In addition, some patients exhibit better written than oral naming (Hier & Mohr, 1977; Bub & Kertesz, 1982a), and in some cases written and spoken output show dramatic differences with respect to syntactic word class (Bub & Kertesz, 1982a; Patterson & Shewell, 1987; Caramazza & Hillis, 1991; Rapp & Caramazza, 1997a).

Taken together, these observations indicate that access to orthography is possible even when the correct phonological word form is unavailable. This is not to deny phonological influences in normal spelling (Wing & Baddeley, 1980; Hotopf, 1980; Ellis, 1982); nor should the documented dissociations be taken to imply that we must postulate completely independent language systems for speaking and writing. In fact, it is generally assumed that high-level pragmatic, semantic, and syntactic operations are shared between the two major forms of linguistic expression. However, the neuropsychological evidence cited above does demonstrate convincingly that the linguistic mechanisms of speaking and writing diverge at the level at which phonological and orthographic forms of words are retrieved, and it suggests that lexical representations for spoken and written words are also neuroanatomically distinct. Complementary functional dissociations between alexia and agraphia have also been documented (Beauvois & Dérouesné, 1981; Bub & Kertesz, 1982b; Newcombe & Marshall, 1984; Goodman & Caramazza, 1986a; Behrmann, 1987), raising the possibility that, contrary to the classic view championed by Déjerine (1891), the orthographic representations used in reading and spelling may also be separate. In summary, it seems justifiable on neuropsychological grounds to consider writing a partially autonomous language skill. From a theoretical point of view, this implies that writing must have a specific cognitive architecture that includes processing components not shared by speech or reading.

In this chapter we review different clinical forms of agraphia encountered in neurological patients, and we attempt to interpret patterns of impairment within the framework of a cognitive information-processing model of writing. Our discussion focuses mostly on evidence obtained from single-case studies, as it is our belief that detailed clinical and experimental investigations in individual patients can provide valuable insights into the neuropsychological mechanisms of spelling and writing, and that such empirical observations can in turn be used to constrain theoretical models of the normal writing process. In the final sections of the chapter, we discuss the clinical assessment of writing disorders and provide a brief overview of the different approaches used in rehabilitation.

TOWARD A COGNITIVE MODEL OF SPELLING AND WRITING

The past three decades have witnessed a significant paradigm shift in aphasiology, characterized by attempts to explain aphasic performance with reference to information-processing models of normal language. As part of this new enterprise, a number of efforts have been made to construct comprehensive functional models of the writing process (Ellis, 1982, 1988; Van Galen, 1980, 1991; Margolin, 1984; Goodman & Caramazza, 1986a; Shallice, 1988; Roeltgen, 1985, 1993; Margolin & Goodman-Schulman, 1992; Rapcsak, 1997). The model of spelling and writing presented in Figure 8.1 is conceptually similar to the ones proposed by Ellis (1982, 1988) and Margolin (1984). Following Ellis (1982, 1988), we distinguish between "central" or linguistic processes that generate spellings for words or nonwords, and a special subset of "peripheral" processes which convert abstract graphemic information into motor commands for writing movements.

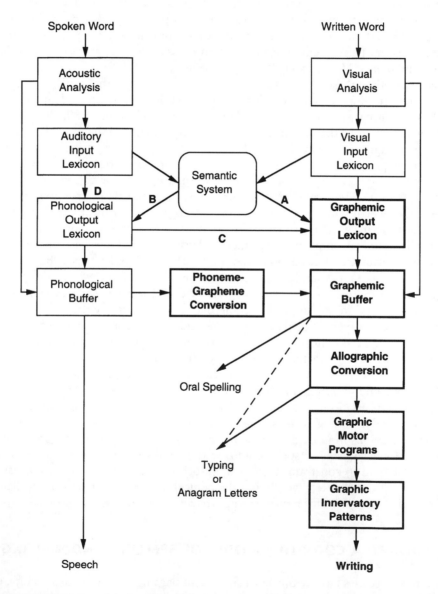

FIGURE 8.1. Cognitive model of spelling and writing. Central and peripheral processing components specific to writing are shown in boldface type.

Central Processes

Our model postulates three potentially independent central spelling routes: "lexical–semantic," "lexical–nonsemantic," and "nonlexical" (Table 8.1). The proposed routes differ with respect to the kinds of linguistic operations they perform and the types of spelling tasks they support.

Lexical routes are used to generate spellings for familiar words. Lexical spelling is accomplished by retrieving the orthographic representation of the word from the "graphemic output lexicon"—the memory store of learned spellings (Figure 8.1). Our knowledge concerning the content and internal organization of the graphemic output lexicon is still incomplete. At the very least, lexical entries must specify the number, identity, and serial ordering of the graphemes that constitute the spelling of a given word. Caramazza and Miceli (1990) have argued that graphemic representations are multidimensional in nature and also contain information about consonant–vowel status, graphosyllabic structure (i.e., the syllabic organization of graphemes in the word, as in "syl-la-ble"), and geminate features (i.e., letter doubling, as in "ru*bb*er"), independent of grapheme identity. It has also been suggested that the graphemic output lexicon is organized in a category-specific fashion with respect to syntactic word class (Baxter & Warrington, 1985; Caramazza & Hillis, 1991; Rapp & Caramazza, 1997a), and there is some evidence that affixed words are represented in morphologically decomposed form (i.e., that the root and affix in such words are represented separately) (Badecker, Hillis, & Caramazza, 1990). Finally, it is generally assumed that lexical entries for high-frequency words have lower activation thresholds than entries for low-frequency words (Morton, 1969).

Access to stored word-specific orthography plays a central role in spelling by both the lexical–semantic and lexical–nonsemantic routes. However, there are critical differences in the way orthographic representations are retrieved by the two routes. In spelling by the lexical–semantic route, a semantic code is used to activate the appropriate orthographic word form. Semantic input to orthography may be direct (pathway A), or indirect via the phonological representation of the word (pathways B and C) (Figure 8.1). Ellis (1982) has proposed that entries in the graphemic output lexicon are activated by simultaneous input through both the direct and indirect routes, providing a unique combination of semantic and phonological specifications for the orthographic target. In our model, the lexical–semantic route provides the only mechanism for incorporating meaning into writing. Therefore, this route plays a critical role in conceptually mediated writing tasks such as written composition and written naming.

Although under normal circumstances the lexical–semantic route is probably used in writing familiar words to dictation, this task can also be accomplished by the lexical–

TABLE 8.1. Central Spelling Routes

Route	Pathway in Figure 8.1
Lexical–semantic	Semantic system → (pathway A) → graphemic output lexicon (*direct route*)
	Semantic system → (pathway B) → phonological output lexicon → (pathway C) → graphemic output lexicon (*indirect route*)
Lexical–nonsemantic	Auditory input lexicon → (pathway D) → phonological output lexicon → (pathway C) → graphemic output lexicon
Nonlexical	Acoustic analysis → phonological buffer → phoneme–grapheme conversion → graphemic buffer

nonsemantic route. Spelling by the lexical–nonsemantic route relies on transcoding between spoken and written forms of the same word, using connections that bypass the semantic system (Figure 8.1). Presumably the heard word first activates its representation in the auditory input lexicon. This leads to the retrieval of the corresponding representation from the phonological output lexicon (pathway D), which in turn activates the appropriate orthographic word form in the graphemic output lexicon (pathway C). An alternative mechanism might involve direct connections between representations in the auditory input lexicon and the graphemic output lexicon (Patterson, 1986; Goodman & Caramazza, 1986a).

In contrast to the lexical procedures discussed above, the nonlexical spelling route is used primarily to compute plausible spellings for novel stimuli not represented in the individual's spelling vocabulary (i.e., unfamiliar words and nonwords). Spelling by the nonlexical route (Figure 8.1) utilizes a subword-level algorithmic procedure based on phoneme–grapheme conversion rules. This computation involves at least two distinct steps: first, the novel auditory stimulus is segmented into its component phonemes, following which each phoneme is converted into the corresponding grapheme. Whether the nonlexical spelling system performs subword-level phonological-to-orthographic translations based on individual phonemes and graphemes only, or whether larger units are also involved, is a subject of debate (Baxter & Warrington, 1987; Patterson, 1988). In addition, it has been suggested that the procedures involved in spelling unfamiliar words and nonwords may not be entirely nonlexical and may instead be based on lexical analogies with familiar words (Campbell, 1983). Developmentally, rule-governed nonlexical procedures are important in learning to spell, but they assume a subsidiary role once a sizable spelling vocabulary is firmly established. The influence of the nonlexical route is revealed by phonologically plausible spelling errors in normal subjects (e.g., "surch" for "search") (Wing & Baddeley, 1980; Hotopf, 1980; Ellis, 1982), suggesting that when precise word-specific orthographic information is unavailable, subjects may rely on a nonlexical strategy to generate candidate spellings. Note that in orthographically opaque languages like English, in which sound-to-spelling relationships are notoriously inconsistent (e.g., consider the different spellings of the long vowel sound /i/ in "she," "mach*i*ne," "n*ea*r," "m*ee*t," "p*ie*r," "rec*ei*ve," "p*eo*ple," "subp*oe*na," and "k*ey*"), the nonlexical procedure can only succeed with unambiguous or regular words that have highly predictable phoneme–grapheme correspondences (e.g., "must"). Ambiguous words in which the same phonology can be realized by using more than one combination of letters (e.g., "brain," "brane," "breyn," "brayne") and irregular words that contain exceptional phoneme–grapheme mappings (e.g., "choir") cannot be spelled correctly by the nonlexical route and require access to stored word-specific orthographic knowledge.

Spellings generated by the lexical and nonlexical central spelling routes, represented as spatially ordered strings of graphemes, are next processed in the "graphemic buffer" (Figure 8.1). The graphemic buffer is a working memory system that temporarily stores abstract graphemic representations while they are being converted into codes appropriate for various output modalities (i.e., writing, oral spelling, typing, spelling with anagram letters) (Miceli, Silveri, & Caramazza, 1985; Caramazza, Miceli, Villa, & Romani, 1987). This cognitive module thus occupies a strategic position between the central and peripheral components of the writing process. Dysfunction of the graphemic buffer results in abnormally rapid decay of information relevant to the identity and serial ordering of stored graphemes. Spelling errors typically take the form of letter substitutions, additions, deletions, and transpositions. Since word length is an important determinant of the amount of time an item needs to be processed in the buffer, errors are expected to be more frequent with longer words. Because information is normally retrieved from the buffer in a serial left-to-right fashion, letters toward the end of a word may be more susceptible to error, since they have to be retained in memory longer than letters at the beginning. It has also been proposed that, due to interference from neighboring items, letters in the middle of the word may be more vulnerable to degradation than letters in initial and terminal positions (Wing & Baddeley, 1980).

Peripheral Processes

Peripheral processing components specific to writing first come into focus below the level of the graphemic buffer (Figure 8.1). Externalizing graphemic information as movements of the pen is accomplished through a number of hierarchically organized computational stages. The first of these, known as the "allographic conversion" process (Goodman & Caramazza, 1986b), involves the selection of the appropriate letter shapes for the string of graphemes held in the graphemic buffer. In handwriting, graphemes can be realized in different cases (upper vs. lower) or styles (print vs. script). The various physical forms each grapheme can take are referred to as "allographs." Ellis (1982) has proposed that allographs are stored in long-term memory as abstract spatial descriptions that specify letter shape but not the absolute size of the letter. Allographic representations do not contain information about the sequence of strokes necessary to create a desired letter form or the specific muscles that are to be used for movement execution. Margolin (1984) has suggested that abstract letter shape representations or "physical letter codes" are also involved in other forms of "visually based" spelling (i.e., typing and spelling with anagram letters). Other investigators (Ellis, 1988; Black, Behrmann, Bass, & Hacker, 1989), however, assume that peripheral mechanisms for writing diverge from those involved in typing and spelling with anagram letters at the level of the graphemic buffer (broken line in Figure 8.1).

The remaining peripheral processing components in our model are directly concerned with the programming and execution of writing movements required to produce the letter shapes designated by the allographic code. It is assumed that abstract motor programs for writing are stored in long-term memory rather than being assembled de novo every time a particular letter is written. Stored "graphic motor programs" are analogous to, but distinct from, the visuokinesthetic engrams (Heilman, 1979; Heilman & Rothi, 1985) that contain abstract spatiotemporal codes for other types of learned, skilled limb movements. According to Ellis (1982), graphic motor programs specify the sequence, direction, and relative size of the strokes necessary to create a given allograph, without specifying absolute stroke size or duration. Although graphic motor programs are letter-specific, they are effector-independent in the sense that they do not determine which muscle groups are to be recruited for movement execution. Writing is typically performed with the distal muscles of the hand and wrist when one is using a pen, but writing on a blackboard is accomplished by the proximal muscles of the shoulder and elbow. One can also write by using different limbs (e.g., dominant vs. nondominant hand or foot), or even by holding a pen with the mouth. The fact that overall letter shape remains remarkably constant when produced by muscle effector systems with different biomechanical properties is consistent with the existence of effector-independent abstract motor programs for writing (Merton, 1972; Wright, 1990).

The final step in the writing process involves translating the information encoded in graphic motor programs into "graphic innervatory patterns" containing sequences of motor commands to specific muscle effector systems. It is at this stage that the appropriate synergies of agonist and antagonist muscles are recruited and concrete movement parameters specifying absolute stroke size, duration, and force are inserted into the program (Ellis,

1982, 1988; Margolin, 1984; Van Galen, 1980, 1991). Since the context of the writing task is never exactly the same, actual movement parameters must be computed "on-line" by the motor system. Once the kinematic parameters for the given biophysical context have been selected, the motor system executes the strokes required to produce the appropriate letters as a sequence of rapid ballistic movements.

Handwriting is a complex perceptual–motor task that requires continuous visual and kinesthetic feedback for maximum speed and accuracy. When feedback provided by afferent control systems is interrupted experimentally, normal subjects make characteristic errors that include a tendency to duplicate or omit letters or strokes when writing sequences of similar items (e.g., they write words with double letters like "street" as "streeet" or "stret"; they add or delete strokes when writing single letters containing repeated stroke cycles, such as "m" or "w") (Van Bergeijk & David, 1959; Smith, McCrary, & Smith, 1960; Kalmus, Fry, & Denes, 1960; Lebrun, 1976; Ellis, Young, & Flude, 1987; Smyth & Silvers, 1987). Margolin (1984) has suggested that sensory feedback plays an important role in updating graphic motor programs as to which strokes have already been executed. Sensory feedback is also needed to maintain the correct spacing between letters and words, and to keep the line of writing straight and properly oriented on the page (Lebrun, 1976, 1985; Smyth & Silvers, 1987).

NEUROPSYCHOLOGICAL DISORDERS OF WRITING

The value of theoretical models is ultimately judged by their ability to account for patterns of abnormal performance observed in the clinical setting. Ideally, different forms of agraphia in neurologically impaired patients should be directly interpretable with reference to specific functional components of the model depicted in Figure 8.1. The validity of this approach is predicated on the assumption that in addition to having psychological reality, the hypothesized processing modules are also neurologically distinct and can therefore be selectively impaired by focal brain damage. It is assumed further that the damaged processing component is identifiable through the careful analysis of impaired and preserved cognitive abilities, and that its putative neural substrate can be inferred from anatomical lesion localization studies. In so-called "pure" cases, only a single processing component is implicated, and observations in such patients can be particularly revealing from a theoretical point of view. However, brain damage does not necessarily respect the functional distinctions of cognitive models, and in clinical practice one frequently encounters patients with simultaneous damage to several processing components.

In our discussion of agraphia, we follow the major theoretical subdivision introduced earlier in the chapter and distinguish between central and peripheral forms. Central agraphias reflect damage to linguistic spelling routes or the graphemic buffer, and are manifested by qualitatively similar spelling difficulties across all possible modalities of output. By contrast, in the peripheral agraphias the damage is distal to the graphemic buffer, and the impairment primarily affects written production.

Central Agraphias

Based on their distinctive linguistic profiles, four major subtypes of central agraphia have been identified: lexical (or surface), phonological, deep, and semantic (Table 8.2). An additional form of central agraphia has been linked to dysfunction of the graphemic buffer.

TABLE 8.2. Central Agraphias

	Lexical	Phonological	Deep	Semantic	Graphemic buffer
Distinctive features	Particular difficulty spelling irregular and ambiguous words	Markedly impaired nonword spelling, with relatively preserved real-word spelling	Prominent semantic errors in writing	Impaired spontaneous writing and written naming; spared writing to dictation without comprehension	Errors of grapheme identity and order, observed in all spelling tasks and affecting all output modalities
Characteristic errors	Phonologically plausible renditions of target	Phonologically incorrect responses that may have visual similarity to targets; functor substitutions; morphological errors	Similar to those in phonological agraphia, plus semantic paragraphias	Special difficulty with homophones	Letter substitutions, deletions, additions, and transpositions
Linguistic influences					
Orthographic regularity	+	0	0	0	0
Word frequency	+	+	+	+	0
Imageability/Concreteness	0	+	+	0	0
Word class (content vs. functor)	0	+	+	0	0
Word length/position within word	0	0	0	0	+
Mechanism	Damage to graphemic output lexicon	Damage to nonlexical route	Damage to all three spelling routes	Damage to lexical–semantic route	Dysfunction of the graphemic buffer; defective short-term storage of graphemic information
Major spelling route used	Nonlexical	Lexical–semantic	Damaged lexical–semantic	Lexical–nonsemantic and nonlexical	All routes
Lesion location	Left posterior temporo-parietal (? angular gyrus)	Left perisylvian (? supramarginal gyrus)	Large left-hemisphere perisylvian	Heterogeneous left-hemisphere sites (often extraperisylvian)	Heterogeneous left-hemisphere sites (? fronto-parietal)

Lexical Agraphia

"Lexical agraphia" reflects the selective impairment of word-specific orthographic knowledge (Beauvois & Dérouesné, 1981; Hatfield & Patterson, 1983; Roeltgen & Heilman,
1984; Goodman & Caramazza, 1986a; Baxter & Warrington, 1987; Behrmann, 1987).
In lexical agraphia, spelling is strongly affected by orthographic regularity. Patients have
significant difficulty spelling irregular and ambiguous words, but they are much more
accurate in spelling regular words that strictly obey phoneme–grapheme correspondence
rules. Spelling performance is influenced by word frequency (worse with low-frequency
words), but not by imageability/concreteness or word class. Spelling errors typically consist of phonologically acceptable renditions of the target word (e.g., "serkit" for "circuit").
The preservation of nonword spelling is a characteristic finding.

The core linguistic features of lexical agraphia are best understood by postulating an
impairment at the level of the graphemic output lexicon. The loss or unavailability of stored
word-specific orthographic information forces patients to rely on the intact nonlexical route
to assemble candidate spellings. The nonlexical route can handle nonwords and even orthographically regular real words, but attempts to spell irregular and ambiguous words via
phoneme–grapheme conversion rules result in phonologically plausible errors. In spelling
by the nonlexical route, the choice of a particular phoneme–grapheme mapping option
may be influenced by the frequency with which that option is used in the language (e.g., in
writing the phoneme /f/, a patient is more likely to chose the grapheme "f" than the grapheme "ph," since the former is more common in English) (Goodman & Caramazza, 1986a).

Lexical agraphia is most commonly associated with left posterior temporo-parietal
lesions (Beauvois & Dérouesné, 1981; Hatfield & Patterson, 1983; Roeltgen & Heilman,
1984; Goodman & Caramazza, 1986a; Behrmann, 1987; Croisile, Trillet, Laurent, Latombe,
& Schott, 1989). Roeltgen and Heilman (1984, 1985) have proposed that the critical lesion
site is located at the junction of the posterior angular gyrus and the parieto-occipital lobule.
Lexical agraphia has also been described in patients with Alzheimer's disease (AD) (Rapcsak,
Arthur, Bliklen, & Rubens, 1989; Smith, Snyder, & Meeks, 1990; Platel et al., 1993; Peniello
et al., 1995; Croisile, Carmoi, Adeleine, & Trillet, 1995; Croisile et al., 1996; Hughes,
Graham, Patterson, & Hodges, 1997) and in patients with semantic dementia (Hodges,
Patterson, Oxbury, & Funnel, 1992; Patterson & Hodges, 1992). The impairment of lexical spelling in AD correlates with reduced metabolic activity in the left angular gyrus, as
revealed by positron emission tomography (PET) (Peniello et al., 1995). Taken together,
the anatomical observations in patients with lexical agraphia suggest that orthographic
representations for familiar words may be stored in or near the dominant angular gyrus,
making this region a possible neural substrate of the graphemic output lexicon.

Phonological Agraphia

"Phonological agraphia" reflects dysfunction of the nonlexical spelling route (Shallice, 1981;
Bub & Kertesz, 1982a; Roeltgen, Sevush, & Heilman, 1983; Roeltgen & Heilman, 1984;
Baxter & Warrington, 1985; Bolla-Wilson, Speedie, & Robinson, 1985; Goodman-Schulman
& Caramazza, 1987; Alexander, Friedman, Loverso, & Fischer, 1992). Clinically, the syndrome is characterized by markedly impaired nonword spelling with relatively preserved
real-word spelling. Errors in nonword spelling typically include phonologically incorrect
nonword responses and real words that have some visual or phonological similarity to the
target (e.g., "flig"–"flag"). The breakdown of nonlexical spelling in phonological agraphia
may be caused by at least two different types of processing deficits. Some patients cannot

write even single letters correctly when given their characteristic sounds, suggesting severe impairment of phoneme–grapheme conversion (Roeltgen et al., 1983). Others can translate individual phonemes into the corresponding graphemes, and in these cases the nonlexical spelling impairment may be related to an inability to segment nonwords into their constituent sounds (Roeltgen et al., 1983; Bolla-Wilson et al., 1985). In some individuals, both functional components are compromised (Shallice, 1981).

Theoretically, the selective impairment of the nonlexical route should only affect nonword spelling. Consistent with this hypothesis, real-word spelling in some cases of phonological agraphia was performed at a fairly high level (Shallice, 1981; Bub & Kertesz, 1982a; Bolla-Wilson et al., 1985). Other patients, however, also had difficulty with familiar words, indicating an additional impairment of lexical spelling (Roeltgen et al., 1983; Roeltgen & Heilman, 1984; Alexander et al., 1992). A number of observations suggest that residual spelling abilities in phonological agraphia are mediated by the lexical–semantic route. For instance, it has been demonstrated that patients are usually unable to write a word correctly unless they have access to its meaning (Shallice, 1981; Bub & Kertesz, 1982a). Furthermore, spelling performance is influenced by lexical–semantic variables such as imageability/concreteness (high-imageability/concrete words > low imageability/abstract words), word class (content words > functors), and frequency (high-frequency words > low-frequency words), whereas orthographic regularity does not have a significant effect. Although in phonological agraphia spelling errors in real words are phonologically implausible, they often retain visual similarity to the target, indicating partial lexical knowledge (e.g., "guitar–guilat") (Ellis, 1982; Roeltgen et al., 1983). Other common error types include morphological errors (e.g., "govern–government") and functor substitutions (e.g., "how–where").

Phonological agraphia is typically seen following left perisylvian lesions (Roeltgen et al., 1983; Roeltgen & Heilman, 1985; Alexander et al., 1992). The location of the damage is usually somewhat anterior to the parietal regions implicated in lexical spelling (Roeltgen & Heilman, 1984, 1985). Roeltgen (1985) concluded that lesions in patients with phonological agraphia overlap in the region of the anterior supramarginal gyrus, suggesting that this perisylvian cortical area plays an important role in spelling by the nonlexical route.

Deep Agraphia

"Deep agraphia" has several linguistic characteristics in common with phonological agraphia, but it is distinguishable from phonological agraphia by the presence of prominent semantic errors in writing (e.g., "igloo–Eskimo") (Assal, Buttet, & Jolivet, 1981; Bub & Kertesz, 1982b; Marshall & Newcombe, 1966; Newcombe & Marshall, 1984; Nolan & Caramazza, 1983; Hatfield, 1985; Van Lancker, 1990; Rapcsak, Beeson, & Rubens, 1991). Nonword spelling in most cases is almost completely abolished. Word spelling is strongly affected by imageability/concreteness (high-imageability/concrete words > low-imageability/abstract words), word class (content words > functors), and frequency (high-frequency words > low-frequency words). Orthographic regularity, however, has no influence on spelling accuracy. In addition to the pathognomonic semantic errors, patients typically produce morphological errors, functor substitutions, and visually similar misspellings indicative of partial lexical knowledge.

In order to explain deep agraphia, it is necessary to postulate multiple processing deficits. The loss of nonword spelling ability is consistent with damage to the nonlexical spelling route. Like patients with phonological agraphia, patients with deep agraphia rely on the lexical–semantic route in spelling; hence the strong effect of lexical–semantic variables on performance. The presence of semantic errors in writing suggests that the lexical–

semantic route itself is dysfunctional, either because of damage to the semantic system or because of impaired transmission of information between the semantic system and the graphemic output lexicon. The proposed breakdown of the lexical–semantic route can account for semantic errors in writing tasks that require obligatory semantic mediation (i.e., spontaneous writing, written naming). To explain semantic errors in writing to dictation, however, we must also postulate an impairment of the lexical–nonsemantic spelling route. If this route were functional, semantic errors would not occur in writing to dictation, since the correct representation in the graphemic output lexicon could be activated directly by the spoken form of the word (pathways D and C in Figure 8.1). In the absence of both the lexical–nonsemantic and the nonlexical spelling routes, writing to dictation in deep agraphia can only be accomplished via the error-prone lexical–semantic route. In conclusion, conditions for semantic errors arise when the output of the dysfunctional lexical–semantic spelling system remains completely unconstrained by orthographic information generated by the lexical–nonsemantic and nonlexical spelling routes.

Given the similarities between phonological and deep agraphia, one might question whether it is justifiable to regard them as distinct entities. The legitimacy of this concern becomes even more apparent when we consider that some patients described in the literature as having phonological agraphia actually produced semantic errors (e.g., Roeltgen et al., 1983; Baxter & Warrington, 1985). The substantial overlap between phonological and deep agraphia suggests that any strict taxonomic separation between the two syndromes is likely to be somewhat arbitrary.

Patients with deep agraphia have large left-hemisphere lesions that typically involve most of the perisylvian language zone. Such extensive damage to left-hemisphere language areas could certainly explain the multiple linguistic processing deficits postulated in this syndrome. However, an intriguing possibility is that in deep agraphia writing is no longer controlled by the damaged left hemisphere, and that the characteristic features of the syndrome reflect the intrinsic functional limitations of the intact right-hemisphere language system. Strong support for this hypothesis is provided by a patient we reported (Rapcsak et al., 1991), who demonstrated deep agraphia after a massive stroke that virtually destroyed the entire left hemisphere.

Semantic Agraphia

Meaning is incorporated into writing via the lexical–semantic route. Damage to the semantic system or the disconnection of the semantic system from the graphemic output lexicon may dissolve the normally tight coupling between word concepts and orthographic word forms. The result is the loss of semantic influence on writing known as "semantic agraphia" (Roeltgen, Rothi, & Heilman, 1986). In semantic agraphia, conceptually mediated writing tasks such as spontaneous writing and written naming may be severely compromised (Patterson, 1986; Rapcsak & Rubens, 1990). Writing to dictation, however, is relatively spared, since this task can also be accomplished via the lexical–nonsemantic or the nonlexical spelling routes. Using spelling routes that bypass the semantic system, patients with semantic agraphia can write familiar words to dictation even when their meaning is not understood (Roeltgen et al., 1986; Patterson, 1986; Kremin, 1987). Although regular words could potentially be spelled by the nonlexical route, correct spelling of ambiguous and irregular words without comprehension of their meaning provides strong evidence of the functional integrity of the lexical–nonsemantic route. Writing to dictation via the intact lexical–nonsemantic route does not show sensitivity to orthographic regularity and is unaffected by linguistic variables typically associated with the use of the lexical–semantic spelling route (e.g., imageability/concreteness and word class). Semantic errors do not occur. However, performance may be influenced by word frequency, since the success of transcoding between spoken and written forms of the same word is likely to depend on the number of times this association has been made previously.

Although writing to dictation in semantic agraphia may be quite accurate, homophonic words create major difficulties for these patients. Homophones have the same sound but different meaning and spelling (e.g., "sea–see"). The correct spelling of a homophonic word depends on the semantic context in which it is used (e.g., "storm at sea" vs. "see the sign"). In semantic agraphia, meaning has little influence on spelling. Consequently, patients cannot use semantic context to disambiguate dictated homophones reliably, and they frequently produce the semantically incorrect member of a pair (Roeltgen et al., 1986; Rapcsak & Rubens, 1990).

Patients with semantic agraphia constitute a heterogeneous group with respect to lesion localization. In the five patients studied by Roeltgen et al. (1986), semantic agraphia was associated with various extraperisylvian lesion sites (both cortical and subcortical) and with transcortical aphasia. However, of the three other patients reported with this syndrome (Patterson, 1986; Kremin, 1987; Rapcsak & Rubens, 1990), two had perisylvian lesions and none had transcortical aphasia. Homophone errors have been observed in patients with lexical agraphia (Hatfield & Patterson, 1983; Roeltgen & Heilman, 1984; Goodman & Caramazza, 1986a; Behrmann, 1987), suggesting that the posterior temporo-parietal lesion sites associated with that condition also have the potential for disrupting semantic influence on writing. Finally, homophone confusions and semantic agraphia have been documented in patients with AD (Schwartz, Marin, & Saffran, 1979; Glosser & Kaplan, 1989; Neils, Roeltgen, & Constantidinou, 1995). In summary, we conclude that at the present time semantic agraphia is better defined by its linguistic characteristics than by its precise neuroanatomical substrate.

Agraphia Due to Impairment of the Graphemic Buffer

In recent years a number of patients have been reported with spelling deficits attributable to dysfunction of the putative graphemic buffer (Miceli et al., 1985; Caramazza et al., 1987; Posteraro, Zinelli, & Mazzucchi, 1988; Hillis & Caramazza, 1989, 1995; Caramazza & Miceli, 1990; Caramazza & Hillis, 1990; Katz, 1991; Cubelli, 1991; Schonauer & Denes, 1994; Trojano & Chiacchio, 1994; Miceli, Benvegnu, Capasso, & Caramazza, 1995). As can be seen in Figure 8.1, the graphemic buffer receives the output of all three central spelling routes. Consequently, errors arising from an impairment of the buffer are observed in all writing tasks (i.e., spontaneous writing, written naming, writing to dictation). Furthermore, damage to the buffer affects the processing of all stored graphemic representations equally, regardless of word status (i.e., words vs. nonwords), lexical–semantic features (i.e., imageability/concreteness, word class, frequency), or orthographic regularity. By contrast, stimulus length has a strong effect on performance (short words are spelled better than long words), since each additional grapheme introduces a potential error by increasing the demand on limited storage capacity. Because the graphemic buffer supports spelling by all possible output modalities, qualitatively similar errors are observed in writing, oral spelling, typing, and spelling with anagram letters. There may be quantitative differences, however, reflecting variations in the processing demands imposed on the buffer by different output tasks.

Damage to the graphemic buffer results in the loss of information about the identity and serial ordering of stored graphemes, leading to errors of letter substitution, deletion, addition, and transposition. Such grapheme-level errors may result in visually similar but phonologically incorrect misspellings (e.g., "secret–securt"). The pattern and distribution of errors, however, are by no means random. Spelling errors may be constrained by consonant–vowel status, graphosyllabic structure, and geminate features (Caramazza & Micheli, 1990; Cubelli, 1991; Schonauer & Denes, 1994; Miceli et al., 1995). Furthermore, the spatial distribution of errors suggests a nonhomogeneous degradation of graphemic information in the buffer. For instance, in some cases more errors were produced on letters at the ends of words (Chédru & Geschwind, 1972; Katz, 1991), consistent with the hypothesized serial left-to-right readout process from a limited-capacity storage system. Errors on terminal letters may decrease in frequency if these patients are asked to spell backward (Katz, 1991), suggesting that the order of retrieval rather than the spatial location of the grapheme within the word is the critical factor. In other cases, errors predominantly involve letters in the middle of the word (Caramazza et al., 1987; Posteraro et al., 1988; Trojano & Chiacchio, 1994), presumably because graphemes in internal positions are more susceptible to interference from neighboring items than are graphemes located at either end (Wing & Baddeley, 1980).

Hemispatial neglect can also contribute to lateralized errors in the readout process from the graphemic buffer. Specifically, some patients with neglect consistently produce more spelling errors on the side of the word opposite their lesion, regardless of stimulus length or output modality (i.e., oral vs. written), and independent of whether they spell in conventional left-to-right order or in reverse (Baxter & Warrington, 1983; Hillis & Caramazza, 1989, 1995; Caramazza & Hillis, 1990). These observations are consistent with a unilateral defect in the distribution of attention over an internal graphemic representation in which the order of graphemes is spatially coded within a word-centered coordinate system (i.e., a spatial coordinate frame whose center corresponds to the midpoint of the word) (Caramazza & Hillis, 1990).

Lesion sites in patients with impairment of the graphemic buffer have been variable. Involvement of left-hemisphere fronto-parietal cortical systems implicated in working memory and spatial attention is common, but more specific localization is not possible at this time. Graphemic buffer deficits have been documented in some patients with AD, and the spelling impairment in these cases correlated with poor performance on tests of visual attention (Neils, Roeltgen, & Greer, 1995). Spelling errors suggestive of graphemic buffer dysfunction have also been observed in patients with generalized attentional deficits during acute confusional states (Chédru & Geschwind, 1972).

Peripheral Agraphias

In the peripheral agraphias, the main difficulty involves the selection and/or production of letters in handwriting. Four clinical subtypes of peripheral agraphia are directly relevant to our model: allographic disorders, apraxic agraphia, nonapraxic disorders of motor execution, and afferent dysgraphia (Table 8.3).

Allographic Disorders

"Allographic disorders" are characterized by an inability to activate or select the letter shapes appropriate for the set of abstract graphemic identities specified by central spelling routes.[1] Since the location of the damage is "downstream" from the graphemic buffer, oral spelling should be spared (Figure 8.1). Consistent with the hypothesis that abstract letter shape representations are also involved in spelling with anagram letters and typing (Margolin, 1984), these modalities of output may be impaired as well (Kinsbourne & Rosenfield, 1974; Levine, Mani, & Calvanio, 1988; Patterson & Wing, 1989; Friedman & Alexander, 1989). This

TABLE 8.3. Peripheral Agraphias

	Allographic disorders	Apraxic agraphia	Nonapraxic disorders of motor execution	Afferent dysgraphia
Distinctive features	Inability to generate or select the correct letter shapes in handwriting, with spared oral spelling	Poor letter formation not attributable to allographic disorder, sensorimotor, cerebellar, or extrapyramidal dysfunction; sparing of oral spelling, typing, spelling with anagram letters	Defective regulation of movement force, speed, and amplitude in handwriting	Duplication or omission of letters or strokes, especially when writing sequences of similar items
Characteristic errors	Writing impairment may be specific to case (upper vs. lower) or style (print vs. cursive); case-mixing errors; substitution of physically similar letter forms	Gross errors of letter morphology; spatial distortions; stroke insertions and deletions; writing may be completely illegible	Micrographia (Parkinson's disease); disjointed and irregular writing movements (cerebellar disorders)	As above, plus inability to write in a straight line and maintain the correct spacing between letters and words; defective spatial organization
Mechanism	Defective assignment of letter shapes to abstract graphemic representations held in the graphemic buffer	Destruction or disconnection of graphic motor programs, or damage to systems responsible for translating these programs into graphic innervatory patterns	Dysfunction of motor systems involved in controlling the kinematic parameters of writing	Inability to use visual and/or kinesthetic feedback to control the execution of writing movements
Lesion location	Left parieto-occipital	Left parietal lobe, dorsolateral premotor cortex (? Exner's area), SMA	Basal ganglia, cerebellum	Right parietal lobe

association, however, could simply reflect simultaneous damage to multiple, functionally independent peripheral conversion mechanisms subserving the various output modalities.

The breakdown of the allographic conversion process can take at least two different clinical forms: "allographic production disorders" and "allographic selection disorders." Some patients may show more than one type of impairment. In allographic production disorders, there may be complete or partial inability to create the appropriate letters, apparently because of a failure to remember letter shapes (Goldstein, 1948; Ellis, 1988; Crary & Heilman, 1988; Patterson & Wing, 1989; Kartsounis, 1992). The inability to retrieve letter shape information in these cases may reflect impaired access or damage to stored allographic representations. In addition to letter production deficits, the unavailability of allographic information may be associated with poor performance on tests of letter shape imagery, even in the absence of significant alexia (Crary & Heilman, 1988; Levine et al., 1988; Friedman & Alexander, 1989). Certain patients with allographic production disorders can write upper-case letters significantly better than lower-case letters (Patterson & Wing, 1989; Kartsounis, 1992), whereas in others the opposite pattern is observed (De Bastiani & Barry, 1986, cited in Patterson & Wing, 1989). These findings argue for distinct representations for upper- and lower-case letter forms within the allographic memory store, which may be selectively disrupted by brain damage. Allographs for different lower-case writing styles may also be represented separately, as suggested by the report of a patient who had difficulty printing lower-case letters but who could produce the same letters in a cursive style (Hanley & Peters, 1996).

Patients with allographic selection disorders produce well-formed but incorrect letters. Different types of selection problems have been described. In a patient reported by De Bastiani and Barry (1989), the disorder manifested as an uncontrollable mixing of upper- and lower-case letters in writing. Other patients produce numerous letter substitution errors but are usually able to keep letter case constant (Kinsbourne & Rosenfield, 1974; Rothi & Heilman, 1981; Kapur & Lawton, 1983; Friedman & Alexander, 1989; Goodman & Caramazza, 1986a; Black et al., 1989; Lambert, Viader, Eustache, & Morin, 1994; Rapp & Caramazza, 1997b). Substitution errors may be influenced by letter frequency (Black et al., 1989) and spatial similarity (Weekes, 1994; Zesiger, Martory, & Mayer, 1997). It has also been proposed that letter substitution errors in general, and those bearing an obvious physical similarity to the intended letter in particular, may actually be postallographic in origin and reflect faulty transmission of information between the allographic store and graphic motor programs (Ellis, 1982, 1988; Margolin, 1984; Friedman & Alexander, 1989; Black et al., 1989; Lambert et al., 1994). Physical similarity effects may be attributable to the fact that graphic motor programs containing similar stroke sequences are more likely to be confused (cf. Rapp & Caramazza, 1997b).

In the majority of patients with allographic disorders due to focal brain damage, the responsible lesion has involved the left parieto-occipital region. These observations suggest that this cortical area may be important for activating and selecting the correct letter shape representations for written production. Allograph-level writing impairments, manifested by defective cross-case transcription of single letters, have also been described in patients with AD (Hughes et al., 1997).

Apraxic Agraphia

"Apraxic agraphia" is a writing disorder characterized by poor letter formation that cannot be attributed to impaired letter shape knowledge or to sensorimotor, extrapyramidal (i.e., basal ganglia), or cerebellar dysfunction affecting the writing limb. Patients with apraxic agraphia are unable to execute the sequence of strokes necessary to produce the letter form specified by the allographic code. In pure cases, oral spelling, typing, and spelling with anagram letters are spared, and letter shape imagery is preserved (Baxter & Warrington, 1986; Alexander, Fischer, & Friedman, 1992; Zettin, Cubelli, Perino, & Rago, 1995).

Within the framework of our model, apraxic agraphia reflects damage to processing components involved in programming the skilled movements of writing. Possible mechanisms include destruction or disconnection of stored graphic motor programs, or damage to systems responsible for translating the information contained in graphic motor programs into graphic innervatory patterns to specific muscles. Apraxic agraphia is dissociable from limb apraxia, providing evidence that motor programs for writing are distinct from programs for other types of skilled movements (Zangwill, 1954; Roeltgen & Heilman, 1983; Margolin & Binder, 1984; Coslett, Rothi, Valenstein, & Heilman, 1986; Baxter & Warrington, 1986; Croisile, Laurent, Michel, & Trillet, 1990; Anderson, Damasio, & Damasio, 1990; Hodges, 1991; Papagno, 1992).

In apraxic agraphia the spatiotemporal attributes of writing are severely disturbed, and the smooth, facile strokes normally used to produce the required spatial trajectory are replaced by hesitant, awkward, and imprecise movements. In severe cases, all attempts at writing may result in illegible scrawls (Figure 8.2). Although individual letters may be difficult to recognize, some distinction between various writing styles and between upper- and lower-case forms may be preserved (Margolin & Binder, 1984; Roeltgen & Heilman, 1983). Characteristic errors of letter morphology include spatial distortions, stroke omissions resulting in incomplete forms, and insertions of anomalous strokes resulting in nonletters (Margolin & Binder, 1984). In some cases, single letters may be produced reasonably well, but performance deteriorates when sequences of letters in words are written (Zettin et al., 1995). When letters are more legible, it may be possible to demonstrate that written spelling per se is intact (Hodges, 1991). The writing difficulty may be specific to letters, since some patients can write numbers correctly (Anderson et al., 1990). Patients with apraxic agraphia can sometimes copy letters better than they can write them spontaneously or to dictation. However, without the processing advantage of stored graphic motor programs, copying is usually carried out in a stroke-by-stroke or "slavish" fashion typical of unskilled motor performance.

Lesions in apraxic agraphia are generally located in the hemisphere contralateral to the hand preferred for writing. Thus, in most right-handers the damage involves the left hemisphere, which is usually also the dominant hemisphere for limb praxis and language. However, in left-handers and in individuals with mixed or atypical cerebral dominance, the hemisphere that controls the skilled movements of writing is not always the hemisphere that is also dominant for language and/or limb praxis (Zangwill, 1954; Heilman, Coyle, Gonyea, & Geschwind, 1973; Heilman, Gonyea, & Geschwind, 1974; Valenstein & Heilman, 1979; Margolin, 1980; Roeltgen & Heilman, 1983; Margolin & Binder, 1984; Rapcsak, Rothi, & Heilman, 1987; Tanaka, Iwasa, & Obayashi, 1990; Rosa, Demiati, Cartz, & Mizon, 1991).

In most cases of apraxic agraphia, the responsible lesion has involved the parietal lobe (Zangwill, 1954; Valenstein & Heilman, 1979; Roeltgen & Heilman, 1983; Coslett et al., 1986; Baxter & Warrington, 1986; Papagno, 1992; Alexander et al., 1992). Alexander et al. (1992) have suggested that the critical lesion site may be in or around the junction of the angular gyrus and the superior parietal lobule. In a smaller number of cases the lesion has been anteriorly placed, centering on a premotor cortical area near the foot of the second frontal convolution (Gordinier, 1899; Anderson et al., 1990; Hodges, 1991). This

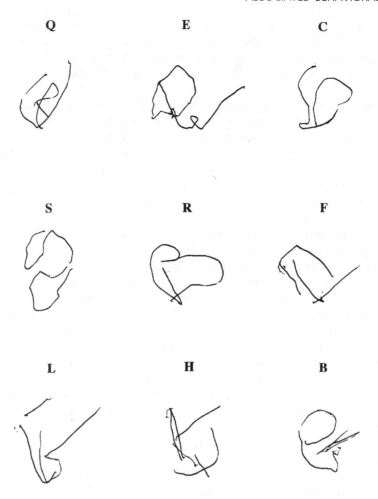

FIGURE 8.2. Attempts to write single letters to dictation by a patient with apraxic agraphia following left parietal damage. The target letters are printed above the patient's productions.

dorsolateral frontal region is known as Exner's writing center, and was considered by many earlier investigators to be the cortical location for the motor memories of writing (Exner, 1881; Pitres, 1884; Henschen, 1922; Nielsen, 1946; Goldstein, 1948). Apraxic agraphia has also been documented in individuals with frontal lesions involving the supplementary motor area (SMA) (Rubens, 1975; Watson, Fleet, Rothi, & Heilman, 1986). Finally, letter production deficits in some patients with AD may also be attributable to apraxic agraphia (Rapcsak et al., 1989; Platel et al., 1993).

Based on the anatomical evidence reviewed above, it is likely that the motor programming of writing is mediated by a distributed neural network that includes both posterior and anterior cortical components with distinct functional roles. Specifically, we propose that graphic motor programs are stored in the parietal lobe, and that frontal premotor areas (dorsolateral premotor cortex and SMA) are involved in translating these programs into graphic innervatory patterns. Parietal lesions cause apraxic agraphia by damaging or destroying stored spatiotemporal representations for writing movements, whereas frontal premotor lesions interfere with the generation of the appropriate motor commands to specific muscle effector systems. Deep white matter lesions (e.g., Croisile et al., 1990) may cause apraxic agraphia by disconnecting the parietal and frontal cortical components of the proposed network. The critical role of parietal and premotor cortex in programming the skilled movements of writing is also supported by functional neuroimaging studies in normal subjects (Petrides, Alivisatos, & Evans, 1995; Seitz et al., 1997).

When right-handers develop agraphia following left-hemisphere lesions, the writing disorder involves both hands, although the right hand may not be testable due to paralysis. Callosal lesions in right-handers should produce unilateral agraphia of the nondominant hand, since writing with the left hand requires the transfer of linguistic and motor information from the left to the right hemisphere across the corpus callosum. Consistent with this prediction, a number of right-handed patients with callosal damage were either completely unable to write with the left hand or produced mostly illegible scrawls (Liepmann & Maas, 1907; Sweet, 1941; Geschwind & Kaplan, 1962; Rubens, Geschwind, Mahowald, & Mastri, 1977; Watson & Heilman, 1983; Graff-Radford, Welsh, & Godersky, 1987; Yamadori, Osumi, Imamura, & Mitani, 1988; Leiguarda, Starkstein, & Berthier, 1989). In some cases, the left hand could spell words correctly when a typewriter was used, suggesting that these patients may have suffered from pure unilateral apraxic agraphia (Watson & Heilman, 1983; Graff-Radford et al., 1987; Leiguarda et al., 1989). Other patients were considered to have a combination of apraxic and linguistic agraphia, since they were also unable to spell with anagram letters or when using a typewriter (Liepmann & Maas, 1907; Geschwind & Kaplan, 1962; Goldenberg, Wimmer, Holzner, & Wessely, 1985).

Unilateral apraxic agraphia is usually associated with ideomotor apraxia of the left hand, and it typically follows lesions involving the anterior two-thirds to four-fifths of the corpus callosum, but sparing the caudal portions of the body and the splenium. In some cases the genu was also partially spared. These anatomical observations support the hypothesis that information critical to the motor programming of skilled limb movements is transferred through fibers located within the body of the corpus callosum (Liepmann, 1920; Geschwind, 1975; Watson & Heilman, 1983). However, the fact that unilateral apraxic agraphia and ideomotor apraxia are occasionally dissociable following callosal damage (Degos et al., 1987; Boldrini, Zanella, Cantagallo, & Basaglia, 1992; Kazui & Sawada, 1993) suggests that motor programs for writing and for other types of skilled movements are transferred through anatomically distinct callosal pathways.

In some right-handed patients with callosal lesions involving the posterior portions of the body and the splenium, unilateral linguistic agraphia of the left hand was observed in the absence of significant limb apraxia (Yamadori, Osumi, Ikeda, & Kanazawa, 1980; Sugishita, Toyokura, Yoshioka, & Yamada, 1980; Gersh & Damasio, 1981; Yamadori, Nagashima, & Tamaki, 1983; Kawamura, Hirayama, & Yamamoto, 1989). Unlike patients with unilateral apraxic agraphia, these patients were generally able to produce legible letters which, however, were linguistically incorrect. Thus, in these individuals the posterior callosal lesion seems to have interfered with the transfer of linguistic information relevant to writing, but motor programs for writing and for other types of skilled movements were presumably able to cross more anteriorly (Gersh & Damasio, 1981; Watson & Heilman, 1983).

Neuropsychological studies of callosal patients offer a rich source of information regarding the hemispheric control of spelling and writing. Detailed case reports of callosal agraphia, interpreted within the theoretical framework provided by information-processing models of writing, are now beginning to emerge (e.g., Zesiger & Mayer, 1992; Zesiger, Pegna, & Rilliet, 1994); however, much additional work is needed.

Nonapraxic Disorders of Motor Execution

Dysfunction of neural systems responsible for generating graphic innervatory patterns may result in defective control of the kinematic parameters of handwriting, leading to nonapraxic errors of movement force, speed, and amplitude. A typical example of this kind of motor execution disorder is the micrographia of patients with Parkinson's disease. Micrographia is characterized by an overall diminution of letter size (Figure 8.3A). Writing size sometimes decreases progressively from the beginning to the end of the line. Patients may be unable to increase letter size voluntarily, or can do so only briefly (McLennan, Nakano, Tyler, & Schwab, 1972). Writing speed is also significantly reduced. Except in severe cases,

A

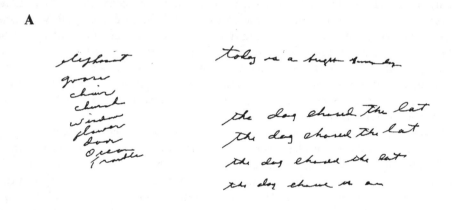

B

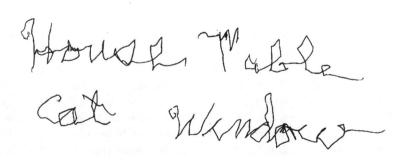

FIGURE 8.3. (A) Handwriting samples from a patient with Parkinson's disease, demonstrating the characteristic features of micrographia, including overall diminution of letter size, progressive decrease of letter size from the beginning to the end of the sentence, and the failure to maintain letter size across repeated productions of the same sentence. (B) Writing produced by a patient with severe cerebellar dysfunction. Poor motor execution and erratic spatial trajectory are related to inadequate control of movement direction, force, speed, and amplitude.

letters remain recognizable and there are no stroke-level errors of the kind seen in apraxic agraphia, attesting to the preservation of information at the level of allographic representations and graphic motor programs. These production features also suggest that the motor system can activate the correct muscles in the appropriate sequence, even though actual movement parameters cannot be calibrated accurately. From a quantitative analysis of handwriting in patients with Parkinson's disease, Margolin and Wing (1983) concluded that their micrographia was primarily attributable to an inability to generate the forces necessary to maintain proper letter size.

Micrographia in Parkinson's disease reflects basal ganglia dysfunction caused by the loss of striatal dopamine. Dopaminergic projections to striatal neurons originate in the substantia nigra of the midbrain. Focal lesions involving the substantia nigra can deprive the ipsilateral striatum of dopaminergic input and may result in micrographia of the contralateral hand (Kim, Im, Kwon, Kang, & Lee, 1998). Contralateral micrographia has also been described following focal damage to the striatum (Lewitt, 1983; Martinez-Vila, Artieda, & Obeso, 1988).

Basal ganglia structures are linked to frontal premotor cortical areas through a major reentrant basal ganglia–thalamo-cortical motor loop (Alexander, DeLong, & Strick, 1986). Specifically, the putamen receives projections from dorsolateral premotor cortex, SMA, and sensorimotor cortex, and projects back through the globus pallidus and the ventrolateral nucleus of the thalamus to the SMA. Operating as a functional unit, the cortical and subcortical components of this neural network play a central role in the programming and initiation of voluntary movements and in controlling movement force, speed, and amplitude (Goldberg, 1985; Alexander et al., 1986; Brooks, 1986). Consistent with this hypothesis, micrographia has also been observed following focal damage to the right SMA (Klatka, Depper, & Marini, 1998). The writing impairment in these patients may be part of the general motor hypometria and hypokinesia associated with damage to this cortical region (Meador, Watson, Bowers, & Heilman, 1986).

Poor motor execution is also characteristic of the writing produced by patients with cerebellar damage (Gilman, Bloedel, & Lechtenberg, 1981; Haggard, Jenner, & Wing, 1994). In cerebellar disorders, the sequence of rapid alternating muscle contractions necessary to produce writing cannot be performed in a smooth and automatic fashion. Writing movements are slow and disjointed, requiring deliberate effort and concentration on a patient's part. Due to the inadequate control of movement direction, force, speed, and amplitude, the writing trajectory is frequently irregular and erratic (Figure 8.3B). Letters with curved shapes tend to be decomposed into a series of straight lines, reflecting abrupt transitions in movement direction (Haggard et al., 1994).

Similar to the basal ganglia, the cerebellum is connected to frontal premotor cortical areas through reentrant neuronal circuitry (Brooks, 1986). The characteristic decomposition of voluntary movements following cerebellar lesions (Holmes, 1939; Gilman et al., 1981) suggests that the cortico-cerebellar motor loop is involved in the selection and implementation of kinematic parameters for skilled movements.

In summary, basal ganglia–thalamo-cortical and cortico-cerebellar motor loops are possible neural substrates of a distributed system that generates and modulates innervatory patterns for skilled limb movements, including graphic innervatory patterns for writing movements. This hypothesis is supported by regional cerebral blood flow and PET studies, which have demonstrated increased metabolic activity in premotor cortex, basal ganglia, cerebellum, and sensorimotor cortex during the performance of various writing tasks (Lauritzen, Henriksen, & Lassen, 1981; Mazziotta, Phelps, & Wapenski, 1985; Decety, Philippon, & Ingvar, 1988; Petrides et al., 1995; Seitz et al., 1997).

Afferent Dysgraphia

Lesions that interfere with the ability to utilize sensory feedback to control the execution of writing movements give rise to a characteristic clinical picture known as "afferent dysgraphia" (Lebrun, 1976, 1985; Ellis, 1982, 1988; Ellis et al., 1987; Ardila & Rosselli, 1993; Silveri, 1996; Croisile & Hibert, 1998). Writing errors in afferent dysgraphia are similar to those observed in normal subjects under experimental conditions that prevent the efficient use of visual and/or kinesthetic feedback. Errors typically include repetitions and omissions that are especially likely to occur when sequences of similar letters or strokes are being produced (Figure 8.4). In addition to the tendency to duplicate or omit letters and strokes, patients may have difficulty keeping the line of writing straight and maintaining the proper spacing between letters and words. On occasion, letters or words may be written on top of each other (Lebrun, 1985; Ardila & Rosselli, 1993). Silveri (1996) has proposed that writing in upper-case print may be more severely affected in afferent dysgraphia than cursive handwriting, presumably because the former task is less automatized and may thus rely more heavily on attention and sensory feedback. Other investigators, however, observed more frequent errors when patients attempted to write in a cursive style (Lebrun, 1985; Ellis et al., 1987; Croisile & Hibert, 1998).

Afferent or "spatial" dysgraphia is usually seen following right parietal lesions, suggesting that this area plays a critical role in monitoring and integrating visual and kinesthetic sensory feedback for the proper control of writing movements (Marcie & Hécaen, 1979; Lebrun, 1985; Ellis, 1982, 1988; Ellis et al., 1987; Ardila & Rosselli, 1993; Silveri, 1996; Croisile & Hibert, 1998). Writing produced by patients with right parietal damage also frequently shows evidence of left-sided spatial neglect (Figure 8.4). However, neglect-related errors (e.g., the tendency to write on the right side of the page, or the failure to dot "i's" and cross "t's" at the beginning of words) and feedback-related errors (e.g., letter and stroke repetitions or omissions) are dissociable (Ellis et al., 1987; Silveri, 1996; Croisile & Hibert, 1998).

Features of afferent dysgraphia have also been observed in association with cerebellar dysfunction (Silveri, Misciagna, Leggio, & Molinari, 1997). Silveri et al. (1997) have suggested that cerebellar lesions may interfere with the use of proprioceptive feedback critical for updating graphic motor programs and for coordinating the multijoint sequential movements of handwriting. This formulation is consistent with the proposed role of the cerebellum in comparing motor commands for intended movements with afferent feedback about the actual movement taking place (Brooks, 1986). Such comparator functions are important for error detection and for adjusting the evolving movement to changing contextual requirements.

CLINICAL EVALUATION OF WRITING DISORDERS

In the diagnostic assessment of agraphia, attention should be given to both the central (linguistic) and the peripheral (motor) components of writing. A comprehensive evaluation includes tests of spontaneous writing, written naming, writing to dictation, and copying. In testing spontaneous writing, patients are asked to compose a written narrative on a given topic. Using a written picture description task has the advantage of keeping the topic narrowly defined and reproducible across different subjects. Writing samples are examined not only for spelling errors and letter production deficits, but also for semantic organization, word choice, and syntactic structure. Standard stimuli for written picture description include the Cookie Theft from the Boston Diagnostic Aphasia Examination (Goodglass &

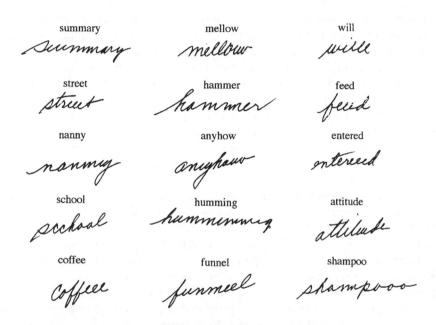

SCENES FROM A KITCHEN MOTHER DRYING DISHES SINIK OVERFLOWING SON TEETERING ON A STOOL TAKING COOKIES FROM FROM COOKIE JAR — WATER IS RUNNING ON KITCHEN FLOOR

summary	mellow	will
street	hammer	feed
nanny	anyhow	entered
school	humming	attitude
coffee	funnel	shampoo

FIGURE 8.4. Written productions of a patient with right temporo-parietal damage. Written picture description shows evidence of increasing neglect of the left side of the page and poor spatial organization. Single-word dictation reveals letter and stroke duplications characteristic of afferent dysgraphia.

Kaplan, 1983) and the Picnic Scene from the Western Aphasia Battery (Kertesz, 1982). Written naming can be assessed with the Boston Naming Test (Kaplan, Goodglass, & Weintraub, 1983) and is compared to oral naming of the same pictures.

Writing to dictation gives the experimenter direct control over a number of linguistic variables known to affect spelling. Test stimuli should allow independent evaluation of the effect of lexical status (words vs. nonwords), imageability/concreteness (high vs. low), word class (content words vs. functors, nouns vs. verbs), frequency (high vs. low), orthographic regularity (regular vs. ambiguous or irregular), word length (short vs. long), and morphology (monomorphemic vs. affixed). The influence of semantic context on homophone spelling should also be assessed. Although investigators may prefer to compile their own materials for testing writing to dictation, there are now also published word lists that permit this type of fine-grained psycholinguistic analysis (Kay, Lesser, & Coltheart, 1992).

The evaluation of patients with agraphia should not be limited to written production. Oral spelling, typing, and spelling with anagram letters should also be investigated in a parallel fashion to identify potential dysfunction of these output modalities. As noted previously, similar difficulties across different modalities are diagnostic of central agraphia, whereas modality-specific deficits suggest peripheral agraphia. Once it is established that a patient suffers from central agraphia, a systematic examination of spelling errors is undertaken. Based on the linguistic profile that emerges from the detailed analysis of impaired and preserved spelling abilities, it should be possible to determine whether the patient fits diagnostic criteria for one of the various central agraphia syndromes outlined earlier (Table 8.2). In addition to identifying the damaged spelling route or processing component, this type of analysis can also yield important clues about residual or compensatory spelling strategies used by the patient.

In evaluating the peripheral components of writing, patients should be asked to write in different cases or styles and to transcode between various allographic forms (e.g., to transcribe from upper- to lower-case or from print to script). In analyzing the motor aspects of writing, attention is paid to overall legibility, letter size, and morphology. Written productions are also examined for evidence of impaired afferent control and defective spatial organization. Poor control of movement speed, force, and amplitude may be readily apparent from simply observing a patient in the act of writing. If possible, writing with both hands should be tested and compared, but allowances have to be made for the normal "clumsiness" of the nondominant hand. Any sensorimotor, basal ganglia, or cerebellar dysfunction affecting the writing limb requires careful documentation, and patients should be examined for limb apraxia.

Assessment of copying should include letters, words, nonwords, and nonlinguistic visual patterns as stimuli. In interpreting performance on these tasks, however, it is important to keep in mind that copying is not a unitary function (Ellis, 1982). For example, some patients may reproduce letters or words in the same way that they copy or draw nonlinguistic visual patterns. Since this type of "pictorial" copying is not mediated by the writing system, performance cannot benefit from stored graphic motor programs. Consequently, copying is slow and fragmented, relying heavily on "closed-loop" visual control typical of unskilled motor behavior. Although patients who use the pictorial copying route exclusively may be able to reproduce letter shapes, they should not be able to transcode between various allographic forms of a letter, since this requires access to allographic memory representations. Damage to the pictorial route is accompanied by defective copying of all types of visual patterns and poor performance on drawing tasks in general. A patient demonstrating impaired pictorial copying of letters with intact writing was described by Cipolotti and Denes (1989).

In contrast to pictorial copying, in "graphemic" and "lexical" copying, input letter strings are first processed by the reading system, and graphic output is subsequently generated by the peripheral components of the writing system. In graphemic copying, a direct link is postulated between letter recognition units located within the visual analysis module and the graphemic buffer (Figure 8.1) (Morton, 1980; Ellis, 1982). Graphemic copying is used primarily to reproduce single letters, unfamiliar words, and nonwords. In copying by the lexical route, the written word first activates its appropriate entry in the visual input lexicon, following which the corresponding spelling is retrieved from the graphemic output lexicon. Orthographic information is then transferred to the graphemic buffer for peripheral conversion. Copying by the graphemic and lexical routes is facile under normal circumstances, since it can take advantage of stored graphic motor programs. Because they share the same output mechanisms, graphemic and lexical copying and writing may show similar patterns of impairment following brain damage.

Although copying is usually tested with the target stimulus in full view, a number of investigators have advocated the use of delayed copying in clinical assessment (Nolan & Caramazza, 1983; Miceli et al., 1985). In delayed copying, the previously viewed target stimulus is removed from sight before the patient is allowed to start writing. Delayed copying requires short-term memory and may thus provide useful information about the functional status of the graphemic buffer.

To date, the relationship between visual imagery and writing has only been examined in a few agraphic patients. The imagery tasks used typically require subjects to answer questions about the physical appearance of letters (e.g., whether or not a letter contains straight or curved lines). Therefore, these tests probe letter shape knowledge that is thought to be represented at the level of the allographic memory store. Consistent with this hypothesis, some patients with presumed allographic writing disorders have an associated impairment of letter shape imagery (see above). However, written production of letters can be preserved even when letter shape imagery is severely defective (Kosslyn, Holtzman, Farah, & Gazzaniga, 1985; Shuren, Maher, & Heilman, 1996), indicating that conscious visualization of letter shapes is not normally required for writing. Mental imagery for writing movements may have more in common with motor production than letter shape imagery. For instance, it has been shown that imagined writing movements and actual graphic motor gestures activate partially overlapping brain regions (Decety et al., 1988; Sugishita, Takayama, Shiono, Yoshikawa, & Takahashi, 1996). Furthermore, execution times for imagined writing movements closely approximate the time required for the overt production of the same movements (Decety & Michel, 1989). These findings suggest that mentally executed and real graphic movements may be controlled by the same central motor representation (i.e., graphic motor programs). If this hypothesis is correct, it may be possible to show that patients with apraxic agraphia have defective motor imagery for writing movements.

TREATMENT OF AGRAPHIA

The goals of agraphia treatment are to maximize the return of premorbid writing skills and to promote the utilization of preserved abilities to substitute for lost or impaired functions. The cognitive model of writing can guide the therapist in identifying the impaired processes and preserved functions that may be exploited to achieve improvement. Treatment generally involves incremental stimulation of the linguistic and motor procedures necessary for writing, the relearning of item-specific associations, and/or the incorporation of strategic compensations. The treatment plan will take into account the time post-onset; the nature of the agraphia profile; and the overall cognitive, linguistic, and pragmatic abilities of the patient.

Acute agraphia may not conform to a specific syndrome, although an identifiable syndrome may emerge during the first several months following brain damage, or as compensatory strategies are employed. For example, the reliance on the nonlexical spelling route that is the hallmark of lexical agraphia may reflect a self-selected strategy to compensate for the loss of access to stored orthographic knowledge. Writing impairment that results from damage to multiple processing components may never fit a specific agraphia profile; however, treatment that is designed to strengthen impaired processes and maximize the use of preserved abilities is a valid approach, whether a patient has a pure or complex agraphia syndrome.

Before we review various treatment approaches, it should be acknowledged that treatment outcomes for similar patients may vary for numerous reasons, including individual variation of brain organization, residual cognitive resources, and motivation. Hillis and

Caramazza (1994) elegantly made this point by comparing several single-subject treatment outcomes. They demonstrated (1) that some patients with the same presumed locus of impairment required different treatment approaches, (2) that different treatment approaches may be equally appropriate for the same impairment, and (3) that a given treatment strategy may affect several different levels of processing impairment. Furthermore, a patient's response to treatment may provide additional information about the specific nature of the underlying functional deficit, and thus the diagnostic process may continue throughout rehabilitation.

Treatment of Acute Agraphia

During the first several months following the onset of brain damage, when physiological restitution is most likely to occur, the natural recovery process may be promoted by systematic stimulation of writing. Large-group studies comparing treatment with no treatment (Basso, Capitani, & Vignolo, 1979) or with deferred treatment (Wertz et al., 1986) have documented significant positive effects of traditional stimulus–response treatment approaches for relatively acute agraphia associated with aphasia. Stimulation techniques involve structured methods of response elicitation and selective reinforcement of correct responses to the exclusion of error responses at controlled levels of difficulty (Peach, 1993; Rosenbek, LaPointe, & Wertz, 1989). Responses may be evoked by a cueing hierarchy that facilitates correct responding and then incrementally reduces the external support provided for successful writing (Hillis, 1989; Linebaugh, 1983). An incremental treatment progression may begin with single words presented for such tasks as tracing, copying, delayed copying, writing to dictation, and sentence completion. If single-word writing is functional, treatment may follow a linguistic progression from single words to phrases to sentences to narrative writing.

The recovery of writing ability may progress at a rapid rate during the first few months following onset of agraphia (assuming that no further neurological damage occurs), as the effects of treatment coincide with physiological recovery. As neurological restitution stabilizes and the more chronic effects of brain damage become evident, treatment should exploit residual cognitive abilities to achieve reorganization and compensation of function. A growing body of well-documented studies provides evidence in support of treatment for relatively chronic agraphia; a representative sample of those studies is reviewed to demonstrate various approaches to rehabilitation.

Treatment for Central Agraphias

In general, treatment for central agraphia syndromes is directed toward strengthening the lexical–semantic route, facilitating use of the nonlexical route (i.e., phoneme–grapheme conversion), or a combination of both (Carlomagno, Iavarone, & Colombo, 1994; Hillis, 1992). Some approaches serve to rebuild writing skills in an item-specific manner (i.e., word by word), whereas other procedures target the remediation of processes that influence spelling for more than one item. Treatments are discussed here as though they were process-specific; however, we acknowledge that there is dynamic interplay among damaged and preserved functional components, and that performance reflects the summation of available visual, semantic, phonological, and graphemic information (Hillis & Caramazza, 1991).

Strengthening the Lexical–Semantic Route

The literature on agraphia rehabilitation suggests that it is possible to improve writing via the lexical–semantic spelling route by intervention at various levels of processing. In some cases, writing may reflect impairment to the semantic system so that lexical retrieval errors are evident in all modalities, not just writing. Hillis (1991) reported that treatment of semantic deficits by means of teaching distinctions among semantically related items resulted in improved written naming; there was also generalization to oral naming and repetition tasks. In other cases, in which semantic representations appeared to be intact, writing improvement has been achieved by strengthening the link between semantics and the graphemic output lexicon and/or by facilitating the restoration of degraded orthographic representations.

A treatment approach described by Carlomagno et al. (1994) was devised to take advantage of residual semantic and partial lexical knowledge in six aphasic individuals with linguistic agraphia of unspecified type. Subjects were presented with pictured items, along with a hierarchy of visual and semantic cues to evoke correct spelling of words. The treatment tasks included direct copying of target words, delayed copying, serial ordering of letters with visual cues provided (e.g., number of letters, word contour, and prepositioning of some letters), and semantic cues (e.g., describing the object's function). As correct written responses were achieved, visual and semantic cues were progressively withdrawn to achieve independent writing of the words in response to the pictures. Carlomagno et al. (1994) found the visual–semantic treatment to be effective for three of their six subjects, whereas the other three subjects benefited from a nonlexical (i.e., phonological) treatment strategy. In this case, the patients' responses to treatment provided clarification of the nature of their impairment and the availability of residual writing processes.

A similar visual and semantic cueing hierarchy for written naming was reported earlier by Hillis (1989) with two aphasic individuals with agraphia. Treatment resulted in improved written naming for both subjects, and there was generalization to oral naming in one patient but not the other. Hillis (1989) attributed the differential outcome to the different loci of impairment: a semantic deficit in the patient with generalization to oral naming, and damage to the graphemic buffer in the other patient.

Aliminosa, McCloskey, Goodman-Schulman, and Sokol (1993) used a delayed copying procedure with an aphasic individual whose spelling deficit reflected multiple impairments to the graphemic output lexicon, the phoneme-to-grapheme conversion process, and possibly the graphemic buffer. Target words were presented for study and then removed from sight for delayed copying. After delayed copying reached criterion, writing to dictation was drilled, and correct spelling was stabilized for a corpus of words. There was no generalization to untrained items, suggesting that training improved the availability of specific stored orthographic representations but did not improve functioning of the graphemic buffer.

Another item-specific approach was described by Seron, Deloche, Moulard, and Rousselle (1980). They used a computer program that prompted typewriting of target words by presenting a series of blank spaces, one for each letter of the word. Error responses were not shown on the screen, and letters selected out of order were shown in their correct location, thus providing errorless learning trials. This approach facilitated improved spelling in five individuals with aphasia and agraphia that appeared to reflect multiple processing deficits. Although this treatment strategy may have strengthened the availability of orthographic representations for the trained words, follow-up testing showed that the improvement was short-lived. Therefore, additional training may be needed to achieve long-lasting effects with this approach, or concomitant semantic stimulation may be required to strengthen the lexical–semantic route adequately.

Beeson (1999) documented a long-lasting effect of a treatment protocol to strengthen graphemic representations in a severely aphasic individual. Treatment included the arrangement of letter anagrams and repeated copying of target words, with a strong emphasis on daily homework that included copying and recall tasks for single written words. A multiple-baseline treatment design documented a significant treatment effect that was specific to treated items; however, the patient was ultimately able to guide his own selection and home treatment of target words, so that his corpus of written words continually grew. Additional intervention facilitated this patient's functional use of his written words for conversational interaction.

Behrmann (1987) reported on the success of a treatment program intended to strengthen the lexical–semantic spelling route in a patient with lexical agraphia. The treatment plan involved the reestablishment of correct spellings for homophonic words—for example, matching the written words "sail" and "sale" with respective pictures. Semantic specification was necessary for the disambiguation of the homophones, thus placing the treatment emphasis on the link between semantics and the graphemic output lexicon. Treatment resulted in improved spelling of the treated homophone pairs and generalization to some untreated irregular words, but there was little generalization to untreated homophones. The carryover to untreated irregular words was attributed to improved use of reading ability to check for spelling errors. In a subsequent treatment phase, whole-word processing of selected irregular words was stressed, with a deemphasis on phonologically based spelling (Behrmann & Byng, 1992). The procedures were similar to those of the homophone treatment and also proved successful for the reestablishment of item-specific links from semantics to orthography.

de Partz, Seron, & Van der Linden (1992) reported a successful treatment for misspelling of ambiguous and irregular words in lexical agraphia that employed a visual imagery strategy. The stimuli in this word-specific treatment approach consisted of semantically related drawings embedded in the orthographic representation of the word in such a way that it provided cues for the correct spelling for their French-speaking patient. For example, the word *pathologie* ("pathology") was misspelled *patologie* (missing the "h"), so it was trained using a drawing that depicted the "H" as a hospital bed, thus highlighting the correct spelling with a semantically related concept.

Several treatment approaches have employed a lexical relay strategy, whereby preserved spelling abilities for specific words have provided a means to cue spelling for other words. Hatfield (1983) demonstrated that retrievable content words could be used as a link to relearning the spelling of functors in individuals with deep agraphia. For example, retrieval of the word "inn" might be used to establish the relearning of the homophone "in." Hatfield (1983) found that even quasi-homophonic words were useful to trigger retrieval of functors (e.g., "Ron" was used to retrieve the spelling for "on"). This strategic approach is necessarily item-specific, but can be successfully used to circumvent retrieval failure for specific functors.

Carlomagno and Parlato (1989) reported a success with a treatment approach that made use of preserved orthographic knowledge in a nonaphasic individual with severe agraphia. They took advantage of the patient's ability to write a small corpus of proper nouns correctly and to segment the words into syllables. With training, the patient was able to use the proper nouns (and some additional proper nouns that were trained) as "code words" to derive the spelling of syllables, which were then used to spell other words. Treatment benefits generalized to spontaneous writing by means of a self-dictation strategy whereby each syllable was spoken, related to the proper code word, and then spelled.

Taking Advantage of the Nonlexical Spelling Route

When the lexical–semantic route is unavailable or impoverished, spelling may be accomplished via the nonlexical route by means of the phoneme–grapheme conversion mechanism. As mentioned previously, Carlomagno et al. (1994) treated six individuals with central agraphia of unspecified type using a nonlexical treatment strategy combined with a visual–semantic approach. The nonlexical procedure was directed toward the reestablishment of sound-to-letter correspondences for selected consonants, consonant–vowel syllables, and nonwords. The authors found that the nonlexical treatment method resulted in significantly improved spelling of real words and nonwords for five of the six agraphic individuals. Two of those subjects also benefited from a visual–semantic strategy, but three subjects were responsive only to the nonlexical treatment approach.

Some individuals have difficulty using the nonlexical route to assist in spelling, but this route may be strengthened through treatment, thus providing at least partial orthographic information to assist in spelling. Hillis and Caramazza (1994) reported on a treatment approach that employed "key words" to reestablish phoneme–grapheme correspondences to assist in written spelling. Their agraphic patient exhibited an impairment of the graphemic output lexicon that was specific to writing verbs, but she had good access to the phonological output lexicon. Thus the patient was typically able to say a verb she could not write, but could not convert the phonemes to graphemes. Treatment involved teaching the graphemic correspondences (i.e., initial letters) for the first sound for 30 phonemes presented in the context of single words. A cueing hierarchy was employed to train the phoneme–grapheme correspondences for the 30 "key words." Once reestablished, the phoneme–grapheme correspondences were used by the patient to self-cue correct orthographic representations for verbs and to self-monitor semantic paragraphias, resulting in increased use of correct verbs in written narratives.

Partial lexical knowledge or relatively preserved phonological knowledge may be adequate to allow self-correction of spelling errors by means of an electronic dictionary. Many inexpensive, commercially available "pocket" dictionaries offer correct spellings for phonologically plausible misspellings, even in cases of incorrect selection of an initial letter, such as "kamil" for "camel." Fluhardy (1993) documented the use of such a device with synthesized speech to provide a successful, quick means of spelling self-correction in an individual with lexical agraphia. For individuals who use word processors, the spell-check function allows for identification of misspelled words and the provision of plausible options.

Other Treatment Approaches to Central Agraphia

One of the most intriguing treatment approaches for central agraphia is the use of a writing prosthesis for the paralyzed right hand in individuals with agraphia associated with aphasia (Leischner, 1983, 1996; Brown, Leader, & Blum, 1983; Lorch, 1995a, 1995b). The common finding in these studies has been superior linguistic content in written composition produced with the aided hemiparetic right hand, when compared to composition produced with the nonparalyzed left hand. Leischner (1983) used a special pen grip and assisted the patient with movement of the hand after each stroke. Brown et al. (1983) used a pen holder in combination with a skateboard device supporting the forearm, which allowed independent movement of the arm by proximal shoulder muscles. Whurr and Lorch (1991) advocated the use of a device that reduced the spasticity of the right hand and wrist, enabling use of the right hand for writing. In all cases, there was evidence of improved written spelling and more elaborate and accurate linguistic production. The precise mechanisms underlying this phenomenon are a matter of discussion and debate (Brown, 1995; Goldberg & Porcelli, 1995; Lorch, 1995a, 1995b; Rothi, 1995; Sasanuma, 1995; Leischner, 1996). It appears, however, that aided right-handed writing is worthy of clinical consideration in cases of large left-hemisphere lesions associated with agraphia and severe aphasia.

Treatment for Peripheral Agraphias

Relatively little attention has been given to the treatment of peripheral agraphias. One explanation may be that intact central language and spelling processes allow individuals with peripheral agraphia to make good use of typewriters or word processors to circumvent their handwriting impairment. It is also likely that some of the procedures described for central agraphias are appropriate for peripheral agraphias. For example, tracing, copying, transcribing, and delayed copying of letters and words may facilitate retraining of the allographic conversion process and the execution of the appropriate motor programs.

In general, treatment for patients with motor production deficits should aim to reestablish the ability to write letters and words, however slow, deliberate, and feedback-dependent it may be. Once graphic motor control is regained, treatment can be redirected toward improving the automaticity of motor programs for writing. Micrographia, which is often observed in Parkinson's disease, may be modified by the provision of parallel lines or a template to guide the writer to increased letter height (Oliveira, Gurd, Nixon, Marshall, & Passingham, 1997). The lines provide an external cue to facilitate the recalibration of the range and force of movement necessary to achieve the target letter size. Treatment includes fading of external cues, and maintenance requires continuous monitoring of writing movements. Oliveira et al. (1997) demonstrated that a constant verbal reminder to "write big" was as effective as the provision of parallel lines; however, there was no documentation that the beneficial effects of this strategy were maintained.

Concluding Remarks about Treatment

In summary, agraphia treatment may consist of highly specific or somewhat intuitive approaches that aim to restore or circumvent processing deficits, and that also capitalize on the dynamic interplay among residual processes. Although treatment should be derived from careful behavioral analysis, the initiation of rehabilitation should not suggest an end to the diagnostic endeavor. A patient's response to treatment may provide further information about the nature of the underlying impairment and serve as a test of the model of writing upon which treatment is based.

ACKNOWLEDGMENT

The writing of this chapter was supported by a Cummings Endowment Fund to the Department of Neurology at the University of Arizona, and by a National Multipurpose Research and Training Center Grant DC-01409 from the National Institute on Deafness and Other Communication Disorders.

NOTE

1. It should be pointed out that not all models distinguish a separate allographic processing stage in writing. According to some theorists (Shallice, 1988; Van Galen, 1991), allographs correspond to different letter-specific graphic motor programs. Within the framework of such models, "allographic disorders" would result from an inability to activate or select the graphic motor programs necessary for externalizing the strings of graphemes held in the graphemic buffer (for further discussion, see Rapp & Caramazza, 1997b).

REFERENCES

Alexander, G. E., DeLong, M. R., & Strick, P. L. (1986). Parallel organization of functionally segregated circuits linking basal ganglia and cortex. *Annual Review of Neuroscience, 9*, 357–381.

Alexander, M. P., Fischer, R. S., & Friedman, R. (1992). Lesion localization in apractic agraphia. *Archives of Neurology, 49*, 246–251.

Alexander, M. P., Friedman, R. B., Loverso, F., & Fischer, R. S. (1992). Lesion localization in phonological agraphia. *Brain and Language, 43*, 83–95.

Aliminosa, D., McCloskey, M., Goodman-Schulman, R., & Sokol, S. (1993). Remediation of acquired dysgraphia as a technique for testing interpretations of deficits. *Aphasiology, 7*, 55–69.

Anderson, S. W., Damasio, A. R., & Damasio, H. (1990). Troubled letters but not numbers: Domain specific cognitive impairments following focal damage in frontal cortex. *Brain, 113*, 749–766.

Ardila, A., & Rosselli, M. (1993). Spatial agraphia. *Brain and Language, 22*, 137–147.

Assal, G., Buttet, J., & Jolivet, R. (1981). Dissociations in aphasia: A case report. *Brain and Language, 13*, 223–240.

Badecker, W., Hillis, A., & Caramazza, A. (1990). Lexical morphology and its role in the writing process: Evidence from a case of acquired dysgraphia. *Cognition, 35*, 205–243.

Basso, A., Capitani, E., & Vignolo, L. A. (1979). Influence of rehabilitation on language skills in aphasic patients. *Archives of Neurology, 36*, 190–196.

Baxter, D. M., & Warrington, E. K. (1983). Neglect dysgraphia. *Journal of Neurology, Neurosurgery, and Psychiatry, 46*, 1073–1078.

Baxter, D. M., & Warrington, E. K. (1985). Category specific phonological dysgraphia. *Neuropsychologia, 23*, 653–666.

Baxter, D. M., & Warrington, E. K. (1986). Ideational agraphia: A single case study. *Journal of Neurology, Neurosurgery, and Psychiatry, 49*, 369–374.

Baxter, D. M., & Warrington, E. K. (1987). Transcoding sound to spelling: Single or multiple sound unit correspondence? *Cortex, 23*, 11–28.

Beauvois, M.-F., & Dérouesné, J. (1981). Lexical or orthographic agraphia. *Brain, 104*, 21–49.

Beeson, P. M. (1999). Treating acquired writing impairment: Strengthening graphemic representations. *Aphasiology, 13*, 767–785.

Behrmann, M. (1987). The rites of righting writing: Homophone mediation in acquired dysgraphia. *Cognitive Neuropsychology, 4*, 365–384.

Behrmann, M., & Byng, S. (1992). A cognitive approach to the neurorehabilitation of acquired language disorders. In D. I. Margolin (Ed.), *Cognitive neuropsychology in clinical practice.* New York: Oxford University Press.

Black, S. E., Behrmann, M., Bass, K., & Hacker, P. (1989). Selective writing impairment: Beyond the allographic code. *Aphasiology, 3*, 265–277.

Boldrini, P., Zanella, R., Cantagallo, A., & Basaglia, N. (1992). Partial hemispheric disconnection of traumatic origin. *Cortex, 28*, 135–143.

Bolla-Wilson, K., Speedie, L. J., & Robinson, R. G. (1985). Phonologic agraphia in a left-handed patient after a right-hemisphere lesion. *Neurology, 35*, 1778–1781.

Brooks, V. B. (1986). *The neural basis of motor control.* New York: Oxford University Press.

Brown, J. (1995). What dissociation should be studied? *Aphasiology, 9*, 277–279.

Brown, J. W., Leader, B. J., & Blum, C. S. (1983). Hemiplegic writing in severe aphasia. *Brain and Language, 19*, 204–215.

Bub, D., & Kertesz, A. (1982a). Evidence for lexicographic processing in a patient with preserved written over oral single word naming. *Brain, 105*, 697–717.

Bub, D., & Kertesz, A. (1982b). Deep agraphia. *Brain and Language, 17*, 146–165.

Campbell, R. (1983). Writing nonwords to dictation. *Brain and Language, 19*, 153–178.

Caramazza, A., Berndt, R. S., & Basili, A. G. (1983). The selective impairment of phonological processing: A case study. *Brain and Language*, *18*, 128–174.

Caramazza, A., & Hillis, A. E. (1990). Spatial representation of words in the brain implied by studies of a unilateral neglect patient. *Nature*, *346*, 267–269.

Caramazza, A., & Hillis, A. E. (1991). Lexical organization of nouns and verbs in the brain. *Nature*, *349*, 788–790.

Caramazza, A., & Miceli, G. (1990). The structure of graphemic representations. *Cognition*, *37*, 243–297.

Caramazza, A., Miceli, G., Villa, G., & Romani, C. (1987). The role of the graphemic buffer in spelling: Evidence from a case of acquired dysgraphia. *Cognition*, *26*, 59–85.

Carlomagno, S., Iavarone, A., & Colombo, A. (1994). Cognitive approaches to writing rehabilitation: From single case to group studies. In M. J. Riddoch & G. W. Humphreys (Eds.), *Cognitive neuropsychology and cognitive rehabilitation*. Hillsdale, NJ: Erlbaum.

Carlomagno, S., & Parlato, V. (1989). Writing rehabilitation in brain damaged adult patients: A cognitive approach. In G. Deloche (Ed.), *Cognitive approaches in neuropsychological rehabilitation*. Hillsdale, NJ: Erlbaum.

Chédru, F., & Geschwind, N. (1972). Writing disturbances in acute confusional states. *Neuropsychologia*, *10*, 343–353.

Cipolotti, L., & Denes, G. (1989). When a patient can write but not copy: Report of a single case. *Cortex*, *25*, 331–337.

Coslett, H. B., Rothi, L. J. G., Valenstein, E., & Heilman, K. M. (1986). Dissociations of writing and praxis: Two cases in point. *Brain and Language*, *28*, 357–369.

Crary, M. A., & Heilman, K. M. (1988). Letter imagery deficits in a case of pure apraxic agraphia. *Brain and Language*, *34*, 147–156.

Croisile, B., Brabant, M.-J., Carmoi, T., Lepage, Y., Aimard, G., & Trillet, M. (1996). Comparison between oral and written spelling in Alzheimer's disease. *Brain and Language*, *54*, 361–387.

Croisile, B., Carmoi, T., Adeleine, P., & Trillet, M. (1995). Spelling in Alzheimer's disease. *Behavioral Neurology*, *8*, 135–143.

Croisile, B., & Hibert, O. (1998). Spatial or afferent agraphia without left-sided neglect. *Aphasiology*, *12*, 147–159.

Croisile, B., Laurent, B., Michel, D., & Trillet, M. (1990). Pure agraphia after deep left hemisphere hematoma. *Journal of Neurology, Neurosurgery and Psychiatry*, *53*, 263–265.

Croisile, B., Trillet, M., Laurent, B., Latombe, B., & Schott, B. (1989). Agraphie lexicale par hématome temporo-parietal gauche. *Revue Neurologique*, *145*, 287–292.

Cubelli, R. (1991). A selective deficit for writing vowels in acquired dysgraphia. *Nature*, *353*, 258–260.

De Bastiani, P., & Barry, C. (1989). A cognitive analysis of an acquired dysgraphic patient with an allographic writing disorder. *Cognitive Neuropsychology*, *6*, 25–41.

Decety, J., & Michel, F. (1989). Comparative analysis of actual and mental movement times in two graphic tasks. *Brain and Cognition*, *11*, 87–97.

Decety, J., Philippon, B., & Ingvar, D. H. (1988). rCBF landscapes during motor performance and motor ideation of a graphic gesture. *European Archives of Psychiatry and Neurological Sciences*, *238*, 33–38.

Degos, J. D., Gray, F., Louarn, F., Ansquer, J. C., Poirier, J., & Barbizet, J. (1987). Posterior callosal infarction: Clinicopathological correlations. *Brain*, *110*, 1155–1171.

Déjerine, J. (1891). Sur un cas de cécité verbale avec agraphie, suivi d'autopsie. *Mémoires de la Société de Biologie*, *3*, 197–201.

Déjerine, J. (1914). *Sémiologie des affections du système nerveux*. Paris: Masson et Cie.

de Partz, M.-P., Seron, X., & Van der Linden, M.V. (1992). Re-education of surface dysgraphia with a visual imagery strategy. *Cognitive Neuropsychology*, *9*, 369–401.

Ellis, A. W. (1982). Spelling and writing (and reading and speaking). In A. W. Ellis (Ed.), *Normality and pathology in cognitive functions*. London: Academic Press.

Ellis, A. W. (1988). Normal writing processes and peripheral acquired dysgraphias. *Language and Cognitive Processes*, *3*, 99–127.

Ellis, A. W., Miller, D., & Sin, G. (1983). Wernicke's aphasia and normal language processing: A case study in cognitive neuropsychology. *Cognition*, *15*, 111–144.

Ellis, A. W., & Young, A. W. (1988). *Human cognitive neuropsychology*. Hillsdale, NJ: Erlbaum.

Ellis, A. W., Young, A. W., & Flude, B. M. (1987). "Afferent dysgraphia" in a patient and in normal subjects. *Cognitive Neuropsychology*, *4*, 465–486.

Exner, S. (1881). *Untersuchungen über die Localisation der Functionen in der Grosshirnrinde des Menschen.* Vienna: Braunmüller.

Fluhardy, G. (1993). Use of an electronic dictionary to compensate for surface dysgraphia. *Journal of Cognitive Rehabilitation, 11*, 28–30.

Friedman, R. B., & Alexander, M. P. (1989). Written spelling agraphia. *Brain and Language, 36*, 503–517.

Gelb, I. J. (1963). *A study of writing.* Chicago: University of Chicago Press.

Gersh, F., & Damasio, A. R. (1981). Praxis and writing of the left hand may be served by different callosal pathways. *Archives of Neurology, 38*, 634–636.

Geschwind, N. (1969). Problems in the anatomical understanding of the aphasias. In A. L. Benton (Ed.), *Contributions to clinical neuropsychology.* Chicago: Aldine.

Geschwind, N. (1975). The apraxias: Neural mechanisms of disorders of learned movement. *American Scientist, 63*, 188–195.

Geschwind, N., & Kaplan, E. (1962). A human cerebral deconnection syndrome: A preliminary report. *Neurology, 12*, 675–685.

Gilman, S., Bloedel, J. R., & Lechtenberg, R. (1981). *Disorders of the cerebellum.* Philadelphia: Davis.

Glosser, G., & Kaplan, E. (1989). Linguistic and nonlinguistic impairments in writing: A comparison of patients with focal and multifocal CNS disorders. *Brain and Language, 37*, 357–380.

Goldberg, G. (1985). Supplementary motor area structure and function: Review and hypotheses. *Behavioral and Brain Sciences, 8*, 567–616.

Goldberg, G., & Porcelli, J. (1995). The functional benefits: How much and for whom? *Aphasiology, 9*, 274–277.

Goldenberg, G., Wimmer, A., Holzner, F., & Wessely, P. (1985). Apraxia of the left limbs in a case of callosal disconnection: The contribution of medial frontal lobe damage. *Cortex, 21*, 135–148.

Goldstein, K. (1948). *Language and language disturbance.* New York: Grune & Stratton.

Goodglass, H., & Kaplan, E. (1983). *Boston Diagnostic Aphasia Examination.* Philadelphia: Lea & Febiger.

Goodman, R. A., & Caramazza, A. (1986a). Aspects of the spelling process: Evidence from a case of acquired dysgraphia. *Language and Cognitive Processes, 1*, 263–296.

Goodman, R. A., & Caramazza, A. (1986b). Dissociation of spelling errors in written and oral spelling: The role of allographic conversion in writing. *Cognitive Neuropsychology, 3*, 179–206.

Goodman-Schulman, R., & Caramazza, A. (1987). Patterns of dysgraphia and the nonlexical spelling process. *Cortex, 23*, 143–148.

Gordinier, H. C. (1899). A case of brain tumor at the base of the second left frontal convolution. *American Journal of Medical Science, 117*, 526–535.

Graff-Radford, N. R., Welsh, K., & Godersky, J. (1987). Callosal apraxia. *Neurology, 37*, 100–105.

Grashey, H. (1885). Über Aphasie und ihre Beziehungen zur Wahrnehmung. *Archiv für Psychiatrie und Nervenkrankheiten, 16*, 654–688.

Haggard, P., Jenner, J., & Wing, A. (1994). Coordination of aimed movements in a case of unilateral cerebellar damage. *Neuropsychologia, 32*, 827–846.

Hanley, J. R., & Peters, S. (1996). A dissociation between the ability to print and write cursively in lower-case letters. *Cortex, 32*, 737–745.

Hatfield, F. M. (1983). Aspects of acquired dysgraphia and implication for re-education. In C. Code & D. J. Muller (Eds.), *Aphasia therapy.* London: Arnold.

Hatfield, F. M. (1985). Visual and phonological factors in acquired dysgraphia. *Neuropsychologia, 23*, 13–29.

Hatfield, F. M., & Patterson, K. (1983). Phonological spelling. *Quarterly Journal of Experimental Psychology, 35A*, 451–468.

Heilman, K. M. (1979). Apraxia. In K. M. Heilman & E. Valenstein (Eds.), *Clinical neuropsychology.* New York: Oxford University Press.

Heilman, K. M., Coyle, J. M., Gonyea, E. F., & Geschwind, N. (1973). Apraxia and agraphia in a left-hander. *Brain, 96*, 21–28.

Heilman, K. M., Gonyea, E. F., & Geschwind, N. (1974). Apraxia and agraphia in a right-hander. *Cortex, 10*, 284–288.

Heilman, K. M., & Rothi, L. J. G. (1985). Apraxia. In K. M. Heilman & E. Valenstein (Eds.), *Clinical neuropsychology* (2nd ed.). New York: Oxford University Press.

Henschen, S. E. (1922). *Klinische und anatomische Beitrage zur Pathologie des Gehirns* (Vol. 7). Stockholm: Nordiska Bokhandeln.

Hier, D. B., & Mohr, J. P. (1977). Incongruous oral and written naming. *Brain and Language, 4*, 115–126.

Hillis, A. E. (1989). Efficacy and generalization of treatment for aphasic naming errors. *Archives of Physical Medicine and Rehabilitation, 70*, 632–636.

Hillis, A. E. (1991). Effects of separate treatments for distinct impairments within the naming process. *Clinical Aphasiology, 19*, 255–265.

Hillis, A. E. (1992). Facilitating written production. *Clinics in Communication Disorders, 2*, 19–33.

Hillis, A. E., & Caramazza, A. (1989). The graphemic buffer and attentional mechanisms. *Brain and Language, 36*, 208–235.

Hillis, A. E., & Caramazza, A. (1991). Mechanisms for accessing lexical representations for output: Evidence from a category-specific semantic deficit. *Brain and Language, 40*, 106–144.

Hillis, A. E., & Caramazza, A. (1994). Theories of lexical processing and rehabilitation of lexical deficits. In M. J. Riddoch & G. W. Humphreys (Eds.), *Cognitive neuropsychology and cognitive rehabilitation*. Hillsdale, NJ: Erlbaum.

Hillis, A. E., & Caramazza, A. (1995). Spatially specific deficits in processing graphemic representations in reading and writing. *Brain and Language, 48*, 263–308.

Hodges, J. R. (1991). Pure apraxic agraphia with recovery after drainage of a left frontal cyst. *Cortex, 27*, 469–473.

Hodges, J. R., Patterson, K., Oxbury, S., & Funnell, E. (1992). Semantic dementia: Progressive fluent aphasia with temporal lobe atrophy. *Brain, 115*, 1783–1806.

Holmes, G. (1939). The cerebellum of man. *Brain, 62*, 1–30.

Hotopf, N. (1980). Slips of the pen. In U. Frith (Ed.), *Cognitive processes in spelling*. London: Academic Press.

Hughes, J. C., Graham, N., Patterson, K., & Hodges, J. R. (1997). Dysgraphia in mild dementia of Alzheimer's type. *Neuropsychologia, 35*, 533–545.

Kalmus, H., Fry, D. B., & Denes, P. (1960). Effects of delayed visual control on writing, drawing and tracing. *Language and Speech, 3*, 96–108.

Kaplan, E., Goodglass, H., & Weintraub, S. (1983). *Boston Naming Test*. Philadelphia: Lea & Febiger.

Kapur, N., & Lawton, N. F. (1983). Dysgraphia for letters: A form of motor memory deficit. *Journal of Neurology, Neurosurgery and Psychiatry, 46*, 573–575.

Kartsounis, L. D. (1992). Selective lower-case letter ideational dysgraphia. *Cortex, 28*, 145–150.

Katz, R. B. (1991). Limited retention of information in the graphemic buffer. *Cortex, 27*, 111–119.

Kawamura, M., Hirayama, K., & Yamamoto, H. (1989). Different interhemispheric transfer of Kanji and Kana writing evidenced by a case with left unilateral agraphia without apraxia. *Brain, 112*, 1011–1018.

Kay, J., Lesser, R., & Coltheart, M. (1992). *Psycholinguistic Assessment of Language Processing in Aphasia (PALPA)*. Hillsdale, NJ: Erlbaum.

Kazui, S., & Sawada, T. (1993). Callosal apraxia without agraphia. *Annals of Neurology, 33*, 401–403.

Kertesz, A. (1982). *The Western Aphasia Battery*. New York: Grune & Stratton.

Kim, J. S., Im, J. H., Kwon, S. U., Kang, J. H., & Lee, M. C. (1998). Micrographia after thalamomesencephalic infarction: Evidence for striatal dopaminergic dysfunction. *Neurology, 51*, 625–627.

Kinsbourne, M., & Rosenfield, D. B. (1974). Agraphia selective for written spelling: An experimental case study. *Brain and Language, 1*, 215–225.

Klatka, L. A., Depper, M. H., & Marini, A. M. (1998). Infarction in the territory of the anterior cerebral artery. *Neurology, 51*, 620–622.

Kosslyn, S. M., Holtzman, J. D., Farah, M. J., & Gazzaniga, M. S. (1985). A computational analysis of mental image generation: Evidence from functional dissociations in split-brain patients. *Journal of Experimental Psychology: General, 114*, 311–341.

Kremin, H. (1987). Is there more than ah-oh-oh?: Alternative strategies for writing and repeating lexically. In M. Coltheart, G. Sartori, & R. Job (Eds.), *The cognitive neuropsychology of language*. Hillsdale, NJ: Erlbaum.

Lambert, J., Viader, F., Eustache, F., & Morin, P. (1994). Contribution to peripheral agraphia: A case of post-allographic impairment? *Cognitive Neuropsychology, 11*, 35–55.

Lauritzen, M., Henriksen, L., & Lassen, N. A. (1981). Regional cerebral blood flow during rest and skilled hand movements by Xenon-133 inhalation and emission computerized tomography. *Journal of Cerebral Blood Flow and Metabolism, 1*, 385–389.

Lebrun, Y. (1976). Neurolinguistic models of language and speech. In H. Whitaker & H. A. Whitaker (Eds.), *Studies in neurolinguistics* (Vol. 1). New York: Academic Press.

Lebrun, Y. (1985). Disturbances of written language and associated abilities following damage to the right hemisphere. *Applied Psycholinguistics, 6*, 231–260.

Leiguarda, R., Starkstein, S., & Berthier, M. (1989). Anterior callosal hemorrhage: A partial inter-hemispheric disconnection syndrome. *Brain, 112*, 1019–1037.

Leischner, A. (1983). Side differences in writing to dictation of aphasics with agraphia: A graphic disconnection syndrome. *Brain and Language, 18*, 1–19.

Leischner, A. (1996). Word class effects upon the intrahemispheric graphic disconnection syndrome. *Aphasiology, 10*, 443–451.

Levine, D. N., Calvanio, R., & Popovics, A. (1982). Language in the absence of inner speech. *Neuropsychologia, 20*, 391–409.

Levine, D. N., Mani, R. B., & Calvanio, R. (1988). Pure agraphia and Gerstmann's syndrome as a visuospatial–language dissociation: An experimental case study. *Brain and Language, 35*, 172–196.

Lewitt, P. A. (1983). Micrographia as a focal sign of neurological disease. *Journal of Neurology, Neurosurgery and Psychiatry, 46*, 1152–1157.

Lhermitte, F., & Dérouesné, J. (1974). Paraphasies et jargonaphasie dans le langage oral avec con-servation du langage écrit: Genése des néologismes. *Revue Neurologique, 130*, 21–38.

Liepmann, H. (1920). Apraxie. *Ergebnisse der Gesamten Medizin, 1*, 516–543.

Liepmann, H., & Maas, O. (1907). Fall von Linksseitiger Agraphie und Apraxie bei Rechsseitiger Lähmung. *Journal für Psychologie und Neurologie, 10*, 214–227.

Linebaugh, C. (1983). Treatment of anomic aphasia. In C. Perkins (Ed.), *Current therapies for communication disorders: Language handicaps in adults*. New York: Thieme-Stratton.

Lorch, M. P. (1995a). Laterality and rehabilitation: Differences in left and right hand productions in aphasic agraphic hemiplegics. *Aphasiology, 9*, 257–271.

Lorch, M. P. (1995b). Language and praxis in written production: A rehabilitation paradigm. *Aphasiology, 9*, 280–282.

Luria, A. R. (1970). *Traumatic aphasia: Its syndromes, psychology, and treatment* (D. Bowen, Trans.). The Hague: Mouton. (Original work published 1947)

Marcie, P., & Hécaen, H. (1979). Agraphia: Writing disorders associated with unilateral cortical lesions. In K. M. Heilman & E. Valenstein (Eds.), *Clinical neuropsychology*. New York: Oxford University Press.

Margolin, D. I. (1980). Right hemisphere dominance for praxis and left hemisphere dominance for speech in a left-hander. *Neuropsychologia, 18*, 715–719.

Margolin, D. I. (1984). The neuropsychology of writing and spelling: Semantic, phonological, motor and perceptual processes. *Quarterly Journal of Experimental Psychology, 36A*, 459–489.

Margolin, D. I., & Binder, L. (1984). Multiple component agraphia in a patient with atypical cerebral dominance: An error analysis. *Brain and Language, 22*, 26–40.

Margolin, D. I., & Goodman-Schulman, R. (1992). Oral and written spelling impairments. In D. I. Margolin (Ed.), *Cognitive neuropsychology in clinical practice*. New York: Oxford University Press.

Margolin, D. I., & Wing, A. M. (1983). Agraphia and micrographia: Clinical manifestations of motor programming and performance disorders. *Acta Psychologica, 54*, 263–283.

Marshall, J. C., & Newcombe, F. (1966). Syntactic and semantic errors in paralexia. *Neuropsychologia, 4*, 169–176.

Martinez-Vila, E., Artieda, J., & Obeso, J. A. (1988). Micrographia secondary to lenticular hematoma. *Journal of Neurology, Neurosurgery and Psychiatry, 51*, 1353–1356.

Mazziotta, J. C., Phelps, M. E., & Wapenski, J. A. (1985). Human cerebral motor system metabolic responses in health and disease. *Journal of Cerebral Blood Flow and Metabolism, 5* (Suppl. 1), S213–S214.

McLennan, J. E., Nakano, K., Tyler, H. R., & Schwab, R. S. (1977). Micrographia in Parkinson's disease. *Journal of the Neurological Sciences, 15*, 141–152.

Meador, K. J., Watson, R. T., Bowers, D., & Heilman, K. M. (1986). Hypometria with hemispatial and limb motor neglect. *Brain, 109*, 293–305.

Merton, P. A. (1972). How we control the contraction of our muscles. *Scientific American, 226*, 30–37.

Miceli, G., Benvegnu, B., Capasso, R., & Caramazza, A. (1995). Selective deficit in processing double letters. *Cortex, 31*, 161–171.

Miceli, G., Silveri, M. C., & Caramazza, A. (1985). Cognitive analysis of a case of pure dysgraphia. *Brain and Language, 25,* 187–212.

Morton, J. (1969). Interaction of information in word recognition. *Psychological Review, 76,* 165–178.

Morton, J. (1980). The logogen model and orthographic structure. In U. Frith (Ed.), *Cognitive processes in spelling.* London: Academic Press.

Neils, J., Roeltgen, D. P., & Greer, A. (1995). Spelling and attention in early Alzheimer's disease: Evidence for impairment of the graphemic buffer. *Brain and Language, 49,* 241–262.

Neils, J., Roeltgen, D. P., & Constantidinou, F. (1995). Decline in homophone spelling associated with loss of semantic influence on spelling in Alzheimer's disease. *Brain and Language, 49,* 27–49.

Newcombe, F., & Marshall, J. C. (1984). Task- and modality-specific aphasias. In F. C. Rose (Ed.), *Advances in neurology: Vol. 42: Progress in aphasiology.* New York: Raven Press.

Nielsen, J. M. (1946). *Agnosia, apraxia, aphasia: Their value in cerebral localization.* New York: Hoeber.

Nolan, K. N., & Caramazza, A. (1983). An analysis of writing in a case of deep dyslexia. *Brain and Language, 20,* 305–328.

Oliveira, R. M., Gurd, J. M., Nixon, P., Marshall, J. C., & Passingham, R. E. (1997). Micrographia in Parkinson's disease: The effect of providing external cues. *Journal of Neurology, Neurosurgery and Psychiatry, 63,* 429–433.

Papagno, C. (1992). A case of peripheral dysgraphia. *Cognitive Neuropsychology, 9,* 259–270.

Patterson, K. (1986). Lexical but nonsemantic spelling? *Cognitive Neuropsychology, 3,* 341–367.

Patterson, K. (1988). Acquired disorders of spelling. In G. Denes, C. Semenza, & P. Bisiacchi (Eds.), *Perspectives on cognitive neuropsychology.* Hillsdale, NJ: Erlbaum.

Patterson, K., & Hodges, J. R. (1992). Deterioration of word meaning: Implications for reading. *Neuropsychologia, 30,* 1025–1040.

Patterson, K., & Shewell, C. (1987). Speak and spell: Dissociations and word-class effects. In M. Coltheart, G. Sartori, & R. Job (Eds.), *The cognitive neuropsychology of language.* Hillsdale, NJ: Erlbaum.

Patterson, K., & Wing, A. M. (1989). Processes in handwriting: A case for case. *Cognitive Neuropsychology, 6,* 1–23.

Peach, R. (1993). Clinical intervention for aphasia in the United States of America. In A. L. Holland & M. M. Forbes (Eds.), *Aphasia treatment: World perspectives.* San Diego, CA: Singular Press.

Peniello, M.-J., Lambert, J., Eustache, F., Petit-Taboué, M. C., Barré, L., Viader, F., Morin, P., Lechevalier, B., & Baron, J.-C. (1995). A PET study of the functional neuroanatomy of writing impairment in Alzheimer's disease: The role of the left supramarginal and angular gyri. *Brain, 118,* 697–707.

Petrides, M., Alivisatos, B., & Evans, A. C. (1995). Functional activation of the human ventrolateral frontal cortex during mnemonic retrieval of verbal information. *Proceedings of the National Academy of Sciences USA, 92,* 5803–5807.

Pitres, A. (1884). Considerations sur l'agraphie. *Revue de Médecine, 4,* 855–873.

Platel, H., Lambert, J., Eustache, F., Cadet, B., Dary, M., Viader, F., & Lechevalier, B. (1993). Characteristic evolution of writing impairment in Alzheimer's disease. *Neuropsychologia, 31,* 1147–1158.

Posteraro, L., Zinelli, P., & Mazzucchi, A. (1988). Selective impairment of the graphemic buffer in acquired dysgraphia: A case study. *Brain and Language, 35,* 274–286.

Rapcsak, S. Z. (1997). Disorders of writing. In L. J. G. Rothi & K. M. Heilman (Eds.), *Apraxia: The neuropsychology of action.* Hove, England: Psychology Press.

Rapcsak, S. Z., Arthur, S. A., Bliklen, D. A., & Rubens, A. B. (1989). Lexical agraphia in Alzheimer's disease. *Archives of Neurology, 46,* 66–68.

Rapcsak, S. Z., Beeson, P. M., & Rubens, A. B. (1991). Writing with the right hemisphere. *Brain and Language, 41,* 510–530.

Rapcsak, S. Z., Rothi, L. J. G., & Heilman, K. M. (1987). Apraxia in a patient with atypical cerebral dominance. *Brain and Cognition, 6,* 450–463.

Rapcsak, S. Z., & Rubens, A. B. (1990). Disruption of semantic influence on writing following a left prefrontal lesion. *Brain and Language, 38,* 334–344.

Rapp, B., & Caramazza, A. (1997a). The modality-specific organization of grammatical categories: Evidence from impaired spoken and written sentence production. *Brain and Language, 56,* 248–286.

Rapp, B., & Caramazza, A. (1997b). From graphemes to abstract letter shapes: Levels of representation in written spelling. *Journal of Experimental Psychology: Human Perception and Performance*, 23, 1130–1152.

Roeltgen, D. P. (1985). Agraphia. In K. M. Heilman & E. Valenstein (Eds.), *Clinical neuropsychology* (2nd ed.). New York: Oxford University Press.

Roeltgen, D. P. (1993). Agraphia. In K. M. Heilman & E. Valenstein (Eds.), *Clinical neuropsychology* (3rd ed.). New York: Oxford University Press.

Roeltgen, D. P., & Heilman, K. M. (1983). Apractic agraphia in a patient with normal praxis. *Brain and Language*, 18, 35–46.

Roeltgen, D. P., & Heilman, K. M. (1984). Lexical agraphia: Further support for the two-system hypothesis of linguistic agraphia. *Brain*, 107, 811–827.

Roeltgen, D. P., & Heilman, K. M. (1985). Review of agraphia and a proposal for an anatomically-based neuropsychological model of writing. *Applied Psycholinguistics*, 6, 205–230.

Roeltgen, D. P., Rothi, L. G., & Heilman, K. M. (1986). Linguistic semantic agraphia: A dissociation of the lexical spelling system from semantics. *Brain and Language*, 27, 257–280.

Roeltgen, D. P., Sevush, S., & Heilman, K. M. (1983). Phonological agraphia: Writing by the lexical–semantic route. *Neurology*, 33, 755–765.

Rosa, A., Demiati, M., Cartz, L., & Mizon, J. P. (1991). Marchiafava–Bignami disease, syndrome of interhemispheric disconnection, and right-handed agraphia in a left-hander. *Archives of Neurology*, 48, 986–988.

Rosenbek, J. C., LaPointe, L. L., & Wertz, R. T. (1989). *Aphasia: A clinical approach*. Austin, TX: Pro-Ed.

Rothi, L. J. G. (1995). Are we clarifying or contributing to the confusion? *Aphasiology*, 9, 271–273.

Rothi, L. J. G., & Heilman, K. M. (1981). Alexia and agraphia with spared spelling and letter recognition abilities. *Brain and Language*, 12, 1–13.

Rubens, A. B. (1975). Aphasia with infarction in the territory of the anterior cerebral artery. *Cortex*, 11, 239–250.

Rubens, A. B., Geschwind, N., Mahowald, M. W., & Mastri, A. (1977). Posttraumatic cerebral hemispheric disconnection syndrome. *Archives of Neurology*, 34, 750–755.

Sasanuma, S. (1995). The missing data. *Aphasiology*, 9, 273–274.

Schonauer, K., & Denes, G. (1994). Graphemic jargon: A case report. *Brain and Language*, 47, 279–299.

Schwartz, M. F., Marin, O. S. M., & Saffran, E. M. (1979). Dissociations of language function in dementia: A case study. *Brain and Language*, 7, 277–306.

Seitz, R. J., Canavan, A. G. M., Yaguez, L., Herzog, H., Tellmann, L., Knorr, U., Huang, Y., & Homberg, V. (1997). Representations of graphomotor trajectories in the human parietal cortex: evidence from controlled processing and automatic performance. *European Journal of Neuroscience*, 9, 378–389.

Seron, X., Deloche, G., Moulard, G., & Rousselle, M. (1980). A computer based therapy for the treatment of aphasic subjects with writing disorders. *Journal of Speech and Hearing Disorders*, 45, 45–58.

Shallice, T. (1981). Phonological agraphia and the lexical route in writing. *Brain*, 104, 413–429.

Shallice, T. (1988). *From neuropsychology to mental structure*. Cambridge, England: Cambridge University Press.

Shuren, J. E., Maher, L. M., & Heilman, K. M. (1996). The role of visual imagery in spelling. *Brain and Language*, 52, 365–372.

Silveri, M. C. (1996). Peripheral aspects of writing can be differentially affected by sensorial and attentional defect: Evidence from a patient with afferent dysgraphia and case dissociation. *Cortex*, 32, 155–172.

Silveri, M. C., Misciagna, S., Leggio, M. G., & Molinari, M. (1997). Spatial dysgraphia and cerebellar lesion: A case report. *Neurology*, 48, 1529–1532.

Smith, S. T., Snyder, W. B., & Meeks, M. L. (1990). *Agraphia in Alzheimer's disease*. Paper presented at the 28th Annual Meeting of the Academy of Aphasia, Baltimore.

Smith, W. M., McCrary, J. W., & Smith, K. U. (1960). Delayed visual feedback and behavior. *Science*, 132, 1013–1014.

Smyth, M. M., & Silvers, G. (1987). Functions of vision in the control of handwriting. *Acta Psychologica*, 65, 47–64.

Sugishita, M., Takayama, Y., Shiono, T., Yoshikawa, K., & Takahashi, Y. (1996). Functional magnetic resonance imaging (fMRI) during mental writing with phonograms. *NeuroReport*, 7, 1917–1921.

Sugishita, M., Toyokura, Y., Yoshioka, M., & Yamada, R. (1980). Unilateral agraphia after section of the posterior half of the truncus of the corpus callosum. *Brain and Language*, 9, 215–225.

Sweet, W. H. (1941). Seeping intracranial aneurysm simulating neoplasm. *Archives of Neurology and Psychiatry*, 45, 86–104.

Tanaka, Y., Iwasa, H., & Obayashi, T. (1990). Right hand agraphia and left hand apraxia following callosal damage in a right-hander. *Cortex*, 26, 665–671.

Trojano, L., & Chiacchio, L. (1994). Pure dysgraphia with relative sparing of lower-case writing. *Cortex*, 30, 499–507.

Valenstein, E., & Heilman, K. M. (1979). Apraxic agraphia with neglect-induced paragraphia. *Archives of Neurology*, 36, 506–508.

Van Bergeijk, W. A., & David, E. D. (1959). Delayed handwriting. *Perceptual and Motor Skills*, 9, 347–357.

Van Galen, G. P. (1980). Handwriting and drawing: A two stage model of complex motor behavior. In G. E. Stelmach & J. Requin (Eds.), *Tutorials in motor behavior*. Amsterdam: North-Holland.

Van Galen, G. P. (1991). Handwriting: Issues for a psychomotor theory. *Human Movement Science*, 10, 165–192.

Van Lancker, D. (1990). Reading and writing without letters: A case of deep dysgraphia attributed to right-hemisphere function. *Journal of Clinical and Experimental Neuropsychology*, 3, 420.

Watson, R. T., Fleet, W. S., Rothi, L. J. G., & Heilman, K. M. (1986). Apraxia and the supplementary motor area. *Archives of Neurology*, 43, 787–792.

Watson, R. T., & Heilman, K. M. (1983). Callosal apraxia. *Brain*, 106, 391–403.

Weekes, B. S. (1994). A cognitive-neuropsychological analysis of allograph errors from a patient with acquired dysgraphia. *Aphasiology*, 8, 409–425.

Wernicke, C. (1874). *Der Aphasische Symptomenkomplex*. Breslau: Cohn & Weigert.

Wernicke, C. (1886). Nervenheilkunde: Die neueren Arbeiten über Aphasie. *Fortschritte der Medizin*, 4, 463–482.

Wertz, R. T., Weiss, D. G., Aten, J. L., Brookshire, R. H., Garcia-Bunuel, L., Holland, A. L., Kurtzke, J. F., LaPointe, L. L., Milianti, F. J., Brannegan, R., Greenbaum, H., Marshall, R. C., Vogel, D., Carter, J., Barnes, N. S., & Goodman, R. (1986). Comparison of clinic, home, and deferred language treatment for aphasia: A Veterans Administration cooperative study. *Archives of Neurology*, 43, 653–658.

Whurr, M., & Lorch, M. (1991). The use of a prosthesis to facilitate writing in aphasia and right hemiplegia. *Aphasiology*, 5, 411–418.

Wing, A. M., & Baddeley, A. D. (1980). Spelling errors in handwriting: A corpus and a distributional analysis. In U. Frith (Ed.), *Cognitive processes in spelling*. London: Academic Press.

Wright, C. E. (1990). Generalized motor programs: Reevaluating claims of effector independence in writing. In M. Jeannerod (Ed.), *Attention and performance* XXIII. Hillsdale, NJ: Erlbaum.

Yamadori, A., Nagashima, T., & Tamaki, N. (1983). Ideogram writing in a disconnection syndrome. *Brain and Language*, 19, 346–356.

Yamadori, A., Osumi, Y., Ikeda, H., & Kanazawa, Y. (1980). Left unilateral agraphia and tactile anomia: Disturbances seen after occlusion of the anterior cerebral artery. *Archives of Neurology*, 37, 88–91.

Yamadori, A., Osumi, Y., Imamura, T., & Mitani, Y. (1988). Persistent left unilateral apraxia and a disconnection theory. *Behavioral Neurology*, 1, 11–22.

Zangwill, O. L. (1954). Agraphia due to a left parietal glioma in a left-handed man. *Brain*, 77, 510–520.

Zesiger, P., Martory, M.-D., & Mayer, E. (1997). Writing without graphic motor patterns: A case of dysgraphia for letters and digits sparing shorthand writing. *Aphasiology*, 14, 743–763.

Zesiger, P., & Mayer, E. (1992). Left unilateral dysgraphia in a patient with an atypical pattern of handedness: A cognitive analysis. *Aphasiology*, 6, 293–307.

Zesiger, P., Pegna, A., & Rilliet, B. (1994). Unilateral dysgraphia of the dominant hand in a left-hander: A disruption of graphic motor selection. *Cortex*, 30, 673–683.

Zettin, M., Cubelli, R., Perino, C., & Rago, R. (1995). Impairment of letter formation: The case of ideomotor apraxic agraphia. *Aphasiology*, 9, 283–294.

9

APRAXIA OF SPEECH: A TREATABLE DISORDER OF MOTOR PLANNING AND PROGRAMMING

MALCOLM R. McNEIL
PATRICK J. DOYLE
JULIE WAMBAUGH

THE GENERAL CONTEXT FOR APRAXIA OF SPEECH

"Apraxia of speech" (AOS), as a viable theoretical construct and as an isolated clinical entity, has attracted beneficent attention for two primary reasons. First, if validated, it would provide insight into the nature of speech motor plans and motor programs. The validation of cognitive modules (representations, rules, or dedicated processors) is consistent with the general goals of neuropsychology, and one method for such validation is the demonstration and careful examination of isolated pathologies resulting from "accidents of nature." The reasoning is such that if a specific impairment can be identified, and this cannot be accounted for by any other hypothesized mechanism, the existence of this module is said to have been demonstrated. This form of instantiation is called a "dissociation." Taken at face value, such verification would provide evidence of a motor program—a construct with a great deal of appeal, and also a great deal of debate surrounding it. The verification of AOS as a disorder of motor programming plays an important role in theories of speech motor control. Indeed, the existence of this clinical entity has attracted the interest of motor theorists such as Gracco (1990), Kelso, Tuller, and Harris (1983), Kent (Kent & Rosenbek, 1983), Munhall (1989), Schmidt (McNeil, Robin, & Schmidt, 1997), Van der Merwe (1997), and others. It is also evident in the examination of the contrasting and complementary motor theories of *coordinative structure theory* (Kelso & Tuller, 1981; Kugler, Kelso, & Turvey, 1980), *action theory* (Kelso et al., 1983), *dynamical theory* (Kelso, Vatikiotis-Bateson, Saltzman, & Kay, 1985), and *generalized motor program theory* (Schmidt, 1976).

Second, there is a well-motivated clinical interest in AOS. This interest derives most directly from Darley's (1967, 1968) influential observations and from the recurring broad-based observations of clinicians from a variety of disciplines. This position holds that certain clinical phenomena of neurological origin do not fit within the generally accepted neurogenic speech production pathologies associated with the dysarthrias and/or with the phonological deficits resulting from aphasia. Broadly recognized and accepted in the literature on speech and language pathology is the subdivision of motor speech disorders into the dysarthrias and AOS (Duffy, 1995). Frequently included are speech production disorders such as "neurogenic stuttering," "cluttering," and "akinetic mutism." More rarely included are the "aprosodias" and the "foreign dialect syndrome" (Ross, 1981). AOS may be of greatest interest, and most widely diagnosed, in children. The diagnosis of AOS is often assigned by default when a child's speech production deficits do not fit within recognized categories of either acquired or developmental speech production disorders (Crary, 1993; Hall, Jordan, & Robin, 1993). Alternative terms include "developmental apraxia of speech," "developmental verbal dyspraxia," "developmental verbal apraxia," "articulatory dyspraxia," and "articulatory apraxia" (see Hall et al., 1993, for a more complete list of synonyms). Though AOS in children is rarely found in isolation from other speech and language disorders, and is perhaps egregiously overdiagnosed, its phenomenology and proposed mechanisms are generally consistent with those in adults. However, AOS in children is usually found without the known or assumed focal left-hemisphere cortical or subcortical lesion, and without the assumed fully learned phonological and phonetic lexicons and motor programs. The importance of the clinical account for AOS in both children and adults is that (1) the clinical entity exists separately from dysarthria, aphasia, and other developmental phonological disorders; and (2) the management of individuals with AOS (assessment, treatment, prognosis) takes a decidedly different form from those of its closest clinical neighbors. The failure to make this differentiation has important consequences for both theory and patient care.

In spite of the theoretical and clinical motivations, three ordinate objections to AOS have arisen. The first is a pervasive and persistent problem with the term "apraxia" applied to speech production. This problem with the term is generally not encountered when the term is applied to other movement structures or systems. Martin (1974) most clearly articulated his objections to the *term* "AOS." These objections centered on the use of the term as applied to the speech production deficits of the specific patients described in the literature at that time. Although his objections are often interpreted as making the claim that "apraxia is actually aphasia," this characterization does not accurately represent the essence of his arguments. In fact, we would argue that the form of the argument— "that AOS is actually aphasia"—is illogical. Apraxia by definition is a motor disorder. The term may be applied to the wrong individuals, or the criteria for its existence may be in dispute, but apraxia cannot be aphasia. Martin did not make that logical error. Martin did *not* object to the notion of AOS or to the existence of the phenomenon. He argued that the evidence presented by Darley and colleagues could be used as evidence for a phonological-level deficit as well as, or better than, it could for a motor deficit. In great measure, we agree with the substance of his objections. However, more precisely developed models of speech production have allowed the further differentiation of AOS from phonological-level production disorders of aphasic origin and have largely obviated Martin's objections.

The second objection to the term, often leveled at the constellation of AOS signs proposed in this chapter, is the absence of a differentiation between *automatic* and *volitional* speech production deficits. This differentiation is an inherent part of most definitions of any apraxia. Specifically, critics of the term as applied to speech have observed that in other apraxias, there may be a quantitative and qualitative difference between movements produced on command (volitionally) and those executed in the commission of an automatic or vegetative act,[1] and that these differences have not been convincingly demonstrated in

AOS. In fact, persons with AOS can be quite debilitated during both highly volitional speech and automatic speech. Oral-nonspeech apraxia ("buccofacial apraxia"), a frequent but not obligatory associate of AOS, provides a nice example of the volitional–automatic dissociation that may be seen with other apraxias (see Square-Storer, Roy, & Hogg, 1990, and the epidemiological discussion of AOS below, for a more thorough review of this subject). Oral nonspeech apraxia co-occurs frequently with both Broca's and conduction aphasias, and with a variety of other communication disorders. It can also be the only sign of a left-hemisphere lesion. It is characterized by trial-and-error attempts to initiate movement, usually with expressed effort, and frequently with verbal augmentation (substituting the word for the intended act, such as saying the word "click" when asked to "click your tongue"). The difference between automatic and volitional performance can often be seen when a clinician requests a patient to "show me how you cough." Upon this request, a person with oral-nonspeech apraxia often displays a variety of movement deviations, including desynchronized breathing, sustained voicing, oral posturing, and (not infrequently) the verbal augmentation of producing the word "cough." These behaviors stand in bold contrast to the situation in which the same patient reflexively coughs for purposes of airway clearance, and does so without observable movement deviations. Another example might occur when a child or adult is unable to lick his or her lips on the prompt "Pretend to lick your lips" or the command "Show me how you lick your lips," but does so without delay or movement discoordination when automatically licking his or her lips to remove food residue. The assumption is that the quality of movement for these acts is *intact* for automatic/nonvolitional movements. This clear difference between oral movements produced to command and those produced in the context of automatic or vegetative acts is a striking feature of most persons with oral-nonspeech apraxia. The argument from some AOS opponents is that any apraxic speech behavior should be observed only under voluntary conditions (executed on command and not restricted to pantomimic actions), and that this clear distinction has not been convincingly demonstrated in AOS. One implication of this seemingly obligatory distinction is that there should be no functional consequences of apraxia, whether limb, oral-nonspeech, agraphic, or speech. However, the observations of De Renzi (1985) and Foundas et al. (1995) that patients with limb apraxia (not including persons with ideational apraxia) have substantive impairments of tool and object use in everyday action call into question the necessity of demonstrating the volitional–automatic distinction. They also call into question the need to demonstrate a difference between those acts performed in response to a command and those elicited naturally. In addition, these observations challenge the volitional–automatic criterion for the diagnosis of apraxia. Rothi and Heilman (1997b) have summarized this point:

> . . . the [compromised] ability of patients with limb apraxia to use tools and objects in natural contexts . . . [has] confirmed our impression that apraxia is not a trivial behavioural disorder only of theoretical interest, but instead apraxia is a common and disabling disorder. (p. 3)

The degree of intentionality, volition, or cognitive effort required for the successful execution of a motor act or a sequence of isolated movements, under various purposive and responsive conditions, is unknown. The psychological construct underlying this differentiation is elusive, and criteria for judging the differences have not been established. In addition, the degree of intentionality, volition, or conscious effort allocated to any particular task may vary from moment to moment within an individual and between individuals, even under the same assessment conditions. Ajuriaguerra and Hécaen (1964; reported by

Brown, 1972) also discuss the impairment of *both* automatic and volitional movements in "limb-kinetic" apraxia. Thus the lack of clear evidence differentiating volitional and automatic speech acts does not appear to be sufficient reason to dismiss the notion of AOS or the proposed mechanism of a motor programming or planning disorder as its basis.

A third argument has been made that it is too difficult to differentiate the speech errors of neurologically impaired patients, and that the use of the term "AOS" should therefore be avoided. The clinical difficulty in distinguishing apraxic speech errors from aphasic or dysarthric errors, as a basis for rejecting either the concept or the term "AOS," is indeed a shallow rationale. This reasoning is akin to the rejection of cortex as an anatomical brain region distinct from subcortex because an isotope scan is incapable of differentiating cortical from subcortical structures or lesions.

In spite of the considerable evidence that AOS is differentiable from its clinical neighbors and that it generally adheres to the theoretically expected phenomenology of a motor planning or programming disorder, a minority of researchers and clinical scientists repudiate the use of the term. This rejection has had the effect of essentially ignoring the voluminous literature describing the clinical entity and its management, as well as its theoretical basis. Some of these skeptics have, however, described what appears to be a syndrome with similar if not identical signs and symptoms, which they term "aphemia" (e.g., Nebes, 1975; Shif, Alexander, Naeser, & Galaburda, 1983; Littlefield, Barresi, & Goodglass, 1998). Although a direct and systematic comparison between AOS and aphemia does not appear to have been undertaken, as a first approximation, we are struck by the similarities and left in search of the differences. The term "aphemia," given by Broca to the severe speech production disorder of his now classic patient, is without theoretical justification and provides no differential diagnostic or treatment direction. Preference for this term over "AOS" is unjustified, and in the interest of advancing clinical science, its continued use should be discouraged.

There does appear to be a disciplinary bias toward using the term "AOS." Speech and language pathologists typically support its use (probably because of the biases established by Darley and colleagues), and neurologists and perhaps neuropsychologists argue against use of the term or omit it as a differential diagnostic category (probably because of the biases established by Geschwind and colleagues). However, these disciplinary biases are not universal. Neurologists such as Brown (1972) and Caplan (Rochon, Caplan, & Waters, 1991; Waters, Rochon, & Caplan, 1992), and neuropsychologists such as Dronkers (1997) find appropriate theoretical and clinical justification for its use.

DIFFERENTIATION OF AOS FROM THE DYSARTHRIAS

Although AOS is considered a motor speech disorder, as are the dysarthrias, its assumed psychophysiological mechanisms and clinical presentation are differentiable from those of the dysarthrias. Dysarthrias are usually associated with abnormal muscle tone or reflexes, paralysis or paresis, and ataxia or involuntary movements, while AOS is not. In addition, persons with AOS are not expected to have abnormal strength, movement (range, speed, or direction), or interarticulator coordination other than during speech, unless a co-occurring dysarthria or oral nonspeech apraxia is present. In persons with dysarthria, there is an assumed correspondence between movement deficits observed during speech and during nonspeech acts (although the correlation is imperfect because of the extreme difficulty in establishing equivalent speech and nonspeech task demands). Wertz, LaPointe, and Rosenbek (1984) have also proposed that AOS can be differentiated from the dysarthrias on anatomical grounds, with AOS resulting from unilateral and anterior lesions, and dysarthria resulting from bilateral cortical lesions or from lesions distributed throughout the cortico-bulbar system, the basal ganglia, and the cerebellum and its pathways. The pattern of speech errors observed in the course of clinical, motor, auditory, and visual examinations is also traditionally believed to differentiate the dysarthrias from AOS.

The recent recognition of unilateral upper-motor-neuron (UUMN) dysarthria as a distinct motor speech disorder has complicated these clinical conventions (see Duffy, 1995, for an excellent discussion of this disorder and its differentiation from AOS). However, well-trained speech-language pathologists can reliably distinguish between AOS and dysarthrias, using perceptual (clinical motor examinations, auditory and visual evaluations), acoustic, and physiological data. Wertz et al. (1984) have suggested that the speech errors of dysarthria can be distinguished from those of AOS. In their view, the errors of the dysarthric speaker are characterized by sound-level distortions, whereas the errors of the apraxic speaker are characterized by phoneme initiation impairments, sound selection (substitution) and sequencing errors with infrequent metatheses, and abnormal prosody. However, McNeil et al. (1997) have argued against this list of speech error types as characterizing, or even being consistent with, AOS. Nonetheless, the general phenomenology of apraxic speech errors is typically differentiable from that of the dysarthrias (except perhaps for the UUMN type). As a motoric disorder, AOS is marked by clear motoric-level deficits. Acoustic and physiological data supporting this assumption have been summarized elsewhere (Kent & McNeil, 1987; McNeil & Kent, 1990; McNeil et al., 1997) and are not reviewed here.

DIFFERENTIATION OF AOS FROM PHONEMIC PARAPHASIA

Code (1998) has recently reviewed the role that the hypothesized phonological–phonetic distinction has played in research on AOS. Indeed, this distinction has motivated the majority of clinical observations, experimental research, and theoretical ruminations about AOS, perhaps inspired by Martin's (1974) challenge to the theoretical and experimental application of the term. The logical and most prevalent approach to the phonological–phonetic distinction has been to describe the patterns of phonological errors produced by individuals diagnosed with AOS but without aphasia or dysarthria, and by individuals with aphasia but without AOS or dysarthria. There are, however, two problems with this approach. One has been the establishment of criteria for assigning subjects to these groups, and the second is the extreme difficulty of finding the "pure" subjects. As discussed by McNeil et al. (1997), it is likely that the majority of the literature on AOS, and on phonemic paraphasia as well, is seriously confounded by the observation and quantification of behaviors implicating both praxic and phonological mechanisms. There was a paucity of speech production models during the early formulations of AOS as a theoretically distinct entity (from 1968 to about 1985), and the majority of descriptive data on AOS were collected during this period. Because of these factors, pioneering AOS researchers have left a legacy of literature that is difficult to interpret with confidence. Typically, the descriptions of subjects selected for study have been so poorly detailed that it is as likely that the subjects were aphasic as apraxic. In the few studies in which subject selection criteria have been described with sufficient detail to determine the nature of their impairment, it appears that the subjects showed signs of both aphasia and AOS. The converse is also true when subjects with phonemic paraphasia have been the object of study. This difficult situation is not unreasonable, given the complexity of the theoretical and clinical problems, and given the fact that these disorders coexist in the overwhelming majority of patients. This difficulty does not, however, mean that the differentiation is theoretically unjustified, clinically unimportant, or impossible.

Another problem with the distinction between AOS and phonological paraphasia has involved the a priori selection of behaviors to be observed and the conditions under which to observe them. Neither has been without bias. That is, observing linguistic variables is likely to yield linguistic interpretations, and observing motor or physiological behaviors is likely to yield motor or physiological interpretations. Rarely have both types of variables been studied simultaneously in the same subjects, and even more rarely have "pure" cases of either disorder been studied. In addition, some speech behaviors that have traditionally been interpreted as evidence for a linguistic-level impairment may be explained best by motoric constructs. For example, Code (1998) has contemplated the role that markedness theory has played in the discussion of the nature of speech errors (both apraxic and aphasic), and the realigning of markedness with phonetic mechanisms rather than with the unrestrained and highly abstract phonological code. This realignment could potentially require reinterpretation of the assignment of linguistic and motoric mechanisms in a number of studies (e.g., Blumstein, 1973; Nespoulous, Joanette, Beland, Caplan, & Lecours, 1984). Similarly, some have challenged the concept that phonemic substitutions, categorized as such with broad phonetic transcription, are automatically generated by phonological mechanisms. Conversely, the assignment of metathetic, anticipatory, and perseveratory phonemic speech errors to a motoric mechanism (Wertz et al., 1984) has also been called into question. It is now fairly clear that patterns of phonological errors alone will not differentiate AOS from phonemic paraphasia (Blumstein, 1981; McNeil et al., 1997). It has also been argued recently (McNeil et al., 1997) that many other features traditionally assigned to AOS are also shared by persons with phonemic paraphasia, including difficulty initiating speech (with trial-and-error searching), variability of errors, and single-feature sound substitutions.

Acknowledging a measure of wisdom in Marshall's (1989) admonition to avoid definitions in neuropsychology, McNeil et al. (1997) have attempted to define the mechanisms of AOS and to specify the kernel or core features that must be present for its diagnosis. They define AOS as

> . . . a phonetic–motoric disorder of speech production caused by inefficiencies in the translation of a well-formed and filled phonologic frame to previously learned kinematic parameters assembled for carrying out the intended movement, resulting in intra- and inter-articulator temporal and spatial segmental and prosodic distortions. It is characterized by distortions of segments and intersegment transitionalization resulting in extended durations of consonants, vowels and time between sounds, syllables and words. These distortions are often perceived as sound substitutions and as the mis-assignment of stress and other phrasal and sentence-level prosodic abnormalities. Errors are relatively consistent in location within the utterance and invariable in type. It is not attributable to deficits of muscle tone or reflexes, nor to deficits in the processing of auditory, tactile, kinesthetic, proprioceptive, or language information. In its extremely infrequently occurring "pure" form, it is not accompanied by the above listed deficits of motor physiology, perception, or language. (p. 329)

The critical clinical features assumed are that the person with AOS will demonstrate (1) distortions (extended durations) of consonant and vowel segments; (2) intersegment transitionalization difficulties, realized as increased time between sounds, syllables, and words, and often described as "sound and syllable segregation"; (3) errors that are relatively consistent in location within the utterance and invariable in type; and (4) prosodic distortions realized as the misassignment of stress and other phrasal and sentence-level abnormalities. This list does not imply that the person with AOS will not also demonstrate broadly transcribed sound substitutions, trial-and-error groping and struggle behaviors, susceptibility to specific motoric or contextual constraints, or any particular phonologically categorized error type. It does, however, provide the theoretically motivated bases and the empirically supported evidence for the differential diagnosis of AOS from other neurogenic speech production disorders including the dysarthrias and phonemic paraphasia. Table 9.1 is a tentative list of prosodic, phonological, kinematic, phenomenological, and treatment response characteristics that differentiate AOS from phonemic paraphasia.

Although AOS as a disorder differentiable from phonemic paraphasia has been only briefly discussed here, it has been reviewed critically elsewhere. The reader is referred to the summaries and critical reviews of Buckingham (1979, 1981, 1992), Keller (1984), Kent and McNeil (1987), LaPointe and Johns (1975), Lebrun (1990), McNeil and Kent (1990), McNeil et al. (1997), Miller (1986), Pierce (1991), Rosenbek, Kent, and LaPointe (1984), Square (1995), Square and Martin (1994), and Wertz et al. (1984).

EPIDEMIOLOGY OF AOS

The etiologies and clinical associations of AOS, like those of most other neurogenic speech and language disorders, have been inadequately investigated. Duffy (1995) provides what are perhaps the most reliable and valid prevalence figures for AOS, although data from smaller studies are also included in this review. Based on the evaluation of 3,417 patients evaluated at the Mayo Clinic for acquired neurogenic communication disorders (aphasia, dysarthria, AOS, other neurogenic speech production disorders, and other cognitive–linguistic disorders), he reported a 4.6% prevalence of AOS. He also reported a 9% prevalence of AOS in a quasi-randomly selected set of motor speech disorder cases from the database at Mayo Clinic. In all of these cases, it is assumed that AOS co-occurred with other motor, language, or cognitive disorders. Of particular clinical importance is the observation from Duffy (1995) that AOS was the first sign of neurological disease in 23% of all patients with neurogenic speech and language disorders, and was one of the initial signs in 70%. Given our assumption that phonemic paraphasia is probably confounded in the diagnosis of at least a portion of these AOS-diagnosed subjects, we believe that these figures are likely to be overestimates in most categories.

Duffy (1995) also reported that AOS can result from a number of neurological diseases (e.g., Creutzfeldt–Jakob disease, leukoencephalopathy) and disorders (e.g., seizure disorders). The most frequent etiology was a single left-hemisphere vascular accident, but degenerative disease, traumatic brain injury (primarily neurosurgically induced) and seizure disorders were also associated with AOS (see Table 9.2). Wertz, Rosenbek, and Deal (1970; cited in Duffy 1995) reported a similar prevalence of associated diseases. Table 9.3, which gives the frequency of different types of apraxias assocated with right- versus left-hemisphere lesions, shows how much more often AOS is linked with left-hemisphere disturbance.

AOS is frequently associated with other apraxias or with aphasia (see Table 9.4). The prevalence of concurrent oral-nonspeech (buccofacial) apraxia has been assessed in a number of studies of AOS. Figures range from a high of 85% reported by LaPointe and Wertz (1974) to a low of 48% reported by Dronkers (1997), with an average of 68%. Among patients with AOS, the prevalence of limb apraxias averaged 67%, limb and oral-nonspeech apraxia 83%, aphasia 81%, and dysarthria 31%.

TABLE 9.1. Tentative List of Characteristics That Differentiate AOS from Phonemic Paraphasia

Apraxia of speech	Phonemic paraphasia

Disturbed prosody

Overall rate:	
Slow rate in phonemically "on-target" or "off-target" phrases and sentences.	*Near normal rate* in phonemically "on-target" phrases and sentences.
Inability to increase rate while maintaining phonemic integrity.	Variable *ability to increase rate*, but *within normal ranges*, while maintaining phonemic integrity.
Microsegmental rate:	
Variable, but *overall prolonged movement transitions*.	Variable, but *normal movement transition durations*.
Variable, but *prolonged interword intervals* in phonemically "on-target" utterances.	Variable, but *normal average interword intervals* in phonemically "on-target" utterances.
Variable, but *abnormally long vowels* in multisyllabic words or words in sentences.	Variable, but *normal vowel duration* in multisyllabic words or words in sentences.
Variable, but *increased movement durations* for individual speech gestures in the production of contextual speech.	Variable, but *average movement durations* within the ranges for normal subjects.
Successive self-initiated trials to repair an error [lead] *no closer to the target*.	Successive self-initiated trials to repair an error [lead] *closer to the target*.
Stress assignment:	
Presence of errors on stressed syllables.	*No clear relationship between syllabic stress and error frequency.*

Phonological characteristics

With *distorted* perseverative, anticipatory, and exchange phoneme or phoneme cluster errors.	With *undistorted* perseverative, anticipatory, and phoneme exchange or phoneme cluster errors.
With phoneme distortions.	*Without phoneme distortions.*
Presence of distorted sound substitutions— primarily of prolonged phonemes and secondarily devoiced phonemes.	*Absence of distorted sound substitutions.*

Other kinematic characteristics

Inability to track predictable movement patterns with speech articulators.	*Ability to track predictable movement patterns* with speech articulators.
Ability to track unpredictable movement patterns with speech articulators.	*Inability to track unpredictable movement patterns* with speech articulators.

Other characteristics

The *location of errors* in the utterance is *consistent* from trial to trial.	The *location of errors* in the utterance is *inconsistent* from trial to trial.
The *types of errors* in the utterance are *not variable* from trial to trial.	The *types of errors* in the utterance are *variable* from trial to trial.

Treatment characteristics

Positive response to "minimal [-contrast] pairs" treatment.	*Negative* response to "minimal [-contrast] pairs" treatment.
Positive response to treatment based on principles of "motor learning."	*Ineffective* response to treatment based on principles of "motor learning."

Note: From McNeil, M. R., Robin, D. A., & Schmidt, R. A. (1997). Apraxia of speech: Definition, differentiation, and treatment. In M. R. McNeil (Ed.), *Clinical management of sensorimotor speech disorders* (p. 327). New York: Thieme.

TABLE 9.2. Etiology of AOS (107 Cases)

Cause	Percent of cases
Vascular	58
Single left-hemisphere stroke	48
Multiple strokes	10
Degenerative	16
Unspecified	9
Associated with dementia	4
Primary progressive aphasia	3
Traumatic brain injury	15
Neurosurgically induced lesions	12
Closed head trauma	3
Left-hemisphere neoplasm	6
Seizure disorder	1
Undetermined and mixed etiology	5

Note: Data from Duffy. (1995).

Among patients with AOS, the prevalence of aphasia ranged from a high of 92% reported by Dronkers (1997) to a low of 78% reported by Duffy (1995), with an average of 81% in the two studies from which data could be extracted. These figures appear to be low, given our collective clinical experience. Whether differences in diagnostic criteria or other factors are responsible is unknown.

Few data estimating the prevalence of "pure" AOS are available. Dronkers (1997) reported an 8% figure, but her study population is unlikely to have been epidemiologically representative. Square-Storer, Roy, and Hogg (1990) found that none of their 23 persons with AOS were without other forms of apraxia.

It is apparent that whereas AOS can result from nearly any disorder affecting the central nervous system, the majority of cases have unilateral left-hemisphere strokes. It is very frequently associated with other disorders, such as oral-nonspeech apraxia, limb apraxia, oral-nonspeech and limb apraxias in combination, or aphasia; it is somewhat less frequently associated with UUMN dysarthria. The prevalence of "pure" AOS is very difficult to estimate. However, it is our experience that "pure" AOS is so rare that practicing clinicians will be unlikely to observe it more than once or twice in the course of their careers. This is likely to be the case even if they are sensitized to its importance and are exposed to a full and continuing caseload of neurogenic communication disorders. It is important to recognize that the data summarized in this section and in Tables 9.2, 9.3, and 9.4 represent

TABLE 9.3. Frequency of Apraxias in Patients with Right- and Left-Hemisphere Lesions

Apraxia type	Percentage of patients	
	Right hemisphere (*n* = 10)	Left hemisphere (*n* = 26)
Limb alone		8
Oral-nonspeech alone	30	
Limb and apraxia of speech	10	
Limb and oral-nonspeech		4
Oral-nonspeech and apraxia of speech		4
Limb, oral-nonspeech, and apraxia of speech		73

Note: Data from Square-Storer, Roy, & Hogg (1990).

TABLE 9.4. Co-Occurrence of Other Disorders in Patients with AOS

	Number of patients	Percent with co-occurring disorders
Oral-nonspeech (buccofacial) apraxia		
Dronkers (1997)	25	48
Duffy (1995)	64	63
Kertesz (1984)	10	80
LaPointe and Wertz (1974)	13	85
Marquardt and Sussman (1984)	15	80
Square-Storer, Roy, and Hogg (1990)	23	83
Total	150	68
Limb apraxia		
Dronkers (1997)	25	52
Square-Storer et al. (1990)	23	83
Total	48	67
Limb apraxias and oral-nonspeech apraxia		
Square-Storer et al. (1990)	23	83
Aphasia		
Dronkers (1997)		
Broca's	13	52
Global	3	12
Anomic aphasia	7	28
Conduction	0	0
Wernicke	0	0
Unclassifiable	0	0
Dronkers (1997) total	25	92
Duffy (1995)	106	78
Total	131	81
Dysarthria		
Dronkers (1997)	25	40
Duffy (1995)	106	29
Total/	131	31

epidemiologically unrepresentative subject samples that were selected for specific studies with specific purposes and goals. Only the data reported by Duffy (1995) represent a relatively large sample of unselected (though not randomly selected) subjects from which some tentative conclusions might reasonably be drawn. Nonetheless, there is actually more coherence among the studies reviewed than might be predicted from the biases inherent in the studies.

AOS LESION DATA

Intimately tied to the notion of AOS, to possible AOS subcategories, and to its theorized mechanisms are beliefs about the lesion locations that cause them. It is frequently held among AOS researchers that lesions in parietal and frontal lobes can cause signs consistent with AOS (Square, Darley, & Sommers, 1982). Some clinical scientists have sought models (Mlcoch & Noll, 1980) and experimental evidence that subcortical lesions, as well as the more traditionally recognized cortical lesions, may underlie the behaviors consistent with AOS (Mohr et al., 1978). Indeed, a lesion pathognomonic of AOS has been elusive.

The distinction between potential frontal lobe and parietal lobe mechanisms has played an important role in the proposed differentiation of AOS from phonological paraphasias, and in the possible subtyping of AOS. The frontal lobe mechanism is thought to be instantiated in Broca's area (Luria, 1966). It is proposed to store and access motor plans or programs for gestures or speech segments (phonemes, syllables, or words). The parietal lobe mechanism is most likely instantiated in the facial region of the postcentral gyrus (Luria, 1966). It is believed to govern the transitionalization between speech segments or between nonspeech gestures (Canter, Trost, & Burns, 1985; Mateer & Kimura, 1977; Poeck & Kerschensteiner, 1975; Square et al., 1982). "Transitionalization" is the coordinated movement from one speech segment to another.

Square-Storer, Roy, and Martin (1997) have hypothesized that AOS can arise from parietal lobe, frontal lobe, or subcortical ("frontal quadralateral space") lesions. Combined frontal cortical–subcortical lesions may additionally be associated with pseudobulbar dysarthria. Square-Storer et al. (1997) have further hypothesized that Broca's area is only one of many brain regions involved in the regulation of speech motor control. They have identified six areas that, when damaged, can cause AOS: (1) nonprimary motor cortex (Brodmann area 6), including both lateral premotor cortex and mesial premotor cortex (supplementary motor cortex); (2) frontal pars opercularis (Brodmann area 44); (3) white matter underlying Broca's area; (4) the insula; (5) the lenticular nucleus; and (6) midparietal cortex. Of note are the speech characteristics associated with midparietal lesions. Square-Storer et al. (1997) describe these as repetitions, reattempts and articulation errors *without slowness* [italics added] as evidenced by normal word, syllable and vocalic nuclei durations.[2] These authors also wisely point out that structural lesions outside of the frontal lobes can cause remote effects on the frontal lobes that can result in behaviors consistent with AOS.

As stated above, one model of AOS implicates lesions of Broca's area in the genesis of such features as lengthened segmental distortions, and lesions of the parietal lobe in the genesis of disorders of transitionalization. The assignment of these behaviors to these specific anatomical regions or lesion sites is not, however, universal. For example, Liepmann (1905, 1913) linked the labored articulation of individual speech sounds and disorders of transitionalization to lesions of Broca's area.

Kertesz (1984) reported computerized tomographic (CT) evidence of subcortical lesions involving the left anterior limb of the internal capsule, putamen, and globus pallidus, in 10 patients with disorders of speech output including dysarthria. Because all patients were aphasic and their speech production was not precisely described, it is difficult to have confidence in any relationships drawn between lesion locus and signs of AOS in these patients. This limitation is, however, not unique to this report. The limpid historical account of AOS by Lebrun (1989) makes clear that poor observation and description of signs and symptoms have contributed as much as inadequate theory to the continuing controversies about AOS and its neuroanatomical substrates. Furthermore, this confusion is evident throughout the contemporary history (now approximately 140 years) of the literature on AOS and related disorders of speech production. Poor description and inadequate theory notwithstanding, the search for the essential lesion producing AOS continues unabated.

Deutsch (1984) was among the first to conduct a prospective investigation of lesion location in patients with AOS. He studied 18 adults with left-hemisphere lesions who displayed two or more of the following speech behaviors that were considered to define AOS: phoneme, syllable, or word segregation/transitionalization (the abnormal separation of speech units, often with the intrusion of a neutral vowel such as /a/ or the schwa); disturbed prosody; initiation deficits, including groping and searching; errors in phonemic and syllabic sequencing; phoneme substitutions, omissions, additions, repetitions, and distortions; error inconsistency; and increased errors with increased word length.[3] Nine of the subjects had frontal lobe lesions, and nine had "posterior" lesions. Thirteen predictor variables were entered into a stepwise discriminant-function analysis. Monosyllabic errors were classified as complex, fluency, articulation, syllable addition, sequencing, and total monosyllabic. Polysyllabic errors were classified as complex, fluency, articulation, syllable addition, syllable omission, sequencing, and total polysyllabic. The model assigned 16 of the 18 subjects to the correct group. The percentages of polysyllabic sequencing errors, monosyllabic articulation errors, and total polysyllabic errors were the best predictor variables, yielding 89% correct subject classification. One subject from each lesion group was misclassified. Overall, the posterior group had 6.3% fewer monosyllabic articulation errors, 5.3% more polysyllabic sequencing errors, and 5.8% more total polysyllabic errors compared to the frontal group.

Marquardt and Sussman (1984) also prospectively studied what their chapter title termed "The Elusive Lesion–Apraxia of Speech Link in Broca's Aphasia." Fifteen individuals with Broca's aphasia and an identifiable lesion on CT scan were studied. Subjects were heterogeneous with respect to age, time since onset, and etiology. AOS was identified and quantified with the Verbal Agility subtest of the Boston Diagnostic Aphasia Exam (Goodglass & Kaplan, 1972) and six subtests from an unpublished protocol. The latter included imitations of (1) 6 multisyllabic words, (2) 12 words of increasing length, (3) 10 words with identical initial and final consonants, (4) 5 sentences, and (5) serial repetition of stop-vowel syllables. Both lesion volumes and centroid values were correlated with these speech production measures and with a variety of oral nonspeech and limb apraxia measures. The diagnosis of Broca's aphasia, according to Marquardt and Sussman's criteria, was not synonymous with the presence of AOS, as only 12 subjects (80%) were judged to demonstrate AOS. Likewise, limb apraxia was present in only 5 subjects, while oral nonspeech apraxia was present in all 15 subjects. The only statistically significant correlation was a negative one between lesion volume and diadochokinetic rate (rapid serial repetition of stop-vowel syllables). Neither the presence nor the severity of AOS was reliably related to the lesion volume, or to the medial–lateral or the superior–inferior center of the lesion. Although lesions were located primarily within the left frontal lobe, they also included the anterior parietal and superior temporal lobes. All subjects demonstrated lesions deep to the cortex, and several of the lesions included the insular cortex and frontal operculum. The examination of individual cases did not reveal a consistent relationship between lesion location (e.g., cortical vs. subcortical) or lesion volume and the presence or absence of AOS.

Perhaps the most often cited and best-controlled study of lesion locations associated with AOS is the prospective neuroimaging investigation by Dronkers (1997). Using a method of overlapping lesion locations identified on CT and magnetic resonance imaging, she reported that 100% of a group of 25 individuals with adult acquired AOS had a discrete left-hemisphere cortical lesion in the precentral gyrus of the insula. A control group of 19 individuals without AOS, but with left-hemisphere lesions in the same arterial distribution as the subjects with AOS, all showed sparing of this specific region of the insula. This double dissociation provides the most compelling evidence for a lesion-specific AOS site to date. However, it must be remembered that, as in most of the rest of the literature on AOS, the behavioral criteria used for subject selection leave the distinct possibility that the subjects displayed phonemic paraphasias as well as (or instead of) AOS.

McNeil, Weismer, Adams, and Mulligan (1990) reported CT lesion data on four carefully studied individuals with "pure" AOS (without aphasia or dysarthria) who met the definition and criteria for AOS described by McNeil et al. (1997). Only two of the four subjects had involvement of the insula. Two of three subjects without AOS but with conduction aphasia also had involvement of the insula. Two of the four subjects with AOS and one of the three subjects with conduction aphasia had partial destruction of Broca's area. The only common lesion location identified among the four subjects with AOS was in the facial region of the postcentral gyrus. Three of the four persons with AOS and one of the persons with conduction aphasia were judged by a neurologist experienced in making these judgments to have substantial destruction of this area. The supramarginal gyrus and the angular gyrus were the only lesion locations common to the three subjects with conduction aphasia.

AOS COMPARED TO OTHER APRAXIAS

The first issue in any comparison of AOS to other apraxias is a theoretical one, focused on a discussion of "apraxia without adjectives" that parallels the debate in the aphasia literature (Darley, 1982). Square-Storer et al. (1990) indicate their reluctance to dissociate oral, limb, and speech apraxia because of an assumed common mechanism subserving all three. Discussing 3 of their 23 individuals who did not demonstrate the presence of all three types of apraxia, they state:

> Just as we would not consider alexia, in the absence of other language modality impairments, a true aphasia but instead an instance of disconnection between visual receptive and association areas, we hesitate to refer to these three instances of apraxia modality dissociations as true apraxias. (p. 466)

Discussing the evidence for a commonality among apraxias, Roy and Square-Storer (1990) proposed three possible factors contributing to their co-occurrence; the presence of aphasia, the location of the lesion, and the nature of the neuromotor control processes. Both lesion location and a common motor control mechanism were discussed as important reasons for the typical co-occurrence of the apraxias. Indeed, a coherent theory that accounts for the dissociation among limb apraxia, oral-nonspeech apraxia, and AOS has not been proposed. Whether the isolated presence of one form of apraxia should be considered apraxia at all may be a legitimate point of discussion.

Darley (1968) and his proteges (Aten, Johns, & Darley, 1971; Deal & Darley, 1972; Johns & Darley, 1970; Rosenbek, Wertz, & Darley, 1973; Shane & Darley, 1978; Square, Darley, & Sommers, 1981, 1982; Square-Storer, Darley, & Sommers, 1988), in applying the term "apraxia" to speech, made the same general assumptions about the nature of the disorder and criteria for its diagnosis that are made in the diagnosis of other apraxias. Like Liepmann (1900, 1905, 1913) in his influential early formulations, and like most apraxia researchers, Darley suggested that the term should be applied only to previously learned speech movements. Furthermore, the term should be applied only when it is reasonably certain that a patient displays the intent (has the understanding of the task and the will to comply), knowledge of the underlying linguistic representation, ability to process the language (i.e., aphasic deficits are not likely to interfere with task performance), and the fundamental sensory and motor ability (i.e., absence of sensory deficits, weakness, paralysis or dyscoordination of the speech musculature when used for nonspeech tasks), and that the patient is disproportionately impaired during volitional activity. These criteria meet those of many definitions of apraxia. For example, Rothi and Heilman (1997b) define apraxia as "a neurological disorder of learned purposive movement skill that is not explained by deficits of elemental motor or sensory systems" (p. 3). Although many disorders fall under the term "apraxia," each with unique cognitive and motoric mechanisms, the criteria listed above do not apply equally to all types of apraxia. There are many published pellucid reviews of the various forms of apraxia, including those in the volumes edited by Hammond (1990), Rothi and Heilman (1997a), and Roy (1985). There are also several newly proposed forms of apraxia, including "dissociation," "conduction," and "conceptual" (Rothi, Ochipa, & Heilman, 1991). However, these forms are not reviewed here.

It is the goal in this part of the chapter to briefly discuss the relationships between AOS and three types of limb apraxia, focusing on coherence between them in their assumed mechanisms and in their clinical and kinematic manifestations. The search for similarities and differences is indeed reasonable. As Roy and Square (1985) suggest, "Given that the motor control processes in speech and limb systems are similar (De Renzi, Pieczuro, & Vignolo, 1966) disruptions to verbal and limb praxis should also follow similar principles" (p. 111). The precise relationship between AOS and the various limb apraxias is difficult to define. The units of disturbed movement vary with type of limb apraxia. Whole conceptual units are said to be impaired in ideational apraxia. Elements of the overall concept are impaired in ideomotor apraxia, perhaps analogous to units operated on in the motor plan in the model of Van der Merwe (1997). Subconceptual elements (perhaps analogous to the elements in the motor program in the model of Van der Merwe, 1997) are involved in limb-kinetic apraxia. The movement "chunks" associated with speech (and writing) are realized as linguistic units of various sizes (phonemes, morphemes, syllables, words, grammar, etc.) and not as kinematic entities. However, impairment of the kinematic entities underlying speech praxis is often indistinguishable from linguistic impairment. That is, it is difficult to define deficits in speech that are mechanistically comparable to deficits in limb praxis, and that cannot be attributed to linguistic dysfunction at the level of the phonological output buffer or lexical–semantic retrieval systems. Segments of speech or writing that are the size of those said to be impaired in ideational apraxia would have to be equivalent to those processed at the lexical–semantic level, the impairment of which would be indistinguishable from aphasia. Speech segments analogous to the movements that are impaired in ideomotor apraxia may be comparable to those produced by the phonological, morphological, and syntactic (sequence) systems, and hence conceptually and functionally inseparable from aphasia. By default, it seems that the limb analogue of AOS is limb-kinetic apraxia, unless the argument is waged that phonological selection and sequencing errors are really apraxic in origin (Buckingham, 1983) . Maintaining the distinction between aphasia and apraxia is clearly warranted on many grounds, but it is sufficiently justified by the fact that aphasia and apraxia can occur completely independently of one another, though they often do co-occur.

"Ideational apraxia" is defined as a sequence of movements that, although correct as individual components (e.g., slicing cheese and buttering bread), do not in aggregate accomplish the desired objective (e.g., making a sandwich). Errors of sequence may be present (e.g., putting the cheese on the sandwich before the bread is buttered). As described by Wertz et al. (1984), these patients may put matches in their mouths, or drink from a cup by leaning over or under it. Poeck (1982, 1985) and Lehmkuhl and Poeck (1981) describe errors such as beating a can with a can opener or stirring water in a cup with a water immersion heater (errors more consistent with conceptual apraxia in current terminology, but see below). Severity of ideational apraxia is related to task complexity. Ideational apraxia can occur in the presence of the ability to name the object correctly and even describe its function, although there is frequently concomitant severe aphasia or dementia that makes this assessment impossible. For Poeck (1985), ideational apraxia is only one of two forms of limb apraxia (along with ideomotor apraxia) that "is the consequence of a disturbance in the conceptual organization of movements" (p. 99). He observed it in only about 4% of patients with dominant parietal lobe lesions (almost always in the left hemisphere). According to Poeck (1985), "All patients with ideational apraxia are aphasic" (p. 105). Ochipa, Rothi, and Heilman (1992) differentiate ideational apraxia (the inability to complete a goal such as making a sandwich) from "conceptual apraxia," which is characterized by an inability to demonstrate knowledge of specific tool use. Nonetheless, most classification systems do not make this distinction, and for the current discussion this possible differentiation is irrelevant.

According to De Renzi (1985), the diagnosis of ideational apraxia requires impaired performance while a patient is using objects (as opposed to deficits in pantomime with or without a stimulus being present). It can be seen even during the imitation of intransitive gestures (symbolic and natural movements intended to express ideas or feelings) (see Heilman, 1973, for a counterargument relative to the impairment of imitation in ideational apraxia).

There is considerable controversy in the literature as to whether ideational apraxia is simply a more severe form of ideomotor apraxia, though several investigators make the case that it is not (e.g., De Renzi, 1985; Heilman, 1973; Poeck, 1985). A precise behavioral characterization of ideational apraxia is difficult to formulate from its diverse descriptions throughout the literature. Because of this diversity, it is difficult to formulate a reasonable analogy to AOS in its behavioral characterization, in the situations under which it is elicited, in its anatomical substrates, or in its hypothesized theoretical (psychological) underpinnings. If a speech or language analogy were to be drawn, one to verbal paraphasia or paragrammatic speech (a substitution or sequencing error of a lexical or morphological form) might be the closest.

"Ideomotor apraxia" is characterized by the impairment of isolated gestures but with preserved overall purpose. Terminology for the various limb apraxias is not universally shared. Nonetheless, Kimura (1977) and Heilman (1979) have described patients with ideomotor apraxia as demonstrating "clumsiness." Poizner, Mack, Verfaellie, Rothi, and Heilman (1990) classified patients as having ideomotor apraxia when they demonstrated errors in the timing and spatial aspects of the movement (see also Ochipa & Rothi, Chapter 10, this volume).

Many authors suggest that the disorder rarely presents itself during spontaneous activity, and is often detected only when execution or imitation of a tool use pantomime is requested. For Poeck (1985), "the inappropriate selection of motor elements within a motor sequence is of equal importance" (p. 99) to sequencing errors involving correctly selected elements. According to Poeck, axial as well as distal movements may be affected. Perseveration of previously correct and incorrect movements is a characteristic behavior.

Heilman, Rothi, and Valenstein (1982) proposed the existence of a motor memory center in the parietal lobe. Here motor programs for skilled movement are stored that instantiate kinesthetic and visual information. They proposed two distinct forms of ideomotor apraxia, depending on whether the lesion has damaged this motor memory center, or whether it has damaged the "innervatory pattern" target of projections from this center (in premotor cortex) or the projections themselves. Damage to the motor memory center itself is hypothesized to cause ideomotor apraxia that includes deficits of both gesture production and recognition/comprehension, as well as impaired learning of new gestural patterns. Damage to the pathways connecting this center to premotor cortex should create ideomotor apraxia (because of difficulty retrieving information from visual–kinesthetic memory), but with preserved recognition/comprehension of limb gestures and unimpaired learning of new movement patterns. Although evidence supporting this contention is sparse, Heilman et al.'s proposal has led to identification of additional subtypes of limb apraxia, a more finely elaborated definition of the behaviors that characterize the disorder, and more precise criteria for diagnosis.

If an analogy to a speech or language disorder were to be postulated for this type of apraxia, it would perhaps be closest to the phonological paraphasia present in all "types" of aphasia, but perhaps most frequently observed in so-called conduction aphasia. It should be remembered that, as Lehmkuhl, Poeck, and Willmes (1983) have found in classical aphasia syndromes (Wernicke's, Broca's, global), the severities of aphasia and limb apraxia appear to be unrelated.

"Limb-kinetic apraxia" is characterized by disturbances in the precise movements of the limb, usually described as impaired "coordination" and "smoothness" of action. Liepmann (1920; quoted in Brown, 1972, p. 180) described the clinical picture of limb-kinetic apraxia as one consisting of "coarse, mutilated simple movements, while complex motion such as sewing may not even get started. Errors resemble those of ataxia, and are not diminished by imitative or transitive movements with objects." Based on a single case with probable diffuse cerebral damage, Kleist (1907; quoted in Brown, 1972, p. 180) reported the movement characteristics of "slowness" and "awkwardness," with particular difficulty in fine isolated or partial movements. Comparable characteristics of AOS have been summarized in the reviews by Kent and McNeil (1987), McNeil and Kent (1990), and McNeil et al. (1997). Kleist also discussed a disturbance in the simultaneous action of separate muscle groups in limb-kinetic apraxia (also reported by Foerster, 1936) quite comparable to the simultaneous agonist–antagonist muscle co-contraction in AOS reported by Fromm, Abbs, McNeil, and Rosenbek (1982), and the lack of smoothness of the over-all movement sequence in AOS discussed by McNeil and Adams (1990) and McNeil, Caliguiri, and Rosenbek (1989). Moreover, Kleist noted that in limb-kinetic apraxia, the severity of the movement disorder is proportional to the general complexity of the movement task. He suggested that limb-kinetic apraxia is often associated with paresis and motor memory impairments, but is mechanistically independent of both. He felt that it cannot be attributed to disorders of "ideation," because the correct movement always appears in the deficient performance. We take this to mean that the movements are distorted, not replaced or omitted, in much the same way as in AOS as described by McNeil et al. (1997). Luria (1966) also described limb-kinetic apraxia as a movement disorder of premotor origin. He viewed it as characterized by normal strength, but with isolation of the actions constituting highly organized and highly skilled movements such as typing and handwriting. It may be that these features are analogous to the sound, syllable, and word segregation abnormalities described by McNeil et al. (1997) as one of the cardinal features of AOS. Brown (1972) describes this constellation of signs as an akinesia of the distal part of the limb that often appears as a remnant of resolving hemiparesis once strength has returned to normal levels.

In contrast to AOS (see reviews by McNeil & Kent, 1990; McNeil et al., 1997), there are relatively few precise and carefully gathered kinematic descriptions of movement impairments in limb-kinetic apraxia. Perhaps this paucity of investigation is due to its tenuous status as a legitimate type of apraxia, whose characteristics are often subsumed under ideomotor apraxia. One kinematic study of patients with ideomotor apraxia by Poizner et al. (1990) demonstrated a variety of temporal–spatial movement distortions. These movement patterns have been compared to those of "purely" apraxic speakers, who were carefully selected for an absence of aphasia or dysarthria of any kind (Forrest, Adams, McNeil, &

Southwood, 1991). Forrest et al. examined the phase plane trajectories (from simultaneous kinematic and electromyographic studies of lower-lip and jaw-closing movements during speech gestures) in normal subjects and in patients with conduction aphasia, ataxic dysarthria, and pure AOS. They reported that the productions of subjects with AOS were decoupled in their temporal–spatial relations (i.e., amplitude–velocity relations) relative to the same gestures in the normal subjects. They also noted the strikingly similar decomposition of multiarticulated movements involved in complex arm trajectories in the individuals with limb apraxia reported by Poizner et al. (1990).

PAST AND EMERGING THEORIES ABOUT AOS

Darley (1968) originally defined AOS as a disturbance of motor programming that results in a disorder of purposeful movement, and that cannot be accounted for by deficits of perception, comprehension, paralysis, or muscular weakness (conditions consistent with Liepmann's definition of apraxia). This definition framed the questions that immediately followed from Darley's observations. It continues to frame most of the theoretical and clinical debate at present. The construct of "motor programs" holds important theoretical and clinical implications for the apraxias of all varieties, including AOS. A number of motor programming conceptual frameworks and models have been proposed and related to AOS. Hall et al. (1993) have reviewed simple open- and closed-loop models, serial order models, Roy's hierarchical model, and schema theory (including the generalized motor program component of schema theory), and related each theory's potential for explaining developmental apraxia of speech. Darley's specification of AOS as a disorder of motor programming (taken from the general explanation of other apraxias, following Liepmann), as opposed to a disorder at the motor "execution" level (dysarthria) or the linguistic level (aphasia), set the general terms of the debate and the paradigms under which AOS would be studied. However, a number of other general constructs, models, and theories about AOS and other apraxias have been postulated since his seminal observations. What follows is a discussion of the past and emerging theories of AOS.

Traditional Explanations: "Motor Programs"

It is important to state at the outset of any discussion of motor programming that substantive arguments *against* the notion of motor programs have been advanced (Reed, 1982; Keele, Cohen, & Ivry, 1990; Kelso, 1995; Kelso & Tuller, 1984). Likewise, arguments and evidence *for* the notion of motor programs have been provided (Harrington & Haaland, 1987, 1991; Schmidt, 1982; Wickens, Hyland, & Anson, 1994; Gracco & Abbs, 1987). It is beyond the scope of this chapter to present the arguments and evidence for or against motor programs, but suffice it to say that the construct of such programs endures, albeit in many forms and with many lineaments.

Rosenbek et al. (1984) reviewed some of the basic tenets and varieties of motor programming and dynamic theories as they may relate to AOS. They included the center-pathway models espoused by Geschwind (1975) and Rothi and Heilman (1997a); the stage models, such as those proposed by Brown and Perecman (1986) for speech and language in general, and by Sternberg, Monsell, Knoll, and Wright (1978) for motor programming of speech and finger movements; Kelso and Tuller's (1981) coalition model; Shaffer's (1982) rhythm and timing model; Roy's (1978) hierarchical model; and Schmidt's (1975) motor schema model. Although these important formulations have motivated considerable experimental work in motor control (including speech motor control), as well as some work in AOS (e.g., Strand, 1987), critical questions about the unit or units of movement or speech that are programmed, coalesced, emergent, or hierarchical remain unanswered and debated. Until this complex but fundamental issue is resolved, the notion of motor programs will remain a very general guiding principle, but one without the power to generate explicit predictions about speech pathologies. Nevertheless, explicit theories, frameworks, and hypotheses of AOS have emerged. The most important recent contributions are reviewed below.

Planning versus Programming

Although the terms "speech planning" and "speech programming" have at times been used synonymously and without careful distinction, Van der Merwe (1997) has made it clear that the distinction is critical in differentiating among neurogenic speech pathologies. Van der Merwe describes the planning phase of speech production as one preceding the initiation of any movements, and one involving the gradual transformation of phonemes into a recognizable code for the motor system. It involves the formulation of an action strategy by specifying motor goals. In this formulation, speech planning is accomplished in the motor association areas. These areas include premotor cortex (lateral area 6), Broca's area, the supplementary motor area (medial area 6), the prefrontal and parietal association areas (including areas 5 and 7), the caudate circuit of the basal ganglia, and Wernicke's area (area 22). Van der Merwe's formulation adheres to MacNeilage's (1970) target-based model, with the assumption that within the context of the specific utterance, the phoneme is the unit of planning and there are invariant spatial and temporal specifications for each phoneme. Sensory–motor memory, in the form of the proprioceptive, tactile, and auditory engrams associated with these learned phonemes, is accessed during speech production. In this formulation, the invariant movement parameters derived from the specific sequence of phonemes being planned are adapted by the context in which they will appear. These adaptations (compensations) include shortening the "chunks" or units of the utterance (sound, syllable, or word segregation), reducing the number of phonological targets within a word, duplicating sounds within a word, and slowing speech rate. Van der Merwe notes that these "compensations" have been reported to occur in AOS, and that the slowed rate also occurs in normal speakers who are confronted with long or unfamiliar speech targets (note the similar observation of Whiteside & Varley, 1998, discussed below).

Central to this view of speech planning is the notion that the motor plans are sequential. The plans are articulator-specific, not muscle-specific. "Motor goals," such as lip rounding, jaw depression, glottal closure, raising or lowering of the tongue tip, and interarticulator phasing (coarticulation) are also specified at this level. Plans are derived for the different sounds and specify the spatial and temporal goals of the planned unit. For normal speakers, the planned unit is usually several words in size. Although the motor plans are derived from invariant sensory–motor memory, the actualization of these goals is susceptible to several sources of variability. These sources include adaptation to the sound environment, coarticulatory requirements, motor equivalence (the ability to achieve an acceptable articulatory/acoustic goal via several movement patterns, such as achieving lip closure by either moving the lower lip to meet the upper, moving the upper lip to meet the lower, or moving both to varying degrees), phonetic and linguistic influences on segmental duration, clear or formal speech requirements, and changes in speech rate. In this model, the motor plan is composed of various "subroutines." Once the motor goals are identified and adapted to the general or "core" plan, the serial and parallel executable subroutines are specified and made available to the motor programmer.

Van der Merwe adheres to Brooks's (1986) comparison of motor plans as being analogous to strategies and motor programs to tactics. She also seems to equate motor plans to what Allen and Tsukahara (1974) and Gracco and Abbs (1987) refer to as "preprogramming," what Evarts (1982) calls "central programs," and what Schmidt (1982) calls "generalized motor programs." Presumably these levels of stored sensory–motor information are mediated at the highest level of the motor control system, composed of the cortical association areas. The motor programs, on the other hand, are mediated by the middle level of the motor hierarchy, which is composed of the basal ganglia (caudate and putamen), lateral cerebellum, supplementary motor area, and premotor and motor cortex.

Van der Merwe (1997) subscribes to the "weak" definition of motor programming offered by Marsden (1984). In this definition, motor programs are sets of muscle commands that are structured and unpacked before movement sequences begin, and can be modified by peripheral feedback, both before the program is unpacked and in real time during movement execution. Thus motor programs supply specific movement parameterization to specific muscles or muscle groups. According to Van der Merwe, motor programs specify muscle tone, direction, force, range, and rate of movement, as well as stiffness of the joints as the movement unfolds. Disorders of the motor programmer, defined as such, cause hypokinetic, hyperkinetic, spastic, and ataxic dysarthria, leaving only flaccid dysarthria for assignment to the "execution" or lower level of the motor hierarchy. For Van der Merwe, therefore, AOS is by default a motor planning disorder. AOS is by definition *not* a motor programming disorder, because the speech musculature must be free from evidence of abnormal muscle tone or reflexes, and it must not be impaired in movement range, rate, direction, timing, and force of muscle contraction when used for nonspeech activities.

A Deficit in the Direct Phonetic Encoding Route?

Whiteside and Varley (1998) have recently proposed what they term a "cognitive-based reconceptualization" of AOS. This theory is based upon Keller's (1987) notion that speech motor memories (verbal motor patterns) can be either retrieved from storage for frequently used syllables and their consequent movements (e.g., generalized motor programs), or recalculated anew for infrequently used syllables/movement patterns each time they are called. This notion is consistent with the dual-route phonetic encoding model of Levelt (1989, 1992) and Levelt and Wheeldon (1994). Whiteside and Varley (1998) review the speech characteristics of normal speakers during the production of infrequently occurring syllables and words, which are presumably accessed through the subsyllabic, indirect phonetic encoding route. They also review the speech production characteristics of high-frequency syllables and words that are accessed through the direct phonetic encoding route. They propose that the characteristics of speech produced via the indirect route are physiologically, acoustically, and perceptually consistent with those of normal speakers using "clear speech" or carefully articulated speech, such as that produced while delivering a lecture or under degraded transmission conditions. The characteristics of speech produced via the indirect route are, at first pass, also consistent with many of the core features of AOS as described by McNeil et al. (1997) and summarized earlier, such as (1) increased consonant and vowel durations (articulatory prolongation), (2) increased durations between segments (syllable segregation), (3) inability to control speech rate, and (4) reduced coarticulatory patterns. Thus patients with AOS appear to be using the indirect route exclusively, and therefore, by inference, have a disorder of the direct phonetic encoding route.

A deficit in the direct phonetic encoding route is an interesting hypothesis that connects current speech production models to AOS, and provides a framework for relating phonology to speech motor control. However, several questions require answers before this account can be embraced. Although normal speakers demonstrate subtle signs consistent with AOS during clear speech (e.g., syllable segregation, increased segment durations, and reduced coarticulation), their productions of novel or low-frequency words or syllables is not likely to be mistaken for those of AOS. Why do normal speakers make fewer narrowly transcribed sound and syllable-level errors (primarily phoneme distortions) than apraxic speakers while so engaging the indirect route? This leads to a question as to whether the effects of indirect route use can be graded, such that patients with AOS have access to fewer or less sophisticated generalized motor programs than do normal speakers producing the same low-frequency targets. This leads to the question of why persons with AOS should have access to less sophisticated motor programs than normal speakers producing the same low-frequency speech targets. In other words, if all AOS behaviors can be explained by exclusive reliance on the indirect phonetic encoding route, what makes an apraxic speaker apraxic if normal speakers are not judged as apraxic when forced to rely on this same route?

Any theory seeking to account for AOS must incorporate a mechanism that would allow inconsistent correct productions of the same target on repeated trials. A simple forced reliance on the indirect phonetic route does not explain the known, though perhaps less pervasive than traditionally described (McNeil, Odell, Miller, & Hunter, 1995), trial-to-trial variability in the responses of apraxic speakers. These and numerous other questions require answers before this rather provocative theory can be endorsed.

The Hypothesis of Reduced Buffer Capacity

Rogers and Storkel (1998, in press) accept stage models of speech production (e.g., phonological encoding, phonetic encoding, and/or speech motor programming), but propose that these encoding activities occur in "processing buffers." They characterize this process as "phonological" encoding through motor programming." They acknowledge the interaction among "premotor planning" stages, as well as the difficulty in separating impairments of different levels and stages. They hypothesize that in AOS, there is a reduced capacity (temporal and spatial) of one or more of the sublexical processing buffers. This hypothesis provides a mechanism for at least one of the core features of AOS (syllable segregation) proposed by McNeil et al. (1997). They specifically hypothesize that in AOS, there is a single-syllable limitation on the capacity of the processing buffers.

Rogers and Storkel (1998) used a response-priming paradigm, in which normal subjects read aloud, as rapidly as possible, word lists or word pairs presented on a computer monitor. They found that "target" words that were phonologically similar to "prime" words (defined by shared phonetic features) were initiated significantly more slowly than words that did not share features (particularly manner) with the prime. Based on this finding, they concluded that premotor processing was delayed when reprogramming of phonologically similar prime–target pairs was required, presumably because the programs were temporarily inactivated following use with the prime. Rogers and Storkel (in press) then used the parameter-remapping paradigm (Rosenbaum, Weber, Hazelett, & Hindorff, 1986), in which both the prime and the target were made available for advanced planning/programming before production onset.

They predicted and confirmed that under these circumstances, the phonological similarity effect disappeared in normal subjects because they could use the same phonological programs for both words, obviating the need for reprogramming. They hypothesized that the phonological similarity effect should not be evident in subjects with AOS if they can program more than one syllable at a time, since the simultaneous availability of both words should eliminate the need for reprogramming. In other words, the word pairs sharing phonetic features should be produced as quickly as word pairs with no shared phonetic features, as long as subjects are able to program two words at a time. Conversely, if individuals with AOS have a reduced processing buffer capacity, then the phonological similarity effect should be evident, even in the context permitting monosyllabic words to be programmed at once. In this case, the speakers should have to program each word independently. That is, they should have to respond in the same way as normal subjects engaged in the response-priming paradigm. Five subjects in each of three groups—aphasia without AOS, aphasia with AOS,[4] and normal controls—were subjected to the parameter-remapping paradigm with and without phonetic features shared between the two words. Results revealed no significant differences between the no-shared-features and the shared-features conditions among the aphasic patients, presumably because they, like the normal controls, could assemble the phonological structure and the motor programs of the words within one set of buffers and with one activation process. However, the patients in the aphasia-plus-AOS group showed significantly longer times (consonant-to-consonant times and a trend for longer interpair intervals) in the shared-feature condition (both voicing and manner and place and manner) relative to the no-shared-feature condition. These results were consistent with the posited reduction in processing buffer capacity and the need to reprogram the buffer for each word in patients with AOS.

It should be noted that while this interesting study adds importantly to the specification of the disordered cognitive architecture of AOS, it also validates one of the proposed kernel features of AOS, syllable segregation. It should also be noted that these observations are consistent with the Whiteside and Varley (1998) hypothesis, even though the hypothesized mechanism is different.

Despite the competing theories in AOS, the inadequate phenomenological description of the disorder and the contexts in which it presents itself, and the lingering controversy about the specific behaviors that are sufficient to define its presence, patients with this devastating impairment have sought relief and remediation. Treatments for AOS, based on varying theoretical perspectives about the underlying disorder, have been proposed and tested. The detailed review and critical analysis of the AOS treatment literature that follows demonstrates the array of approaches that have been taken. It also makes clear that there are few data meeting the minimal criteria for proof of efficacy. It indicates the need for continued careful experimental evaluation of AOS treatments.

Following this critical review of AOS treatment and its efficacy, we present a detailed map of the treatment of AOS that is based upon theory and clinical evidence. This map includes a discussion of motor learning principles applicable to AOS treatment, concepts of treatment efficacy, principles of treatment target selection, and general treatment options.

REVIEW OF AOS TREATMENT

As stated above, the rationale for treatment of AOS in contemporary speech and language pathology has been grounded in the clinical observations and conceptualization of the disorder as reported by Darley (1968). Since that time, clinical management of the disorder

(Rosenbek, 1978), and several specific treatment programs and facilitative techniques (Rosenbek, Lemme, Ahern, Harris, & Wertz, 1973; Sparks & Holland, 1976; Deal & Florance, 1978; Stevens & Glaser, 1983; Square, Chumpelik, Morningstar, & Adams, 1986; Wambaugh, Doyle, Kalinyak, & West, 1996), have been described (cf. Wertz et al., 1984). Square-Storer (1989) reviewed many of the traditional treatment programs and techniques reported in the literature to that point and classified them according to whether they addressed articulatory/kinematic aspects of speech production at the segmental and/or syllable levels, or sequencing of segments in longer utterances. These categories represent two primary aspects of the disorder as originally specified by Darley: difficulty in positioning the speech musculature accurately, and difficulty in sequencing and coordinating multiple speech movements. Indeed, with few exceptions (Florance, Rabidoux, & McCauslin, 1980; Lane & Samples, 1981; McNeil, Prescott, & Lemme, 1976), most studies reporting the effects of a specific treatment on the speech production performance of persons with AOS have targeted one of these broad categories, or components of both. As many of the specific treatments (e.g., PROMPT, MIT, Eight-Step Continuum) and facilitative techniques (e.g., key word, phonetic placement, integral stimulation, rate control, contrastive stress) have been described elsewhere and are well known to most clinicians and students of the discipline, they are not reiterated in great detail here. Rather, our purpose is to critically evaluate the literature of the past four decades on the use of these programs and techniques to effect change in the speech production performance of individuals with AOS. Having set this goal, we must state at the outset that to our knowledge, no treatment studies have been reported in which the subjects were diagnosed with AOS in the absence of aphasia and/or dysarthria. The subjects on whom this review is based had AOS and coexisting aphasia. In reviewing the literature, we address the rationale, implementation, and evidence supporting each treatment and/or technique. In addition, we examine the characteristics of the subjects for whom treatment effects have been reported, the behaviors targeted for intervention, and the levels of outcome at which treatments have been examined.

Prospective between-group studies in which treated and nontreated AOS subjects have been compared have, to our knowledge, yet to be reported. However, Wertz (1984) conducted a *retrospective* analysis of the response to treatment of persons diagnosed with AOS and aphasia who participated in the Veterans Administration Cooperative Study comparing individual and group treatment for aphasia (Wertz et al., 1981). He reported that 19 of 67 subjects meeting predetermined study selection criteria were judged to demonstrate AOS coexisting with aphasia at study entry. The diagnosis of AOS was based upon a motor speech evaluation adapted from Wertz and Rosenbek (1971). Precise diagnostic criteria were not specified, nor were descriptions of the selected subjects' speech characteristics. The severity of AOS for those subjects receiving the diagnosis was quantified via a 7-point rating scale, with 1 representing mildly impaired and 7 representing severely impaired performance. In addition to the 19 subjects receiving a definitive diagnosis of AOS at study entry, another 10 subjects were included in the analysis who were suspected of having AOS but for whom the diagnosis could not be unequivocally determined. Of these 29 patients, 17 (59%) completed a 48-week treatment trial, with 9 subjects receiving individual treatment and 8 receiving group treatment.

Subjects randomly assigned to the individual treatment group received 4 hours per week of direct therapist contact, during which both their language deficits (aphasia) and their speech deficits (apraxia) were targeted. Tactics employed to address AOS included retraining of articulatory postures and sequences of movements; the use of visual cues to program articulatory movements; and the use of compensatory movements, such as placing equal stress on each syllable and inserting the schwa between sounds, syllables, or words (e.g., "newspaper" pronounced as "news/a/pa/a/per," with /a/ pronounced as the vowel in "but"). Drills involved repetition and reading of words, phrases, and sentences of graded difficulty with respect to length of utterance and distance between successive articulatory targets. In this way, treatment may have focused on articulatory/kinematic accuracy at the segmental and/or syllable level, and/or sequencing of segments in longer utterances. However, whether AOS was indeed a focus of intervention, and the extent to which any of these techniques was utilized in treating the subjects, were not reported.

Subjects randomly assigned to the group treatment protocol also received 4 hours per week of direct clinician contact with groups of three to seven patients, among whom conversation was encouraged. However, no direct manipulation of speech or language variables was provided. Response to treatment was examined at 4, 15, 26, 37, and 48 weeks after onset. Effects evaluated were (1) changes in the diagnosis and severity of AOS, (2) changes in the severity of aphasia as measured by the Porch Index of Communicative Abilities (PICA), and (3) the relationship between changes in the two disorders. With regard to the diagnosis of AOS, Wertz (1984) stated that "change . . . was rampant during the treatment trial" (p. 263). Indeed, of the 17 subjects who completed the study, 6 changed diagnosis (some as many as three times), and 2 subjects continued to be judged as "AOS undetermined" over the five successive evaluation points of the 44-week treatment trial. The remaining 9 subjects were judged to have AOS at study entry and at each successive evaluation point. AOS severity ratings revealed a mean change of 1 scale point (3.50 to 2.50) from the first to the last evaluation period for subjects assigned to the individual treatment group. A mean change of 0.40 scale points (3.40 to 3.00) was observed for subjects assigned to the group treatment protocol. Both study groups improved their scores on the PICA at evaluation points 1 through 4, and changes in PICA performance were not significantly correlated with changes in the severity of AOS.

This study did not employ a no-treatment control group. It had a high rate of subject attrition and a large range of reported interjudge reliability coefficients for diagnosis (+.69– +.87) and for rating the severity of the disorders (+.65–+.93). There was also an absence of information regarding which disorder (aphasia vs. AOS) was targeted, and to what extent, in any particular subject diagnosed with both disorders. It is therefore difficult to assert with confidence that the AOS treatment tactics described in this investigation were in any systematic way related to the reported outcomes. Indeed, Wertz et al. (1984) concluded that these findings neither support nor refute the efficacy of treatment for AOS. Furthermore, they do not lend themselves to an analysis of subject characteristics or treatment variables that may have affected the measures reported.

In contrast to the paucity of group designs evaluating the effects of AOS interventions, the literature is replete with small-sample and single-subject experimental design investigations. These small-sample studies have examined specific treatment programs and techniques, as well as their effects on speech and nonspeech behaviors in adults with AOS and aphasia. Such studies permit an examination of subject characteristics, target behaviors, interventions, and treatment effects. These studies should ultimately address the types of interventions that are most efficacious for specific patient types, and they should offer predictions about which outcomes may be expected. It is to this literature that we now turn.

Studies Evaluating Articulatory/Kinematic Approaches to Treatment

Several studies in the literature have examined, in isolation and/or in various combinations, the effects of the facilitative techniques of modeling, imitation, integral stimulation, and phonetic placement. These studies have used auditory and/or visual stimulus presentation modes (Deal & Florance, 1978; Holtzapple & Marshall, 1977; LaPointe, 1984; Rosenbek, Lemme, et al., 1973; Wambaugh, West, & Doyle, 1998). The goal of these techniques, as explicitly stated by Rosenbek, Lemme, et al. (1973), and Wambaugh, West, and Doyle (1998), was to influence articulatory/kinematic aspects of movement and/or to facilitate the coordination or sequencing of articulatory gestures in subjects whose primary deficit involved disrupted articulatory programming. For example, Rosenbek, Lemme, et al. (1973) provided a detailed rationale for their eight-step treatment program, which employed modeling, imitation, integral stimulation, and repeated practice (repetition), supported by both auditory and visual cues. Specifically, they viewed AOS as a nonlinguistic sensory–motor disorder of articulation, which is sensitive to and influenced by a number of phonetic conditions. They stated that treatment should focus on retraining points of articulation and sequencing of articulatory gestures. Interestingly, long before certain principles of motor learning theory (Schmidt, 1982) were employed as a framework for the treatment of AOS (McNeil et al., 1997), Rosenbek and colleagues emphasized the importance of hierarchical task difficulty, systematic intensive drill, knowledge of performance and results, and the parallel development of a strong visual memory for correct articulatory postures. They recommended that manner and place of articulation, speech sound position, difficulty of initial speech sounds, distance between successive speech sounds within words, and word length be taken into consideration in constructing individual treatment hierarchies. Although other investigators (Deal & Florence, 1978; Holtzapple & Marshall, 1977; LaPointe, 1984) were much less explicit in their rationale for treatment, there was clear agreement among the studies cited that the condition being treated was an acquired sensory–motor disturbance of articulation that was substantively different in its clinical manifestations and underlying mechanisms from aphasia. All authors referred to these individuals as having AOS.

Rosenbek, Lemme, et al., (1973) applied their eight-step treatment program to three subjects with chronic and severe AOS and coexisting aphasia. They examined its effects on the intelligible production of five meaningful words and/or phrases that varied in length from one to seven words. As was typical of the early treatment reports, little information regarding the speech characteristics of the subjects was provided. However, all subjects were apparently extremely limited in generating or repeating even the simplest of utterances. Whether this reflected the severity of their AOS, their aphasia, or the interaction of the two cannot be determined. Nevertheless, the paucity of speech manifested by these patients may account for the authors' decision to target and measure the intelligibility of longer, functionally relevant segments, as opposed to the accuracy of specific phonemes or classes of phonemes. This report summarized the number of trials required of each subject to reach criterion at each level of the eight-step hierarchy. Although all subjects were reported to have achieved intelligible production of their targeted utterances, the authors noted that these productions were at times distorted. Facilitators were employed, in addition to those formally constituting the reported treatment package. These included manipulations of rate of stimulus presentation, intersyllable and interword pauses, prolongation of consonants and vowels, and insertion of an intrusive schwa within consonant clusters. Many of these techniques are included in those identified by Square-Storer (1989) as facilitating the temporal schemata of speech and the sequencing of segments in longer utterances, and may have had a substantive influence on the reported outcomes. However, the extent to which these facilitators interacted with other components of the treatment program in facilitating intelligible production of words and phrases cannot be determined.

Deal and Florence (1978) administered the eight-step continuum to an additional four patients, with only slight modification. All patients were reported to have severe chronic

AOS and coexisting aphasia. Each subject was reported to have acquired a limited, functional set of utterances over therapy durations that ranged from 3 weeks to 5 months. Thus a total of seven patients with chronic and severe AOS and coexisting aphasia were reported to gain volitional control over the intelligible production of a limited set of functionally relevant utterances following application of the eight-step treatment program. Although the individual contribution of the many facilitative techniques employed in these investigations cannot be determined, these reports provide some of the first *descriptive* data regarding the positive effects of treatment for AOS.

Holtzapple and Marshall (1977) also employed integral stimulation supplemented with visual and auditory cues to target phoneme production. However, the terminal behavior reported in this investigation was sound production in isolation. The treatment program consisted of combining all facilitators in the initial steps of sound production treatment and systematically fading each cue until correct sound production was achieved in response to the presentation of the grapheme alone. The program was applied to five subjects with AOS, with positive results. However, these authors provided data for only one subject with AOS and coexisting aphasia, whose speech was described as unintelligible and perseverative, with frequent inconsistent sound substitutions. Treatment was provided for 1 hour per week in the context of 9 additional hours of speech and language therapy, the nature of which was not specified. As Rosenbek, Lemme, et al. (1973) and Deal and Florence (1978) did, Holtzapple and Marshall provided uncontrolled acquisition data describing the accuracy of sound production at each of three levels of stimulus support. Correct sound production was reported for 21 of 24 phonemes trained over the 30-week treatment trial. The criteria for correct versus incorrect responding were not specified. Although the authors cautiously interpreted these findings as supporting the effectiveness of the program, several alternative explanations of the data (including physiological recovery, alternative treatment carryover, and measurement error) cannot be ruled out.

Thompson and Young (1983) investigated within- and across-class generalization of consonant cluster reacquisition in a single well-described patient with AOS and aphasia. The purpose of their study was to examine whether the subject's cluster reduction errors represented breakdown of a phonological process (Ferguson, 1978). This question was addressed within the context of a multiple-baseline design in which treatment was applied sequentially across different consonant clusters. Generalization was examined by probing production of those clusters in the initial position of untrained words, and of other nontrained consonant clusters in words. It was hypothesized that if the subject's cluster reduction errors represented a phonological process, there should be generalization from trained to untrained clusters.

Treatment consisted of modeling, repetition, and the insertion of an intrusive schwa between the clustered phonemes, and was provided for a total of 22 sessions. The results revealed robust improvement in the production of trained clusters in initial positions in trained words, but no generalization to untrained clusters or untrained words. Thompson and Young concluded that there was no evidence to support the hypothesis that the cluster reduction errors of this subject represented a phonological process. Indeed, the subject's failure to generalize his production of acquired clusters to untrained contexts (i.e., different words) may be explained by the differences in the phonetic environment between trained and untrained words. Such an explanation is consistent with the view of AOS as disrupting spatial targeting/phasing of segments. Finally, the lack of generalized responding may also have been related to the nature of the treatment itself. Specifically, the facilitative techniques employed were limited to primarily modeling and repetition, with the use of the intrusive schwa limited to one presentation per trial following an erroneous response to the clinician's model. As such, it provided few opportunities for practice, as well as limited contexts for learning.

LaPointe (1984) employed a multiple-baseline design to examine the effects of a treatment program combining modeling, imitation, integral stimulation, and phonetic placement. He measured the accuracy of phoneme production in treated and untreated words in a single patient who was described as having "nonfluent" aphasia, complicated by severe phonological selection and sequencing impairment (AOS). Thirty-four treatment sessions were conducted over a 210-day period, during which two lists of 25 words each were trained sequentially. Each treatment session consisted of applying the treatment program to the 25 words in the treated list. However, each treatment trial allowed for multiple (five) repetitions of correctly produced words. Results revealed that the learning curves of the treated lists progressed significantly faster and reached significantly higher levels of accuracy than did that of the untreated lists.

The use of both "phonological selection impairment" and "AOS" as terms to describe this subject's speech disorder is quite curious, as the former implies a disturbance of linguistic processes while the latter implies a sensory–motor articulatory disturbance (see discussion of this issue in McNeil et al., 1997). Unfortunately, LaPointe provided virtually no descriptive information regarding the subject's speech characteristics that would permit judgment of whether the subject's production impairment resulted from disrupted linguistic or motor mechanisms. As such, whether the effects of this well-controlled single-subject investigation represent the response to treatment of a subject with a phonological-level impairment, a motor planning/programming impairment, or both is unknown.

Wambaugh, West, and Doyle (1998) used a multiple-baseline design to examine the effects of a treatment package combining modeling, repetition, integral stimulation, visual cueing, and response-contingent feedback. They measured phoneme production accuracy in sentences loaded with fricatives, stops, and liquids/glides, and in sentences consisting of combinations of each sound class. They administered a total of 33 treatments consisting of 40 trials per session, three sessions per week, to a subject with mild aphasia and AOS as defined by McNeil et al. (1997). Results revealed increased accuracy of sound production during probes for all sound groups and for both trained and untrained exemplars within each class. Maintenance data collected 6 weeks after treatment demonstrated stable treatment effects. In addition, durational measures of each sentence type (fricatives, stops, glides) obtained during the first and third baseline sessions were found to be significantly longer than those obtained during the last two probe sessions of the treatment trial. Thus, in addition to the improvement of sound production in sentence contexts, sentence durations declined toward normal levels.

The foregoing studies included 11 subjects whose speech characteristics were described in varying degrees of detail (LaPointe, 1984; Rosenbek, Lemme, et al., 1973; Thompson & Young, 1983; Wambaugh, West, & Doyle, 1998). Other studies merely stated that their subjects had AOS (Deal & Florance, 1978; Holtzapple & Marshall, 1977). Only Wambaugh, West, and Doyle (1998) and Wambaugh, Kalinyak-Fliszar, West, and Doyle (1998) provide a sufficiently detailed subject description to allow the reader to differentiate their subject from subjects with phonological-level impairments according to the criteria specified by McNeil et al. (1997).

Many of the same facilitative techniques were employed in the studies described above. However, they were applied in different combinations, intensities, and durations to different classes of target behaviors, and to subjects with differing levels of AOS severity. It is possible that the patient reported by LaPointe (1984) may have had a phonological-level impairment and not AOS. In addition, the facilitative techniques employed among the reported studies were evaluated under more or less rigorously controlled experimental conditions. It is apparent from the foregoing review that early reports examining the effects of interventions on speech production in AOS focused on utterance-level behaviors and provided essentially uncontrolled descriptive data. More recent reports have examined the effects of treatment packages on changes in the accuracy of phoneme production within word and sentence contexts. They have applied experimental controls in the form of extended multiple baselines and evaluation of measurement reliability. Finally, while all studies reported positive outcomes for treated behaviors, only LaPointe (1984), Thompson and Young (1983), and Wambaugh, West, and Doyle (1998) examined the effects of treatment on untreated behaviors. Clearly, additional controlled investigations are needed to establish the efficacy of the facilitative techniques discussed in achieving meaningful change in the speech production performance of persons with AOS.

Wambaugh and colleagues have reported a series of studies examining the effects of a minimal-contrast pairs treatment for AOS (Wambaugh et al., 1996; Wambaugh, Kalinyak-Flizar, West, & Doyle, 1998; Wambaugh, Martinez, McNeil, & Rogers, in press; Wambaugh & Cort, 1998). These studies report findings for six well-described subjects with AOS and coexisting aphasia who were administered this treatment program under well-controlled experimental conditions. Acquisition, response generalization, stimulus generalization, and maintenance effects were reported for targeted phonemes. For all subjects, the treatment consisted of modeling and imitation of minimal-contrast pairs, with a repetition of this step if a subject's response was incorrect. If modeling was not sufficient to elicit a correct response, the modeled production was then paired with orthographic representations of the sounds, and imitation was again requested. Subsequent steps of the hierarchy included integral stimulation, modeling with the use of a silent juncture, articulatory placement cues, and response-contingent feedback. For all subjects, accurate phoneme production was the target behavior. Wambaugh et al. (1996) reported robust acquisition effects in one subject for imitative production of /sh/, /r/, and /sw/ in words. Furthermore, despite long-standing impairment, this AOS subject generalized production of sounds to untrained words and phrases to well above baseline levels. The subject also maintained these effects at a 6-week follow-up probe.

A follow-up investigation (Wambaugh, Kalinyak-Flizar, et al., 1998) replicated the earlier study with an additional three subjects, all of whom had chronic AOS and coexisting aphasia. The results revealed robust effects for targeted sounds in trained and untrained word-initial locations. However, two of the subjects performed at much lower levels and with greater response variability for sounds trained in word-final positions. Generalization to phrase-level productions occurred in only one subject, but did so in all sounds trained. Maintenance effects remained at acquisition levels at 6-week follow-up probes for all sounds trained in word-initial positions in all subjects.

Another single-subject replication (Wambaugh et al., in press) produced similar results. That is, acquisition of trained items and response generalization were achieved. However, maintenance probes during training of subsequent sounds revealed decreased response accuracy and highly variable performance. A detailed analysis of maintenance data for each sound revealed a pattern of overgeneralization, whereby sounds undergoing training were substituted for sounds acquired earlier in the treatment sequence.

Generalization to untrained sounds (as opposed to similar sounds in untrained words) was not achieved in any of the previously reported investigations. Wambaugh and Cort (1998) examined the effects of the minimal-contrast pairs treatment on across-sound generalization in a patient with chronic AOS and coexisting aphasia. This subject consistently produced voiced stops and affricates that were perceived as their voiceless cognates.

Previous research with this subject revealed that these sound errors were not sound substitutions, but distorted productions of the intended voiced phoneme. This was evidenced by significantly shorter voice onset times (VOTs) for the substituted sounds than for the intended voiceless productions (Wambaugh, West, & Doyle, 1997). That is, the apparent loss of the voiced–voiceless distinction was specifically viewed as phonetic rather than phonemic in nature. Nevertheless, this consistent error pattern allowed an examination of whether practicing of the voiced–voiceless distinction within the minimal-contrast pairs treatment paradigm would promote across-sound generalization. The results revealed that when the first sound (/b/) was entered into training, productions of /dz/, /d/, and /g/ increased in accuracy. Subsequent VOT analyses revealed that significant changes in VOT values corresponded with perceptual judgments of sound production.

The findings from this series of investigations represent the first systematic, experimental, and replicated examination of the acquisition, generalization, and maintenance effects of a specific treatment designed to enhance articulatory/kinematic aspects of AOS speech at the segmental and syllable level. Together, they provide initial experimental evidence that treatment strategies designed to promote improved postural shaping and phasing of the articulators are efficacious in improving sound production in treated and untreated words, phrases, and sentences. Furthermore, there is limited evidence that for some patients and some sounds, generalization to untrained sounds and contexts may be expected.

Studies Evaluating the Facilitative Effects of Rhythm, Rate, and Stress

Numerous studies have reported the effects of treatments in which the rate, rhythm, and stress contours of longer utterances have been manipulated to enhance speech production. It is hypothesized that these techniques facilitate speech motor control by providing a temporal schema for the organization of multiple speech movements (Square-Storer, 1989). The empirical evidence supporting their effectiveness is examined here.

Perhaps the best-known treatment program employing rhythm, rate, and stress manipulation as facilitators for the production of word- and phrase-level utterances is melodic intonation therapy (MIT). MIT has been described in great detail by a number of authors, including Albert, Sparks, and Helm (1973), Sparks and Deck (1986), Sparks, Helm, and Albert (1974), and Sparks and Holland (1976). Although the program was not originally developed to target mechanisms underlying AOS (i.e., disrupted motor planning and programming), it has since been suggested that in view of the criteria for determining MIT candidacy, patients with AOS should benefit from the program (Tonkovich & Marquardt, 1977). Indeed, given the descriptions of the original patients reported by Albert et al. (1973), Sparks et al. (1974), and Naeser and Helm-Estabrooks (1985), it is likely that many of them had AOS and coexisting aphasia. Nevertheless, these early clinical reports, like so many others of the time (e.g., Keith & Aronson, 1975; Rosenbek, Lemme, et al., 1973; Deal & Florence, 1978; Holtzapple & Marshall, 1977), provided little more than anecdotal clinical observations and uncontrolled descriptive data in evaluating subjects' response to treatment. Responses to MIT have been reported for 20 subjects (Albert et al., 1973; Sparks et al., 1974; Naeser & Helm-Estabrooks, 1985). Little information is available regarding these subjects' speech characteristics or the frequency and duration of treatment administered. No data have been provided regarding the effects of MIT on targeted utterances or untrained exemplars of the same form. Although these early studies provide little empirical evidence to support the effectiveness of MIT for improving speech production in persons with aphasia and/or AOS, they do assist in the identification of potentially robust independent variables. They also provide an impetus for the systematic examination of these variables in patients in whom disrupted motor speech planning and programming mechanisms are recognized as the primary deficits accounting for their speech production impairment. Several such studies are described below; these have examined the effects of rate control, rhythmic tapping and/or pacing, and emphatic stress on the speech production skills of subjects with AOS.

Dworkin, Abkarian, and Johns (1988) employed a multiple-probe design to examine the efficacy of a hierarchically arranged treatment program employing metronomic pacing. These investigators trained sequentially (1) nonspeech movements; (2) alternating /pa/, /ta/, /ka/; (3) bisyllabic words; (4) trisyllabic words; and (5) sentences. These targets were trained to a preestablished acquisition criterion in a subject with AOS without accompanying aphasia or dysarthria, 16 months after a left-hemisphere intracerebral hemorrhage. It should be noted however, that no aphasia test performance scores were reported for this subject, who in the acute stages of her stroke was reported to have global aphasia. Furthermore, the presence of many of the speech characteristics reported (i.e., phonemic metathesis, highly inconsistent articulatory omissions and substitutions, word-finding difficulties on confrontation naming, and lexical transpositions) and the absence of others (sound-level distortions) requires cautious interpretation of the diagnosis of pure AOS. Treatment consisted of having the subject synchronize production of targeted oral motor movements and speech productions to a metronome rhythm. Rates were systematically increased toward normal for each task. The final phase of treatment withdrew the metronome and employed emphatic stress in sentence contexts as a facilitator. Detailed procedural information was provided. This included descriptions of each program level, the sequence in which stimuli were delivered, the criteria for advancing to successive steps of the program, the actual number of trials required to reach criterion at each step, the steps that proved difficult or easy to master, and treatment duration. The results revealed acquisition and maintenance of all targeted behaviors at the preestablished acquisition criterion levels. However, there was no generalization of these treatment effects to untreated behaviors.

In a follow-up study, Dworkin and Abkarian (1996) applied the metronomic pacing treatment to another subject who was diagnosed with coexisting apraxia of phonation and UUMN dysarthria secondary to a severe closed head injury. This patient's vocal behaviors were characterized by uncontrollable pitch fluctuations, squeals, episodic whispering, and vocal arrest, all judged to be the result of a motor planning disturbance. No motor execution deficits or anatomical abnormalities of the vocal apparatus were noted. Articulatory behaviors were described as slow and imprecise, with numerous false starts, restarts, abnormal intersyllabic pausing, and anticipatory sound transpositions. Metronomic pacing was sequentially applied, within the context of a multiple-probe design, to three target behaviors: production of isolated vowels, three-vowel sequences, and alternating vowel and glottal (h) consonant sequences. Target mastery, defined as the volitional control of phonation, was set at 95% correct production in each of two successive treatment sessions. Criterion was achieved and maintained for all targeted behaviors within the 44 treatment sessions. Consistent with the Dworkin et al. (1988) report, generalization to nontrained behaviors was not attained.

Wambaugh and Martinez (2000) assessed the effect of combined metronomic pacing and hand tapping on consonant production in sets of trained and untrained three-syllable words differing in primary stress placement. One subject with mild to moderate AOS and coexisting agrammatic aphasia was trained to produce one syllable per beat while tapping his hand in unison with a metronome providing both an audible click and a flashing red light. Initial rates were set at 93 beats/minute, but were increased to 110 beats/minute as the subject progressed through a treatment hierarchy. This hierarchy included (1) a visual schematic of stress placement in words; (2) clinician modeling of words while tapping in unison with the metronome; (3) subject tapping in unison with the metronome in the absence of verbal responses; (4) repeated practice (three trials), with the clinician and subject tapping and verbalizing in unison with the metronome; and (5) subject tapping and verbalizing in unison with the metronome. Finally, response-contingent feedback was provided regarding the correspondence between the number and timing of the subject's tappings relative to the syllables in the word and the rate of the metronome. No feedback was provided regarding the articulatory accuracy of consonant production in the words. The findings revealed increased levels of responding over baseline for measures of (1) the number of words containing no sound errors, and (2) the percentage of correct consonants in treated and untreated words.

Southwood (1987) reported results similar to those of Wambaugh and Martinez (2000) in a study of the effects of prolonged speech and manipulation of speaking rate on the accuracy of consonant production during paragraph readings in two subjects with mild AOS and aphasia. In three separate experiments using single-subject withdrawal and changing criterion designs, this investigator demonstrated that prolonged speech resulted in decreased speaking rates and decreased sound errors. Furthermore, sound errors remained well below baseline levels when prolonged speech was employed as speaking rate was systematically increased. However, neither reduced speaking rates, the use of prolonged speech, nor the reduction in sound errors was observed to generalize to a spontaneous speech task condition.

Rubow, Rosenbek, Collins, and Longstreth (1982) used a vibrotactile stimulus to provide afferent cues regarding the rhythm and stress patterns of multisyllabic words. They examined the effects of this stimulus on the articulatory accuracy of these words in a subject with AOS and coexisting aphasia. A 50-Hz vibratory stimulus was applied to the volar surface of the subject's right index finger, in unison with each syllable of polysyllabic words spoken by the examiner. High-intensity vibrations were delivered for syllables with primary stress, and low-intensity vibrations were applied for syllables carrying secondary and tertiary stress. Each trial consisted of the examiner's saying the word while applying the vibrotactile stimulus. The subject was then required to repeat the word while the examiner once again applied the vibrotactile stimulus to indicate the rhythm and stress patterns of the word. Treatment of 10 words was carried out over a 7-day period (100 trials/session). Performance with the treated words was compared to performance with an equivalent list of 10 words on which the subject had received the same amount and duration of training using a simple modeling and repetition method, in the absence of the tactile stimulus. Results of pretest–posttest comparisons for each list revealed substantial improvement in the articulatory accuracy of words treated with vibrotactile stimulation, but little improvement in the articulatory accuracy of words treated under the repetition condition.

Simmons (1978) reported the effects of a simple rhythmic pacing technique, similar in principle to the metronomic/tapping and vibrotactile cueing strategies discussed above. She trained a subject with chronic AOS and coexisting aphasia to "finger-count" in unison with the production of each word of subject–verb–prepositional phrase sentence frames. Simmons stated that the finger counting was designed to punctuate the rhythm and stress patterns of the sentences. The program was hierarchically organized, with the clinician's modeling the sentence and demonstrating the technique in the initial step of the program. In subsequent steps, the clinician's participation was gradually faded. Although no direct measures of the articulatory accuracy or intelligibility of the targeted sentences were provided, an improvement of 21 percentile points on PICA verbal scores was reported.

Just as there are few studies reporting the effects of techniques designed to enhance segmental articulation, there are few studies reporting techniques directed toward other aspects of speech at the segmental level. Likewise, the empirical evidence supporting the facilitative effects of rhythmic pacing, rate control, and stress manipulations on articulatory accuracy and production of longer speech units in adults with AOS is limited. To our knowledge, only five subjects have been studied under conditions allowing for an examination of the functional relationship between the treatment delivered and the dependent measures reported (Dworkin et al., 1988; Dworkin & Abkarian, 1996; Wambaugh et al., in press; Southwood, 1987). It is difficult to make direct cross-study comparisons because of differences among studies in the severity of the subjects's AOS and aphasia; the frequency, duration, and context in which the various facilitative techniques have been applied; the behaviors targeted for intervention; and the extent to which important aspects of treatment (e.g., generalization) have been controlled or assessed. Nevertheless, the limited available evidence suggests that facilitative techniques serving to reduce the rate of articulatory movements and to highlight rhythmic and prosodic aspects of speech production may be efficacious in improving the articulatory accuracy, the subjective quality of the speech, and perhaps the intelligibility of speech in some persons with AOS.

Another treatment program that employs components of both articulatory/kinematic and rhythmic/rate control strategies in the treatment of AOS is the Prompts for Restructuring Oral Muscular Phonetic Targets (PROMPT) treatment program (Square-Storer & Hayden, 1989). The authors describe the treatment as a dynamic tactile–kinesthetic oral–facial cueing system that uses a combination of proprioceptive, pressure, and kinesthetic cues. It is designed to provide apraxic patients with sensory input regarding the place of articulatory contact, extent of mandibular opening, voice, tension, relative timing of segments, and manner of articulation and coarticulation. The treatment itself has not, to our knowledge, been described in sufficient detail to permit replication of the technique by other clinicians. Indeed, in the most comprehensive description of the treatment reported to date (Square-Storer & Hayden, 1989), the authors state that extensive training is required in order to administer the program competently and efficiently, and that learning the system based upon its published description would be impossible. Responses to PROMPT treatment have been reported for only four adults with AOS and coexisting aphasia (Square et al., 1985; Square et al., 1986). In these studies, PROMPT treatment was used to train subjects to produce minimally contrastive phonemes, polysyllabic words, and short phrases. Positive results were reported for all target behaviors for two of the three subjects, but as pointed out by Freed, Marshall, and Frazier (1997) in the only trial of the technique conducted by other investigators, these studies are problematic. Specifically, Square et al. (1985) used an uncontrolled simultaneous-treatment design that did not permit isolation of the reported outcomes to either treatment.

The strongest evidence to date of the program's effectiveness comes from the study reported by Freed et al. (1997). These investigators employed a multiple-baseline design in a single patient with severe AOS and coexisting aphasia. They examined the effects of PROMPT treatment on the production accuracy of a core vocabulary consisting of 30 words and short phrases that played an important role in the person's daily communication. Treatment was delivered sequentially for six separate lists of five words each. Each treatment session consisted of 20 training trials for each word in the set. Results revealed robust acquisition effects for all 30 items, and maintenance effects remained well above baseline levels for all trained items, despite some variability across lists. Generalization to untrained words did not occur. These data provide some initial, albeit limited, evidence supporting the clinical observations provided by Square and colleagues regarding the program's efficacy. Nevertheless, reported outcomes have been restricted to very limited sets of target behaviors.

In summary, the literature addressing the effects of treatments and/or specific facilitative techniques on the speech production performance of persons with AOS and coexisting aphasia raises more questions than it answers. There is some limited evidence from well-conducted small-sample and single-subject studies to support the general efficacy of treatment for AOS. However, additional systematic research is needed to isolate those subject, treatment, and measurement variables that will more directly address questions as to which facilitative techniques are most effective for achieving specific outcomes in specific patients. The following section describes a general framework for the treatment of AOS, based upon concepts derived from motor learning theory and upon principles extracted from the AOS treatment efficacy literature.

PRINCIPLES OF TREATMENT FOR AOS

The specific suggestions for treating AOS provided here are based upon the developing framework and assumptions about this disorder that have been reviewed earlier in this chapter, as well as by McNeil et al. (1997). This framework suggests that AOS is not a phonological disorder, and that sound errors occur because of problems in translating an accurately filled phonological frame into the kinematic parameters necessary for executing speech movements. Therefore, treatment for AOS in its rare pure form need not involve techniques to facilitate frame building or phonological processes of sound selection. Furthermore, in the course of translating the filled phonological frame, it may be the case that previously learned motor programs have become less reliably accessible (at least in their previously generalized program forms), resulting in intra- and interarticulator timing and positioning problems. Consequently, it is suggested that the objective of treatment for AOS should be to improve the ability to specify the kinematic parameters necessary for adequate production of speech sounds and prosody, with a resultant increase in effective segment and prosodic production. To this end, principles of motor learning and treatment efficacy as they apply to AOS management, including selection of treatment targets and treatment strategies, are discussed.

Principles of Motor Learning

Because problems with speech sensory–motor control underlie the disordered speech behaviors of AOS, principles of motor learning should be applicable to the treatment of these behaviors. General principles of motor learning have been discussed by Schmidt (1982) and have been explicated in terms of motor speech learning by Clark and Robin (1996) and McNeil et al. (1997). The principles most pertinent to AOS treatment include (1) the necessity of intensive and repeated practice; (2) the use of carefully controlled feedback and feedback delay intervals; (3) the importance of prepractice issues (e.g., motivating patients, providing instructions, establishing referents for correctness); (4) the systematic control of variability in practice; and (5) the organization of hierarchies of tasks according to difficulty. These principles are discussed briefly, and the reader is encouraged to refer to the preceding references for more thorough discussions of these important issues.

Research in motor learning has shown that maximizing the number of treatment trials is important (Schmidt, 1991). As indicated by Duffy (1995), "virtually every specific behavioral treatment approach for AOS emphasizes drill" (p. 421). Intensive and repeated practice appears to be essential for the reestablishment of accurate and effectively implemented motor programs. Therefore, AOS treatment sessions should be structured to allow the maximum number of treatment trials and targeted productions possible, given the constraints of preventing undue fatigue and boredom.

Feedback may take the form of what Schmidt (1982) terms "knowledge of results" (KR) or "knowledge of performance" (KP). KR is an indication of the correctness or incorrectness of the overall response (e.g., "Not quite," "That's correct"), and KP is a specification about the movement pattern performed (e.g., "Your tongue wasn't raised"). Although it is clear that information about errors is critical for motor learning, it is not as clear what schedule of KR is most effective, particularly for facilitating motor speech learning. Upon reviewing the motor learning literature, Schmidt (1982, 1988, 1991) argued that too much feedback may be detrimental to motor learning, in that it may foster a reliance on KR by the performer. He suggested that a relatively high-frequency schedule of KR may be needed in initial learning trials, but that the frequency schedule should be reduced as the performer's proficiency increases. Similarly, behavior analysts indicate that intermittent reinforcement schedules are more likely to strengthen generalization over time (Stokes & Baer, 1977).

In addition to considering the type and frequency of feedback provided during AOS treatment, the clinician should systematically control the timing of the application of KR. The time between the production of a response and the administration of KR is called the "KR delay interval." During this time interval, it is probable that the learner must retain the sensory aspects of the movement in order to associate these aspects with the KR (Schmidt, 1988). McNeil et al. (1997) have suggested that a large delay in applying KR could impair motor speech learning. In addition, motor learning research has indicated that the KR delay interval should be kept free of other movements, because these movements may interfere with learning of the desired movement pattern (Schmidt, 1988). McNeil et al. (1997) advocate maintaining an unfilled interval of time (i.e., at least 3 seconds) following the provision of KR ("post-KR delay interval"), to allow the learner to process information before the next movement trial.

Several issues related to preparing the learner for practice have been identified as being potentially important in facilitating motor learning. These "prepractice" considerations, as discussed by Schmidt (1982, 1988, 1991) and McNeil et al. (1997), center around motivating the learner and clarifying the tasks to be undertaken in practice. More specifically, these authors have suggested that the performer's motivation may be enhanced if the importance of the task is made clear and if specific practice goals are set. Task understanding may be promoted by using simple, clear instructions; providing observational learning experiences (e.g., modeling desired behaviors, showing videos of performance); and establishing clear referents for determining performance correctness.

The structuring of tasks within a practice session also deserves careful attention and should take into account principles of motor learning. Practice should allow for the desired movement to be performed in systematically varying conditions, to increase the probability that the learner will be able to perform the desired movement in novel situations. For example, if an apraxic speaker is asked to practice production of a specific sound, he or she should be given the opportunity to practice that sound in several different phonetic contexts. This notion speaks directly to the issue of generalization, which is discussed in the next section. Practice should also be structured hierarchically, so that the learner begins with motorically less complex tasks and proceeds to more complex tasks. This may necessitate practicing nonspeech tasks (e.g., oral nonspeech motor movements) prior to practicing speech tasks. Currently there is little evidence to indicate whether or not improvement in nonspeech movements will result in improved speech movements. Schmidt (1982), in fact, suggests that practicing components of movement patterns may not result in acquisition of the desired overall movement pattern. However, there may be occasions with apraxic speakers when practice of speech movements is not possible and components of speech behaviors should be targeted (Rosenbek, 1978). In general, practice should begin at a level at which a speaker can achieve some measure of initial success and should progress systematically to motorically more difficult levels (Rosenbek et al., 1984).

With the exception of the use of hierarchies, it appears that motor learning principles have not been sufficiently utilized or specified in the majority of reported treatments for AOS. These principles can be relatively easily applied with most AOS treatment approaches, and should receive careful consideration as part of the process of designing an apraxic patient's treatment regime.

Concepts of Treatment Efficacy

AOS speakers may be more consistent in the location of their errors and less variable in the type of errors on repeated trials of an utterance than was previously believed (McNeil et al., 1995). However, it is still critical to obtain an indication of speech production variability prior to instituting treatment. This requires applying the tenets of single-subject research and obtaining repeated measurements of the behaviors of interest before beginning treatment. Ideally, stable baselines ought to be obtained for all behaviors under treatment and should be readily achieved with patients with chronic AOS. Although baseline stability may not be possible with patients with recently acquired AOS, establishing baselines for behaviors will provide trend lines and estimates of variability, which may then be used to define changes in trends and variability during treatment.

Treatment data and probe data may be used to determine the effects of treatment. "Treatment data" are data that are obtained during the treatment process itself (e.g., performance during practice trials designed, through principles of learning, to change the behavior). "Probe data" are data obtained at a time other than when treatment is occurring. Probe data are collected either prior to or following a treatment session. Whereas both types of data are essential for efficient and effective administration of treatment, probe data constitute the more stringent measure of treatment effectiveness. Probe data reflect performance without the benefits of feedback and treatment recency effects, and therefore may provide a more accurate portrayal of generalized and maintained treatment gains than treatment data. Although treatment data may not be the best indicators of treatment effectiveness, they may show changes in behavior before changes are evident in probe data. Treatment data are certainly critical for determining whether treatment requires modification. Obtaining probe and treatment data on a regular basis may appear to be a time-consuming task, but both types of data are essential if one wishes to determine whether treatment is effective. Although little is known about the relationship between probe and treatment data, there is not necessarily a strong correlation between the two types of data (Wambaugh et al., 1996). Therefore, it is recommended that clinicians not rely on only one form of data, but routinely collect both treatment and probe data.

Response generalization is another crucial aspect of treatment effectiveness. Response generalization may be assessed in untrained contexts of trained behaviors, as well as in untrained, related behaviors. It appears that response generalization may be expected to occur when speakers with AOS are trained in sound productions (see Wambaugh et al., (in press, for a review). However, given the paucity of data available, it is not safe to assume that generalization will occur; rather, it should be actively promoted and measured. This may be easily accomplished by including untrained items with trained items during probes. For example, if /k/, /s/, and /t/ were each trained in 10 different contexts, then the probe would incorporate these same 10 contexts and add 5 novel contexts for each phoneme, for a total of 45 items. Improved performance with untrained items is indicative of effective treatment. Performance with untrained items should be comparable to performance with trained items. If response generalization effects are not as strong as acquisition effects, then the clinician may consider extending treatment with the trained items (i.e., promoting overlearning may facilitate generalization) or training the target items in even more contexts.

Stimulus generalization occurs when the trained behavior is utilized under conditions that differ from those used in training (i.e., different speaking contexts, different conversational participants, different speaking locations, etc.). One cannot assume that stimulus generalization will be an automatic result of treatment. Researchers have rarely addressed the issue of stimulus generalization in treatment of AOS (see Wambaugh & Doyle, 1994, for a review), so it is prudent to assume that correct responses in different stimulus conditions are unlikely to occur without specific intervention. Therefore, a systematic and thorough assessment of speech production in the conditions to which generalization is desired is necessary. This will entail deciding upon the stimulus generalization measurement conditions prior to the start of treatment and obtaining baseline data in those conditions. Those measurements can then be repeated periodically throughout the course of treatment to determine whether or not generalization is occurring. If generalization is not evident, a number of strategies may be employed to promote stimulus generalization. Tactics such as training sufficient stimulus exemplars, mediating generalization, and sequentially modifying treatment have been specifically discussed for AOS (Wambaugh, West, & Doyle, 1998), although empirical verification of such approaches is currently unavailable.

In addition to striving to assure adequate response generalization and stimulus generalization, the clinician should be aware of the potential for undesirable overgeneralization effects. We (Wambaugh et al., in press) have reported that sounds receiving treatment were produced inappropriately in lieu of other experimental sounds (both untrained and previously trained) by a single apraxic–aphasic speaker. Although the overgeneralization reported in this case was extreme, and overgeneralization has not been objectively documented in other cases, clinicians should be prepared for the possibility of overgeneralization. For example, if maintenance of a previously learned behavior becomes problematic, overgeneralization of other behaviors should be examined as a possible contributing factor. We found that reinstituting treatment with previous behaviors appeared to be effective in thwarting the adverse overgeneralization effects. Overgeneralization may be avoided by training a sufficient number of different behaviors for stimulus discrimination to be achieved. That is, training one behavior at a time may provide an environment in which overgeneralization is likely to occur, because there are not opportunities for the learner to develop stimulus discrimination. Although we (Wambaugh et al., in press) provided minimal-contrast pairs practice as part of our treatment, this practice was not sufficient to prevent overgeneralization to other sounds. Unfortunately, at the present time there are limited data to guide the clinician in determining the optimal method for presenting stimuli to facilitate generalization and minimize overgeneralization.

The determination of maintenance effects of treatment is perhaps the most stringent measure of treatment efficacy. This area has been largely overlooked in the AOS treatment literature. There are a few findings suggesting that maintenance of treatment gains may require follow-up therapy (Square et al., 1985; Wambaugh, Kalinyak-Fliszar, et al., 1998; Wambaugh et al., in press). Maintenance cannot be assumed and should be assessed routinely several weeks and several months following the completion of treatment.

Selection of Treatment Targets

A number of deviant speech behaviors have been identified as typifying AOS (McNeil et al., 1997; Square & Martin, 1994; Wertz et al., 1984), and any of these behaviors can be potential targets for treatment: perceived sound distortions, substitutions, and omissions; increased segmental durations and movement transitions; increased interword intervals; dysprosody; articulatory groping; and slow rate. Each apraxic speaker should be considered individually in terms of the presence or absence of particular deviant behaviors and their relative contribution to his or her communication disruption. That is, each apraxic speaker will present with his or her own relatively unique combination of deviant speech behaviors, and each will require a thorough assessment to determine the impact of those behaviors on overall communication abilities. Furthermore, the selection and ordering of behaviors to receive treatment should be individualized and should include consideration of the assumed underlying pathophysiology.

Misarticulation of speech sounds has frequently been noted with apraxic speakers (Dunlop & Marquardt, 1977; LaPointe & Johns, 1975; Trost & Canter, 1974). These misarticulations commonly take the form of perceived distortions and/or substitutions (Odell, McNeil, Rosenbek, & Hunter, 1990, 1991). A thorough evaluation of the production of all speech sounds should be conducted as part of the process of identifying behaviors for treatment. The examiner should sample all sounds in all word positions, using formal or informal assessment instruments. Several exemplars of each sound in each position, in different phonetic contexts, should be elicited (e.g., to examine /k/ in the word-final position, the examiner can elicit "beak," "sake," "rock," "chick," and "perk"). The examiner should phonetically transcribe the speaker's productions, preferably using narrow phonetic transcription, in order to obtain as precise a description of any sound errors as possible. The sound assessment may be conducted at the single-word level, phrase level, multisyllabic word level, or sentence level, depending upon the proficiency of the speaker's sound production. Similarly, the samples may be elicited through repetition, oral reading, or picture description, or may be self-generated (e.g., "Tell me a sentence using the word 'beak'"), depending upon the capabilities of the speaker.

The elicited sample should be analyzed for patterns of errors within and across sounds. Specifically, the examiner should determine which sounds are most frequently in error. The errors on sounds found to be frequently misarticulated should be examined to determine whether there is any predictability to the error pattern (e.g., /r/, when in error, is always "replaced" by /w/; /k/, when in error, is usually produced as /t/ or /d/). A generative analysis should be considered to determine whether error patterns cross groups of sounds (e.g., /b/ → /p/, /d/ → /t/, and /g/ → /k/ represent a pattern of devoicing of stops). The sound error analysis may then be used to guide selection of sounds to be targeted for treatment.

There are limited data to direct clinicians in the most efficient and effective selection and ordering of sounds to be targeted for treatment. A few investigations have indicated that simultaneously training multiple sound targets may be an effective approach with apraxic speakers (Holtzapple & Marshall, 1977; Wambaugh, West, & Doyle, 1998). Other studies have shown postive effects of training sounds sequentially (Wertz et al., 1984; Raymer & Thompson, 1991; Wambaugh & Cort, 1998; Wambaugh et al., in press). Our investigation (Wambaugh et al., in press) reported interference effects from training sounds sequentially. Although the data are not yet clear regarding this issue, it is suggested that more than one sound be targeted for treatment at a given time, if possible. As suggested by Wertz et al. (1984), maximally contrasting sounds may be considered first for selection. However, if a consistent error pattern is seen with a group of similar sounds (e.g., /g/ → /k/; /d/ → (/t/; /b/ → /p/; /dz/ → /tS/), then it may be more efficient to treat similar sounds simultaneously. This approach of treating several sounds simultaneously is consistent with the motor learning literature, in that systematic variability in practice is considered to be important. Because of the limited and somewhat conflicting data regarding number of sounds to treat simultaneously, trial therapy employing groupings or ordering of sounds may be warranted.

There are a number of other factors to consider in selecting sound targets for treatment. The importance of these factors in determining treatment targets will certainly vary across individual patients. Impact upon speech intelligibility is an important consideration and encompasses issues such as error frequency (i.e., how often is this sound in error?), degree of homonymy created by error(s) (i.e., do errors cause target words to sound like other words?), and frequency of occurrence in the language (i.e., is the error sound a frequently or infrequently occurring sound?). Priority should be given to sounds or error patterns that, when corrected, are most likely to have the greatest impact upon intelligibility. Level or frequency of correct production is also an essential point. Specifically, the motor learning literature indicates that motor learning may be more successful if the learner experiences a relatively high level of success during practice. Therefore, it may be more appropriate to initially select sounds that are only moderately or infrequently misarticulated. Of course, error sounds may not occur with different frequencies; in this case, a period of trial therapy may be utilized to determine which sound(s) may be more responsive to treatment, so that high levels of success can be achieved. Trial therapy may also be useful in determining which sounds have the most potential for correction. Sounds that are more amenable to correction should be considered early in the treatment process. Adjustments in outcome expectations may need to be made for sounds that are resistant to treatment. That is, improvement rather than normalization may be a more appropriate goal for some sounds. For example, if an apraxic speaker produces fricative sounds as stops or affricates, and appears to be incapable of accurate fricative productions, distorted fricatives may represent acceptable goals, since such productions would be likely to improve speech intelligibility or achieve qualitative acceptability.

Improvements in sound productions need not be measured only in terms of perceived phonetic accuracy. As indicated previously, subphonemic aspects of speech production that differentiate AOS from other neuromotor and phonological disorders and have provided the core definitional features of AOS, such as segmental and intersegmental durations, segmental transitions, and variability of durations and transitions, may also serve as indicators of improved sound production.

Suprasegmental aspects of speech production that may or may not be positively impacted by improvements in sound production include durations of interword intervals and other prosodic variables. Treatments that manipulate timing (Dworkin et al., 1988; Dworkin & Abkarian, 1996; Simmons, 1978) and prosody (Wertz et al., 1984) have been advocated for AOS. Currently there are few treatment data available regarding the relationship between segmental and suprasegmental aspects of speech production. Suprasegmental variables may be manipulated to facilitate speech production in AOS (Wambaugh & Martinez, 2000) and may also serve as the direct targets of treatment. Lengthening of interword intervals is thought to be a defining feature of AOS (McNeil et al., 1997) and will certainly deserve attention in most speakers with AOS. Disruptions in the production of the prosodic parameters of fundamental frequency and intensity may be observed in some, but not all, patients with AOS (Square-Storer, 1989); therefore, a prosodic assessment should be considered for all such patients. Robin, Klouda, and Hug (1991) have developed a protocol that incorporates perceptual and acoustic measures of prosody. Sentence-level productions are elicited to assess emotive intonation (e.g., production of sentences with happy, sad, and angry intonations), conveyance of emphatic stress (e.g., production of sentences with stress placed on a particular word in response to a question posed by the examiner), production of linguistic stress to distinguish questions and statements, and use of syntactic juncture to clarify sentence meaning (e.g., production of sentences for which pausing is crucial for interpretation). This protocol may require modification, depending upon the degree of severity of co-occurring aphasia.

Other variables to consider in selecting treatment targets and in measuring treatment progress include such fluency-disrupting behaviors as articulatory groping, false starts and revisions, use of hesitations and fillers, and prearticulatory rehearsals. In addition, overall speech rate may be an appropriate dependent measure. At the present time, there are no data concerning such variables in relation to treatment effectiveness.

Treatment Options

As discussed previously in this chapter, as well as by others (Square & Martin, 1994), there has been a tendency to group the majority of aphasias that involve speech production difficulties into the single diagnostic category of AOS. The differences in behaviors are usually attributed to varying severity of AOS. It has also been suggested that treatment strategies be assigned by severity level (Wertz et al., 1984). Unfortunately, at the current time it is not clear how various deviant speech behaviors seen in AOS relate to perceived severity (Haley, Wertz, & Ohde, 1998). Given the relatively wide array of behaviors possible in apraxic speech, it is likely that different combinations of behaviors may result in similar severity ratings across speakers. Therefore, like Square and Martin (1994), we suggest that perceived severity not be used as the main determinant in selecting a treatment approach. Instead, the probable pathophysiology underlying the disordered speech behaviors should be considered the most important variable in treatment selection.

NOTES

1. Other investigators/theorists (e.g., Whiteside & Varley, 1998—see discussion below) make the distinction between automatic and volitional speech acts according to whether there is forced selection of the direct or the indirect phonetic encoding route in AOS. In this account, access to the direct encoding route is automatic and requires few processing resources. Selection of the indirect phonetic encoding route, whether done volitionally or by default because of an impaired direct route, is controlled and requires additional processing resources compared to use of the direct route. In this account, the distinction between "volitional" and "vegetative" is not necessary to account for differences in production accuracy, although the constructs do share similarities.

2. This description of one form of AOS associated with parietal lobe lesions is specifically excluded as AOS in the definition proposed by McNeil et al. (1997) and reproduced here. It is argued that although articulation errors, repetitions, and reattempts do occur in AOS, these signs do not differentiate AOS from aphasia with phonemic paraphasias in the absence of a fundamental deficit of segmental and intersegmental rate. As such, the presence of these signs cannot be considered sufficient evidence for the diagnosis of AOS per se.

3. It should be recognized in regard to this study, as well as most others in the area of AOS, that some of these features have been argued as being consistent with phonemic paraphasia (e.g., sound substitutions, groping and searching, initiation deficits, and error inconsistency), while others have been argued as being pathognomonic of phonemic paraphasia (e.g., phonemic and syllabic sequencing errors). Thus these data, on the whole, may not serve as the purest form of evidence supporting the lesion–behavioral correlation for AOS.

4. It is difficult to be confident that the subjects selected demonstrated AOS without phonological paraphasias, as the subjects with aphasia and AOS were described as having a "predominance of sound level errors and literal paraphasias"—a characteristic typically used to characterize the speech of a person with phonological-level sound selection and sequencing deficits.

REFERENCES

Ajuriaguerra, J., & Hécaen, H. (1964). *Le cortex cerebrale.* Paris: Masson.

Albert, M. L., Sparks, R., & Helm, N. (1973). Melodic intonation therapy for aphasia. *Archives of Neurology, 29,* 130–131.

Allen, G. I., & Tsukahara, N. (1974). Cerebrocerebellar communication systems. *Physiological Review, 54,* 957–997.

Aten, J. L., Johns, D. F., & Darley, F. L. (1971). Auditory perception of sequenced words in apraxia of speech. *Journal of Speech and Hearing Research, 14,* 131–143.

Blumstein, S. (1973). *A phonological investigation of aphasic speech.* The Hague: Mouton.

Blumstein, S. (1981). Phonological aspects of aphasia. In M. T. Sarno (Ed.), *Acquired aphasia* (pp. 129–155). New York: Academic Press.

Brooks, V. B. (1986). *The neural basis of motor control.* New York: Oxford University Press.

Brown, J. W. (1972). *Aphasia, apraxia and agnosia.* Springfield, IL: Thomas.

Brown, J. W., & Perecman, E. (1986). Neurological basis of language processing. In R. Chapey (Ed.), *Language intervention strategies in adult aphasia* (2nd Ed., pp. 12–27). Baltimore: Williams & Wilkins.

Buckingham, H. W. (1979). Explanations in apraxia with consequences for the concept of apraxia of speech. *Brain and Language, 8,* 202–226.

Buckingham, H. W. (1981). Explanations in apraxia with consequences for the concept of apraxia of speech. In M. T. Sarno (Ed.), *Acquired aphasia* (2nd. ed., pp. 271–301). New York: Academic Press.

Buckingham, H. W. (1983). Apraxia of language vs. apraxia of speech. In R. A. Magill (Ed.), *Memory and control of action* (pp. 275–292). Amsterdam: North-Holland.

Buckingham, H. W. (1992). Phonological production deficits in conduction aphasia. In S. E. Kohn (Ed.), *Conduction aphasia* (pp. 77–116). Hillsdale, NJ: Erlbaum.

Cantor, G. J., Trost, J. E., & Burns, M. S. (1985). Contrasting speech patterns in apraxia of speech and phonemic paraphasia. *Brain and Language, 24,* 204–222.

Clark, H., & Robin, D. A. (1996). Sense of effort during a lexical decision task: Resource allocation deficits following brain damage. *American Journal of Speech–Language Pathology, 4,* 143–147.

Code, C. (1998). Models, theories and heuristics in apraxia of speech. *Clinical Linguistics and Phonetics, 12*(1), 47–65.

Crary, M. A. (1993). *Developmental motor speech disorders.* San Diego, CA: Singular Press.

Darley, F. L. (1967). Lacunae and research approaches to them: IV. In C. H. Millikan & F. L. Darley (Eds.), *Brain mechanisms underlying speech and language* (pp. 236–290). New York: Grune & Stratton.

Darley, F. L. (1968). *Apraxia of speech: 107 years of terminological confusion.* Paper presented at the annual convention of the American Speech and Hearing Association, Denver, CO.

Darley, F. L. (1982). *Aphasia.* Philadelphia: Saunders.

Deal, J. L., & Darley, F. L. (1972). The influence of linguistic and situational variables on phonemic accuracy in apraxia of speech. *Journal of Speech and Hearing Research, 15,* 639–653.

Deal, J. L., & Florance, C. L. (1978). Modification of the eight-step continuum for treatment of apraxia of speech in adults. *Journal of Speech and Hearing Disorders, 43,* 89–95.

De Renzi, E. (1985). Methods of limb apraxia examination and their bearing on the interpretation of the disorder. In E. A. Roy (Ed.), *Neuropsychological studies of apraxia and related disorders* (pp. 45–64). Amsterdam: Elsevier.

De Renzi, E., Pieczuro, O., & Vignolo, L. A. (1966). Oral apraxia and aphasia. *Cortex, 2*, 50–73.

Deutsch, S. (1984). Prediction of site of lesion from speech apraxic error patterns. In J. C. Rosenbek, M. R. McNeil, & A. Aronson (Eds.), *Apraxia of speech: Physiology, acoustics, linguistics, management* (pp. 113–134). San Diego, CA: College-Hill Press.

Dronkers, N. F. (1997). A new brain region for coordinating speech coordination. *Nature, 384*, 159–161.

Duffy, J. R. (1995). *Motor speech disorders: Substrates, differential diagnosis and management.* St. Louis, MO: Mosby.

Dunlop, J. M., & Marquardt, T. P. (1977). Linguistic and articulatory aspects of single word production in apraxia of speech. *Cortex, 13*, 17–29.

Dworkin, J. P., & Abkarian, G. G. (1996). Treatment of phonation in a patient with apraxia and dysarthria secondary to severe closed head injury. *Journal of Medical Speech–Language Pathology, 4*, 105–115.

Dworkin, J. P., Abkarian, G. G., & Johns, D. F. (1988). Apraxia of speech: The effectiveness of a treatment regimen. *Journal of Speech and Hearing Disorders, 53*, 280–294.

Evarts, E. V. (1982). Analogies between central motor programs for speech and for limb movements. In S. Grillner, B. Lindblom, J. Lubker, & A. Persson (Eds.), *Speech motor control* (Vol. 36, pp. 19–41). Oxford: Pergamon Press.

Ferguson, C. A. (1978). Learning to pronounce: The earliest spaces of phonological development. In F. Minifie & L. Lloyd (Eds.), *Communicative and cognitive abilities in early behavioral assessment* (pp. 273–297). Baltimore: University Park Press.

Florance, C. L., Rabidoux, P. L., & McCauslin, L. S. (1980). An environmental manipulation approach to treating apraxia of speech. *Clinical Aphasiology, 14*, 285–293.

Foerster, O. (1936). Symptomatologie der Erkrankungen des Gehirns. In O. Bumke & O. Foerster (Eds.), *Handbook der Neurologie*. Berlin: Springer.

Forrest, K., Adams, S., McNeil, M. R., & Southwood, H. (1991). Kinematic, electromyographic, and perceptual evaluation of speech apraxia, conduction aphasia, ataxic dysarthria and normal speech production. In C. A. Moore, K. M. Yorkston, & D. R. Beukelman (Eds.), *Dysarthria and apraxia of speech: Perspectives on management* (pp. 147–171). Baltimore: Brookes.

Foundas, A., Macauley, B. L., Raymer, A. M., Maher, L. M., Heilman, K. M., & Rothi, L. J. G. (1995). Ecological implications of limb apraxia: Evidence from mealtime behavior. *Journal of the International Neuropsychological Society, 1*, 62–66.

Freed, D. B., Marshall, R. C., & Frazier, K. E. (1997). The long-term effectiveness of PROMPT treatment in a severely apractic–aphasic speaker. *Aphasiology, 11*, 365–372.

Fromm, D., Abbs, J. H., McNeil, M. R., & Rosenbek, J. C. (1982). Simultaneous perceptual–physiological method for studying apraxia of speech. *Clinical Aphasiology, 10*, 155–171.

Geschwind, N. (1975). The apraxias: Neural mechanisms of disorders of learned movement. *American Scientist, 63*, 188–195.

Goodglass, H., & Kaplan, E. (1972). *The assessment of aphasia and related disorders.* Philadelphia: Lea & Febiger.

Gracco, V. L. (1990). Characteristics of speech as a motor control system. In G. E. Hammond (Ed.), *Cerebral control of speech and limb movements* (pp. 3–28). Amsterdam: North-Holland.

Gracco, V. L., & Abbs, J. H. (1987). Programming and execution processes of speech movement control: Potential neural correlates. In L. E. Keller & M. Gopnik (Eds.), *Motor and sensory processes of language* (pp. 165–218). Hillsdale, NJ: Erlbaum.

Haley, K. L., Wertz, R. T., & Ohde, R. N. (1998). Single word intelligibility in aphasia and apraxia of speech. *Aphasiology, 12*(7–8), 715–730.

Hall, P. K., Jordan, L. S., & Robin, D. A. (1993). *Developmental apraxia of speech.* Austin, TX: Pro-Ed.

Hammond, G. E. (Ed.). (1990). *Cerebral control of speech and limb movements.* Amsterdam: North-Holland.

Harrington, D. L., & Haaland, K. Y. (1987). Programming sequences of hand postures. *Journal of Motor Behavior, 19*, 77–95.

Harrington, D. L., & Haaland, K. Y. (1991). Hemispheric specialization for motor sequencing: Abnormalities in levels of programming. *Neuropsychologia, 29*, 147–163.

Heilman, K. M. (1973). Ideational apraxia: A re-definition. *Brain, 96*, 861–864.

Heilman, K. M. (1979). Apraxia. In K. M. Heilman & E. Valenstein (Eds.), *Clinical neuropsychology* (pp. 159–185). New York: Oxford University Press.

Heilman, K. M., Rothi, L. J. G., & Valenstein, E. (1982). Two forms of ideomotor apraxia. *Neurology*, *32*, 342–346.

Holtzapple, P., & Marshall, N. (1977). The application of multiphonemic articulation therapy with apraxic patients. *Clinical Aphasiology*, *5*, 46–58.

Johns, D. L., & Darley, F. L. (1970). Phonemic variability in apraxia of speech. *Journal of Speech and Hearing Research*, *13*, 556–583.

Keele, S.W., Cohen, A., & Ivry, R. (1990). Motor programs: Concepts and issues. In M. Jeannerod (Ed.), *Attention and performance XIII: Motor representation and control* (pp. 77–110). Hillsdale, NJ: Erlbaum.

Keith, R., & Aronson, A. E. (1975). Singing as therapy for apraxia of speech and aphasia: Report of a case. *Brain and Language*, *2*, 483–488.

Keller, E. (1984). Simplification and gesture reduction in phonological disorders of apraxia and aphasia. In J. C. Rosenbek, M. R. McNeil, & A. Aronson (Eds.), *Apraxia of speech: Physiology, acoustics, linguistics, management* (pp. 221–256). San Diego, CA: College-Hill Press.

Keller, E. (1987). The cortical representations of motor processes of speech. In E. Keller & M. Gopnik (Eds.), *Motor and sensory processes of language* (pp. 125–162). Hillsdale, NJ: Erlbaum.

Kelso, J. A. S. (1995). *Dynamic patterns: The self organization of brain and behavior.* Cambridge, MA: MIT Press.

Kelso, J. A. S., & Tuller, B. (1981). Toward a theory of apractic syndromes. *Brain and Language*, *12*, 224–245.

Kelso, J. A. S., & Tuller, B. (1984). A dynamical basis for action systems. In M. S. Gazzaniga (Ed.), *Handbook of cognitive neuroscience* (pp. 321–356). New York: Plenum Press.

Kelso, J. A. S., Tuller, B., & Harris, K. S. (1983). A "dynamic" pattern perspective on the control and coordination of movement. In P. F. MacNeilage (Ed.), *The production of speech* (pp. 137–173). New York: Springer-Verlag.

Kelso, J. A. S., Vatikiotis-Bateson, E., Saltzman, E. L., & Kay, B. (1985). A qualitative dynamic analysis of reiterant speech production: Phase portraits, kinematics, and dynamic modeling. *Journal of the Acoustical Society of America*, *77*, 266–280.

Kent, R. D., & McNeil, M. R. (1987). Relative timing of sentence repetition in apraxia of speech and conduction aphasia. In J. H. Ryalls (Ed.), *Phonetic approaches to speech production in aphasia and related disorders* (pp. 181–220). Boston: College-Hill Press.

Kent, R. D., & Rosenbek, J. C. (1983). Acoustic patterns of apraxia of speech. *Journal of Speech and Hearing Research*, *26*, 231–249.

Kertesz, A. (1984). Subcortical lesions and verbal apraxia. In J. C. Rosenbek, M. R. McNeil, & A. Aronson (Eds.), *Apraxia of speech: Physiology, acoustics, linguistics, management* (pp. 73–90). San Diego, CA: College-Hill Press.

Kimura, D. (1977). Acquisition of motor skill after left hemisphere damage. *Brain*, *100*, 527–542.

Kleist, K. (1907). Kortikale (innervatorische) Apraxie. *Jahrb. f. Psychiat. U. Neurol.*, *28*, 46–112. (Reported in J. W. Brown, (1972). *Aphasia, Apraxia and Agnosia*. Springfield: C. C. Thomas.)

Kugler, P. N., Kelso, J. A. S., & Turvey, M. T. (1980). On the concept of coordinative structures as dissipative structures: I. Theoretical lines of convergence. In G. E. Stelmach (Ed.), *Tutorials in motor behavior* (pp. 1–47). Amsterdam: North-Holland.

Lane, V. W., & Samples, J. M. (1981). Facilitating communication skills in adult apraxics: Application of Blisssymbols in a group setting. *Journal of Communication Disorders*, *14*, 157–167.

LaPointe, L. L. (1984). Sequential treatment of split lists: A case report. In J. C. Rosenbek, M. R. McNeil, & A. Aronson (Eds.), *Apraxia of speech: Physiology, acoustics, linguistics, management* (pp. 277–286). San Diego, CA: College-Hill Press.

LaPointe, L. L., & Johns, D. F. (1975). Some phonemic characteristics in apraxia of speech. *Journal of Communication Disorders*, *8*, 259–269.

LaPointe, L. L., & Wertz, R. T. (1974). Oral movement abilities and articulatory characteristics of brain-injured adults. *Perceptual and Motor Skills*, *39*, 39–46.

Lebrun, Y. (1989). Apraxia of speech: History of a concept. In P. Square-Storer (Ed.), *Acquired apraxia of speech in aphasic adults* (pp. 3–19). London: Taylor & Francis.

Lebrun, Y. (1990). Apraxia of speech: A critical review. *Neurolinguistics*, *5*(4), 379–406.

Lehmkuhl, G., & Poeck, K. (1981). A disturbance in the conceptual organization of the motor system in the monkey. *Cortex*, *17*, 153–158.

Lehmkuhl, G., Poeck, K., & Willmes, K. (1983). Ideomotor apraxia and aphasia: An examination of types and manifestations of apraxic symptoms. *Neuropsychologia*, *21*, 199–212.

Levelt, W. J. M. (1989). *Speaking: From intention to articulation*. Cambridge, MA: MIT Press.

Levelt, W. J. M. (1992). Accessing words in speech production: Stages, processes, representation. *Cognition, 42,* 1–22.

Levelt, W. J. M., & Wheeldon, L. (1994). Do speakers have access to a mental syllabary? *Cognition, 50,* 239–269.

Liepmann, H. (1900). Das Krankheitsbild der apraxie (motorischen asymboli) auf Grund eines Falles von einseitiger apraxie. *Monatschrift für Psychiatrie und Neurologie, 9,* 15–40.

Liepmann, H. (1905). Die linke hemisphaere und das handeln. *Muchener Medizinische Wochenschift, 52,* 2322–2326, 2375–2378.

Liepmann, H. (1913). Motor aphasia, anarthria and apraxia. *Transactions of the 17th International Congress of Medicine, Section XI, Part II,* 97–106.

Liepmann, H. (1920). Apraxie. *Ergbn. der ges. Med., 1,* 516–543. Reported in: Brown, J. W. (1972). *Aphasia, Apraxia and Agnosia.* Springfield: C. C. Thomas.)

Littlefield, C., Barresi, B. A., & Goodglass, H. (1998). Verbal short-term memory in an aphemic patient: Effects of encoding and retrieval modalities. *Brain and Language, 65*(1), 233–236.

Luria, A. R. (1966). Morg Čeloveka i psixičeskie Processy, Moscow, Acad. Ped. nauk, 1963. *Human brain and psychological processes.* New York: Harper.

MacNeilage, P. F. (1970). Motor control of serial ordering of speech. *Physiological Review, 77,* 182–196.

Marquardt, T., & Sussman, H. (1984). The elusive lesion–apraxia of speech link in Broca's aphasia. In J. C. Rosenbek, M. R. McNeil, & A. E. Aronson (Eds.), *Apraxia of speech: Physiology, acoustics, linguistics, management* (pp. 91–112). San Diego, CA: College-Hill Press.

Marsden, C. D. (1984). Which motor disorder in Parkinson's disease indicates the true motor function of the basal ganglia? In D. Evered & M. O'Connor (Eds.), *Functions of the basal ganglia* (Ciba Foundation Symposium No. 107, pp. 225–237). London: Pitman.

Marshall, J. (1989). Commentary: Carving the cognitive chicken. *Aphasiology, 3,* 735–740.

Martin, A. D. (1974). Some objections to the term apraxia of speech. *Journal of Speech and Hearing Disorders, 39,* 53–64.

Mateer, C. K., & Kimura, D. (1977). Impairment of nonverbal oral movements in aphasia. *Brain and Langauge, 4,* 262–276.

McNeil, M. R., & Adams, S. (1990). A comparison of speech kinematics among apraxic, conduction aphasic, ataxic dysarthric and normal geriatric speakers. *Clinical Aphasiology, 18,* 279–294.

McNeil, M. R., Caliguiri, M., & Rosenbek, J. C. (1989). A comparison of labiomandibular kinematic durations, displacements, velocities and dysmetrias in apraxic and normal adults. *Clinical Aphasiology, 17,* 173–193.

McNeil, M. R., & Kent, R. D. (1990). Motoric characteristics of adult aphasic and apraxic speakers. In G. E. Hammond (Ed.), *Cerebral control of speech and limb movements* (pp. 349–386). Amsterdam: North-Holland.

McNeil, M. R., Odell, K. H., Miller, S. B., & Hunter, L. (1995). Consistency, variability, and target approximation for successive speech repetitions among apraxic, conduction aphasic, and ataxic dysarthric speakers. *Clinical Aphasiology, 23,* 39–55.

McNeil, M. R., Prescott, T. E., & Lemme, M. L. (1976). An application of electromyographic biofeedback to aphasia/apraxia treatment. *Clinical Aphasiology, 4,* 151–171.

McNeil, M. R., Robin, D. A., & Schmidt, R. A. (1997). Apraxia of speech: Definition, differentiation, and treatment. In M. R. McNeil (Ed.), *Clinical management of sensorimotor speech disorders* (pp. 311–344). New York: Thieme.

McNeil, M. R., Weismer, G., Adams, S., & Mulligan, M. (1990). Oral structure nonspeech motor control in normal dysarthric aphasic and apraxic speakers: Isometric force and static position control. *Journal of Speech and Hearing Research, 33,* 255–268.

Miller, N. (1986). *Dyspraxia and its management.* Rockville, MD: Aspen.

Mlcoch, A., & Noll, J. D. 1980. Speech production models as related to the concept of apraxia of speech. In N. J. Lass (Ed.), *Speech and language: Advances in basic research and practice* (Vol. 4, pp. 201–238). New York: Academic Press.

Mohr, J. P., Pessin, M. S., Finkelstein, S., Funkenstein, H., Duncan, G. W., & Davis, K. R. (1978). Broca aphasia: Pathological and clinical. *Neurology, 28,* 311–324.

Munhall, K. G. Articulatory variability. In P. Square-Storer (Ed.), *Acquired apraxia of speech in aphasic adults* (pp. 64–83). London: Taylor & Francis.

Naeser, M. A., & Helm-Estabrooks, N. (1985). CT scan lesion localization and response to melodic intonation therapy with nonfluent aphasia cases. *Cortex, 21,* 203–233.

Nebes, R. D. (1975). The nature of internal speech in a patient with aphemia. *Brain and Language*, 2, 489–497.

Nespoulous, J. L., Joanette, Y., Beland, R., Caplan, D., & Lecours, A. R. (1984). Phonological disturbances in aphasia: Is there a "markedness" effect in aphasic phonemic errors? In F. C. Rose (Ed.), *Advances in neurology: Vol. 42. Progress in aphasiology* (pp. 203–214). New York: Raven Press.

Ochipa, C., Rothi, L. J. G., & Heilman, K. M. (1992). Conceptual apraxia in Alzheimer's disease. *Brain*, 115, 1061–1072.

Odell, K., McNeil, M. R., Rosenbek, J. C., & Hunter, L. (1990). Perceptual characteristics of consonant production by apraxic speakers. *Journal of Speech and Hearing Disorders*, 55, 345–359.

Odell, K., McNeil, M. R., Rosenbek, J. C., & Hunter, L. (1991). Perceptual characteristics of vowel and prosody production in apraxic, aphasic, and dysarthric speakers. *Journal of Speech and Hearing Research*, 34, 67–80.

Pierce, R. S. (1991). Apraxia of speech versus phonemic paraphasia: Theoretical, diagnostic and treatment considerations. In D. Vogel & M. P. Cannito (Eds.), *Treating disorders of speech motor control: For clinicians by clinicians* (pp. 185–216). Austin, TX: Pro-Ed.

Poeck, K. (1983). Ideational apraxia. *Journal of Neurology*, 230, 1–5.

Poeck, K. (1985). Clues to the nature of disruptions to limb praxis. In E. A. Roy (Ed.), *Neuropsychological studies of apraxia and related disorders* (pp. 99–110). Amsterdam: North-Holland.

Poeck, K., & Kerschensteiner, M. (1975). Analysis of the sequential motor events in oral apraxia. In K. J. Zulch, O. Creutzfeldt, & G. C. Galbraith (Eds.), *Cerebral localization* (pp. 98–109). Berlin: Springer-Verlag.

Poizner, H., Mack, L., Verfaellie, M., Rothi, L. J. G., & Heilman, K. M. (1990). Three-dimensional computer graphic analysis of apraxia. *Brain*, 113, 85–101.

Raymer, A. M., & Thompson, C. K. (1991). Effects of verbal plus gestural treatment in a patient with aphasia and severe apraxia of speech. *Clinical Aphasiology*, 19, 285–298.

Reed, E. S. (1982). An outline of a theory of action systems. *Journal of Motor Behavior*, 14, 98–134.

Robin, D. A., Klouda, G. V., & Hug, L. N. (1991). Neurogenic disorders of prosody. In D. Vogel & M. P. Cannito (Eds.), *Treating disordered speech motor control: For clinicians by clinicians* (pp. 241–271). Austin, TX: Pro-Ed.

Rochon, E., Caplan, D., & Waters, G. S. (1991). Short-term memory processes in patients with apraxia of speech: Implications for the nature and structure of the auditory verbal short-term memory system. *Journal of Neurolinguistics*, 5, 237–264.

Rogers, M. A., & Storkel, H. (1998). Reprogramming phonologically similar utterances: The role of phonetic features in pre-motor encoding. *Journal of Speech and Hearing Research*, 41, 258–274.

Rogers, M. A., & Storkel, H. L. (in press). Planning speech one syllable at a time: The reduced buffer capacity hypothesis in apraxia of speech. *Aphasiology*.

Rosenbaum, D. A., Weber, R. J., Hazelett, W. M., & Hindorff, V. (1986). The parameter remapping effect in human performance: Evidence from tongue twisters and finger fumblers. *Journal of Memory and Language*, 25, 710–725.

Rosenbek, J. C. (1978). Treating apraxia of speech. In D.F. Johns (Ed.), *Clinical management of neurogenic communicative disorders* (pp. 191–241). Boston: Little, Brown.

Rosenbek, J. C., Kent, R. D., & LaPointe, L. L. (1984). Apraxia of speech: An overview and some perspectives. In J. C. Rosenbek, M. R. McNeil, & A. E. Aronson (Eds.), *Apraxia of speech: Physiology, acoustics, linguistics, management* (pp. 1–72). San Diego, CA: College-Hill Press.

Rosenbek, J. C., Lemme, M. L., Ahern, M. B., Harris, E. H., & Wertz, R. T. (1973). A treatment for apraxia of speech in adults. *Journal of Speech and Hearing Disorders*, 38, 462–472.

Rosenbek, J. C., Wertz, R. T., & Darley, F. L. (1973). Oral sensation and perception in apraxia of speech and aphasia. *Journal of Speech and Hearing Research*, 16, 22–36.

Ross, E. (1981). The aprosodias: Functional–anatomic organization of the affective components of language in the righ hemisphere. *Archives of Neurology*, 38, 561–569.

Rothi, L. J. G., & Heilman, K. M. (Eds.). (1997a). *Apraxia: The neuropsychology of action*. Hove, England: Psychology Press.

Rothi, L. J. G., & Heilman, K. M. (1997b). Introduction to limb apraxia. In L. J. G. Rothi & K. M. Heilman (Eds.), *Apraxia: The neuropsychology of action* (pp. 1–6). Hove, England: Psychology Press.

Rothi, L. J. G., Ochipa, C., & Heilman, K. M. (1991). A cognitive neuropsychological model of limb praxis. *Cognitive Neuropsychology, 8,* 443–458.

Roy, E. A. (1978). Apraxia: A new look at an old syndrome. *Journal of Human Movement Studies, 4,* 191–210.

Roy, E. A. (Ed.). (1985). *Neuropsychological studies of apraxia and related disorders.* Amsterdam: North-Holland.

Roy, E. A., & Square, P. A. (1985). Common Consideration in the study of limb, verbal and oral apraxia. In E. A. Roy (Ed.), *Neuropsychological studies of apraxia and related disorders* (pp. 111–161). Amsterdam: North-Holland.

Roy, E. A., & Square-Storer, P. A. (1990). Evidence for common expressions of apraxia. In G. Hammond (Eds.), *Cerebral control of speech and limb movements* (pp. 477–502). Amsterdam: North Holland.

Rubow, R. T., Rosenbek, J. C., Collins, M. J., & Longstreth, D. (1982). Vibrotactile stimulation for intersystemic reorganization in the treatment of apraxia of speech. *Archives of Physical Medicine and Rehabilitation, 63,* 150–153.

Schmidt, R. A. (1975). A schema theory of discrete motor skill learning. *Psychological Review, 82,* 225–260.

Schmidt, R. A. (1976). The schema as a solution to some persistent problems in motor learning theory. In G. E. Stelmach (Ed.), *Motor control: Issues and trends* (pp. 41–64). New York: Academic Press.

Schmidt, R. A. (1982). *Motor control and learning: A behavioral emphasis.* Champaign, IL: Human Kinetics.

Schmidt, R. A. (1988). *Motor control and learning: A behavioral emphasis, 2nd ed.* Champaign, IL: Human Kinetics.

Schmidt, R. A. (1991). *Motor learning and performance: From principles to practice.* Champaign, IL: Human Kinetics.

Shaffer, L. H. (1982). Rhythm and timing in skill. *Psychological Review, 89,* 109–122.

Shane, H. C., & Darley, F. L. (1978). The effect of auditory rhythmic stimulation on articulatory accuracy in apraxia of speech. *Cortex, 14,* 444–450.

Shif, H. B., Alexander, M. P., Naeser, M. A., & Galaburda, A. M. (1983). Aphemia: Clinical–anatomic correlations. *Archives of Neurology, 40,* 720–727.

Simmons, N. N. (1978). Finger counting as an intersystemic reorganizer in apraxia of speech. *Clinical Aphasiology, 6,* 174–179.

Southwood, H. (1987). The use of prolonged speech in the treatment of apraxia of speech. *Clinical Aphasiology, 15,* 277–287.

Sparks, R. W., & Deck, J. W. (1986). Melodic intonation therapy. In R. Chapey (Ed.), *Language intervention strategies in adult aphasia* (2nd ed., pp. 320–332). Baltimore: Williams & Wilkins.

Sparks, R., Helm, N., & Albert, M. (1974). Aphasia rehabilitation resulting from melodic intonation therapy. *Cortex, 10,* 303–316.

Sparks, R., & Holland, A. L. (1976). Method: Melodic intonation therapy for aphasia. *Journal of Speech and Hearing Disorders, 41,* 287–297.

Square, P. A. (1995). Apraxia of speech reconsidered. In F. Bell-Berti & L. J. Raphael (Eds.), *Producing speech: Contemporary issues for Katherine Safford Harris* (pp. 375–386). New York: AIP Press.

Square, P. A., Chumpelik, D., & Adams, S. (1985). Efficacy of the PROMPT system of therapy for the treatment of acquired apraxia of speech. *Clinical Aphasiology, 13,* 319–320.

Square, P. A., Chumpelik, D., Morningstar, D., & Adams, S. (1986). Efficacy of the PROMPT system of therapy for the treatment of acquired apraxia of speech: A follow-up investigation. *Clinical Aphasiology, 14,* 221–226.

Square, P. A., Darley, F. L., & Sommers, R. I. (1981). Speech perception among patients demonstrating apraxia of speech, aphasia, and both disorders. *Clinical Aphasiology, 9,* 83–88.

Square, P. A., Darley, F. L., & Sommers, R. I. (1982). An analysis of the productive errors made by pure apractic speakers with differing loci of lesions. *Clinical Aphasiology, 10,* 245–250.

Square, P. A., & Martin, R. A. (1994). The nature and treatment of neuromotor speech disorders in aphasia. In R. Chapey (Ed.), *Language intervention strategies in adult aphasia* (3rd ed., pp. 467–499). Hillsdale, NJ: Erlbaum.

Square-Storer, P. A. (1989). Traditional therapies for apraxia of speech—Reviewed and rationalized. In P. A. Square-Storer (Ed.), *Acquired apraxia of speech in aphasic adults* (pp. 145–161). London: Taylor & Francis.

Square-Storer, P. A., Darley, F. L., & Sommers, R. I. (1988). Speech processing abilities in patients with aphasia and apraxia of speech. *Brain and Language, 33*(1), 65–85.

Square-Storer, P. A., & Hayden, D. C. (1989). PROMPT treatment. In P. Square-Storer (Ed.), *Acquired apraxia of speech in aphasic adults* (pp. 190–219). London: Taylor & Francis.

Square-Storer, P. A., Roy, E. A., & Hogg, S. C. (1990). The dissociation of aphasia from apraxia of speech, ideomotor limb, and buccofacial apraxia. In G. E. Hammond (Ed.), *Cerebral control of speech and limb movements* (pp. 451–476). Amsterdam: North-Holland.

Square-Storer, P. A., Roy, E. A., & Martin, R. E. (1997). Apraxia of speech: Another form of praxis disruption. In L. J. G. Rothi & K. M. Heilman (Eds.), *Apraxia: The neuropsychology of action* (pp. 173–206). Hove, England: Psychology Press.

Sternberg, S., Monsell, S., Knoll, R. L., & Wright, C. E. (1978). The latency and duration of rapid movement sequences: Comparisons of speech and typewriting. In G. E. Stelmach (Ed.), *Information processing in motor control and learning* (pp. 117–152) New York: Academic Press.

Stevens, E., & Glazer, L. (1983). Multiple input phoneme therapy: An approach to severe apraxia and expressive aphasia. *Clinical Aphasiology, 11*, 148–155.

Stokes, T., & Baer, D. M. (1977). An implicit technology of generalization. *Journal of Applied Behavior Analysis, 10*, 349–367.

Strand, E. A. (1987). *Acoustic and response time measures in utterance production: A comparison of apraxic and normal speakers.* Unpublished doctoral dissertation, University of Wisconsin.

Thompson, C. K., & Young, E. C. (1983). *A phonological process approach to apraxia of speech: An experimental analysis of cluster reduction.* Paper presented at the annual convention of the American Speech Language and Hearing Association, Cincinnati, OH.

Tonkovich, J., & Marquardt, T. (1977). The effects of stress and melodic intonation on apraxia of speech. *Clinical Aphasiology, 5*, 97–102.

Trost, J. E., & Canter, G. J. (1974). Apraxia of speech in patients with Broca's aphasia: A study of phoneme production accuracy and error patterns. *Brain and Language, 1*, 63–79.

Van der Merwe, A. (1997). A theoretical framework for the characterization of pathological speech sensorimotor control. In M. R. McNeil (Ed.), *Clinical management of sensorimotor speech disorders* (pp. 1–25). New York: Thieme.

Wambaugh, J. L., & Cort, R. C. (1998). *Treatment for AOS: Perceptual and VOT changes in sound production.* Paper presented at the biennial Motor Speech Conference, Tucson, AZ.

Wambaugh, J. L., & Doyle, P. J. (1994). Treatment for acquired apraxia of speech: A review of efficacy reports. *Clinical Aphasiology, 22*, 231–243.

Wambaugh, J. L., Doyle, P. J., Kalinyak, M. M., & West, J. E. (1996). A minimal contrast treatment for apraxia of speech. *Clinical Aphasiology, 24*, 97–108.

Wambaugh, J. L., Kalinyak-Fliszar, M. M., West, J. E., & Doyle, P. J. (1998). Effects of treatment for sound errors in apraxia of speech and aphasia. *Journal of Speech, Language, and Hearing Research, 41*, 725–743.

Wambaugh, J. L., & Martinez, A. L. (1999). Effects of rate and rhythm control treatment on sound production in apraxia of speech. *Aphasiology, 14*, 603–617.

Wambaugh, J. L., Martinez, A. L., McNeil, M. M., & Rogers, M. A. (1999). Sound production treatment for apraxia of speech: Overgeneralization and maintenance effects. *Aphasiology, 13*, 821–837.

Wambaugh, J. L., West, J. E., & Doyle, P. J. (1997). A VOT analysis of apraxic/aphasic voicing errors. *Aphasiology, 11*, 521–532.

Wambaugh, J. L., West, J. E., & Doyle, P. J. (1998). Treatment for apraxia of speech: Effects of targeting sound groups. *Aphasiology, 12*, 731–743.

Waters, G. S., Rochon, E., & Caplan, D. (1992). The role of high-level speech planning in rehearsal: Evidence from patients with apraxia of speech. *Journal of Memory and Language, 31*, 54–73.

Wertz, R. T. (1984). Response to treatment in patients with apraxia of speech. In J. C. Rosenbek, M. R. McNeil, & A. E. Aronson (Eds.), *Apraxia of speech: Physiology, acoustics, linguistics, management* (pp. 257–276). San Diego, CA: College-Hill Press.

Wertz, R. T., Collins, M. J., Weiss, D., Kurtzke, J. F., Friden, T., Brookshire, R. H., Pierce, J., et al. (1981). VA co-operative study on aphasia: A comparison of individual/group treatment. *Journal of Speech and Hearing Research, 24*, 580–594.

Wertz, R. T., LaPointe, L. L., & Rosenbek, J. C. (1984). *Apraxia of speech in adults: The disorder and its management.* Orlando, FL: Grune & Stratton.

Wertz, R. T., & Rosenbek, J. C. (1971). Appraising apraxia of speech. *Journal of the Colorado Speech and Hearing Association, 5*, 18–36.

Wertz, R. T., Rosenbek, J. C., & Deal, J. (1970). *A review of 228 cases of apraxia of speech: Classification, etiology and localization.* Paper presented at the annual convention of the American Speech and Hearing Association, New York.

Whiteside, S. P., & Varley, R. A. (1998). A reconceptualisation of apraxia of speech: A synthesis of evidence. *Cortex, 34,* 221–231.

Wickens, J., Hyland, B., & Anson, G. (1994). Cortical cell assemblies: A possible mechanism for motor programs. *Journal of Motor Behavior, 26,* 66–82.

10

LIMB APRAXIA

CYNTHIA OCHIPA
LESLIE J. GONZALEZ ROTHI

"Limb apraxia" is defined as a disorder of learned, skilled, purposeful movement not caused by weakness, akinesia, deafferentation, abnormalities of tone or posture, movement disorders, intellectual deterioration, or impaired comprehension (Heilman & Rothi, 1993). The spatial, temporal, and/or conceptual errors observed in the gestural performance of individuals with limb apraxia are thought to represent a disruption in the praxis system, which is responsible for storing skilled motor information about purposeful movement. The neural networks that mediate praxis are represented in the left hemisphere of most right-handed individuals (Heilman, Rothi, & Valenstein, 1982; Liepmann, 1900/1977, 1905/1980).

Limb apraxia has been considered a neuropsychological syndrome of theoretical significance with some value in lesion localization, but with little practical importance (Basso, Capitani, Sala, Laiacona, & Spinnler, 1987; Poeck, 1985). However, recent studies have demonstrated the negative impact of limb apraxia on activities of daily living (Foundas et al., 1995; Ochipa, Rothi, & Heilman, 1989; Schwartz et al., 1995; Schwartz, Reed, Montgomery, Palmer, & Mayer, 1991; Sundet, Finset, & Reinvang, 1988). Another area of particular clinical relevance is the treatment of persons with aphasia or dysarthria, for whom gesture is often an important component of the individuals' compensatory communicative strategies.

This chapter reviews the neuroanatomical correlates of limb apraxia, and presents a model of praxis processing that may account for the variety of deficits seen in apraxic individuals. Finally, implications of the model for assessment and treatment of limb apraxia are discussed.

NEUROANATOMICAL CORRELATES OF LIMB APRAXIA

Liepmann (1900/1977, 1920/1980) is credited with the original description of the mechanism underlying limb apraxia. In his review of the gestural performance of 83 patients with left or right hemiparesis, Liepmann noted that it was rare to see a patient with left hemiparesis who had impaired gestural ability. He proposed that in right-handed subjects, the guidance for performing skilled movements with both the right and left arms is provided by the left hemisphere. Specifically, Liepmann proposed that the left-hemisphere sensory–motor cortex guides not only the right arm, but also the left arm via the corpus callosum. He suggested that the left hemisphere holds motor representations for learned, skilled movement, which he described as "movement formulae" containing the "time–space–form picture of the movement." Liepmann concluded that a lesion of the left sensory–motor cortex should result in a limb apraxia in both arms (though it may be masked in the right arm by hemiparesis). A lesion of the corpus callosum should cause a unilateral, left-arm apraxia, as this lesion should disconnect the praxis-dominant left hemisphere from the motor areas of the right hemisphere that control fine movements of the left arm. Although Liepmann and Maas first reported "callosal apraxia" in 1907, similar cases have been reported in recent times (Boldrini, Zanella, Cantagallo, & Basaglia, 1992; Geschwind & Kaplan, 1962; Watson & Heilman, 1983).

Following Liepmann, Geschwind (1965) also believed that the left hemisphere of right-handed subjects guides skilled movements of both arms. He proposed a neuronal network for the mediation of learned, skilled movements. Geschwind suggested that pantomime to verbal command requires information to flow sequentially from the auditory pathway to Heschl's gyrus and to Wernicke's area. Information then flows to the motor association cortex, where the motor movements are programmed and sent to the primary motor area for the control of the right hand. For left-handed movements, information proceeds to the right-hemisphere premotor areas via the corpus callosum. According to Geschwind's schema, lesions of the supramarginal gyrus or the arcuate fasciculus should yield an apraxia by disconnecting the posterior language comprehension areas from the anterior motor association area. However, the schema does not fully explain the inability of some apraxic individuals to imitate visually presented gestures. Geschwind suggested that visual information may also be processed through this pathway (visual association cortex to premotor cortex via the arcuate fasciculus). Still, the difficulty that some apraxic persons have in demonstrating tool use, even when the actual implement is held, cannot be fully accounted for by Geschwind's schema.

Heilman et al. (1982) specifically proposed that movement memories, or "visual–kinesthetic motor engrams," are stored in the left inferior parietal lobe. These authors suggested that the destruction or disconnection of these movement memories from other areas critical to praxis processing can explain the various disassociations seen in apraxic patients. According to their schema, pantomime to verbal command engages the posterior language areas; then information flows to the inferior parietal lobe, where the movement memories are accessed. Information subsequently flows to the premotor and motor areas of the left hemisphere for the control of the right arm. Information crosses the corpus callosum to the motor areas of the right hemisphere for control of the left arm. Visual information may also gain access to the stored visual–kinesthetic engrams in the left inferior parietal lobe.

Heilman et al. (1982) tested 20 patients with unilateral left-hemisphere lesions, using tasks of gesture to verbal command and gesture discrimination. For gesture discrimination, subjects were shown a film of a man performing a pantomime, and they had to choose which of three choices represented the target pantomime named by the examiner. Two groups were distinguished: those who had apraxia and could not discriminate gestures, and those who had apraxia but spared gesture discrimination. Those subjects with lesions of the left parietal lobe had gesture discrimination problems, attributed by Heilman et al. (1982) to a degraded memory trace. That is, they could not recognize gestures because there was damage to the representations for learned, skilled, purposeful movements. Subjects with anterior lesions not involving the left parietal lobe had production difficulties but not a gesture discrimination problem, suggesting destruction of more anterior premotor or motor areas or disconnection of these areas from the parietal lobe, but not degraded visual–kinesthetic engrams within the parietal lobe. That these representations for learned, skilled movements could be disconnected from visual input was demonstrated by Rothi, Mack, and Heilman (1986), who reported two patients with left occipito-temporal lesions who could not comprehend or discriminate visually presented gestures, yet could perform gestures normally. These patients were considered to have "pantomime agnosia."

A COGNITIVE-NEUROPSYCHOLOGICAL MODEL OF APRAXIA

The evidence for the separability of praxis production from praxis reception, along with evidence of other dissociations, led to the development of a model of praxis processing to account for the variety of behavioral disturbances noted in the performance of apraxic individuals (Rothi, Ochipa, & Heilman, 1991). Similar to models that have been developed to illustrate language processing (see Nadeau, Chapter 3; Wilshire & Coslett, Chapter 4; Raymer & Rothi, Chapter 5; and Chatterjee & Maher, Chapter 6, this volume), this model attempts to explain how impairment of the complex, multicomponent praxis system may result in a variety of deficits, presumably depending upon which components of the system are compromised. Support for this model is provided by describing a series of functional dissociations observed in neurologically impaired adults.

The Praxicon

In the study of language, the term "lexicon" is used to describe that portion of the language system that provides a processing advantage for words that the language user has previously experienced. Heilman and Rothi (1993) have proposed that the "movement formulae" of Liepmann may be analogous to the stored representations for words found in the lexicon. Heilman and Rothi (1993) have used the term "praxicon" for these movement memories, and suggested that these praxis representations provide a processing advantage in the performance of complex movement. That is, if the central nervous system stores information about purposeful movements that an individual has previously experienced, it can call upon this information to reconstitute previously constructed programs rather than reconstructing the process de novo with each experience (Rothi et al., 1991).

As described previously, at least two mechanisms have been proposed to account for the performance of apraxic patients (Heilman et al., 1982; Rothi, Heilman, & Watson, 1985). A degraded memory trace (see Figure 10.1, lesion A), involving the movement formulae of the praxicon, should cause difficulties in both the discrimination and the production of gestures. This pattern of performance is noted in individuals with lesions of the left parietal lobe. Disconnection of the praxicon from its projection targets, or damage to those targets (see Figure 10.1, lesion B), should yield only a gesture production deficit. Here, the movement memories that allow one to recognize viewed gestures are intact, but can no longer interact with the parts of the brain responsible for motor implementation. Lesion C (Figure 10.1) is proposed to account for pantomime agnosia (Rothi et al., 1986) wherein patients can produce gestures to verbal command, but are unable to comprehend or discriminate visually presented gestures.

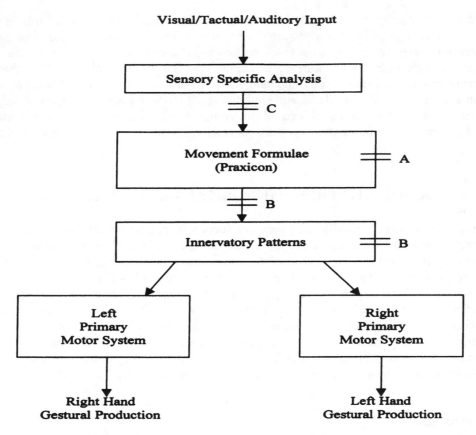

FIGURE 10.1. A model of praxis processing accounting for deficits of gesture production and gesture reception.

The Innervatory Patterns

Liepmann (1920/1988) suggested that in addition to the movement formulae, there is a separate component of the action system, the "innervatory pattern system," which is thought to transform the movement representation into a motor plan. It has been posited that the movement formulae (the visual–kinesthetic engrams) are coded in a three-dimensional supramodal code (Heilman, Watson, & Rothi, 1989). These representations must be transcoded into an innervatory pattern that in turn is fed to the motor cortex. The supplementary motor area (SMA) has connections with the primary motor cortex and the parietal lobe (Jurgens, 1984). It is activated prior to motor cortex activation (Brinkman & Porter, 1979), and it becomes activated during the performance of learned, skilled movements (Roland, Larsen, Lassen, & Skinhoj, 1980). It therefore may be the site of the transcoding of the praxis representations into motor programs for execution by the motor cortex. Watson, Fleet, Rothi, and Heilman (1986) described several patients with SMA lesions who had bilateral apraxia but could comprehend and discriminate gestures. Thus a gesture production deficit in the absence of a gesture reception deficit may occur when the praxis representations can no longer interact with the innervatory patterns, or the innervatory patterns cannot gain access to the motor area (Figure 10.1, lesion B).

Input versus Output Praxicons

Differences in the ability of some patients to imitate gestures have called for further refinement of the model presented in Figure 10.1. The model in Figure 10.1 may appear to be sufficient to account for the gesture reception and production deficits of both hands in response to visual, tactual, or auditory–verbal input. However, Bell (1994) found that performance on tasks of pantomime recognition and imitation did not correlate in aphasic subjects, suggesting that these tasks may rely on separate processing mechanisms, which may be independently impaired with brain damage. In addition, there have been a few reported cases of patients whose imitation of limb movements was significantly worse than their production of these movements to verbal command, even though gesture comprehension was spared (Mehler, 1987; Ochipa, Rothi, & Heilman, 1994). To account for spared gesture comprehension in the context of impaired gesture imitation, the model shown in Figure 10.2 incorporates separate processing components for praxis input and output: the "input praxicon" and the "output praxicon." Thus spared gesture comprehension in the presence of impaired gesture imitation is accounted for by dysfunction at some point downstream from the input praxicon. The input praxicon allows one to recognize previously viewed gestures. The finding that pantomime to verbal command can be superior to pantomime imitation suggests that spoken language can access the output praxicon (allowing one to produce known gestures) without engaging the input praxicon. Gesture imitation worse than pantomime to verbal command can be accounted for by damage to the input praxicon. Alternatively, this pattern of impairment may imply more than one level of deficit, such as a problem at the level of the output praxicon as well as between the

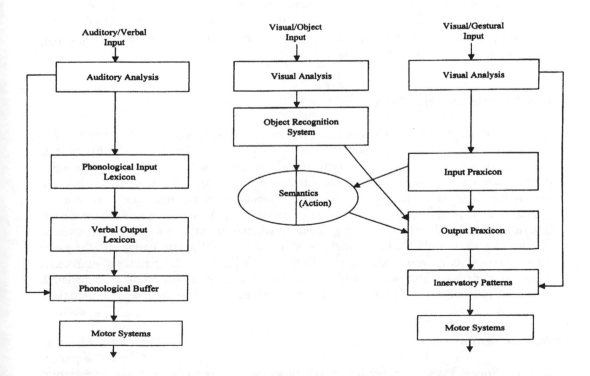

FIGURE 10.2. A model of praxis processing and its relationship to semantics and language.

input and output praxicons, resulting in relatively worse gesture imitation. Impairment in pantomiming to verbal command that is as severe as impairment of pantomime imitation suggests dysfunction at or beyond the output praxicon.

The Nonpraxical Route

In addition to a route that accesses the stored movement representations of the praxicon, there may be a route available for pantomime imitation that bypasses these stored representations. Rothi et al. (1986) reported patients who could imitate gestures they could not comprehend or discriminate. A parallel type of information processing is evident in language—in patients with transcortical sensory aphasia, who can repeat without comprehending spoken language. This has led some investigators (Coslett, Roeltgen, Rothi, & Heilman, 1987; McCarthy & Warrington, 1987) to suggest both a "lexical" route (which accesses stored word representations) and a "nonlexical" route for repetition. The model in Figure 10.2 depicts a corresponding "nonpraxical" route for action processing, wherein the innervatory patterns may be accessed directly from analysis of visual input, bypassing the praxicon. That such a route exists is supported by the ability of normal subjects to imitate meaningless gestures, which by definition have no movement memories to address. The selective impairment of this nonpraxical route was suggested by Mehler (1987), whose patients had deficits of imitation limited to unfamiliar movements. Additional evidence that this route may be selectively impaired has been provided by Goldenberg and Hagmann (1977); these authors described two patients with damage of the left angular gyrus who demonstrated impaired imitation of meaningless gestures but spared production of meaningful gestures on verbal command and in imitation. We (Rothi et al., 1991) have suggested that the selective sparing of this nonpraxical action route may account for the finding that some patients with apraxia have superior gestural imitation ability, compared to their ability to produce gestures to verbal command.

Input Modality Selectivity

A number of cases provide evidence that there may be fractionations of performance, depending upon the sensory modality of the input to the praxicons. Rothi et al. (1986) reported two patients who were able to gesture to verbal command but could not comprehend or discriminate visually presented gestures (pantomime agnosia). The left occipito-temporal lesions in these cases may have prevented visual information from gaining access to the input praxicon, or may have damaged the input praxicon itself. Many other investigators have described differential performance, depending on whether the stimulus was verbal or visual (Coslett & Saffran, 1989; De Renzi, Faglioni, & Sorgato, 1982; Kaplan, Verfaellie, & Caplan, 1990; Raymer, Greenwald, Richardson, Rothi, & Heilman, 1992). Failure of gesture to somesthetic input has also been described (De Renzi et al., 1982). The model in Figure 10.2 allows for possible fractionations of gestural performance based on input sensory modality.

Action Semantics

Roy and Square (1985) suggest that praxis processing is mediated by a two-part system involving both conceptual and production components. Thus far, this chapter has dealt with what Roy and Square would call the production component of action processing—the sensory–motor component of action knowledge, including the information contained in action programs and the translation of the programs into action. The errors generated by disruption of the production component are usually spatial or temporal in nature. A disruption of the production component of praxis processing corresponds to what Liepmann called "ideomotor apraxia."

According to Roy and Square (1985), the praxis conceptual system involves three kinds of knowledge: knowledge of the functions of tools and objects, knowledge of action independent of tools, and knowledge about the organization of single actions into sequences. Failure of the praxis conceptual system should result in content errors in gesture production (such as gesturing a hammering motion for a spoon), as opposed to the spatial and temporal errors seen in ideomotor apraxia. In addition, a disruption of the praxis conceptual system may result in the failure to recognize the mechanical advantages afforded by tools, or the misselection of tools for particular applications (Ochipa et al., 1989).

Liepmann (1905/1980) described a patient who used a razor as a comb and who put glasses on his outstretched tongue. Liepmann felt that this behavior reflected difficulty in the ideation of tool use and termed this "ideational apraxia." The term "ideational apraxia" has since been used in two ways: as a term for impairment in the sequencing of tool use (Poeck, 1983), and as a term for the failure to use single tools appropriately (De Renzi, Pieczuro, & Vignolo, 1968). To avoid confusion arising from these multiple uses, we employ the term "conceptual apraxia" to refer to the behaviors arising from impairment of the praxis conceptual system—that is, failure to use single tools appropriately (Ochipa, Rothi, & Heilman, 1992).

We (Ochipa et al., 1989) reported a patient whose behavior suggested impairment of the praxis conceptual system. This man, who was left-handed and had had a right-hemisphere stroke, was noted to use objects inappropriately. For instance, he was observed to eat with a toothbrush and brush his teeth with a comb. He was not agnosic, as he could name these tools and point to them on verbal command. However, he could not identify tools when their function was described, nor could he verbally describe tool function. His deficit could not be attributed to language comprehension difficulties, as he could follow commands that did not involve tool function. His inability to use tools appropriately could not be solely accounted for by a production deficit (severe ideomotor apraxia), because he could not even match tools with the objects on which they are used. His impairment was felt to be in the appreciation of the functional relationship between tools and the objects they act upon. Thus his inability to use tools suggested an impairment of the conceptual praxis system, represented in Figure 10.2 as "action semantics." Conceptual apraxia has also been described following focal, unilateral left-hemisphere lesions (Heilman, Maher, Greenwald, & Rothi, 1995), although it is most commonly associated with diffuse disease (Ochipa et al., 1992).

The model in Figure 10.2 draws a distinction between action semantics and other forms of conceptual knowledge. The existence of multiple semantic systems has been proposed to account for the behavior of patients with optic aphasia. These individuals can gesture the function of viewed tools that they are unable to name, suggesting a fractionation of action and verbal semantics, with differential impairment of verbal semantics (Beauvois & Saillant, 1985; Shallice, 1987). We (Ochipa et al., 1992) and Raymer (1992), in studies of groups of patients with Alzheimer's disease, found support for the notion of an action semantic system that is at some level dissociable from other forms of semantic knowledge. In a study of 24 subjects with Alzheimer's disease (Ochipa et al., 1992), some subjects were found to have preserved lexical–semantic abilities in a word comprehension task, but impaired performance on tasks of action knowledge and tool function.

Raymer, Rothi, and Heilman (1995) found that some patients with Alzheimer's disease were able to gesture tool use and name tools when these tools were visually presented, but were unable to gesture tool use or name tools when tool functions were verbally described. Acting from verbal description is thought to require access to semantics. This finding suggested that gesture may be made possible in such cases by accessing nonsemantic information about tools (such as perceptual attributes or stored structural knowledge). Thus the model of praxis processing (Figure 10.2) indicates a direct connection between the object recognition system (housing stored structural information about objects and tools) and the output praxicon. (See Raymer & Rothi, Chapter 5, this volume, for a further discussion of the potential fractionations of the semantic system.)

CLINICAL IMPLICATIONS

What are the clinical implications of a cognitive-neuropsychological model of praxis processing? A theoretical discussion of the mechanisms underlying limb apraxia may not directly inform the rehabilitation of apraxic patients. However, an understanding of the cerebral processes underlying limb praxis may help the clinician discern the underlying basis for a given patient's deficit. The ability to identify deficits at specific levels of processing should in turn lead to the development of intervention strategies that are specific to the deficit.

Assessing Limb Praxis

There are few standardized tests commercially available for the assessment of limb apraxia (see Helm-Estabrooks, 1992, for one exception). None are available that test limb apraxia in a manner suitable for detecting all of the possible behavioral fractionations that may occur. This section reviews some of the assessment techniques that have been used in our clinical practice and research with neurologically impaired adults (Rothi et al., 1992). For a more comprehensive review of limb praxis assessment, the reader is referred to Rothi, Raymer, and Heilman (1997), or to De Renzi (1985) for another view.

By analyzing patient performance across tasks that contrast praxis input, praxis output, and praxis semantic processing demands, we generate converging evidence to support hypotheses about the cognitive mechanisms underlying praxis impairment in a given patient. We draw all stimuli from a single corpus so that comparisons across tasks can be made. When possible, we test the dominant hand. Because hemiparesis tends to preclude this, the nondominant, ipsilesional hand is often tested.

We have found that both our normal and apraxic subjects often produce pantomimes that lack sufficient precision and elaboration. For this reason, we have found it helpful to spend time beforehand instructing subjects to produce the gesture as one would while actually holding the imagined tool (e.g., a hammer). We also ask subjects to imagine the object (e.g., a nail) they are acting upon.

Videotaping responses for later scoring is recommended, as praxis performance by nature is dynamic and difficult to score on-line. We use the scoring system described by Rothi and colleagues (Rothi, Mack, Verfaellie, Brown, & Heilman, 1988; Rothi et al., 1997), which is based on a system used by Klima and Bellugi (1979) in their research with deaf signers using American Sign Language. See Table 10.1 for error type definitions.

TABLE 10.1. Praxis Error Types

I. Content

P = Perseverative—a response that includes all or part of a previously produced pantomime.

R = Related—an accurately produced pantomime semantically associated with the target, such as pantomiming playing a trombone for the target bugle.

N = Nonrelated—an accurately performed pantomime not associated in content with the target, such as pantomiming playing a trombone for using a razor.

H = Hand error—the subject performs the action without benefit of a real or imagined tool. For example, when asked to cut a piece of paper with scissors, the subject pretends to rip the paper.

II. Temporal

S = Sequencing—any perturbation of the characteristic sequence of movements in a gesture, including addition, deletion, or transposition of elements, as long as the overall movement structure remains recognizable.

T = Timing—any alteration from the typical timing or speed of a pantomime, including increased, decreased, or irregular rate of production.

O = Occurrence—any multiplication of single cycles or reduction of a characteristically repetitive cycle to a single event.

III. Spatial

A = Amplitude—any amplification, reduction, or irregularity of the characteristic amplitude of a target pantomime.

IC = Internal configuration—any abnormality of the required finger/hand posture and its relationship to the target tool.

BPT = Body part as tool—the subject uses his or her finger, hand, or arm as the imagined tool of the pantomime.

EC = External configuration—errors in orienting the gesture to the imagined object receiving the tool's action.

M = Movement—any disturbance of the characteristic movement associated with the pantomime.

C = Concretization—the subject performs a transitive pantomime not on an imagined object, but instead on a real object not normally used in the task. For example, when asked to pretend to saw some wood, the subject pantomimes sawing on his or her leg.

IV. Other

NR = No response.

UR = Unrecognizable response.

Note. Adapted from Rothi, L. J. G., Mack, L., Ver Faillie, M., Brown, P., & Heilman, K. M. (1988). Ideomotor apraxia: Error pattern analysis. *Aphasiology, 2,* 381–388. Copyright 1988. Adapted with permission.

We use at least two judges and arrive at a consensus score. We have found that novice judges tend to accept errors of movement that do not obscure a gesture's meaning. That is, as long as the gesture is recognizable, a novice judge may score it as correct. Clinicians are discouraged from using "content recognizability" as a criterion for correct gestural production, because even very aberrant gestures may still be decipherable.

The influence of a language disorder on performance during praxis assessment must be considered. Many apraxic individuals are also aphasic, making it difficult to distinguish an apraxic disorder from a language disorder. If a patient performs poorly when given a limb command, but can adequately answer yes–no questions or can adequately describe the task he or she was asked to perform, impaired gestural performance is likely to be due to apraxia and not to impaired comprehension (Heilman & Rothi, 1993). Flexibility in evaluating verbal responses may be required (such as accepting paraphasia or circumlocution). The use of an alternative response mode may be necessary in some cases. For example, in a gesture comprehension task, if expressive language ability is impaired, the patient may be permitted to select the correct tool from an array of choices.

Assessing Gesture Reception

Measures of gesture reception are designed to assess the integrity of praxis mechanisms involved in processing viewed gestures, including the input praxicon, action semantics, and the connection between these components of praxis processing (Rothi et al., 1997). In our studies we use videotaped gestures and present them on a monitor for viewing. Two tasks are gesture naming and gesture recognition. For gesture naming, subjects are asked to name the action or tool corresponding to a viewed pantomime. Gesture recognition requires the subject to view a series of three gestures (one is the target and two are foils) and to select the gesture that matches a target tool named by the examiner.

Assessing Gesture Production

Measures of gesture production are designed to assess the praxis processing mechanisms involved in producing familiar gestures, including the semantic system (or action semantics), the output praxicon, and the connections between these components of praxis processing (Rothi et al., 1997). Testing different input modalities (gesture to verbal command, gesture to visually presented tools, gesture to tactually presented tools) can reveal whether deficits are related to sensory-specific input processing mechanisms. To assess pantomime to verbal command, we use a 30 item task with stimulus items that can be performed using only one hand (see Table 10.2). The items include 20 transitive gestures involving tool use (e.g., "Show me how to use a hammer . . .") and 10 intransitive gestures not involving tool use (e.g., "Show me how you salute"). Gesture to visual and tactual presentation of tools can then be performed for the transitive items. Gesture to visual presentation of tools is performed by showing the subject a tool and asking, "Show me how you use this." Gesture to tactual presentation of tools is performed with the subject's eyes covered. The subject inspects the tool by hand while the examiner says, "Show me how you use this tool." The tool is removed prior to performance. All gesture production tasks are videotaped and scored using the system of error types listed in Table 10.1.

Assessing Gesture Imitation

Tasks of gesture imitation are designed to assess the praxicon and nonpraxical routes for imitating gestural movements. One gesture imitation task requires the subject to imitate familiar gestures viewed on videotape. The examiner says, "I will produce a gesture and I want you to do it the same way I do it. Don't name the gesture, and don't produce your gesture until I am finished." This task may be processed by either the praxicon or nonpraxical routes. Another gesture imitation task, nonsense gesture imitation, presumably can only be performed with an intact nonpraxical route. Here the subject imitates nonfamiliar, nonsense

TABLE 10.2. Stimuli Used in the Florida Apraxia Screening Test—Revised

Show me:
 1. how you salute
 2. how to use scissors to cut a piece of paper out in front of you
 3. how to use a saw to cut a piece of wood out in front of you
 4. how you hitchhike
 5. how to use a bottle opener to remove a cap on a bottle out in front of you
 6. how to use wire cutters to snip a wire out in front of you
 7. stop
 8. how to use a salt shaker to salt food on a table out in front of you
 9. go away
10. how to use a glass to drink water
11. how to use a spoon to stir coffee on a table out in front of you
12. how to wave goodbye
13. how to use a hammer to pound a nail into a wall in front of you
14. how to use a comb to fix your hair
15. how to use a knife to carve a turkey on a table in front of you
16. how to use a brush to paint a wall out in front of you
17. come here
18. how to use a screwdriver to turn a screw into a wall out in front of you
19. how to use a pencil to write on a paper on a table out in front of you
20. someone is crazy
21. how to use a key to unlock a doorknob on a door out in front of you
22. be quiet
23. how to use an iron to press a shirt out in front of you
24. how to use a razor to shave your face
25. OK
26. how to use an eraser to clean a chalkboard out in front of you
27. how to use a vegetable peeler to shred a carrot
28. how to make a fist
29. how to use an ice pick to chop ice out in front of you
30. how to use a scoop to serve ice cream

Note. From Rothi, L. J. G., Raymer, A. M., Ochipa, C., Maher, L. M., Greenwald, M. L., & Heilman, K. M. (1992).

gestures. Responses are scored using the coding system (Rothi et al., 1988, 1997) as it applies to inaccuracies in the temporal and spatial dimensions of the target movement.

Assessing Action Semantics

Performance patterns during tasks of gesture reception and gesture production may provide converging evidence for a deficit in action semantics. For example, a subject who produces errors in the content of the gesture (such as pantomiming a hammering movement for a spoon) may have a deficit of the praxis conceptual system. In addition, we have found a tool selection task to be sensitive to deficits of action semantics. In this task, the subject views a partially completed task (such as a screw partially driven into a piece of wood). The subject must choose, from an array of three tool choices, which tool would complete the task. The response is scored as correct if the subject points to the appropriate tool.

Observation of Praxis in the Natural Environment

It has long been believed that apraxia has little impact on a patient's functional independence; however, recent studies suggest otherwise (Foundas et al., 1995; Ochipa et al., 1989;
Schwartz et al., 1995). Therefore, the clinician may want to observe tool use in natural
settings. Often during the acute phase of recovery and rehabilitation of stroke patients,
activities of daily living are structured and monitored, thereby limiting opportunities to
detect difficulties with tool and object selection and use. Foundas et al. (1995) conducted
a study involving the mealtime observation of hospitalized patients. Each patient was
videotaped while eating lunch from a standard hospital tray. In addition to the appropriate eating utensils, tool foils (including a toothbrush, comb, and pencil), were placed on
the tray. These investigators found that normal controls always exhibited a three-phase
meal infrastructure: preparation, eating, and cleanup. Apraxic subjects showed a disorga-
nization of this meal structure, inaccurate selection of utensils, and inefficient and inaccurate action sequencing. Apraxic subjects also used fewer tools and produced fewer tool
actions than the control group. Some patients, such as the man previously described (Ochipa
et al., 1989) who used a toothbrush to eat and a comb to brush his teeth, present serious
safety concerns, as the inability to select appropriate tools for tasks may lead to accidents
(e.g., the selection of a razor for brushing teeth can cause serious injury).

Recovery in Limb Apraxia

Relatively little is known about the pattern and extent of recovery in limb apraxia. Some
investigators have reported that patients with this deficit recover spontaneously (Basso et al.,
1987). Recent studies, however, indicate that although some aspects of limb praxis improve over time, other aspects of the disorder persist (Foundas, Raymer, Maher, Rothi, &
Heilman, 1993; Maher, Raymer, Foundas, Rothi, & Heilman, 1994). Maher et al. (1994),
in a study of the evolution of limb apraxia over a 6-month period, found different patterns
of recovery for intransitive and transitive gestures. For intransitive gestures, there was a
decrease over time in the number of content errors (in which the meaning representations
of gestures were incorrect). For transitive gestures, there was a decrease over time in the
number of perseverations, unrecognizable responses, and failures to respond. For both
transitive and intransitive gestures, spatial and temporal errors persisted. These results
suggest that recovery in limb apraxia may involve improvements in the recognizability of
gestures, while the spatial and temporal aspects of the gesture may remain inaccurate.

Management and Treatment of Limb Apraxia

Very little has been written about the management or treatment of limb apraxia. One reason why the rehabilitation of limb praxis has not been well studied may be many clinicians' belief that this disorder is only apparent in the artificial context of the clinical
examination of pantomime. Because apraxic patients may improve with actual tool use,
apraxia is generally believed to have a negligible impact on daily life. However, McDonald,
Tate, and Rigby (1994) found that of 17 subjects with apraxia, all but two subjects made
the same types of errors in actual tool use as they did in pantomime tasks. A study by Sundet
et al. (1988) evaluated the dependency of right- and left-hemisphere stroke patients on
caregiver assistance in activities of daily living 6 months after stroke. They found that

patients with limb apraxia required more assistance with tasks of daily living than patients with other neuropsychological deficits did. These studies suggest that limb apraxia may have a greater impact on functional activities than previously believed.

Another area in which limb apraxia may have particular clinical relevance is the treatment of aphasic individuals. Gesture is often used as a facilitator of spoken output (Hanlon, Brown, & Gerstman, 1990; Kearns, Simmons, & Sisterhen, 1982), or as an alternative or augmentative communication system for aphasic adults (Kirshner & Webb, 1981). Specifically, Amer-Ind gesture training (Skelly, 1979) is commonly used in aphasia therapy with individuals who have difficulty producing adequate verbal output. Helm-Estabrooks, Fitzpatrick and Barresi (1982) promote the use of pantomime training to circumvent the language deficits of patients with severe aphasia. They consider their visual action therapy for globally aphasic patients a treatment approach for limb apraxia.

Although severely apraxic patients may be able to learn gestures, the presence of limb apraxia has been reported to adversely affect the quality of communicative gestures (Feyereisen, Barter, Goossens, & Clerebaut, 1988) and the ease of communicative gesture acquisition (Rothi & Heilman, 1984). In addition, the presence of limb apraxia may partially account for the findings of gestural training studies reporting poor generalization of learned gestures to other communicative contexts, and little generalization of gestural improvement to gestures not specifically targeted in treatment (Coelho, 1990; Ochipa, Maher, & Rothi, 1995; Pilgrim & Humphreys, 1994). Because limb apraxia may negatively affect the acquisition and use of gestures by aphasic individuals, and may have a negative impact on their activities of daily living, it seems important to consider the rehabilitation of this deficit.

The clinician wishing to treat limb apraxia has two options: management of the functional impairment and direct treatment of the deficit (Rothi, 1995). Management of limb apraxia involves altering the environment so that the negative impact of the apraxia on activities of daily living is minimized, and the risk of injury is eliminated (Maher & Ochipa, 1997). This may include removing dangerous implements from the patient's access, limiting the tools available for a particular task, avoiding tasks involving tool use in novel contexts, and avoiding tasks involving the use of multiple tools.

Few studies have reported the direct treatment of apraxic deficits (Maher, Rothi, & Greenwald, 1991; Ochipa, Maher, & Rothi, 1995; Pilgrim & Humphreys, 1994). We (Ochipa et al., 1995) describe the direct treatment of apraxia in a study in which we attempted to eliminate three error types made by two subjects: internal configuration errors, external configuration errors, and movement errors (see Table 10.1). The subjects were systematically trained (one error type at a time was targeted) in the appropriate hand posture, the appropriate orientation in space, and the appropriate joint movements for selected gestures. Both subjects showed considerable improvement in producing the trained gestures; that is, the occurrence of a particular error type decreased to criterion when specifically addressed in treatment. However, the observed effects were treatment-specific: The frequency of a given error type did not decline to criterion until it was targeted in treatment. In addition, treating one error type did not lead to improvement of any other error type, and generalization to untreated gestures did not occur. Pilgrim and Humphreys (1994) also found a lack of generalization in a study in which they used a modified form of "conductive education," which consisted of "a task analysis of the movements involved in using common objects, and verbalized articulation of the goal directed task" (p. 280). The lack of generalization noted in these studies of apraxia treatment suggests that gestures chosen for training should be carefully selected for their functional value to the patient.

More studies are needed to determine whether limb apraxia is amenable to treatment and, if so, which treatment approaches are most efficacious. Rothi (1995) conceptualizes treatment approaches as being either "restitutive" or "substitutive" in nature. Restitutive treatments aim to address the underlying deficit and encourage maximal return of function by reconstructing the impaired deficit in the manner that the function was performed premorbidly. In contrast, substitutive treatments aim to achieve the behavioral goal in a new way. One type of substitutive approach, "vicariation," attempts to facilitate functional reorganization by having unimpaired functions support the performance of impaired functions. Rothi (1995) suggests that both restitutive and substitutive approaches may be appropriate in the acute phases of recovery when the brain is capable of physiological recovery, while substitutive approaches alone may be most appropriate later.

If one wishes to "reconstruct" an impaired gestural representation, a restitutive approach designed to address the visual/iconic aspects of target gestures may be appropriate. For example, such a treatment may require an apraxic patient to image or view accurate gestural performance prior to production, or to distinguish poorly performed and well-performed viewed gestures. Another restitutive treatment may target the kinesthetic/motor aspects of gestures. For example, the clinician can correct flawed gestural responses by providing "hands-on" physical prompts to the apraxic patient. Feedback in the form of physical manipulation of the limb to adjust for spatial or movement errors, and practice in performing the gesture after correcting for errors, may result in a "reconstructed" gestural representation. Alternatively, a vicariative approach, such as a verbally mediated task analysis and verbal description of the movements involved in the use of common tools, may also facilitate improved gestural performance. The choice of treatment approach, restitutive or vicariative, may depend upon whether the clinician decides to recruit intact praxis processing abilities to support the impaired function, or to restore the integrity of the impaired function directly.

Theoretically, a model-driven analysis of an individual's praxis performance may identify those components of the process that need to be reconstructed, modified, or circumvented to improve performance. For instance, if a patient's errors are thought to stem from underspecified semantic representations, treatment may be directed toward teaching specific features of action and tool function that distinguish related tool items. Alternatively, teaching the patient to analyze the structural and perceptual attributes of tools (e.g., scissors' blades open and close; the flat, heavy end of a hammer may be good for pounding), and relating that information to the action goal, may help to support disturbed action semantic processing.

If poor gesture reception suggests an impairment of the input praxicon, attempts to improve gestural production may be better supported by verbal cueing than by the visual cues presented in a gestural imitation task. Alternatively, if assessment reveals relative sparing of the nonlexical route for praxis processing, imitating viewed gestures and perhaps breaking gestures down into their constituent parts may be more appropriate strategies to employ in treatment. Both of these approaches are considered vicariative in nature, whereas a treatment approach that attempts to reconstruct the representations for gesture in both the input and output praxicons is a restitutive approach to treating impaired gestural performance.

Clearly, this is not an exhaustive list of the possible treatment approaches for limb apraxia. Although the application of a cognitive-neuropsychological model to the assessment and treatment of limb apraxia seems to have theoretical appeal, the efficacy of treatments based on this approach has not been established. Furthermore, little is known about how this approach may compare to a more functional, pragmatic treatment approach applied in the natural environment. Answers to these questions await further study.

REFERENCES

Basso, A., Capitani, E., Sala, S. D., Laiacona, M., & Spinnler, H. (1987). Recovery from ideomotor apraxia. *Brain, 110,* 747–760.

Beauvois, M. F., & Saillant, B. (1985). Optic aphasia for colours and colour agnosia: A distinction between visual and visuo-verbal impairments in the processing of colours. *Cognitive Neuropsychology, 2,* 1–48.

Bell, B. D. (1994). Pantomime recognition impairment in aphasia:An analysis of error types. *Brain and Language, 47,* 269–278.

Boldrini, P., Zanella, R., Cantagallo, A., & Basaglia, N. (1992). Partial hemispheric disconnection syndrome of traumatic origin. *Cortex, 28,* 135–143.

Brinkman, C., & Porter, R. (1979). Supplementary motor areas in the monkey: Activity of neurons during performance of a learned motor task. *Journal of Neurophysiology, 42,* 681–709.

Coelho, C. A. (1990). Acquisition and generalization of simple manual sign grammars by aphasic subjects. *Journal of Communication Disorders, 23,* 383–400.

Coslett, H. B., Roeltgen, D. P., Rothi, L. J. G., & Heilman, K. M. (1987). Transcortical sensory aphasia: Evidence forsubtypes. *Brain and Language, 32,* 362–378.

Coslett, H. B., & Saffran, E. M. (1989). Preserved object recognition and reading comprehension in optic aphasia. *Brain, 112,* 1091–1110.

De Renzi, E. (1985). Methods of limb apraxia examination and their bearing on the interpretation of the disorder. In E. A. Roy (Ed.), *Neuropsychological studies of apraxia and related disorders* (pp. 45–64). Amsterdam: Elsevier.

De Renzi, E., Faglioni, P., & Sorgato, P. (1982). Modality specific and supramodal mechanisms of apraxia. *Brain, 101,* 301–312.

De Renzi, E., Pieczuro, A., & Vignolo, L. A. (1968). Ideational apraxia: A quantitative study. *Neuropsychologia, 6,* 41–52.

Feyereisen, P., Barter, D., Goossens, M., & Clerebaut, N. (1988).Gesture and speech in referential communication by aphasic subjects: Channel use and efficiency. *Aphasiology, 2,* 21–32.

Foundas, A. L., Macauley, B. C., Raymer, A. M., Maher, L. M., Heilman, K. M., & Rothi, L. J. G. (1995). Ecological implications of limb apraxia: Evidence from mealtime behavior. *Journal of the International Neuropsychological Society, 1,* 62–66.

Foundas, A. L., Raymer, A. M., Maher, L. M., Rothi, L. J. G., & Heilman, K. M. (1993). Recovery in ideomotor apraxia. *Journal of Clinical and Experimental Neuropsychology, 15,* 44.

Geschwind, N. (1965). Disconnexion syndromes in animals and man: Parts I and II. *Brain, 88,* 237–294, 585–644.

Geschwind, N., & Kaplan, E. (1962). A human cerebral disconnection syndrome: A preliminary report. *Neurology, 12,* 675–685.

Goldenberg, G., & Hagmann, S. (1997). The meaning of meaningless gestures: A study of visuo-imitative apraxia. *Neuropsychologia, 35,* 333–341.

Hanlon, R. E., Brown, J. W., & Gerstman, L. J. (1990). Enhancement of naming in nonfluent aphasia through gesture. *Brain and Language, 38,* 298–314.

Heilman, K. M., Maher, L. M., Greenwald, M. L., & Rothi, L. J. G. (1995). Conceptual apraxia from lateralized lesions [Abstract]. *Neurology, 45,* A266.

Heilman, K. M., & Rothi, L. J. G. (1993). Apraxia. In K. M. Heilman & E. Valenstein (Eds.), *Clinical neuropsychology* (3rd ed., pp. 141–163). New York: Oxford University Press.

Heilman, K. M., Rothi, L. J. G., & Valenstein, E. (1982). Two forms of ideomotor apraxia. *Neurology, 32,* 342–346.

Heilman, K. M., Watson, R. T., & Rothi, L. J. G. (1989). Limb apraxia. *Current Neurology, 9,* 179–190.

Helm-Estabrooks, N. (1992). *Test of Oral and Limb Apraxia.* Chicago: Applied Symbolix.

Helm-Estabrooks, N., Fitzpatrick, P., & Barresi, B. (1982).Visual action therapy for global aphasia. *Journal of Speech and Hearing Disorders, 44,* 385–389.

Jurgens, U. (1984). The efferent and afferent connections of the supplementary motor area. *Brain Research, 300,* 63–81.

Kaplan, R. F., Verfaellie, M., & Caplan, L.R. (1990). Visual anomia and visual apraxia in a patient with a left occipital brain lesion. *Journal of Clinical and Experimental Neuropsychology, 12,* 89.

Kearns, K. P., Simmons, N. N., & Sisterhen, C. (1982). Gestural sign (Amer-Ind) as a facilitator of verbalization in patients with aphasia. In R. Brookshire (Ed.), *Clinical Aphasiology Conference proceedings* (Vol. 12, pp. 183–191). Minneapolis, MN: BRK.

Kirshner, H. S., & Webb, W. G. (1981). Selective involvement of the auditory–verbal modality in an acquired communication disorder: Benefit from sign language therapy. *Brain and Language, 13,* 161–170.

Klima, E., & Bellugi, U. (1979). *The signs of language.* Cambridge, MA: Harvard University Press.

Liepmann, H. (1977). The syndrome of apraxia (motor asymboly)based on a case of unilateral apraxia. In D. A. Rottenburg & F. H. Hochberg (Eds. and Trans.), *Neurological classics in modern translation* (pp. 155–182). New York: Macmillan. (Original work published 1900)

Liepmann, H. (1980). The left hemisphere and action. In *Translations from Liepmann's essays on apraxia* (Research Bulletin No. 506). London, Ontario, Canada: Department of Psychology, University of Western Ontario. (Original work published 1905)

Liepmann, H. (1988). Apraxia. In J. W. Brown (Ed. and Trans.), *Agnosia and apraxia: Selected papers of Liepmann, Lange and Potzl* (pp. 3–39). Hillsdale, NJ: Erlbaum. (Original work published 1920)

Liepmann, H., & Maas, O. (1907). Fall von linksseitger agraphie und apraxie bei rechtsseitiger lahmung. *Journal für Psychologie und Neurologie, 10,* 214–227.

Maher, L. M., & Ochipa, C. (1997). The management and treatment of limb apraxia. In L. J. G. Rothi & K. M. Heilman (Eds.), *Apraxia: The cognitive neuropsychology of action.* Hove, England: Psychology Press.

Maher, L. M., Raymer, A. M., Foundas, A. L., Rothi, L. J. G., & Heilman, K. M. (1994). *Patterns of recovery in ideomotor apraxia.* Paper presented at the annual meeting of the International Neuropsychological Society, Cincinnati, OH.

Maher, L. M., Rothi, L. J. G., & Greenwald, M. L. (1991).Treatment of gesture impairment: A single case. *ASHA, 33,* 195.

McCarthy, R. A., & Warrington, E. K. (1987). The double dissociation of short-term memory for lists and sentences. *Brain, 110,* 1545–1563.

McDonald, S., Tate, R. C., & Rigby, J. (1994). Error types in ideomotor apraxia: A qualitative analysis. *Brain and Cognition, 25,* 250–270.

Mehler, M. F. (1987). Visuo-imitative apraxia. *Neurology, 37,* 129.

Ochipa, C., Maher, L. M., & Rothi, L. J. G. (1995). Treatment of ideomotor apraxia. *Journal of the International Neuropsychological Society, 2,* 149.

Ochipa, C., Rothi, L. J. G., & Heilman, K. M. (1989). Ideational apraxia: A deficit in tool selection and use. *Annals of Neurology, 25,* 190–193.

Ochipa, C., Rothi, L. J. G., & Heilman, K. M. (1992). Conceptual apraxia in Alzheimer's disease. *Brain, 115,* 1061–1071.

Ochipa, C., Rothi, L. J. G., & Heilman, K. M. (1994). Conductionapraxia. *Journal of Neurology, Neurosurgery and Psychiatry, 57,* 1241–1244.

Pilgrim, E., & Humphreys, G. W. (1994). Rehabilitation of a case of ideomotor apraxia. In M. J. Riddoch & G. W. Humphreys (Eds.), *Cognitive neuropsychology and cognitive rehabilitation* (pp. 271–285). Hillsdale, NJ: Erlbaum.

Poeck, K. (1983). Ideational apraxia. *Journal of Neurology, 230,* 1–5.

Poeck, K. (1985). Clues to the nature of disruptions to limbpraxis. In E. A. Roy (Ed.), *Neuropsychological studies of apraxia and related disorders* (pp. 99–109). Amsterdam: Elsevier.

Raymer, A. M. (1992). *Dissociations of semantic knowledge: Evidence from Alzheimer's disease.* Unpublished doctoral dissertation, University of Florida.

Raymer, A. M., Greenwald, M. L., Richardson, M. E., Rothi, L. J. G., & Heilman, K. M. (1992). Optic aphasia and optic apraxia: Theoretical interpretations. *Journal of Clinical and Experimental Neuropsychology, 14,* 396.

Raymer, A. M., Rothi, L. J. G., & Heilman, K. M. (1995).Nonsemantic activation of lexical and praxis output systems in Alzheimer's subjects. *Journal of the International Neuropsychological Society, 1,* 147.

Roland, P. E., Larsen, B., Lassen, N. A., & Skinhoj, E. (1980). Supplementary motor area and other cortical areas inorganization of voluntary movements in man. *Journal of Neurophysiology, 43*(1), 118–136.

Rothi, L. J. G. (1995). Behavioral compensation in the case of treatment of acquired language disorders resulting from brain damage. In R. A. Dixon & L. Backman (Eds.), *Psychological compensation: Managing losses and promoting gains* (pp. 219–230). Hillsdale, NJ: Erlbaum.

Rothi, L. J. G., & Heilman, K. M. (1984). Acquisition and retention of gestures by apraxic patients. *Brain and Cognition, 3,* 426–437.

Rothi, L. J. G., Heilman, K. M., & Watson, R. T. (1985). Pantomime comprehension and ideomotor apraxia. *Journal of Neurology, Neurosurgery and Psychiatry, 48*, 207–210.

Rothi, L. J. G., Mack, L., & Heilman, K. M. (1986). Pantomime agnosia. *Journal of Neurology, Neurosurgery and Psychiatry, 49*, 451–454.

Rothi, L. J. G., Mack, L., Verfaellie, M., Brown, P., & Heilman, K. M. (1988). Ideomotor apraxia: Error pattern analysis. *Aphasiology, 2*, 381–388.

Rothi, L. J. G., Ochipa, C., & Heilman, K. M. (1991). A cognitiveneuropsychological model of limb praxis. *Cognitive Neuropsychology, 8*, 443–458.

Rothi, L. J. G., Raymer, A. M., & Heilman, K. M. (1997). Praxis assessment. In L. J. G. Rothi & K. M. Heilman (Eds.), *Apraxia: The cognitive neuropsychology of action*. Hove, England: Psychology Press.

Rothi, L. J. G., Raymer, A. M., Ochipa, C., Maher, L. M., Greenwald, M. L., & Heilman, K. M. (1992). *Florida apraxia battery: Experimental edition*. Gainesville: University of Florida, Department of Neurology.

Roy, E. A., & Square, P. A. (1985). Common considerations in the study of limb, verbal, and oral apraxia. In E.A. Roy (Ed.), *Neuropsychological studies of apraxia and related disorders* (pp. 111–161). Amsterdam: Elsevier.

Schwartz, M. F., Montgomery, M. W., Fitzpatrick-DeSalme, E. J., Ochipa, C., Coslett, H. B., & Mayer, N. H. (1995). Analysis of a disorder of everyday action. *Cognitive Neuropsychology, 12*(8), 863–892.

Schwartz, M. F., Reed, E. S., Montgomery, M. W., Palmer, C., & Mayer, N. H. (1991). The quantitative description of action disorganisation after brain damage: A case study. *Cognitive Neuropsychology, 8*, 381–414.

Shallice, T. (1987). Impairments of semantic processing: Multiple dissociations. In M. Coltheart, G. Sartori, & R. Job (Eds.), *The cognitive neuropsychology of language* (pp. 111–127). Hillsdale, NJ: Erlbaum.

Skelly, M. (1979). *Amer-Ind gestural code based on universal American Indian hand talk*. New York: Elsevier/North-Holland.

Sundet, K., Finset, A., & Reinvang, I. (1988). Neuropsychological predictors in stroke rehabilitation. *Journal of Clinical and Experimental Neuropsychology, 10*, 363–379.

Watson, R. T., Fleet, W. S., Rothi, L. J. G., & Heilman, K. M. (1986). Apraxia and the supplementary motor area. *Archives of Neurology, 43*, 787–792.

Watson, R. T., & Heilman, K. M. (1983). Callosal apraxia. *Brain, 106*, 391–403.

11

LANGUAGE USE

LEE XENAKIS BLONDER

The study of aphasic disorders has afforded neurolinguists an opportunity to examine both the cognitive and neuroanatomical representation of language. This large body of research has focused on the breakdown of phonology, morphology, syntax, and semantics in brain-damaged patients, and on what these syndromes reveal about the mechanisms that underlie language processing in neurologically intact individuals.

This emphasis on language form and structure and on the breakdown of each in individual aphasic patients has been the dominant focus of neurolinguistic research for the past century. Consistent with formal approaches in linguistics, these studies have focused on an individual in isolation, rather than on a speaker interacting with others. The methods typically used by those studying brain and language relations stress this concept of language as represented in the individual. In particular, neurolinguistic research has been heavily dominated by quantitative assessment methods favored in the psychological and clinical sciences. These standardized measures provide a structured and reproducible method of eliciting linguistic competencies. Aphasia batteries are designed to furnish detailed information on a patient's fluency, comprehension, repetition, naming, reading, and writing. Spontaneous speech is typically assessed by a picture elicitation task.

Within the last couple of decades, an interest in examining "discourse," or language at the suprasentential level, has permeated the field of aphasiology (see Joanette & Brownell, 1990). This shift in focus by a relatively small but growing number of researchers has been influenced by developments in several fields, including linguistics, psychology, sociology, anthropology, and philosophy. Emphasis on language use as opposed to language structure was introduced by the French linguist Ferdinand de Saussure, when he made the often-cited distinction between *langue*, the language system shared by speakers, and *parole*, the utterances produced by speakers in situations. This distinction foreshadowed Noam Chomsky's concepts of "linguistic competence" (the system of rules mastered by speakers that enables them to comprehend and generate an infinite number of sentences) and "linguistic performance" (the specific utterances produced by a speaker). Chomsky's interest lay largely in the realm of linguistic competence (see Searle, 1974, for further discussion). He sought to replace descriptive and structural linguistics and their preoccupation with the classification of formal properties of language with a theory that would identify the rules governing sentence generation. Yet the emphasis of the transformational linguists was on language structure, broadly defined, and the innate or "rational" properties of the individual mind that would make possible such phenomena. In a discussion of the historical antecedents to discourse analysis in linguistics, Patry and Nespoulous (1990, p. 3) describe the focus of Chomskyan linguists as follows: "These researchers are interested in the internal functioning of grammars seen as nearly closed systems, that is, as systems defined and discussed as largely independent of contingencies observed in everyday language use."

The emergence of the fields of sociolinguistics and the ethnography of speaking represents in part a reaction to the preoccupation with linguistic competence. This research is characterized by its concentration on what Dell Hymes (1972) has termed "communicative competence." Hymes has argued that Chomsky's concept of linguistic competence is too narrowly focused on grammatical knowledge. According to Hymes and others, linguists ought to consider the ability of speakers to use language in sociocultural context and the capacity of speakers to produce socially appropriate utterances.

Studies of language use constitute a substantial body of literature in the behavioral sciences. These include analyses of speech events, such as greetings, jokes, narratives, and ritual insults (Hymes, 1974; Labov, 1972), as well as of the organization of conversation (Sacks, Schlegloff, & Jefferson, 1974). Sociolinguists tend to use the "utterance" or "turn" as the unit of analysis. A "turn" is defined as one person's conversational discourse bounded by that of another. The methodology is both inductive and empirical in its focus on the analysis of spontaneous discourse.

The view of language as a socially embedded phenomenon that occurs within the context of interpersonal interaction has not yet fully penetrated neurobehavioral research. Although there are many studies of spontaneous speech in aphasic patients, there are few studies of the effects of aphasia on everyday language use. This is made apparent in the chapter on narrative and procedural discourse by Ulatowska, Allard, and Chapman (1990). They note that several types of discourse have been identified, including "narrative," "procedural," and "conversational." Narrative discourse is discourse that recounts past events and includes descriptions of a setting, an action, and a resolution. Procedural discourse describes the steps necessary to complete a task, or how something is done. Conversational discourse is talk produced in the context of an interchange between two or more people. To date, however, the majority of studies of aphasic patients' discourse have focused on the narrative and procedural varieties. This is a logical outgrowth of the prevalent paradigm in neurolinguistics, which is quantitative and concerned with cognitive processing within an individual. Assessment of spontaneous speech is often limited to a patient's response to a picture elicitation task. There now exist several published studies in which aphasic patients' discourse produced in the context of a communicative event is analyzed. In this chapter I review studies of discourse in aphasia, with an emphasis on those studies that have focused on aphasic patients' communication in the context of spontaneous social interaction.

PRAGMATICS AND APHASIA

The term "pragmatics" has had varying meanings in linguistics that have changed over time. It has been adopted by neurolinguists as a term that connotes a speaker's use of language and the effects of this use on conversational interactants. Several early studies of the effects of aphasia on conversation focused on repair strategies. In general, investigators found that aphasic patients are often able to use repairs appropriately following breakdowns in conversation (Lubinski, Duchan, & Weitzner-Lin, 1980; Newhoff, Tonkovich, Schwartz, & Burgess, 1982; Linebaugh, Marguiles, & Mackisack, 1985). According to

Ulatowska, Allard, Reyes, Ford, and Chapman (1992), these studies demonstrate that communicative competence is preserved in aphasia.

Following British linguist M. A. K. Halliday (1977), Guilford and O'Connor (1982) define language that satisfies a speaker's own needs as "pragmatic." They explored pragmatic, mathetic, and informative functions in elicited and nonelicited conversation and in response to picture presentation. "Mathetic" language consists of requests for names, language used to obtain details about the environment, and verbal recall. "Informative" language is that which relates experiences not shared by the listener. Halliday distinguishes these as Phase II functions in his research on child language acquisition. Phase II represents the transition from child to adult language and is characterized by learning to engage in dialogue and assuming adult social roles. Guilford and O'Connor's sample consisted of two patients with fluent aphasia and four patients with nonfluent aphasia, as determined by performance on the Boston Diagnostic Aphasia Examination (BDAE; Goodglass & Kaplan, 1972). Results showed that all six patients used pragmatic, mathetic, and informative functions in their speech, although there was intersubject variation in the proportion of responses in each category. Furthermore, regardless of aphasia severity, each patient produced all three speech functions, suggesting that each had retained Phase II pragmatic behaviors.

Bates, Hamby, and Zurif (1983) sought to determine whether aphasia is limited to disruptions in grammatical and lexical processing, or whether it also affects knowledge of the conditions necessary for an utterance to be understood. They chose to assess the sensitivity of aphasic patients to the topic–focus distinction, a component of pragmatic processing. The topic–focus distinction, expressed through a variety of grammatical devices, denotes the juxtapositions and linkages between the new information focus and the established topic of the discourse. Bates et al. (1983) asked five patients with Broca's aphasia and five patients with Wernicke's aphasia to describe what was happening in a three-frame set of pictures. Both groups of patients retained sensitivity to the topic–focus distinction, suggesting a possible dissociation between pragmatic aspects of language processing and syntax and semantics.

Meuse and Marquardt (1985) studied communicative effectiveness in patients with Broca's aphasia, as measured by a referential task and a conversation task. The referential task consisted of a real-objects task, a realistic-blocks task, a geometric-blocks task, and a novel-blocks task. Subjects were first required to name the objects (real-objects task) and the line drawings depicting plants, animals, or geometric forms (remaining tasks). Each participant was then required to function as both speaker and listener, describing and matching the objects and the various types of blocks. The conversation task consisted of conversational discussion of a series of vocational, social, and educational topics introduced by the examiner. The subjects were five patients with Broca's aphasia as determined by performance on the BDAE. They were studied 10 to 176 months after brain injury (stroke or trauma). Results indicated that the aphasic patients produced more grammatical and lexical errors on both referential and conversation tasks than did normal controls, although error frequencies were higher for the referential task. However, the aphasic patients compensated for these impairments by requesting information of the examiner, employing elimination strategies in lieu of direct naming, or using alternate forms of communication such as singing or spelling aloud. From these findings, the authors concluded that aphasic patients maintain communicative effectiveness in spite of documented impairments in linguistic competence.

This conclusion is supported by many investigations of aphasic discourse. In a study comparing interview transcripts of patients with fluent language disorders caused by stroke,

Alzheimer's disease (AD), and closed head injury, Glosser and Deser (1991) found a dissociation between microlinguistic capabilities (e.g., syntax and phonology) and macrolinguistic capabilities (e.g., thematic coherence). Patients with fluent aphasias caused by focal lesions (stroke) showed greater impairment in microlinguistic abilities, whereas patients with AD demonstrated preserved microlinguistic abilities but disturbed macrolinguistic abilities. Patients with closed head injury were impaired in both realms. These findings are consistent with other studies in both aphasic patients and subjects with AD. In particular, two studies (Ripich & Terrell, 1988; Blonder, Kort, & Schmitt, 1994) showed that the discourse produced by patients with AD lacked thematic coherence, even though it was fluent, syntactically normal speech. Glosser and Deser (1991) conclude that separate neural systems underlie the production of micro- and macrolinguistic abilities, and that the latter may be either more diffusely distributed or mediated by right-hemisphere structures.

Psycholinguistic models have been used to guide studies of pragmatic functions in aphasic speakers. Blanken, Dittman, Haas, and Wallesch (1987) studied spontaneous speech (produced during semistructured interviews) by patients with AD, patients with Wernicke's aphasia due to stroke, and normal controls. From previous work in psycholinguistics and neurolinguistics, these investigators proposed a model of language production that delineates three apparatuses. These include a pragmatic–conceptual apparatus that generates the conceptual structure of the speech act; a formulation apparatus that includes lexicalization, grammaticalization, and prearticulatory segmental processing; and an articulatory apparatus that is responsible for planning and executing articulatory movements. In this study, the authors proposed that the existence of separate pragmatic–conceptual and formulation apparatuses could be proven by demonstrating a double dissociation between respective impairments in patients with AD and patients with fluent aphasia. Each patient and control subject participated in a 10-minute interview during which an interviewer posed questions regarding personal data, biography, health, and family. The researchers then examined lexical and grammatical usage and response characteristics (e.g., fragmentary, vague, evasive, confabulated, etc.) in the transcribed interviews. Results indicated that both patients with AD and patients with Wernicke's aphasia produced sentences that were shorter and syntactically simpler than those of controls; however, when error patterns were examined more closely, the investigators found no evidence for morphosyntactic disturbances (i.e., formulation deficits) in patients with AD. Furthermore, the word-finding difficulties of the patients with AD were less pervasive than those of the patients with Wernicke's aphasia, who tended to give up in searching for a word. Both patient groups exhibited deficits in responding behavior. Patients with AD tended to confabulate, while patients with Wernicke's aphasia gave fragmentary responses due to word-finding difficulties. The authors concluded that the pragmatic–conceptual apparatus is disturbed in patients with AD, whereas their language formulation abilities remain relatively intact. In contrast, patients with Wernicke's aphasia primarily demonstrate pathology in the realm of language formulation.

In a study of discourse in aphasia using concepts derived from conversation analysis, Ulatowska et al. (1992) videotaped conversations between patients with aphasia (four had nonfluent and one had fluent aphasia) and either an aphasic or a nonaphasic partner. The investigators examined word production, speech rate, turn taking, speech act production (e.g., requesting, asserting, evaluating, committing, greeting), and script knowledge. They found that aphasic patients produced fewer words and less complex language than normal subjects, but that the distributions of "substantive" turns (turns that add new information), "management" turns (turns that keep the conversation going), and speech acts (assertions, evaluations, and requests) were comparable. Again, these results suggest that conversational structure is preserved in aphasia despite the presence of sentence-level deficits.

My colleagues and I (Blonder, Burns, Bowers, Moore, & Heilman, 1993) performed a series of semistructured videotaped interviews with seven aphasic patients who had left-hemisphere damage (LHD), seven patients who had right-hemisphere damage (RHD), and seven neurologically normal control participants. The poststroke durations for the aphasic patients ranged from 24 to 179 months. Four patients had Broca's aphasia (two mildly), one patient had conduction aphasia, one had anomia, and one had Wernicke's aphasia. Although the primary purpose of the study was to examine facial expressivity as a function of hemispheric side of lesion, we also tabulated and compared the production of various speech acts. We found that the aphasic patients with LHD produced fewer words during the interview than did the patients with RHD or the normal subjects. Furthermore, aphasic patients produced fewer utterances that contained narratives and direct quotes than did normal controls. There were no between-group differences in the percentages of turns containing requests for information, arguments, interruptions, self-initiated comments, elaborations, or taboo words. These results suggest that aphasia may affect one's capacity to produce speech acts referring to events that are displaced in time and location. However, the implicit knowledge of rules governing conversational discourse was left reasonably intact by LHD, as was the capacity of the patients with LHD to express emotion on the face.

All of the studies cited thus far have identified pragmatic or suprasentential variables, quantified their use by aphasic patients and a control group, and used statistical analyses to determine impairment. However, sociolinguists engaged in field studies of natural conversation rarely employ a quantitative approach. Rather, these researchers emphasize qualitative analyses that focus on the context in which utterances are produced, the interactive nature of the discourse, and its content. Perkins (1995) provides a detailed discussion of these issues in her study of conversational discourse in three aphasic patients, using methods derived from conversation analysis (Schlegoff, 1988). Perkins undertook a detailed assessment of each patient's linguistic competence, then identified a communicative partner in the patient's social network with whom he or she regularly discussed daily life. Each participant was given a tape recorder and instructed to record one of these conversations; each participant was also taped engaging in conversation with the researcher. Using first a quantitative strategy, Perkins determined that two of the three aphasic patients shared the conversational floor equally with their partners, while the third patient produced only about 30% of major utterances. Perkins then undertook qualitative analysis as a means of better understanding this finding. She was able to show that the maintenance of turn taking in a conversation occurred in part via the mechanism of "collaborative repair," an attempt made by both conversational participants to correct real or perceived "trouble spots" in aphasic discourse. The third patient's difficulties in lexical retrieval made it difficult for her to hold the floor in conversations with her relative. When this patient was conversing with the researcher, a more collaborative effort was made that sustained her turn-taking behavior. Perkins determined that the phonemic paraphasias produced by the first two patients were not as detrimental to their continued participation in the conversation as were the failures in lexical retrieval characteristic of the third patient's speech. This pairing of quantitative and qualitative analysis represents a significant step in demonstrating how various types of linguistic impairment affect everyday discourse. In addition, these results have implications for therapy, in that a partner who is sensitized to strategies useful in collaborative repair should be more likely to enhance the communicative effectiveness of aphasic speakers (see Milroy & Perkins, 1992).

We (Burns, Blonder, & Heilman, 1991) published a report examining the conversational strategies used by aphasic patients to maintain discourse. We gave as one example the use of metaphor ("yellow streak down the back") by a patient with transcortical motor aphasia to communicate his feelings of fear and cowardice experienced during an event on a submarine that had occurred some years prior. This patient's nonfluent aphasia, combined with the retention of his ability to sing religious songs, also gave him special status in his church: He was perceived as having a unique ability to communicate with God. In a second example, a patient with Broca's aphasia had preserved intention to communicate in the presence of impaired syntax and semantic function. With the assistance of the patient's wife, who paraphrased and simplified the interviewer's questions, this patient succeeded in explaining the sequence of events that preceded and followed his stroke. This study demonstrates that communicative competence can be present in spite of linguistic incompetence. Like the study by Perkins (1995), these results also suggest that interpersonal communication in aphasic patients may require more collaboration from neurologically intact partners than does communication between healthy interlocutors.

We (Manzo, Blonder, & Burns, 1995) also utilized the method of conversational analysis to examine the social-interactional organization of narrative among patients with LHD or RHD (following a stroke) and their spouses. We examined the conversational techniques used by patients and spouses during in-home interviews that were taped and transcribed. The analysis examined the interaction of each patient and spouse during their response to a request to describe the illness. We observed a loss of agency by the stroke patients, characterized by such acts as giving up the floor to their spouses and orienting to their spouses for approval and assistance in telling the story. Spouses of stroke patients were observed to question the accuracy of the patients' narration, to correct the patients' responses, and in some instances to compete with the patients. These behaviors did not characterize the interactions of the control couples. We (Manzo et al., 1995) stress that the process by which spouses of stroke patients assume the floor is a collaborative one that occurs in a step-by-step manner, and that loss of agency characterizes the interaction of these stroke patients, regardless of the hemisphere of lesion or the presence or absence of aphasia. We also suggest that the interpersonal interactions of brain-damaged patients with their spouses contain communicative markers of powerlessness, such as the use of tag questions by patients to elicit spousal agreement and the prevalence of interruptions of the patients' narrations by spouses. We emphasize that power in these cases is defined by "situated" identities (i.e., those that are context-dependent and related to stroke-associated disability), not "demographic" identities (i.e., those derived from stable characteristics, such as gender, ethnic background, occupation, etc.). These results suggest that stroke patients may not be able to maintain status in relationships because status is negotiated during interpersonal interaction, and therefore may be a function of communicative competence.

PRAGMATIC FUNCTIONS AND THE RIGHT HEMISPHERE

Several studies reviewed in the preceding section support the conclusion that pragmatic functions are relatively preserved in aphasia (e.g., Bates et al., 1983; Meuse & Marquardt, 1985; Glosser & Deser, 1991; Ulatowska et al., 1992). By contrast, anecdotal and experimental studies suggest that pragmatic communication is impaired in nonaphasic patients with RHD. For example, Eisenson (1962) noted that the speech of patients with RHD contained "more circumlocutions" and a greater "looseness of verbalization" (tangential communication) than is normally observed. Gainotti, Caltigironi, and Miceli (1983) summarized the language of patients with RHD as excessive and tangential, and as characterized by primitive and inappropriate humor. Joanette, Goulet, Ska, and Nespoulous (1986) and Joanette and Goulet (1990) found that in comparison to the stories of neurologically intact controls, the stories of patients with RHD lacked information content. Independent studies of discourse production in aphasic patients have shown that although these patients tend to preserve the sequence of steps that make up the structure of a narrative (setting, complicating action, and resolution), they include only information that is essential to the content of the story (Ulatowska, North, & Macaluso-Haynes, 1981; Ulatowska, Freedman-Stern, & Weiss-Doyel, 1983; Ulatowska & Bond, 1983). Unlike pragmatic disturbances in patients with RHD, this simplification of narrative content by aphasic patients may represent a strategy designed to compensate for impairments in syntactic processing.

EMOTIONAL COMMUNICATION

In discussing the communicative competence of aphasic patients, one must consider the large body of literature showing dissociation after brain damage between linguistic processing and emotional communication. Most studies comparing the emotional verbal, facial, and prosodic expression of patients with LHD and aphasia to that of patients with RHD have found that the performance of the aphasic patients is comparable to that of controls, whereas the performance of patients with RHD is impaired (see Heilman, Bowers, & Valenstein, 1993, for a review).

Verbal Expression of Emotion

Bloom, Borod, Obler, and Koff (1990) studied the production of emotional discourse in a small number of patients with RHD or LHD and in normal control subjects, and found that the patients with RHD produced words of lower emotional intensity than the words produced by the other two groups. Cimino, Verfaillie, Bowers, and Heilman (1991) found that patients with RHD generated less emotional content than normal controls did in stories produced in response to single-word cues. In a study evaluating the extent to which emotional content mediates pragmatic function in patients with RHD, Bloom, Borod, Obler, and Gerstman (1993) found a double dissociation: Aphasic patients were less impaired in narrative responses to a picture depicting an emotional event than on an equivalent task that lacked emotional content. The opposite pattern was found among patients with RHD. These results suggest that the emotional deficits observed in patients with RHD encompass verbal channels, and that the semantic domain of emotion may be represented in the right hemisphere (see Borod, 1993).

Emotional Facial Expression

In an early experimental study of the effects of brain damage on spontaneous facial expression, Buck and Duffy (1980) videotaped normal control subjects and patients with RHD, LHD, or Parkinson's disease while each individual watched a set of emotionally laden slides. Raters then viewed the videotapes, categorized the subjects' expressions, and rated their expressivity on a 7-point scale. Patients with RHD or Parkinson's disease were rated as significantly less expressive than aphasic patients and normal controls. These results were confirmed in several studies by Borod and colleagues (see Borod, 1993, for a review), who also found reduced emotional facial expressivity following unilateral RHD but not LHD.

We (Blonder et al., 1993) studied the production of facial expressions during video-taped interviews with aphasic patients and their partners, patients with RHD and their partners, and control patients and their partners. We found that patients with RHD were less expressive than were aphasic patients with LHD and controls. In particular, the patients with RHD smiled less than the other two groups. Aphasic patients were statistically comparable in expressivity to normal controls. On the other hand, Mammucari et al. (1988) found no differences between patients with LHD and patients with RHD in spontaneous facial responsivity to emotional movies. However, in comparison to patients with LHD and normal subjects, patients with RHD did show reduced gaze aversion to an unpleasant movie. These results suggest that they failed to process the negative emotions depicted.

Emotional Prosodic Expression

Within the last 25 years, research in American, Chinese, Danish, French, German, and Italian populations has indicated that the right hemisphere plays a dominant role in emotional prosodic expression. Clinical research has shown that patients with RHD lack emotional prosodic variation in speech (Tucker, Watson, & Heilman, 1977; Ross & Mesulam, 1979; Ross, 1981; Weintraub, Mesulam, & Kramer, 1981; Hughes, Chan, & Su, 1983; Borod, Koff, Lorch, & Nicholas, 1985). However, unlike the research on facial expressivity cited above, there are few studies of prosodic expression during the production of spontaneous discourse; moreover, those studies that exist tend to use clinicians' impressions of prosodic impairments. This is partly a result of methodological difficulties. In studies of facial expression, it is possible to isolate the facial–visual channel on videotape and to perform ratings using a variety of coding systems. In the case of prosodic expression, one cannot separate prosody from verbal content without masking the verbal signal. If one does not mask the verbal content, then ratings may be influenced by "leakage." If one does mask the verbal content, some distortion of the prosodic features may result. Some investigators have tried to circumvent these problems and obtain greater objectivity by performing acoustic analysis of prosodic features (see Ryalls & Behrens, 1988). However, it is difficult to use this method to distinguish emotions in spontaneous speech, because it simply quantifies fundamental frequency range, contour, and syllable duration, rather than quantifying emotional content per se. Studies have shown restrictions in fundamental frequency range following RHD but not LHD, and this finding has been used as an indicator of reduced emotional expressivity. For example, we (Blonder, Pickering, Heath, Smith, & Butler, 1995) performed acoustic analysis of spontaneous prosody in audiotapes of interviews with a 77-year-old woman recorded 6 months before and 6 weeks after she experienced a right-hemisphere stroke. We found that after the stroke, the patient had a more restricted fundamental frequency contour, an increased rate of speech, and less variability in pause duration. These results provide acoustic correlates of the syndrome of flat affect often observed following RHD.

Taken together, the findings reviewed in this section suggest that emotional communication is typically impaired in patients with RHD and relatively intact in aphasic patients. One can speculate that relatively intact emotional processing by aphasic patients enhances their communicative competence. Likewise, impairments in these functions may reduce the communicative competence of individuals with RHD, in spite of their intact propositional language. As a result of this dissociation in verbal and nonverbal competencies, however, the messages sent by patients who have had a unilateral stroke may contain discrepant if not contradictory information. To investigate this, we (Langer, Pettigrew, Wilson, &

Blonder, 2000) had two raters view videotapes of 10 patients with LHD, 11 patients with RHD, and 6 neurologically normal controls engaged in interviews with an experimenter. The raters made judgments concerning the positivity of the message conveyed via the verbal channel (based on transcripts), and the positivity of the message conveyed via the facial channel (based on silent viewing of videotapes). Analysis of word–face difference scores revealed a significant linear trend, such that the messages of patients with LHD were judged as more positive in facial expression than in verbal content, and the messages of patients with RHD were judged as more positive in verbal content than in facial expression. Messages of the control subjects were judged as similar in valence across verbal and facial channels. These results suggest that patients who have had a unilateral stroke are sending channel-inconsistent messages (i.e. messages in which verbal and nonverbal messages are not matched in emotional valence).

A second study (Langer, Pettigrew, & Blonder, 1998) was designed to examine the degree to which observers liked patients who had had a unilateral stroke; likeability ratings were based on perceptions of the patients' verbal and nonverbal behavior. We found that the likeability ratings for aphasic patients were significantly lower than those for patients with RHD and normal controls when these ratings were based on verbal communication. Conversely, the likeability ratings of patients with RHD were reduced when these judgments were based on facial expressivity. These results suggest that both aphasia associated with LHD and flat affect associated with RHD can place an individual at interpersonal risk. Finally, in a study of judgments (based on videotaped interviews) of the personality and social competence of patients who had had a unilateral stroke, we (Langer, Pettigrew, Wilson, & Blonder, 1998) found that aphasic patients were judged as less socially competent than were patients with RHD or normal controls. This suggests that the verbal channel of communication may be particularly important in maintaining effective social interaction.

CONCLUSION

The major focus of this chapter has been on language use, with a particular emphasis on aphasic patients. The majority of such studies suggest that aphasic patients are capable of communicating through discourse in spite of impairments in phonology, morphology, syntax, and semantic function. These patients have retained knowledge of what constitutes appropriate conversational behavior (e.g., turn taking), and when interacting with sensitive partners, they participate in collaborative repair to compensate for their linguistic deficits. Studies have also suggested that communicative impairments may function to elevate or reduce a patient's status and power as negotiated in an interaction. Research on language use by aphasic patients has shown that they may rely on communicative strategies that remain intact, such as the use of metaphor or nonverbal communication, to enhance their message-sending capabilities. Right-hemisphere regions not typically involved in the mediation of propositional language may subserve these compensatory functions.

This discussion has brought to light approaches that are traditionally neglected in aphasiology but have the potential to further our understanding of the effects of brain damage on communicative competence. These include the use of qualitative methods such as conversation analysis to examine everyday social interaction. In employing a combined approach of clinical assessment and analysis of social-interactional abilities, one can determine the relationship between linguistic competence and communicative competence, as well as the adaptive strategies employed by patients and their partners to overcome communicative breakdowns. Lastly, every communicative event consists of a sender and a receiver. Little is known of the impressions that neurologically healthy interactants form concerning patients with aphasia or RHD who manifest verbal or nonverbal communicative deficits. Whereas an experienced clinician has an understanding of the varying types of communicative disorders that co-occur with brain damage, and can adjust his or her expectations and responses accordingly, a naive interactant may judge these patients negatively as a function of their verbal or nonverbal deficits or their channel-inconsistent communication. Such negative judgments may place communicatively impaired brain-damaged patients at risk for diminished self-esteem and feelings of social isolation. Thus pervasive psychosocial dysfunction may arise as a direct consequence of brain damage and its effects on communicative competence.

REFERENCES

Bates, E., Hamby, S., & Zurif, E. (1983). The effects of focal brain damage on pragmatic expression. *Canadian Journal of Psychology, 37*(1), 59–84.

Blanken, G., Dittman, J., Haas, J. C., & Wallesch, C. W. (1987). Spontaneous speech in senile dementia and aphasia: Implications for a neurolinguistic model of language production. *Cognition, 27,* 247–274.

Blonder, L. X., Burns, A., Bowers, D., Moore, R. W., & Heilman, K. M. (1993). Right hemisphere facial expressivity during natural conversation. *Brain and Cognition, 21*(1), 44–56.

Blonder, L. X., Kort, E. D., & Schmitt, F. A. (1994). Conversational discourse in patients with Alzheimer's disease. *Journal of Linguistic Anthropology, 4*(1), 50–71.

Blonder, L. X., Pickering, J. E., Heath, R. L., Smith, C., & Butler, S. (1995). Prosodic characteristics of speech before and after right hemisphere stroke. *Brain and Language, 51*(2), 318–335.

Bloom, R. L., Borod, J. C., Obler, L. K., & Gerstman, L. J. (1993). Suppression and facilitation of pragmatic performance: Effects of emotional content on discourse following right and left brain damage. *Journal of Speech and Hearing Research, 36,* 1227–1235.

Bloom, R. L., Borod, J. C., Obler, L. K., & Koff, E. (1990). A preliminary characterization of lexical emotional expression in right and left brain-damaged patients. *International Journal of Neuroscience, 55,* 71–80.

Borod, J. (1993). Cerebral mechanisms underlying facial, prosodic, and lexical emotional expression: A review of neuropsychological studies and methodological issues. *Neuropsychology, 7,* 445–463.

Borod, J. C., Koff, E., Lorch, M. P., & Nicholas, M. (1985). Channels of emotional expression in patients with unilateral brain damage. *Archives of Neurology, 42,* 345–348.

Buck, R., & Duffy, R. J. (1980). Nonverbal communication of affect in brain-damaged patients. *Cortex, 16,* 351–362.

Burns, A., Blonder, L. X., & Heilman, K. M. (1991). Sociolinguistics and aphasia. *Journal of Linguistic Anthropology, 1*(2), 165–177.

Cimino, C. R., Verfaellie, M., Bowers, D., & Heilman, K. M. (1991). Autobiographical memory: Influence of right hemisphere damage on emotionality and specificity. *Brain and Cognition, 15,* 106–118.

Eisenson, J. (1962). Language and intellectual modifications associated with right cerebral damage. *Language and Speech, 5,* 49–53.

Gainotti, G., Caltagironi, C., & Miceli, G. (1983). Selective impairment of semantic–lexical discrimination in right brain-damaged patients. In E. Perecman (Ed.), *Cognitive processing in the right hemisphere* (pp. 149–167). New York: Academic Press.

Glosser, G., & Deser, T. (1991). Patterns of discourse production among neurological patients with fluent language disorders. *Brain and Language, 40*(1), 67–88.

Goodglass, H., & Kaplan, E. (1972). *The assessment of aphasia and related disorders.* Philadelphia: Lea & Febiger.

Guilford, A. M., & O'Connor, J. K. (1982). Pragmatic functions in aphasia. *Journal of Communication Disorders, 15*(5), 337–346.

Halliday, M. A. K. (1977). *Learning how to mean: Explorations in the development of language.* New York: Elsevier.

Heilman, K. M., Bowers, D., & Valenstein, E. (1993). Emotional disorders associated with neurological disease. In K. M. Heilman & E. Valenstein (Eds.), *Clinical neuropsychology* (3rd ed., pp. 461–497). New York: Oxford University Press.

Hughes, C. P., Chan, J. L., & Su, M. S. (1983). Aprosodia in Chinese patients with right cerebral hemisphere lesions. *Archives of Neurology, 40,* 732–736.

Hymes, D. (1972). On communicative competence. In J. B. Pride & J. Holmes (Eds.), *Sociolinguistics* (pp. 269–285). Harmondsworth, England: Penguin.

Hymes, D. (1974). Ways of speaking. In R. Bauman & J. Sherzer (Eds.), *Explorations in the ethnography of speaking* (pp. 433–452). Cambridge, England: Cambridge University Press.

Joanette, Y., & Brownell, H. H. (Eds.). (1990). *Discourse ability and brain damage: Theoretical and empirical perspectives.* New York: Springer-Verlag.

Joanette, Y., & Goulet, P. (1990). Narrative discourse in right-brain-damaged right-handers. In Y. Joanette & H. H. Brownell (Eds.), *Discourse ability and brain damage: Theoretical and empirical perspectives* (pp. 131–149). New York: Springer-Verlag.

Joanette, Y., Goulet, P., Ska, B., & Nespoulous, J. (1986). Informative content of narrative discourse in right brain damaged right handers. *Brain and Language, 29,* 81–105.

Labov, W. (1972). Rules for ritual insults. In D. Sudnow (Ed.), *Studies in social interaction* (pp. 120–169). New York: Free Press.

Langer, S. L., Pettigrew, L. C., & Blonder, L. X. (1998). Observer liking of unilateral stroke patients. *Neuropsychiatry, Neuropsychology, and Behavioral Neurology, 11*(4), 218–224.

Langer, S. L., Pettigrew, L. C., Wilson, J. F., & Blonder, L. X. (1998). Personality and social competency following unilateral stroke. *Journal of the International Neuropsychological Society, 4,* 447–455.

Langer, S. L., Pettigrew, L. C., Wilson, J. F., & Blonder, L. X. (2000). Channel-consistency following unilateral stroke: An examination of patient communication and non-verbal domains. *Neuropsychologia, 38,* 337–344.

Linebaugh, C. W., Marguiles, C. P., & Mackisack, E. L. (1985). Contingent queries and revisions used by aphasic individuals and their most frequent communication partners. In R. H. Brookshire (Ed.), *Clinical Aphasiology Conference proceedings* (pp. 229–236). Minneapolis, MN: BRK.

Lubinski, R., Duchan, J., & Weitzner-Lin, B. (1980). Analysis of breakdowns and repairs in aphasic adult communication. In R. H. Brookshire (Ed.), *Clinical Aphasiology Conference proceedings* (pp. 111–116). Minneapolis, MN: BRK.

Mammucari, A., Caltagirone, C., Ekman, P., Friesen, W., Gainotti, G., Pizzamiglio, L., & Zoccolotti, P. (1988). Spontaneous facial expression of emotions in brain-damaged patients. *Cortex, 24,* 521–533.

Manzo, J. F., Blonder, L. X., & Burns, A. F. (1995). The social-interactional organization of narratives and narrating among stroke patients and their spouses. *Sociology of Health and Illness, 17*(3), 307–327.

Meuse, S., & Marquardt, T. P. (1985). Communicative effectiveness in Broca's aphasia. *Journal of Communication Disorders, 18*(1), 21–34.

Milroy, L., & Perkins, L. (1992). Repair strategies in aphasic discourse: Towards a collaborative model. *Clinical Linguistics and Phonetics, 6*(1–2), 27–40.

Newoff, M., Tonkovich, J. D., Schwartz, S. L., & Burgess, E. K. (1982). Revision strategies in aphasia. In R. H. Brookshire (Ed.), *Clinical Aphasiology Conference proceedings* (pp. 83–84). Minneapolis, MN: BRK.

Patry, R., & Nespoulous, J. L. (1990). Discourse analysis in linguistics: Historical and theoretical background. In Y. Joanette & H. H. Brownell (Eds.), *Discourse ability and brain damage: Theoretical and empirical perspectives* (pp. 3–27). New York: Springer-Verlag.

Perkins, L. (1995). Applying conversation analysis to aphasia: Clinical implications and analytic issues. *European Journal of Disorders of Communication, 30,* 372–383.

Ripich, D. N., & Terrell, B. Y. (1988). Patterns of discourse cohesion and coherence in Alzheimer's disease. *Journal of Speech and Hearing Disorders, 53*(1), 8–15.

Ross, E. (1981). The aprosodias. *Archives of Neurology, 38,* 561–569.

Ross, E., & Mesulam, M. M. (1979). Dominant language functions of the right hemisphere?: Prosody and emotional gesturing. *Archives of Neurology, 35,* 144–148.

Ryalls, J. H., & Behrens, S. J. (1988). An overview of changes in fundamental frequency associated with cortical insult. *Aphasiology, 2,* 107–115.

Sacks, H., Schegloff, E. A., & Jefferson, G. (1974). A simplest systematics for the organization of turn-taking for conversation. *Language, 50*(4), 696–735.

Saussure, F. (1966). *Course in general linguistics*. New York: McGraw Hill.

Schegloff, E. A. (1988). Discourse as an interactional achievement: II. An exercise in conversation analysis. In D. Tannen (Ed.), *Linguistics in context: Connecting observation and understanding* (pp. 135–158). Norwood, NJ: Ablex.

Searle, J. (1974). Chomsky's revolution in linguistics. In G. Harman (Ed.), *On Noam Chomsky: Critical essays* (pp. 1–33). Garden City, NY: Doubleday/Anchor.

Tucker, D. R., Watson, R., & Heilman, K. M. (1977). Discrimination and evocation of affectively intoned speech in patients with right parietal disease. *Neurology, 27,* 947–950.

Ulatowska, H. K., Allard, L., & Chapman, S. B. (1990). Narrative and procedural discourse in aphasia. In Y. Joanette & H. H. Brownell (Eds.), *Discourse ability and brain damage: Theoretical and empirical perspectives* (pp. 180–198). New York: Springer-Verlag.

Ulatowska, H. K., Allard, L., Reyes, B. A., Ford, J., & Chapman, S. (1992). Conversational discourse in aphasia. *Aphasiology, 6*(3), 325–331.

Ulatowska, H. K., & Bond, S. A. (1983). Aphasia: Discourse considerations. *Topics in Language Disorders, 3,* 21–34.

Ulatowska, H. K., Freedman-Stern, R., & Weiss-Doyel, A. (1983). Production of narrative discourse in aphasia. *Brain and Language, 19,* 317–334.

Ulatowska, H. K., North, A. J., & Macaluso-Haynes, S. (1981). Production of narrative and procedural discourse in aphasia. *Brain and Language, 19,* 317–334.

Weintraub, S., Mesulam, M. M., & Kramer, L. (1981). Disturbances in prosody: A right hemisphere contribution to language. *Archives of Neurology, 38,* 742–744.

PART IV

Emerging Alternative Approaches

12

CONNECTIONIST MODELS AND LANGUAGE

STEPHEN E. NADEAU

Although the study of "connectionist" or "parallel-distributed-processing" (PDP) models has become widespread only within the last 15 years, the importance of this area of research is so great that it has become essential knowledge for every behavioral neuroscientist. In this chapter I seek to provide an introduction for the novice. The first section of the chapter is devoted to defining PDP models and delineating some of their most important features. The second section focuses on specific attributes of PDP that are particularly relevant to language. The third section describes the importance of relating PDP models to neural structure, as well as some major problems we currently face in this task. The fourth section deals with the issue of neural plausibility of computational models. The final section consists of what is effectively an annotated bibliography to guide the reader to specific research of potential interest. For other reviews, see McClelland and Plaut (1993), Quinlan (1991), and Small (1994). The two-volume set by McClelland, Rumelhart, and their colleagues (McClelland, Rumelhart, & the PDP Research Group, 1986; Rumelhart, McClelland, & the PDP Research Group, 1986), though slightly dated, is still a very useful introductory text to this field.

CONNECTIONIST MODELS

Definition

A "connectionist" model is based upon a large array of processing units, each performing a simple function, and each connected to many if not all of the other units in the array. The capability of the array for processing sophistication lies in the interaction of many units operating in parallel. Figure 12.1 depicts an example of a simple network. Units in an array may stand for anything, including hypotheses (e.g., about the presence or absence of letters in a display, or about the syntactic roles of words in a sentence), goals, or features. Thus a room may be defined in terms of its contents, in which case the contents represent features of the room. In this example, each unit represents an item likely to be found in a particular room. In many models, the units are not defined beforehand but are permitted to evolve a definition as the model processes.

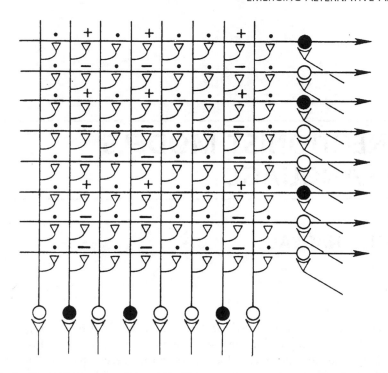

FIGURE 12.1. A simple PDP network (specifically, a pattern associator network). Each unit on the right receives input from each unit at the bottom. The connection strengths between the units at the bottom and the units on the right are depicted as •, −, or +, indicating zero, inhibitory, or excitatory, respectively. Given this "matrix" of connection strengths, the pattern of activation at the bottom elicits the pattern of activation at the right. From Rumelhart, D. E., & McClelland, J. L. (1986). On learning the past tenses of English verbs. In J. L. McClelland, D. E. Rumelhart, & the PDP Research Group (Eds.), *Parallel distributed processing: Explorations in the microstructure of cognition. Vol. 2. Psychological and biological models* (pp. 216–271). Cambridge, MA: MIT Press. Copyright 1986 by the MIT Press. Reprinted with permission.

Schemas, or concepts, are not represented by specific units but by a pattern of activation of a large number of units; a pattern of activation delineates the cluster of features that define a particular concept or schema. This is called a "distributed representation." If we view the brain as a connectionist network, then in biological reality features themselves would not be represented by units but by distributions of activity over other sets of units, which in turn would be distributed representations. However, for purposes of modeling networks on computers, it is not practical to employ such successive hierarchies of units. At some point, local representations are employed as a matter of computational convenience and economy. Figure 12.2 provides an example of an entirely local and a partly distributed representation of some words.

Processing in PDP networks is massively parallel. In fact, unlike conventional digital computers, in which there is one or at most several central processing units, in PDP every unit is a processor. Information processing takes place through the interactions of large numbers of simple processing units, each sending excitatory and inhibitory signals to other units. A concept is not stored, but exists only as long as a particular pattern of activation persists. What is stored is the ability to regenerate that pattern of activation, given an appropriate input cue. *The knowledge that underlies the concept is represented in the strengths of connections between units in the network.* This makes it possible to regener-

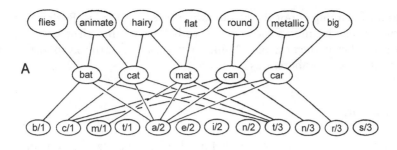

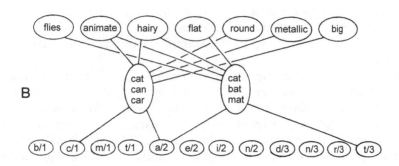

FIGURE 12.2. A three-layered network defining some word representations. The top network (A) uses entirely local representations. Each unit corresponds to a single discrete entity. Thus, for example, the word "cat" has an orthographic representation as "c" in the first position, "a" in the second position, and "t" in the third position. It has a semantic representation as "animate" and "hairy." The bottom network (B) uses a distributed representation at the intermediate or word level. The unit "cat can car" has no readily interpretable meaning. However, all of its components have an orthographic representation incorporating "c" in the first position and "a" in the second position and together they have a broad semantic representation as "animate," "hairy," "round," "metallic," and "big." The meaning of the second intermediate unit "cat bat mat" is similarly inscrutable. However, if both these intermediate units are activated, the one entity they have in common is "cat": The units in the orthographic layer that are activated are "c" in the first position, "a" in the second position, and "t" in the third position, and the two units in the semantic layer that get double activation are "animate" and "hairy," the semantic features of "cat." Thus the bottom model achieves the same results as the top model in a way that actually is somewhat more economical. From Hinton, G. E., McClelland, J. L., & Rumelhart, D. E. (1986). Distributed representations. In D. E. Rumelhart, J. L. McClelland, & the PDP Research Group (Eds.), *Parallel distributed processing: Explorations in the microstructure of cognition. Vol. 1. Foundations* (pp. 77–109). Cambridge, MA: MIT Press. Copyright 1986 by the MIT Press. Reprinted with permission.

ate a pattern of activation corresponding to an entire concept, even if we are capable of directly activating only a fraction of the units in the network (something called "content-addressable memory"). To the extent that the brain may be represented as a connectionist network, connections are entirely hardware in the sense that they exist as synapses, but they are entirely software in that they are modifiable through learning or input from other neural systems that alter the weights of connections.

Learning is the development of the right connection strengths, so that the right pattern of activation will be produced under the right circumstances. If a model is equipped with a learning device, it can learn, by tuning its connections, to capture interdependencies between activation patterns to which it is exposed in the course of processing.

The goal of learning is not the instantiation of explicit rules. Rather, the acquisition of connection strengths allows the network to behave as though it knew the rules. The rules become *implicit* in the network. A single network can learn to support many patterns of activity that are each coherent as concepts.

Implementation

Connectionist models have been a tour de force because they can be implemented on computers and can produce voluminous, detailed, explicit, and testable predictions about behavior. In this chapter I am considering PDP models almost exclusively at the conceptual level, but it is important for the reader to have a sense of the computer implementation of these models. This requires mathematical representation of the notions being discussed here at the conceptual level. Figure 12.3 provides examples of the mathematical representations commonly employed.

One of the most interesting aspects of PDP models—an aspect of particular relevance to the neural structures they may emulate—is their learning behavior. Because PDP models are typically complex, their developers typically choose to focus on specific problems and to make use of simplifying assumptions in areas that are not the focus of interest. Thus not all models are given a learning capability. Tanzi (1893) and Ramón y Cajal (1923) were the first to propose that physical changes in neural connections might underlie learning, but it was Donald Hebb (1949) who really developed this idea. Some learning algorithms in PDP models actually incorporate Hebb's proposal that changes in connection strengths should occur to the degree that connected units are simultaneously active. Hebbian learning recapitulates the well-studied neural learning process of long-term potentiation, and it provides a plausible basis for the organization of a number of neural systems, such as ocular dominance columns and orientation-selective cells in visual cortex (Elman et al., 1996). However, because it has so far been difficult to employ Hebbian learning in a fruitful way in PDP models of cognitive function, most investigators have developed learning algorithms that produce weight changes according to the discrepancy between actual network output and targeted output. The following formula captures this concept; it defines the changes in the weights of connections that are to occur with each processing cycle:

$$\Delta \omega_{ij} = \eta(t_i(t) - a_i(t))o_j(t)$$

This says that the change in the weight (strength of connection) between unit i and unit j should be the product of a constant (η), the difference between the targeted activity of unit i and the actual activity of unit i, and the output of unit j. Various other learning algorithms have been studied. Models employing such teaching functions often make use of "backpropagation," a procedure that propagates signals related to the magnitude of the output error back through all the layers of the model, indicating how connection weights should be changed. The patterns of connectivity emerging in intermediate layers of networks that have been trained with the backpropagation algorithm often exhibit important patterns or regularities in the data. For example, Small (1994) and colleagues constructed a very simple four-layer model to associate objects with their features. The input units encoded features of objects (e.g., number of limbs, size, color, texture, and shape), and the output units coded the objects themselves. The network was trained to take a collection of features and to associate it with a single object. Analysis of the intermediate layers in the

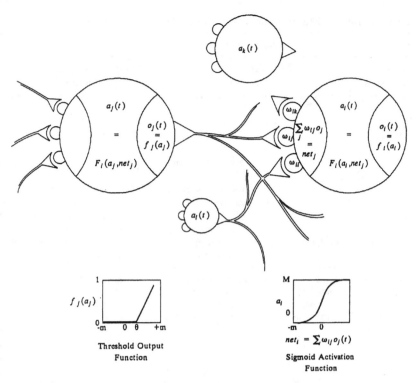

FIGURE 12.3. The basic components of a PDP system. The brain itself functions as an analog computer: Computational processes involving tens of billions of neurons are taking place simultaneously. However, PDP models are implemented on digital computers, so the state of the units has to be updated one at a time. This figure depicts the mathematical formulae for updating those states. Thus the new activation level of unit j, $a_j(t)$, is calculated as some function of its present activation level, a_j, and its net input, net_j. The output of this same unit, $o_j(t)$, is then computed as a function of its newly recalculated activation level. The input to unit i is computed as the sum of the outputs of all the units "synapsing" on it, each output being multiplied by the strength of the connection between the unit that generated it and unit i (ω_{ij}). The graphs at the bottom of the figure illustrate the types of output and activation functions that are often employed in these models. The output function depicted exhibits a threshold feature; that is, the output of this unit will be zero unless its activation level exceeds a minimum, θ, whereupon it becomes a linear function of that activation level. This type of output function achieves two purposes. First, it helps to squelch random, low-level noise in the system. Second, it gives the unit a nonlinear feature, enabling it to support a symbolic representation; thus the particular feature represented by this unit is either absent or present, depending on whether the activation level is below or above θ. The sigmoid activation function depicted at the right (another nonlinear feature) is a convenient way of making an activation level highly sensitive to input even while it is constrained between a minimum, $-m$, and a maximum, M. From Rumelhart, D. E., Hinton, G. E., & McClelland, J. L. (1986). A general framework for parallel distributed processing. In D. E. Rumelhart, J. L. McClelland, & the PDP Research Group (Eds.), *Parallel distributed processing: Explorations in the microstructure of cognition. Vol. 1. Foundations* (pp. 45–76). Cambridge, MA: MIT Press. Copyright 1986 by the MIT Press. Reprinted with permission.

trained network revealed that they had "learned" the difference between animate and inanimate objects, tools and animals, and fruits and vegetables.

From here on this chapter considers connectionism exclusively in conceptual terms, but it is important to recognize that the rapidly expanding connectionist literature is based upon the mathematical implementation of these models. Connectionist models can be readily conceived in neural-like, mathematical, or conceptual terms (Table 12.1).

TABLE 12.1. Neural, Mathematical, and Conceptual Equivalence in PDP

Neural	Mathematical	Conceptual
Neurons	Units	Hypotheses, features
Spiking frequency	Activation	Degree of confidence
Spread of depolarization	Spread of activation	Propagation of confidence: inference
Synaptic contact	Connection	Inferential relations
Excitation/inhibition	Positive/negative weight	Positive/negative inferential relations
Approximate additivity of depolarizations	Summation of inputs	Approximate additivity of evidence
Spiking thresholds	Threshold for spread of activation	Independence from irrelevant information; basis for symbolic representation
Limited dynamic range	Sigmoidal function	Limited range of processing strength

Note. From Smolensky, P. (1986). Neural and conceptual interpretation of PDP models. In J. L. McClelland, D. E. Rumelhart, & the PDP Research Group (Eds.), *Parallel distributed processing: Explorations in the microstructure of cognition. Vol. 2. Psychological and biological models* (pp. 390–431). Cambridge, MA: MIT Press. Copyright 1986 by the MIT Press. Reprinted with permission.

The Fundamental Appeal of Connectionism

PDP models have elicited a great deal of enthusiasm among experimental psychologists because of their appealing computational properties, their ability to produce voluminous output that can be compared with behavioral data, and their success in accounting for empirical observations. PDP models have an additional source of appeal to the behavioral neuroscientist: their brain-like character. For over a century, behavioral neuroscientists have systematically studied complex behavior with a simple faith that one day it would be possible to relate this vast database to the neural architecture of the brain in a systematic and scientifically plausible fashion. Connectionism has validated that faith by providing the explicit means for linking neural microstructure to complex behavior.

The brain-like character of PDP models is worth considering in somewhat greater detail. These models employ a massively parallel processor architecture with extensive interconnectivity that bears a potentially direct correspondence to neural cytoarchitecture. Their employment of a large number of units emulates the large number of neurons in the brain (10^{10}–10^{11}). In PDP models, each unit functions in a relatively simple manner. The function of neurons in the brain is not quite so simple, but it does appear that processing sophistication in the brain, as in PDP models, derives primarily from the interaction of large numbers of neurons linked together into functional neural networks. The relatively slow firing rate of single neurons to any given stimulus is strong evidence of distributed encoding involving networks, as opposed to information coding in firing rates. Learning in PDP models and in the brain involves the modification of connection strengths. The currency of PDP models, as of the brain, consists of excitation and inhibition rather than symbols. On the other hand, units in PDP models may be given both threshold and ceiling properties (nonlinearities). These nonlinear properties provide the basis for nonlinear network behavior, such as categorical responses (necessary to support symbolic representations) and sudden transitions in network behavior as networks accumulate information in the course of training. Functional imaging studies suggest that whereas synaptic activity in primary cortices is proportional to the rate of stimulus presentation or motoric response, synaptic activity in association cortices is relatively insensitive to rate effects (Price et al., 1992; Sadato et al., 1996), suggesting a greater tendency to an all-or-none, on-or-off response (i.e., a nonlinear, categorical response).

Nonlinear properties have implications for development as well. Such disparate phenomena as Piagetian stages in childhood development, periods of special susceptibility to uniocular visual deprivation in kittens, and the sudden emergence of schizophrenic symptoms can potentially be accounted for entirely in terms of the natural evolution of such nonlinear dynamic systems. PDP models are optimal in reconciling nativist (cognitive capacities are hard-wired at birth) and empiricist (cognitive capacities are exclusively learned) views of neurological development. Information, whether genetically determined or learned, is represented in the strengths of neural connections. The prolonged developmental period of humans provides great opportunities for experience to shape the rough neurodevelopmental processes set in motion and constrained by genetic factors. In this way, the modest brain-relevant information in the human genome can be parlayed into a structure that contains several orders of magnitude more information (Elman et al., 1996).

PDP models reveal how the brain might transcend the processing limitations imposed by the slowness of neuronal function through massive parallelism. The sophistication of function achievable by very modest PDP networks provides a sense of how the brain might plausibly achieve the levels of sophistication it does. In PDP models, output is continuously available, just as it is in the brain. PDP models exhibit a property known as "graceful degradation"; that is, a network's performance deteriorates gradually as units are destroyed or input becomes noisy or degraded. There is no single point when performance breaks down. Despite network dysfunction, output continues to reflect the processing principles implicit in the original network, albeit with some loss of reliability or signal strength. This is also true of the brain. In contrast, with serial processing models, disruption of a single step can catastrophically affect the performance of the system. In PDP models, as in the brain, central control is not required. There is no part of a model or of the cerebral cortex upon which all other parts depend. There are no subroutines, but rather subsystems that modulate the behavior of other subsystems. Behavior emerges from the dynamic interaction of multiple networks, the relative role of any given network at any given time being autodefined by the requirements of the situation. PDP provides a means for systematically studying how such emergent properties arise. In PDP models, information processing and both immediate and long-term memory share the same circuitry. There is rapidly accumulating evidence that this holds true for the brain as well (Ungerleider, 1995).

PDP models have now been applied to a number of more elemental brain processes, including olfactory learning in rats (Granger, Ambros-Ingerson, Antón, & Lynch, 1990), the development of the "barrels" in somatosensory cortex of rats that are organized around vibrissae input (Montague, Gally, & Edelman, 1991), the organization of somatosensory cortex in primates (Finkel, 1990), the development of ocular dominance columns in visual cortex (Miller & Stryker, 1990), and the conversion of retinotopic to hemispheric visual coordinates (Zipser & Andersen, 1988). Movement direction, saccade direction, and auditory localization are defined by distributed representations in motor cortex, the superior colliculus, and auditory cortex, respectively (see review by Singer, 1994).

Examples

In this section I review several PDP models to illustrate particular processing principles or attributes and to give the reader a more concrete sense of PDP.

A Simple Pattern Associator

A "pattern associator network" is a model in which a pattern of activation over one set of units can elicit a pattern of activation over another set of units without any intervening units to stand for either pattern as a whole. For example, a pattern associator may be capable of associating a pattern of activation in one set of units corresponding to the appearance of an object with a pattern in another set corresponding to the aroma, such that when the object is "seen," the pattern of its aroma is evoked. Figure 12.4 depicts a visual–olfactory pattern associator that I use here to demonstrate two important PDP properties: graceful degradation and storage capacity. In Figure 12.5, left, 50% of the input to the rose pattern associator has been lost. Nevertheless, the pattern of output of the associator is the same, albeit less strong; in effect, a "glimpse" of a rose still yields a "whiff" of a rose. In Figure 12.5, right, the rose pattern associator has been damaged; one-third of the units have been lost. Once again, however, given a rose visual input, the network yields an output pattern similar to that of the intact network, although again somewhat less strong. Figure 12.5 illustrates the phenomenon of graceful degradation. Note in these examples that network output in degraded states, though qualitatively the same, is quantitatively less. Thus, if the ability of the network to produce two distinguishable output patterns is dependent on the quantitative difference between those patterns, degraded states will tend to result in near-misses. A familiar neurobehavioral example of this is semantic paraphasias.

In Figure 12.6, the connection matrices of the rose and steak pattern associators are added to each other. The resulting combination matrix will yield the rose aroma when given a rose visual image, and a steak aroma when given a steak visual image. In fact, a given pattern associator can represent up to N independent (i.e., orthogonal) patterns simultaneously, where N is the number of input units. As we shall see, such a network can represent many more patterns if they are to some degree related to each other.

An Autoassociator Network and the Instantiation of Schemas

In this section I discuss a simple example (originally developed by Rumelhart, Smolensky, McClelland, & Hinton, 1986) that exemplifies how a PDP network represents information and how that information can be extracted, as well as the capability of PDP networks for inference.

The rooms of a house contain different items and have particular features that enable us to define each room in terms of its contents and features. Table 12.2 lists 40 room descriptors, each of which labels a unit in this PDP model. These room descriptors can be viewed as features, and in this case the features are locally represented, since each feature corresponds to one unit. Each unit is connected to every other unit in the network. The connection strengths or weights of each of these connections were determined by asking two raters to imagine an office and then to say, for each of the 40 descriptors, whether it was appropriate for the office. This process was repeated for living room, kitchen, bathroom, and bedroom. This cycle was repeated 16 times, yielding a total of 16 judgments on each descriptor for each of 5 rooms. This provided the corpus of material that was "taught" to the network. In this particular instance, the weights of the connections in the network

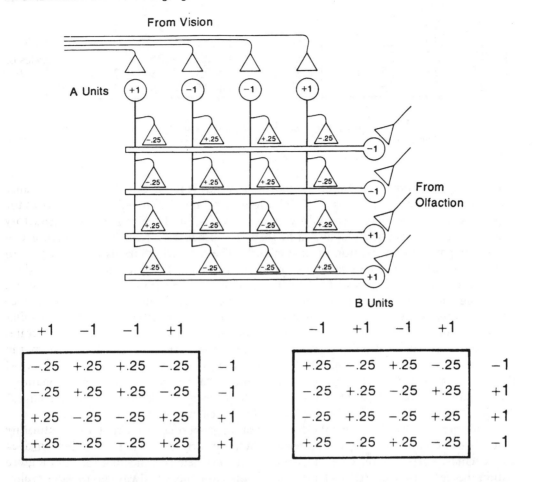

FIGURE 12.4. A visual–olfactory pattern associator network. The pattern of input in the units at the top, multiplied by the respective weights in the connection matrix immediately below and summed, results in the pattern of activation in the units at the right. The two matrices below exemplify a shorthand means of representing patterns of input and output and connection strengths. The left matrix replicates the information in the pattern associator network above; this is designated as the "rose" pattern associator. On the right is the "steak" pattern associator. From McClelland, J. L., Rumelhart, D. E., & Hinton, G. E. (1986). The appeal of parallel distributed processing. In D. E. Rumelhart, J. L. McClelland, & the PDP Research Group (Eds.), *Parallel distributed processing: Explorations in the microstructure of cognition. Vol. 1. Foundations* (pp. 3–44). Cambridge, MA: MIT Press. Copyright 1986 by the MIT Press. Reprinted with permission.

were actually set according to the probability that any two particular features would occur in conjunction, based upon the corpus of judgments rendered by the raters. Figure 12.7 depicts the connection weight matrix that resulted.

In effect, we now have a miniature brain that operates on the basis of PDP. This brain can be operated by clamping one or more units at 1 (in effect, stating that these features are present) and letting the system run until activation spreads from these units throughout the network and the network eventually reaches a steady state. There are 2^{40} possible states of this network, but it settles into one of only five different states. Figure 12.8 depicts that pattern of activation as it evolves and ultimately stabilizes when the features "oven"

+ 1	- 1			
- .25	+.25	+.25	- .25	- .5
- .25	+.25	+.25	- .25	- .5
+.25	- .25	- .25	+.25	+.5
+.25	- .25	- .25	+.25	+.5

+ 1	- 1	- 1	+ 1	
- .25	+.25			- .5
- .25	+.25			- .5
+.25	- .25	- .25		+.75
+.25	- .25	- .25	+.25	+ 1

FIGURE 12.5. The effects of degraded input (left) or network damage (right) on the function of a pattern associator network.

and "ceiling" are turned on. As can be seen, in the steady state that finally emerges, "oven," "coffee-pot," "cupboard," "toaster," "refrigerator," "sink," "stove," "drapes," "coffee-cup," "clock," "telephone," "small," "window," "walls," and "ceiling" are activated. This cluster of features implicitly defines a kitchen. The schema "kitchen" thus emerges as a particular pattern of activation of the network. The network contains in its connection weights the knowledge that enables us to elicit this schema. The kitchen schema is instantiated as a "distributed representation." The capability for eliciting this schema simply by activating one or more features constitutes "content-addressable memory." We do not have to know where the kitchen schema is stored; indeed, it is stored throughout this network. We simply have to evoke a feature of the schema and the schema comes to life, albeit in ephemeral form as a pattern of activation. By activating other features in this same network, we can elicit other schemas. For example, if we clamp "ceiling" and "desk," a pattern of activation emerges that includes "computer," "ash-tray," "coffee-cup," "picture," "desk-chair," "books," "carpet," "bookshelf," "typewriter," "telephone," "desk," "large," "door," "walls," and "ceiling"—unmistakably the schema of an office.

This network exhibits several other interesting properties. It is capable of supporting a number of completely different patterns of activity corresponding to completely different schemas. Furthermore, schemas can contain subschemas, reflecting the connectivity within the network (e.g., "easy-chair" and "floor-lamp" nearly always go together, as do "desk" and "desk-chair," and "window" and "drapes"). Schemas can blend: For example, if we clamp both "bed" and "sofa," we eventually activate "television," "dresser," "drapes," "fire-place," "easy-chair," "sofa," "floor-lamp," "picture," "clock," "books," "carpet," "bookshelf," "bed," "large," "window," "door," "walls," and "ceiling." This is in effect

$$
\begin{bmatrix} - & + & + & - \\ - & + & + & - \\ + & - & - & + \\ + & - & - & + \end{bmatrix}
+
\begin{bmatrix} + & - & + & - \\ - & + & - & + \\ - & + & - & + \\ + & - & + & - \end{bmatrix}
=
\begin{bmatrix} & & ++ & -- \\ -- & ++ & & \\ & & -- & ++ \\ ++ & -- & & \end{bmatrix}
$$

FIGURE 12.6. A single network can represent multiple patterns of information. The weight matrices for the two networks depicted in Figure 12.4 can be added to yield a matrix that will capture both the rose and steak pattern associations. From McClelland, J. L., Rumelhart, D. E., & Hinton, G. E. (1986). The appeal of parallel distributed processing. In D. E. Rumelhart, J. L. McClelland, & the PDP Research Group (Eds.), *Parallel distributed processing: Explorations in the microstructure of cognition. Vol. 1. Foundations* (pp. 3–44). Cambridge, MA: MIT Press. Copyright 1986 by the MIT Press. Reprinted with permission.

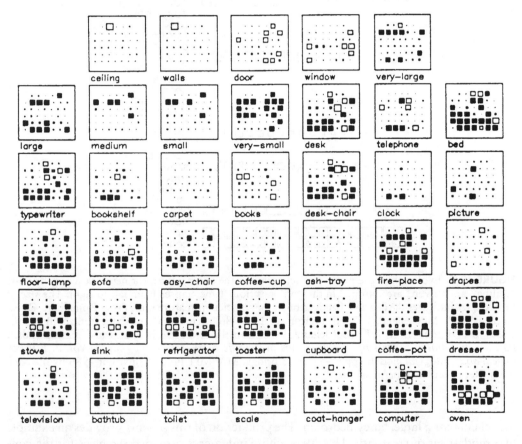

FIGURE 12.7. Matrix of connection weights in the room descriptor model. Small dark squares signify inhibitory connections; white squares indicate excitatory connections. The size of a small square is proportional to the strength of the connection. The descriptor layout in each small square precisely replicates the descriptor layout in the entire figure. Referring to the large square in the bottom right corner, one can see that "oven" (bottom right location within this large square) has a strong negative connection to its neighbor immediately to the left, "computer," but a strong positive connection to its diagonal neighbor, "coffee-pot." From Rumelhart, D. E., Smolensky, P., McClelland, J. L., & Hinton, G. E. (1986). Schemata and sequential thought processes in PDP models. In J. L. McClelland, D. E. Rumelhart, & the PDP Research Group (Eds.), *Parallel distributed processing: Explorations in the microstructure of cognition. Vol. 2. Psychological and biological models* (pp. 7–57). Cambridge, MA: MIT Press. Copyright 1986 by the MIT Press. Reprinted with permission.

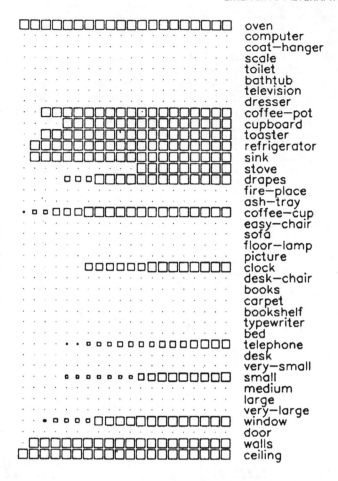

oven
computer
coat—hanger
scale
toilet
bathtub
television
dresser
coffee—pot
cupboard
toaster
refrigerator
sink
stove
drapes
fire—place
ash—tray
coffee—cup
easy—chair
sofa
floor—lamp
picture
clock
desk—chair
books
carpet
bookshelf
typewriter
bed
telephone
desk
very—small
small
medium
large
very—large
window
door
walls
ceiling

FIGURE 12.8. Evolution of the pattern of activation in the room descriptor network when the units "ceiling" and "oven" are clamped in the "on" position. Time elapses from left to right. The size of each square indicates the degree of activation of that particular feature unit. From Rumelhart, D. E., Smolensky, P., McClelland, J. L., & Hinton, G. E. (1986). Schemata and sequential thought processes in PDP models. In J. L. McClelland, D. E. Rumelhart, & the PDP Research Group (Eds.), *Parallel distributed processing: Explorations in the microstructure of cognition. Vol. 2. Psychological and biological models* (pp. 7–57). Cambridge, MA: MIT Press. Copyright 1986 by the MIT Press. Reprinted with permission.

the schema for a large, fancy bedroom. The production of this schema provides an example of a modest bit of creativity. The raters whose judgments provided the basis for the connection weights were never asked what items were appropriate to a large, fancy bedroom. Rather, the network *inferred* this schema from the knowledge it had been provided about more conventional rooms in a house. Viewed in another way, the model *shaded* the meaning of "bedroom," given the additional information that the bedroom contained a sofa.

The capacity for inference underlies the ability of PDP models to generalize—to provide specific predictions about a more general situation, based upon knowledge of one or more specific aspects of the situation. Because living organisms are unlikely to encounter exactly the same situation more than once, the capacity for inference latent in the PDP nature of their brains both makes it possible always to generate some sort of response, and maximizes the probability that this response will be appropriate. Presumably the same capacity underlies the human ability to generate rules and generalizations, despite the fact that people actually experience a series of special instances. However, there are negative aspects to the capacity for inference and generalization. For example, the room descriptor network may make errors of guilt by association: Shown an easy chair, it will assume that there is a floor lamp nearby, even if in a particular instance there is none. More generally, it will confabulate (e.g., if "oven" is clamped it will tell you it "saw" a refrigerator, coffee pot, toaster, etc., even though it only actually "saw" the oven). In fact, the room descriptor network, and indeed PDP networks in general, have no intrinsic way of distinguishing between elements they have seen and elements they have inferred. Humans also tend to make errors of guilt by association and to "remember" what they would have expected, even if it was not really there. This suggests that discriminating fact from inference requires, at least in part, transcendent cerebral mechanisms that are not intrinsic to the networks storing information and break down easily. Such specific instance information constitutes the episodic component of declarative memory.

The concept of distributed representation is often misconstrued as incompatible with evidence of localization of cerebral function. Distributed representations and localization of function are easily reconciled if one recognizes that the brain is made up of an enormous number of variously interconnected neuronal networks, each supporting distributed representations based on net-specific features. Thus a given concept such as "dog" may have a distributed representation in dominant perisylvian cortex based upon the articulatory motor features required to say /dog/; another distributed representation in visual association cortex based on visual features; and still other distributed representations in auditory association cortex, somatosensory cortex, and limbic cortex. A dominant perisylvian lesion may eliminate the capacity for generating the appropriate articulatory motor schema (/dog/) without affecting other distributed representations of "dog."

The room descriptor network, humble as it is, nevertheless can provide some insight into cerebral processes that may underlie thinking (Rumelhart, Smolensky, et al., 1986). A schema or concept in the network is a static representation, but because it represents a pattern of activation, it is intrinsically ephemeral. The replacement of one pattern by another (i.e., one schema by another) instantiates a serial process. Successive "clamps" on units of the network, either by external stimuli (e.g., as the network "walks" from room to room), or by output from other connected networks (as the network "contemplates" moving around the house), may elicit successive schemas. If the brain is viewed as a large collection of variously interconnected networks, then consciousness may correspond to the total complex of schemas corresponding to the current pattern of activation in the cortex. In this view, successive stimuli in the environment serve to clamp the brain networks in different ways, leading to the instantiation of new schemas. An interpretation of a situation often leads to an action, which in turn leads to an alteration in the constellation of schemas, another action, and so on. Therefore, the necessarily serial nature of motor activity entrains a serial change in schemas.

Suppose we postulate the existence of two networks—one supporting a schema corresponding to the present situation, and the other supporting a schema that is a model of the present situation. In the model, the inputs or clamps include both external stimuli and our own internal specification of some component (our internal clamp) that allows us to see what schema emerges given that clamp, and to compare it with the schema corresponding to the actual state of affairs. By such mental modeling, we can anticipate the consequences of our actions—constrained, of course, by the limits of our knowledge, which is stored in the connection strengths within the networks. We can also solve complex problems in our heads by serially altering a given schema in precise ways *as if* those changes were actually being effected in the environment. Thinking, in this conceptualization, corresponds to imagining we are doing the process externally by manipulating an internal network model of the external world. Our ability to solve problems depends in great part on the availability of external representations of those problems, which we can then internalize as model networks with their implicit schemas. External representations, it seems, are difficult to develop, and are in good part culture-bound and evolve only gradually. A major aspect of schooling is teaching representational schemes. It may be that true creativity lies in developing internal model networks that implicitly support novel schemas and in turn enable us to ask unprecedented "what if" questions about the external world.

Learning by a Complex Pattern Associator Model

In this section I review a rather famous PDP model developed by Rumelhart and McClelland (1986) that was successfully trained to produce the past tense of English verbs, given the present tense or root form. The success of the model and the byproducts of its learning experience have provided a very potent demonstration of the power of PDP models in general. However, some of the assumptions built into the model have inflamed critics, who have used the investigation as a basis for questioning the validity of PDP itself. I discuss the model here not only because it demonstrates the power of PDP, but also because it serves as a good introduction to learning by PDP networks.

The goal of the past-tense model development was not just to achieve correct conversion from present to past tense, but also to reproduce the pattern of past-tense learning exhibited by children during normal language development. It was assumed, based on data from a number of investigations of language development, that the normal learning process occurs in three phases:

1. Relatively few past-tense verbs are used—all very high-frequency, most irregular, and some highly idiosyncratic (e.g., "came," "got," "gave," "looked," "needed," "took," "went"). There is no evidence of rule use, and children simply seem to know a small number of items.

2. Evidence of implicit knowledge of a linguistic rule emerges. Children use a much larger number of verbs in the past tense, the majority regular (e.g., "wiped," "pulled"). Children can now generate a past-tense form for an invented verb (e.g., "rick" → "ricked"). They also incorrectly supply regular past-tense endings for words they used correctly in phase 1 (e.g., "come" → "comed" or "camed").

3. Regular and irregular forms coexist, and children retain the implicit rule but reacquire the irregular forms.

The basic structure of the past-tense-learning pattern associator network is shown in Figure 12.9. The units in the network are based on the concept of a "Wickelphone" triad. The following are Wickelphone representations of "cook" and its past-tense form, "cooked":

"cook"   /cuk/ $_{\#}c_{u\ c}u_{k\ u}k_{\#}$
"cooked"   /cukt/ $_{\#}c_{u\ c}u_{k\ u}k_{t\ k}t_{\#}$

The reason for using Wickelphone triads is that they were necessary to capture the prevalent relationships between a given phoneme and its surrounding phonemes.[1]

One major practical problem with assigning units in the network to Wickelphones was that with 35 phonemes, there are $35^3 = 42{,}875$ Wickelphones, requiring a connection matrix

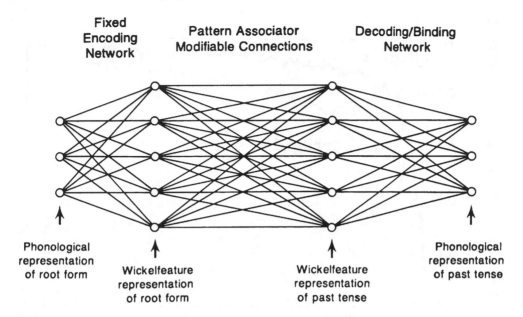

Fixed
Encoding
Network

Pattern Associator
Modifiable Connections

Decoding/Binding
Network

Phonological
representation
of root form

Wickelfeature
representation
of root form

Wickelfeature
representation
of past tense

Phonological
representation
of past tense

FIGURE 12.9. The present-tense–past-tense pattern associator model. See text for explanation. From Rumelhart, D. E., & McClelland, J. L. (1986). On learning the past tenses of English verbs. In J. L. McClelland, D. E. Rumelhart, & the PDP Research Group (Eds.), *Parallel distributed processing: Explorations in the microstructure of cognition. Vol. 2. Psychological and biological models* (pp. 216–271). Cambridge, MA: MIT Press. Copyright 1986 by the MIT Press. Reprinted with permission.

of $2 \cdot 10^9$ connections—an impractical number. For this reason, each phoneme in the Wickelphones was incorporated as a distributed representation over a set of four distinctive features (in the linguistic sense). When this was done, and some sources of redundancy were eliminated, the entire corpus of 500 verbs and past tenses employed in testing this model could be produced without duplication as a distributed representation over 460 Wickelfeatures (distinctive-feature triads). The final model consisted of 460 input and 460 output Wickelfeature units with 211,600 connections between them. The model was trained by giving it a series of paired input and output phoneme strings corresponding to the present-tense and past-tense forms of successive verbs. With each presentation, the model was designed to compare the actual pattern of activation in its output units with the targeted pattern of activation (corresponding to the correct past-tense form) and to adjust its connection weights incrementally, such that the recomputed output would more closely resemble the desired target.

The network was presented with 10 cycles of 10 high-frequency verbs ("come," "get," "give," "look," "make," "take," "go," "have," "live," "feel" [8 irregular, 2 regular]), and then with 190 cycles of 410 medium-frequency verbs (most regular). Responses early in the period of training the medium-frequency verbs-were taken to correspond to childhood phase 2, and responses at the end of a total of 200 cycles were assumed to correspond to childhood phase 3. The network was then tested (but not trained) on 86 low-frequency verbs to which it had never been exposed. The network's response to training is demonstrated in Figure 12.10. Performance on high-frequency irregular verbs dropped as large numbers of regular verbs were introduced, as observed in children, but ultimately it recovered, as also seen in children. The model learned from experience and incorporated an implicit rule. The model also learned a number of unexpected things, such as the fact that

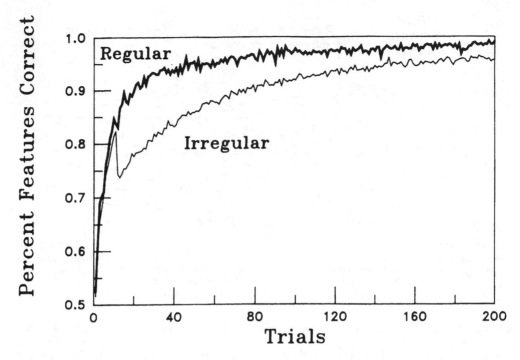

FIGURE 12.10. The percentage of correct features for regular and irregular high-frequency verbs as a function of trials completed. From Rumelhart, D. E., & McClelland, J. L. (1986). On learning the past tenses of English verbs. In J. L. McClelland, D. E. Rumelhart, & the PDP Research Group (Eds.), *Parallel distributed processing: Explorations in the microstructure of cognition. Vol. 2. Psychological and biological models* (pp. 216–271). Cambridge, MA: MIT Press. Copyright 1986 by the MIT Press. Reprinted with permission.

verbs ending in "t" or "d" frequently have an identical past-tense form (Table 12.3), as children do (Table 12.4). The model predicted a particularly high likelihood of regularization errors (adding "ed") for verbs that undergo a vowel change to produce the past tense and end in a diphthong sequence (e.g., "blow" → "blew," "fly" → "flew") and verbs that undergo change of an internal /i/ or /a/ to achieve the past tense (e.g., "sting" → "stung," "hang" → "hung"). This too has been borne out in studies of language in young children (Bybee & Slobin, 1982). The model also provided richly detailed predictions about various classes of irregular verbs (see Rumelhart & McClelland, 1986, for further details). Its responses to unfamiliar verbs were frequently incorrect but usually plausible (Tables 12.5 and 12.6).

This past-tense pattern associator model has received a great deal of criticism on a number of grounds (Jaeger et al., 1996; Pinker, 1991; Pinker & Prince, 1988), most notably because it fails to instantiate morphemes; because patients with posterior brain lesions exhibit particular difficulty in forming the past tense of irregular verbs, while patients with anterior lesions exhibit particular difficulty with regular verbs (Ullman et al., 1997); and because other studies of verb exposure and use in children suggest that they do not follow the precise pattern hypothesized by Rumelhart and McClelland (1986). Many of the specific objections have been addressed through studies of more sophisticated (hidden-unit) versions of the original model (Daugherty & Seidenberg, 1992; Hoeffner, 1992; MacWhinney & Leinbach, 1991).

TABLE 12.3. Average Simulated Strengths of Regularized and No-Change Responses for Verbs Ending in "t" or "d" and Other Verbs

Time period	Verb ending	Regularized	No change
11–15	Not t/d	0.44	0.10
	t/d	0.35	0.27
21–30	Not t/d	0.52	0.11
	t/d	0.32	0.41

Note. From Rumelhart, D. E., & McClelland, J. L. (1986). On learning the past tenses of English verbs. In J. L. McClelland, D. E. Rumelhart, & the PDP Research Group (Eds.), *Parallel distributed processing: Explorations in the microstructure of cognition. Vol. 2. Psychological and biological models* (pp. 216–271). Cambridge, MA: MIT Press. Copyright 1986 by the MIT Press. Reprinted with permission.

TABLE 12.4. Regular and No-Change Response to Verbs Ending in "t" or "d" and Other Verbs

Verb ending	Regular suffix	No change
Not t/d	203	34
t/d	42	157

Note. Data from Bybee and Slobin (1982).

TABLE 12.5. The Model's Responses to Unfamiliar Low-Frequency Irregular Verbs

Presented word	Phonetic input	Phonetic response	English rendition	Response strength
bid	/bid/	/bid/	bid	0.55
thrust	/Tr^st/	/Tr^st^d/	thrusted	0.57
bend	/bend/	/bend^d/	bended	0.28
lend	/lend/	/lend^d/	lended	0.70
creep	/krEp/	/krEpt/	creeped	0.51
weep	/wEp/	/wEpt/	weeped	0.34
		/wept/	wept	0.33
catch	/kaC/	/kaCt/	catched	0.67
breed	/brEd/	/brEd^d/	breeded	0.48
grind	/grInd/	/grInd/	grind	0.44
wind	/wInd/	/wInd/	wind	0.37
cling	/kliN/	/kliNd/	clinged	0.28
		/kl^N/	clung	0.23
dig	/dig/	/digd/	digged	0.22
stick	/stik/	/stikt/	sticked	0.53
tear	/ter/	/terd/	teared	0.90

Note. From Rumelhart, D. E., & McClelland, J. L. (1986). On learning the past tenses of English verbs. In J. L. McClelland, D. E. Rumelhart, & the PDP Research Group (Eds.), *Parallel distributed processing: Explorations in the microstructure of cognition. Vol. 2. Psychological and biological models* (pp. 216–271). Cambridge, MA: MIT Press. Copyright 1986 by the MIT Press. Reprinted with permission.

TABLE 12.6. The Model's Responses to Unfamiliar Low-Frequency Regular Verbs

Verb type	Presented word	Phonetic input	Phonetic response	English rendition	Response strength
End in t/d	guard	/gɑrd/	/gɑrd/	guard	0.29
			/gɑrd^d/	guarded	0.26
	kid	/kid/	/kid/	kid	0.39
			/kid^d/	kidded	0.24
	mate	/mAt/	/mAt^d/	mated	0.43
			/mAd^d/	maded	0.23
	squat	/skw*t/	/skw*t^d/	squated	0.27
			/skw*t/	squat	0.22
End in unvoiced consonant	carp	/kɑrp/	/kɑrpt/	carped	0.28
			/kɑrpt^d/	carpted	0.21
	drip	/drip/	/dript^d/	dripted	0.28
			/dript/	dripped	0.22
	shape	/SAp/	/SApt/	shaped	0.43
			/Sipt/	shipped	0.27
	sip	/sip/	/sipt/	shipped	0.42
			/sept/	sepped	0.28
	slip	/slip/	/slept/	slept	0.40
	snap	/snap/	/snapt^d/	snapted	0.40
End in voiced consonant	brown	/brwn/	/brwnd/	browned	0.46
			/br*nd/	brawned	0.39
	hug	/h^g/	/h^g/	hug	0.59
	mail	/mA^l/	/mA^ld/	mailed	0.38
			/memb^ld/	membled	0.23
	tour	/tUr/	/tUrd^r/	toureder	0.31
			/tUrd/	toured	0.25

Note. From Rumelhart, D. E., & McClelland, J. L. (1986). On learning the past tenses of English verbs. In J. L. McClelland, D. E. Rumelhart, & the PDP Research Group (Eds.), *Parallel distributed processing: Explorations in the microstructure of cognition. Vol. 2. Psychological and biological models* (pp. 216–271). Cambridge, MA: MIT Press. Copyright 1986 by the MIT Press. Reprinted with permission.

The failure to incorporate morphemes cannot be considered a serious shortcoming, as the exact role of morphemic representations in the neural generation of language remains an open scientific question (see "PDP Models and Neural Structure," below).

The double dissociation between regular and irregular past-tense formation in patients with brain lesions has been seized upon with particular enthusiasm by linguists as a clear demonstration that parts of the brain instantiate a grammatical rule (adding "ed"), as opposed to "memorized associations." Of course the Rumelhart and McClelland model *implicitly* instantiates a number of rules, while the association of a capability for forming regular past-tense forms with anterior perisylvian cortex is perfectly consistent with another *implicitly* generated rule and in no way proves a generative rule, in the formal linguistic sense. Moreover, the double dissociation can fairly readily be accounted for by a graded interaction between two distributed connectionist mechanisms—one more anterior and involved in processes roughly subsumed under morphological grammar, the other posterior and semantically related. In this way, the learning of irregular past-tense endings (which actually represent varying degrees of irregularity) could depend to a greater (and variable) extent on posterior (semantic) input. Such an interactive process has provided the basis for a successful connectionist model of the various forms of dyslexia (Plaut, McClelland, Seidenberg, & Patterson, 1996; see "Dyslexia" under "A Synopsis of PDP studies of Language," below).

Recently developed modifications of the Rumelhart and McClelland (1986) model have successfully recapitulated children's behavior (currently better understood in view of further studies motivated by the model) at the same time that they incorporate better approximations of the language exposure of children (Plunkett & Marchman, 1991, 1993).

Modeling of Complex Behavioral Processes with Structured Pattern Associator Models

The preceding section has examined the learning capability of a two-level pattern associator model with no defined internal structure. However, there are many circumstances in which learning is of less interest than is the ability of a "knowledgeable" neural network to account for observed behavior. Moreover, for many types of behavior there is evidence of complex hierarchical structure instantiated by the brain, motivating studies of hierarchical models. Perhaps the best example of this type of behavior is language. In Chapter 3 of this volume, I have considered the potential applicability of PDP models to language output. Here I consider in some detail a model of auditory language decoding—the TRACE model developed by McClelland and Elman (1986)—in order to illustrate the power of a hierarchical pattern associator to account for observed behavior and the mechanisms by which it does so.

Figure 12.11 demonstrates the essential features of the model. It consists of three major levels: a word level, a phoneme level, and a distinctive-feature level. The model actually incorporates seven "distinctive features" as needed to uniquely define the phonemes in its vocabulary: power, degree of vocalicness, diffuseness, acuteness, consonantal, voicing, and burst amplitude (stops only). Only three of these are shown in Figure 12.11. Distinctive features are the discrete attributes of the oral–lingual–pharyngeal apparatus that in different combinations serve to define the phonemes available to us (see Nadeau, Chapter 3, this volume). The model incorporated 15 phonemes: /b/, /p/, /d/, /t/, /g/, /k/, /s/, /S/ ("sh" as in "ship"), /l/, /r/, /a/ (as in "pot"), /i/ (as in "beet"), /u/ (as in "boot"), /^/ (as in "but" and the second vowel of "target"), and /–/ for silence. Each phoneme was given a particular value (from 1 to 8) on each of the seven distinctive-feature dimensions. The model incorporated 211 words, made up of the phonemes available to it.

Each small rectangle in Figure 12.11 corresponds to a single unit in the TRACE network. Units within one level that are inconsistent with each other (i.e., their temporal spans overlap) are connected by mutually inhibitory connections, and units in different levels that are consistent with each other are connected by mutually excitatory connections. All connections are bidirectional. Units in any one level connect only to units in their own or the immediately adjacent levels. Activation is fed to the network only at the feature level one 25-millisecond slice at a time, beginning at the leftmost vertical slice at the feature level and moving successively toward the right. Thus there is no input in the first slice. In the succeeding seven time slices, progressively higher-amplitude input that is low in vocalic and acuteness features (arbitrarily assigned to interword silence in TRACE) is injected. At the eighth time slice, additional input that is high in acuteness and diffuseness and low in vocalicness (corresponding to /t/) is fed into TRACE with gradually increasing amplitude, at the same time that input corresponding to "silence" gradually dies out. Thus successive phonemes overlap, just as in real speech. This input actually represents "mock" speech because the sound of phonemes in this model, unlike in real speech, is not influenced by their phonetic environment. The entire sequence of input at the feature level for the word

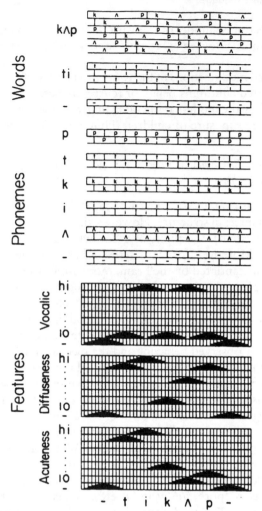

FIGURE 12.11. A subset of units from the TRACE model of auditory speech perception. See text for explanation. From McClelland, J. L., & Elman, J. L. (1986). Interactive processes in speech perception: The TRACE model. In J. L. McClelland, D. E. Rumelhart, & the PDP Research Group (Eds.), *Parallel distributed processing: Explorations in the microstructure of cognition. Vol. 2. Psychological and biological models* (pp. 58–121). Cambridge, MA: MIT Press. Copyright 1986 by the MIT Press. Reprinted with permission.

/tik^p/ ("teacup") is illustrated in Figure 12.11. At each slice, activity spreads up from the feature level to the phoneme level and thence to the word level, and subsequently back down from higher levels to lower levels for each phoneme. Input at the feature level continues over 11 time slices. Input to each phoneme unit from the feature level continues over 6 time slices, and input to each word unit continues over many time slices, depending on the length of the word. The multiple staggered but partially overlapping representations of each phoneme serve to distribute the influence of these units appropriately over time. Overall activity in the network is limited by investing each unit with a gradual-decay function. Even though input is only fed to one feature slice at any given time, spreading of activation occurs throughout the network, even after input ceases.

In general terms, TRACE contains three subnetworks containing local representations of features, phonemes, and words, respectively, and interconnected such that words are linked to their distributed representations at the phoneme and feature levels, and phonemes are linked to their distributed representations at the feature level. Thus words are represented as schemas corresponding to transient patterns of activation distributed over the units in the phoneme and feature levels. Long-term memory is represented in the connections between the various units, but working memory is represented as the transient pattern of activation of the units.

TRACE exhibits a number of important properties that accurately emulate behavior observed in empirical studies of human subjects:

1. Phonemic ambiguity is effectively resolved by the context in which it occurs. Figure 12.12 illustrates the results of input of /b–pl^g/ (interpretable as "blug" or "plug"), in which the feature pattern for the initial phoneme is intermediate between /b/ and /p/ (i.e., noisy input). The figure illustrates the amount of activation delivered to various phoneme and word units during "snapshots" taken at various times in the course of input of the feature stream, as indicated at the bottom of the graph by the ^ marks. As shown in the lower square on the left, /b/ and /p/ are initially given equal amounts of activation. Eventually the only four words in TRACE's vocabulary that begin with /pl/ or /bl/ are activated: "plug," "plus," "blush," and "blood." However, as the terminal /g/ is processed, it delivers activation only to "plug," which in turn delivers top-down activation to /p/ but not /b/, leading to the pattern of phoneme activation seen in the bottom right square.

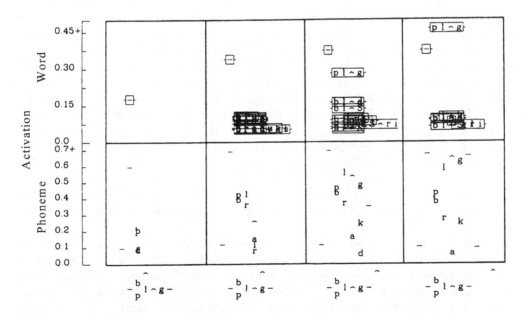

FIGURE 12.12. The time course of activation of various phoneme and word units following injection into TRACE of a distinctive-feature representation of "plug," in which the initial phoneme is ambiguous between /b/ and /p/. See text for explanation. From McClelland, J. L., & Elman, J. L. (1986). Interactive processes in speech perception: The TRACE model. In J. L. McClelland, D. E. Rumelhart, & the PDP Research Group (Eds.), *Parallel distributed processing: Explorations in the microstructure of cognition. Vol. 2. Psychological and biological models* (pp. 58–121). Cambridge, MA: MIT Press. Copyright 1986 by the MIT Press. Reprinted with permission.

2. Lexical influences are exerted on initial phonemes only when they are ambiguous; they are maximal on word-final segments; and lexical effects in general can be eliminated by time pressure. All three phenomena have been demonstrated in psychological studies and find a ready explanation in the fact that it takes time for lexical effects to take place as activation spreads from the bottom up to the top and back down again. If the initial phoneme is unambiguous, it will spread activation only to words beginning with this same phoneme, providing further top-down reinforcement of the phoneme regardless of subsequent phonemes. Only when the first phoneme is ambiguous does the top-down influence of words first activated by the initial phonemic alternatives and later culled by word-final phonemes serve to resolve the ambiguity. TRACE produces stronger lexical effects when a phoneme comes late in the word, simply because top-down activation of that phoneme is already occurring at the time the distinctive-feature units corresponding to that later phoneme are being activated at the bottom. Thus the response strength for the final /t/ in /sikrˆt/ ("secret") builds faster than in the nonword /gˆldˆt/, because the former provides top-down activation of /t/ while the latter, not in TRACE's vocabulary, does not.

3. Phonotactic rules are implicitly instantiated. TRACE does not include any explicit rules about which phonemic sequences are acceptable and which are not. However, in its behavior it reveals implicit knowledge of such restrictions—knowledge that is stored in connections between word and phoneme levels, and exerted via top-down spread of activation from the word level to the phoneme level. For example, the sequence /sli/ is permissible in English, but /sri/ is not. TRACE recognizes this fact because it has two words in its vocabulary incorporating /sli/, "sleep" and "sleet," and none incorporating /sri/; thus it will provide top-down reinforcement only of the phonotactically acceptable /sli/. The hypothesis that knowledge of phonotactic rules is lexically based leads to the prediction that certain sequences should be supported even if they violate phonotactic rules, because they receive activation from closely related words. In a test of this hypothesis, ambiguous phonemes halfway between /b/ and /d/ were presented to experimental subjects in three different contexts. When a legal word competed with an illegal nonword (e.g., "*b–d*windle," interpretable as "dwindle" or "bwindle"), subjects tended to hear the initial /b–d/ as /d/ (i.e., "dwindle") 63% of the time. Thus they favored the phonotactically legal sequence because of the top-down influence of "dwindle." When a legal nonword competed with an illegal nonword (e.g., "*b–d*wiffle"), subjects were as likely to hear /b/ as /d/, even though one was in an illegal phonotactic sequence, reflecting the fact that neither received top-down reinforcement. If the brain *explicitly* incorporated phonotactic rules (as opposed to implicitly incorporating them through lexical effects), subjects would have uniformly favored "dwiffle." When a legal nonword competed with an illegal near-word (e.g., "*b–d*wacelet"), subjects heard /b/ 55% of the time, reflecting the top-down influence of the near-miss "bracelet" even though /bw/ is phonotactically incorrect.

TRACE exhibits a variety of other properties that space limitations do not allow me to detail. Nevertheless, I have shown the ability of this hierarchical model to account in a systematic fashion for a number of empirically observed effects, some quite unexpected. This success of the model can be credited to its PDP nature. TRACE has a number of serious deficiencies, the solution to which is not simple or obvious. Most obvious is the need to reduplicate units and connections many times over, in order to capture an entire segment of the acoustic stream—a feature crucial to providing the opportunity for top-down effects to develop, and absolutely necessary to account for anticipatory and retroactive effects on interpretation of the acoustic stream. How the brain actually instantiates such serial order effects remains unclear. One idea is to incorporate delay units into the model, such that hidden units carry information about both the present and prior stimuli (Norris,

1992) (see "Phonological Processing" under "A Synopsis of PDP Studies of Language," below). The version of TRACE reviewed here is oversimplistic, in that it does not modify the features of phonemes according to their context. Finally, to the extent that learning algorithms can be incorporated into a model like TRACE, such learning will not generalize to other parts of the model. How the brain accommodates learning in complex hierarchical structures remains unclear, although I touch on this briefly later in the chapter.

PDP ATTRIBUTES OF PARTICULAR RELEVANCE TO LANGUAGE

Connectionist models display a number of properties that are relevant to language and other cognitive processes.

Distributed Representations

PDP models often employ local representations to one extent or another, both to accommodate computational limitations and to facilitate interpretation. However, their major source of power in modeling cognitive processes lies in distributed representations, because these provide the basis for nearly infinite shades of meaning or shades of interrelationship between schemas (discussed below), as well as such phenomena as graceful degradation, content-addressable memory, and inference (discussed later).

Consider a domestic pets network modeled on the room descriptor network. In this case the units may be various visual, auditory, tactile, and behavioral features of dogs, cats, guinea pigs, birds, fish, snakes, turtles, and iguanas. Given local representations of these creatures, assume that we clamp a given feature or set of features, such as "warm-blooded," less than 1 foot tall, "wags its tail," "fetches sticks," and "is loyal to its owner" (e.g., a Chihuahua). The network will activate the "dog" unit sufficiently to indicate a substantial probability that the creature is a dog. However, because the model has been taught that dogs are large, it will be dissuaded from a certain conclusion that the creature is a dog and indicate some probability that it is a cat or a guinea pig. An external observer will have to look at the relative degrees of activation of the various creature units and decide whether the activation of the "dog" unit is sufficiently high to be compelling. On the other hand, if the creatures are instantiated as distributed representations, the model will make this decision itself, settling into "dog" on the faith of its tail wagging, fetching sticks, and loyalty to its owner. In addition, it may activate the feature "high-pitched sound," since there are strong connections between "small" and "high-pitched sound" (derived from experience with birds, cats, and guinea pigs). Thus the model has correctly identified a creature it has never encountered before as a dog, demonstrating its sense of "dogness," as well as its ability to accept shadings in the meaning of "dog." It has also, unlike the model with local creature representations, transcended its ambivalence about such alternatives as "cat" and "guinea pig" *without external help* (by settling into the "dog" state), and it has made a correct inference about the quality of sound produced by Chihuahuas.

Distributed representations readily capture not just shades of meaning but shades of relationship. Thus the verb past-tense model captures a number of the subtle irregularities present in English past-tense forms. A model developed by McClelland and Kawamoto (1986) to assign thematic roles to major lexical items in sentences captures the notion that in the sentence "The bat broke the window," "bat" is potentially the agent (a flying bat) or an instrument (a baseball bat)—an ambiguity that would naturally be resolved by context.

This same model captures the shading of meaning that occurs when words are used in different contexts. Although "ball" was coded as a distributed representation over a number of features including "soft," when given the sentence "The ball broke the vase," the model generated a distributed representation essentially identical to "ball" except that it incorporated the feature "hard." It had learned from experience that breaking instruments are generally hard. So, too, we would naturally infer that the type of ball that can break a vase is hard, as opposed to a beach ball, which may break but only by knocking the vase over— a different concept. Thus distributed representations readily capture the subtle shadings of word meaning and role that derive from context.

Graceful Degradation

A lesion does not produce fundamental reorganization or production of a novel system. Errors tend to be near-misses, whether they reflect degraded input or damage to the network (e.g., phonemic and semantic paraphasias, errors in selection of inflectional morphemes). Network damage increases the probability of error rather than fundamentally altering function. Systems tend to work well in the face of ambiguity, incomplete data, or false information. In contrast, information-processing models have had to postulate such things as filters to account for the relative absence of phonological or morphological errors in aphasic individuals that violate rules of phonological sequencing (phonotactic constraints).

Because memories in PDP are also represented in distributed fashion, they tend to be resistant to the effects of discrete lesions. However, in the brain, whereas memories in general are defined as distributed representations over cortices representing many different modalities (visual, somatosensory, auditory, motoric, limbic), any given memory is likely to be represented to a greater degree in cortices supporting one or more particular modalities. For examples, as Warrington and colleagues have suggested, memories for living things are likely to be defined to a greater degree by their visual representations, whereas memories for nonliving things are likely to be defined to a greater degree by their functional or motoric representations (Warrington & McCarthy, 1983; Warrington & Shallice, 1984). Thus, in a brain conceived as a PDP machine, all memories will tend to degrade gracefully with focal lesions; however, there will be differential rates of degradation, depending on the locus of the lesion and the preponderant modalities of representation of particular memories. Lesions of visual cortices will produce greater degradation of memories for living things than for nonliving things. Because the various modality-specific portions of the distributed representations of memories are linked, they tend to be mutually supportive. Thus, while damage to visual association cortex will severely impair ability to describe the visual aspects of living things, it will also, to a lesser degree, degrade the ability to describe the functional attributes of living things because the functional distributed subrepresentation is no longer getting supportive input from the visual distributed subrepresentation. (See Farah & McClelland, 1991, for a review of this literature and a successful recapitulation of patient data by damage inflicted on a simple PDP model employing two-modality [visual and functional] distributed representations of memories.)

Associative Properties

Connectionist models are built on associative principles: Because strong connections between units facilitate the spread of activation between them, when one unit is activated the other will become activated as well. However, as I have discussed above under "Imple-mentation," these associations are explicitly nonlinear. The nonlinear properties of dynamic systems (systems that steadily evolve over time) are what enable them to achieve a multi-tude of discrete states and to define categorical outcomes. When nonlinearities incorpo-rate threshold functions and noise is introduced into these systems, their function assumes a probabilistic element, often referred to as "stochastic." When there is a great deal of redundancy built into a network, the probability will always be close to 100% that the desired output will be achieved. However, when substantial parts of a system are operat-ing at close to threshold levels, nonresponses or incorrect responses may occur. Damage to a system or noisy input increases the likelihood of such aberrant responses. Thus neuronal networks supporting language show evidence of operating close to threshold levels, as errors are fairly common in the spoken language of all of us—whether these are phonological slips, having a word "on the tip of the tongue," making semantic paraphasias, or using incorrect grammar. Damage to the brain enhances the probability of such errors.

Information does not flow from one part of a connectionist model to another or from one part of the brain to another. Rather, the spread of activation through a network asso-ciates certain units or representations with other units or representations. Thus, in one cerebral pattern associator network, a word meaning represented as a pattern of activa-tion in the semantic field becomes associated with a pattern of activity in phonological cortex that corresponds to the articulatory representation of the phonemes in that word. Other types of association may be discerned in language. Associations may reflect the simi-larity of underlying features. Thus, within semantic representations, "horse," "mule," and "donkey" are associated by virtue of their similarities in appearance, behavior, and use. Because of these similarities in underlying features, modest errors in a distributed repre-sentation of one entity (e.g., "mule") may lead to the selection of a word associated with another entity (e.g., "horse")—a semantic paraphasia. Within networks supporting pho-nological function, similar-sounding words are associated by virtue of the phonemes, joint phonemes, rhymes, and syllables they share; hence verbal paraphasias or malapropisms (word substitutions unrelated by meaning). Associations may also reflect the frequency with which two things co-occur. Thus, in the room descriptor model discussed earlier, "easy-chair" and "floor-lamp" were strongly associated, reflecting the fact that in the experi-ence of the raters whose judgments provided the basis for the connection weights, these two items commonly co-occur in living rooms. Associations may also reflect the frequency with which two things are used together. Thus function words (e.g., articles, prepositions, and auxiliary verbs) are uncommonly affected by phonemic paraphasias, suggesting enor-mous strength of association between the representations of these words and their compo-nent phonemes.

Even in realms of language whose fundamental neural principles are more elusive, such as grammar, associative properties can be discerned. For example, the more sources of grammatical association that favor a given (correct) response, the more likely that response is to occur. In a comprehension study in Serbo-Croatian agrammatical patients, case and gender markers and word order were opposed to animacy. All grammatical factors lost their efficacy in determining sentence interpretation; gender markers and word order alone became completely ineffective but could potentiate case, such that when the three were concordant, the correct interpretation was made most of the time (Smith & Bates, 1987; Smith & Mimica, 1984). Other observations suggest that the larger the grammatical lexi-con appropriate to a given circumstance, the less likely an omission error is to occur, but the more likely a misselection error is to occur. Thus the tendency to omit articles is inversely proportional to the number of grammatical constraints governing article selection in a speaker's native language. In Italian, articles are marked for number and gender; in German, they are marked for number, gender, and case; and in both languages, they are marked for definiteness or indefiniteness. Because of the multitude of article forms available in these languages, articles are less often omitted by Italian- or German-speaking patients with Wernicke's or Broca's aphasia than by English-speaking patients with these aphasias. At the same time, the number of inflectional forms produces a greater opportunity for selection errors; hence the greater frequency of paragrammatical errors in German- and Italian-speaking patients with either Wernicke's or Broca's aphasia than in English-speaking patients (Bates, Friederici, & Wulfeck, 1987).

As these examples illustrate, language involves a problem in "parallel-constraint satisfaction." That is, in any given linguistic circumstance, multiple nonlinear associative forces are brought to bear. These include context; the number and frequency of various meanings of the word; the frequency of the various grammatical opportunities posed by a sentence; and, in the case of language comprehension, the presence or absence of ambiguous orthographic or phonological forms (e.g., "rose," verb vs. noun; "wind," to "wind a watch" vs. "the wind blows"; "plain" vs. "plane"). The potential influence of context is nicely illustrated in the following:

"The horse raced past the barn fell."

Most readers will have trouble comprehending this sentence, and most will conclude that it is ungrammatical. However, if it is preceded by the sentence "The trainer raced one horse in the pasture and the other horse in the barnyard," it becomes clear that the proper interpretation of the sentence is this:

"The horse *that was* raced past the barn fell."

The interaction of semantics, grammar, and frequency is optimally posed in what are called "main verb/reduced relative clause" sentences, because the first verb in the sentence may appear to be the main verb but turns out to be the verb of a relative clause, the main verb appearing later. For this reason, these sentences have been the subject of extensive study (Trueswell, Tanenhaus, & Garnsey, 1994). Here are examples of such sentences:

"The defendant examined by the lawyer turned out to be unreliable."
"The evidence examined by the lawyer turned out to be unreliable."

The most frequent syntactic interpretation of "examined" is as an active verb for which the preceding noun or noun phrase is the agent. If the preceding noun is unambiguously agent-like, as is usually the case with animate objects (e.g., "defendant"), the preponderant syntactic interpretation is reinforced: One concludes that the defendant was studying something. This interpretation becomes manifestly incorrect when one progresses to "by the lawyer," which informs one that "examined" is in the passive voice (the less common syntactic structure for this verb) and that "defendant" is the object (or theme), not the agent. On the other hand, in the second sentence, "evidence" is inanimate and rarely agentive; this leads to immediate interpretation of "examined" as the passive form, in which case "by the lawyer" poses no surprises. Eye movement studies of reading have shown that readers will fixate significantly longer on "by the lawyer" when the sentence begins "The defendant" than when it begins "The evidence" (Trueswell *et al.*, 1994). The semantic–syntactic–frequency discordance in a sentence like "The defendant . . ." may be so extreme that the reader becomes lost on encountering "by the lawyer" and has to return to the beginning of the sentence—in which case it is often called a "garden path" sentence. Reading this sentence is facilitated if it is written:

"The defendant *who was* examined by the lawyer turned out to be unreliable."

Connectionist models are optimal devices for solving problems of parallel-constraint satisfaction. Furthermore, they naturally incorporate frequency effects in the form of the relative strengths of various connection weights achieved through variable experience with different representations. Although no truly satisfactory PDP model has yet been developed that incorporates the disparate linguistic parameters in a neurologically plausible architecture, research in connectionism is focusing strongly on this problem (MacDonald, Pearlmutter, & Seidenberg, 1994; Seidenberg, 1997) (Also, see "Sentence Comprehension" and "Lexical Ambiguity" under "A Synopsis of PDP Studies of Language," below).

Implicit Rule Learning

As has clearly been demonstrated in the past-tense pattern associator model, learning occurs through exposure to data, but networks, like the brain, ultimately behave as if they have learned rules. Connectionist networks are capable of learning both a common pattern—a central tendency of multiple stimuli (e.g., the past-tense rule of adding "ed")—and particular instances (e.g., "go–went").

Memory

In PDP, information processing and memory share the same circuitry. Thus knowledge or long-term memory about phonemes is represented in networks in dominant perisylvian cortex that subserve phonological processing. Within a network, there is no basis for distinguishing between loss of memory due to degradation of memory stores and loss of memory due to loss of access to memory stores. Loss of access in a PDP system can refer only to results of disconnection of one network from another. Thus a disconnection between semantic representations and phonological representations denies access of these representations to each other, even when the actual neural substrates for the representations are intact. Long-term memory, in PDP networks and in the brain, is represented in the strengths of connections between units and neurons, respectively. It is convenient to represent immediate or working memory in PDP models as the current pattern of activation, and our current understanding of neural function suggests that working memory is supported in similar fashion in the brain. However, working memory reflects complex processes that are as yet poorly understood, and simple activation representations will not support such features of immediate memory as primacy and serial order.

The learning algorithms employed in PDP, as exemplified in the past-tense model, most closely emulate procedural and associative memory in the brain (Squire, 1992; Squire & Zola-Morgan, 1991). Single-exposure learning and long-term consolidation are features of declarative memory that are attributable to functions of the hippocampal system but have not yet been implemented in PDP systems. Most models exhibit a serious shortcoming, in that learning a new data set results in catastrophic decline in performance on previously learned material (McCloskey & Cohen, 1989). McClelland, McNaughton, and

O'Reilly (1995) have shown that the problem of catastrophic interference can be circumvented by "interleaved learning"—the gradual introduction of new material as old material is being rehearsed. They propose that the hippocampus, perhaps in conjunction with superficial layers of the cerebral cortex, both serves to preserve new material until it is gradually learned, and provides the mechanisms for the interleaved learning process. This process—memory consolidation—take place in humans over more than a decade (humans with bilateral hippocampal lesions exhibit graded retrograde amnesia, maximal over the most recent 2–3 years but evident to some degree as far back as 13 years). They suggest, after David Marr (1971), that the hippocampally mediated interleaved learning process occurs at night, perhaps marked by hippocampal sharp waves. The problem of catastrophic interference has also been substantially circumvented by employing models with sparse representations (low ratio between units supporting a distributed representation and total number of units in the model; modest overlap between distributed representations), binary activation states (any given unit is either on or off), and Hebbian learning algorithms (Chappell & Humphreys, 1994). See Rolls and Treves (1998) for a full reconciliation of connectionist and neurophysiological knowledge in this area.

Clinicians often try to distinguish memory encoding from memory retrieval deficits by providing subjects with multiple choices after they have made an attempt at free recall. If performance improves with multiple choices, it is commonly concluded that the problem lies in retrieval. However, viewed in PDP terms, the provision of multiple choices adds additional selective activation (priming) to the network supporting the memory in question—activation that can compensate for the inadequacy of the representations that were established in the first place. Thus encoding and retrieval deficits cannot be distinguished in this simple fashion.

In a digital computer, memory contents are accessed by address or serial search through the entire memory. In connectionist networks, selection of a few features will activate a schema if that schema is latent in the network (i.e., memory is content-addressable). Content-addressable memory provides the basis for recognition. Input of a few clues leads to instantiation of a schema or concept (as a pattern of activity). The capacity for generating that schema was previously learned, and its instantiation by the clues lends meaning to the clues (i.e., recognition). A digital computer might be made to emulate content addressability by storing lists of locations of memories that share particular attributes. Obviously this would be a somewhat cumbersome arrangement, and it would contrast sharply with the intrinsic content addressability of PDP systems.

Inference

The content addressability of memory provides the basis for inference, recognition, and generalization. Incomplete information will lead to the activation of a limited number of units, which in turn may instantiate a schema by activating closely associated units. The generated schema is an inference based upon partial data. If correct, it may represent recognition (in the case of memory) or a warranted conclusion (in the case of hypotheses). However, it may be incorrect. Because the network has no intrinsic way of knowing it is incorrect, confabulation results. The blurring of the distinction between veridical recall and confabulation or plausible reconstruction seems to be characteristic of human memory. Another aspect of inference is generalization. Activation of certain units corresponding to a member of a group defined by a distributed representation may activate other units associated with that group that correspond to features of that group, even though all members of the group may not share those features (i.e., guilt by association).

Inferences can occur only to the extent that representations overlap. If there is no overlap (i.e., the representations are orthogonal), then inferences between representations cannot occur, even when they are generated in the same network. Thus, in the room descriptor model, the kitchen schema provides no basis for inferences about the bedroom schema. Although the presence of overlapping representations carries with it a sense of sloppiness, it provides the fundamental basis for inference and generalization.

To the extent that different stimuli elicit the same schema, their differences will tend to be minimized and overlooked. To the extent that different stimuli elicit different schemata, their differences will be maximized and reliably detected.

Top-Down and Bottom-Up Processing

PDP models differ fundamentally from serial order models not only in that multiple processes occur in parallel, but that multiple processing steps in a sequence may be carried out with substantial temporal overlap, and processing may proceed forward and backward as activation spreads and evolves through a network (note that this feature is consistently built into structured PDP models, but it is a variable feature of unstructured models developed to learn from experience through backpropagation algorithms). Activation originating at the bottom of a network (e.g., in acoustic representations) spreads up to the top of a network (e.g., acoustic word forms), and as it begins to produce activations at higher levels, these in turn begin to propagate activation back down, thereby shaping the emerging pattern of activation at the acoustic level. In this way, ambiguous information at the level of acoustic representations (due to noisy input or damage to the network) is selectively shaped through top-down excitation and inhibition, such that it tends to assume a comprehensible pattern corresponding to an acoustic word form. A homologous process in orthographic systems readily accounts for our tendency to overlook typographical errors, as top-down spread of activation actually alters our perception of ambiguous or conflicting material. This bottom-up and top-down processing facility instantiates what is in effect a filter that tends to eliminate "impermissible sequences"—namely, sequences that are not represented at upper levels of a hierarchical network. Viewed in another way, it instantiates in concrete, computational terms the interpretation of a stimulus within an environmental context.

Because bottom-up and top-down spread of activation takes time, it provides an opportunity for successive segments within a temporal language stream to interact as well. These processes are discussed at length in Chapter 3 of this volume.

PDP MODELS AND NEURAL STRUCTURE

The PDP models discussed in this chapter (and, indeed, the models in much of the PDP literature) are based on a highly simplistic, really cartoon-like conceptualizations of neurons or aggregations of neurons as "units." The claim that these models are neural-like thus rests on the degree to which they recapitulate the fundamental organizing principles of neural structures, rather than the detailed properties of neurons.

I have described two very different PDP models in the present book: interactive-activation models (IAMs) such as TRACE and the Dell-inspired model of phonological function (see Chapter 3), and distributed-representation models (DRMs) fundamentally similar to the past-tense verb model. IAMs are generally complex multilayer models that incorporate structure derived from our detailed knowledge of some brain function such as language. They incorporate local representations, and they generate output as they settle into a stable state in the course of bottom-up and top-down flow of activation. There is generally no capability for learning. IAMs were the first PDP models developed, and their enormous success in accounting for observed behavior (as well as their transparency) has contributed a great deal to their popularity and to the general appeal of PDP in behavioral neuroscience. DRMs are a more recent development. They tend to be shallower structures, incorporating layers of input and output units like the past-tense model, and typically an intermediate layer of hidden units (unlike the past-tense model). In early versions, flow of activation was strictly from the bottom up. Newer models incorporate two-way interlevel interactions (see below). During the learning phase, an error measure is computed, typically as the sum of the squared differences between each generated activity and its correct value; a mathematical algorithm (backpropagation) is used to calculate how each weight throughout the network contributes to the error; and the weights are changed incrementally to reduce the error (Rumelhart, Hinton, & Williams, 1986). The contemporaneous development of inexpensive but very powerful desktop computers has enabled simulation studies of DRMs sufficiently sophisticated to address complex and interesting behavioral issues.

IAMs have historically played a very useful role, because (1) their transparency—derived in good part from using local representations—facilitates understanding of PDP processes; (2) they have demonstrated very successfully the ramifications of spreading-activation dynamics; and (3) they have provided dramatic evidence of the power of bottom-up and top-down processing interactions to account for a large number of behavioral phenomena. However, DRM simulations have demonstrated the remarkable power of distributed representations in accounting for some of the most fundamental aspects of behavior, such as inference, generalization, content-addressable memory, and graceful degradation. They are much more realistic, because clearly the brain employs distributed, not local representations. Finally, they have enabled studies of learning.

With the evolution that has occurred from IAMs to DRMs, it is natural to ask about the problems that afflict DRMs. In the most general sense, their shortcomings correspond precisely to our lack of understanding of brain network structure and function—a lack that these models are helping to address. However, I focus here on several very specific problems.

Both TRACE and the phonology model developed in Chapter 3 (IAMs) incorporate multilevel hierarchies based on local representations. One crucial question arises: If the ontogenesis of the brain networks supporting these processes is constrained strictly at the input and output layers, why should the intervening hidden-unit levels in DRMs evolve to define recognizable entities? Take the much simpler model of Figure 12.13. Given sufficient training, such a model can learn to convert words to distinctive-feature representations. However, the hidden units that emerge will not have any obvious meaning. A given word will be represented as a distributed representation across these hidden units, as will any given feature. Recognizable intermediate constructs, such as phonemes or syllables, can only emerge as a different set of distributed representations over these hidden units, as in Figure 12.14. For the network to learn such a representational scheme, it will have to be trained using both phonemes and words as input. This is feasible (Norris, 1992). However, let us consider more fully the implications of this line of thinking. Were we to reconceive the PDP network of phonological output processing (Chapter 3) in these terms, the result would be that depicted in Figure 12.15. Because the various intermediate forms depicted in Figure 12.15 (affixes, syllables, rhymes, joint phonemes) have no meaning, it does not seem likely that they evolved out of neural networks supporting meaning (seman-

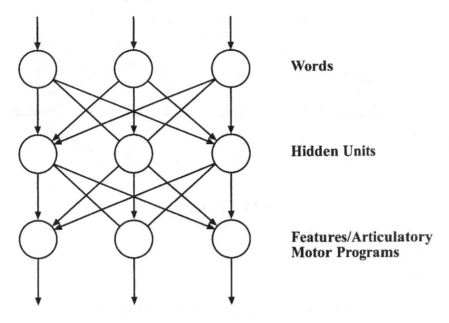

FIGURE 12.13. See text for explanation.

tics). By the same token, if we view language as fundamentally representing phonemic processing, it is not at first clear how such structures could emerge from networks supporting articulatory and acoustic processing. However, the process of repetition involves the conversion of *sequences* of acoustic patterns into *sequences* of articulatory patterns. Hidden units in a PDP processor learning this conversion routine will learn the regularities in correspondences between acoustic and articulatory sequences (see "Dyslexia" under "A Synopsis of PDP Studies of Language," below). It is precisely these regularities that are

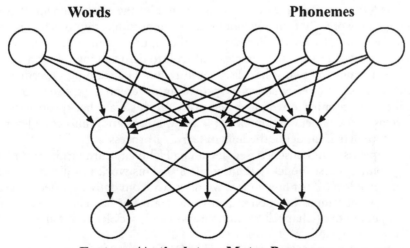

FIGURE 12.14. See text for explanation.

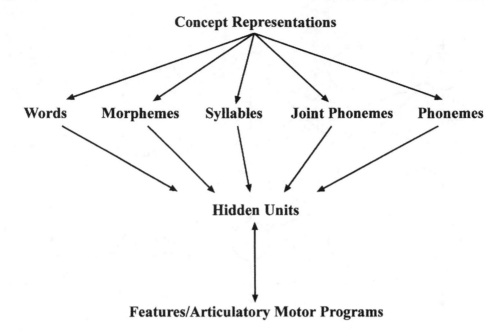

FIGURE 12.15. See text for explanation.

captured by the intermediate forms. To fully capture the relationships depicted in Figure 12.15 in a neurally and developmentally plausible way, we need only posit connections between neural networks supporting semantics and the hidden units in the acoustic–articulatory PDP processor, as depicted in Figure 12.16.

Other problems with DRMs as they are usually instantiated are (1) that they employ a learning device that is most unnatural in that it is minutely supervised, and (2) they require a huge number of interactions (unlike the one-time-only instantiation of declarative memory mediated by the hippocampal system). The great advantage of the backpropagation algorithm that has led to its widespread use is that it enables the establishment of connection weights in large networks that employ thousands of connections, thus precluding the setting of connection weights "by hand." Furthermore, the input–output relationships implicit in these connection weights are often complex, difficult to define in logical terms, and apparent only after a trained network has discovered them. The training procedure can also incorporate stimulus frequency effects by providing differential exposure to the various stimuli in the large number of training iterations. In this way, backpropagation can be viewed more as an extremely useful way of loading information into complex networks, rather than as an actual model of the human learning process.

Various supervised and unsupervised (including Hebbian) learning algorithms are being explored by connectionist modelers (Hinton, 1989). This work has directed renewed attention to the problem of just how in fact we do learn from daily experience. The precise mechanism of hippocampal function remains uncertain but has been reviewed from the connectionist perspective (Chappell & Humphreys, 1994; McClelland et al., 1995; O'Reilly & McClelland, 1994; Rolls & Treves, 1998).

Recent connectionist research has turned to DRMs that incorporate two-way activation flow. Figure 12.17 depicts a typical organization of a standard DRM, employed in this particular case as a model of reading aloud. All representations are distributed, and a

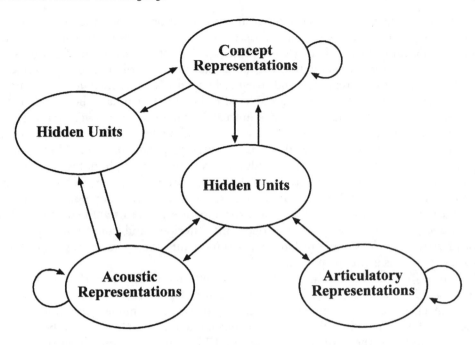

FIGURE 12.16. Hypothetical alternative model of phonological processing.

standard backpropagation algorithm is employed to adjust the connection weights gradually over 300 training passes through the vocabulary, until an input graphemic sequence corresponding to a single-syllable English word is translated into the appropriate phonological sequence with a criterion degree of accuracy. As an aid to understanding, the ultimate outcome may be viewed as matching points in two planes: an input plane on which scattered points correspond to orthographic representations, and an output plane on which

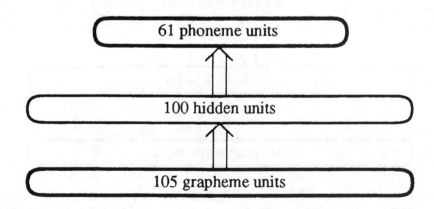

FIGURE 12.17. A typical backpropagation network model, employed to simulate reading aloud. From Plaut, D. C., McClelland, J. L., Seidenberg, M. S., & Patterson, K. (1996). Understanding normal and impaired word reading: Computational principles in quasi-regular domains. *Psychological Review*, *103*, 56–115. Copyright © 1996 by the American Psychological Association. Reprinted with permission.

scattered points correspond to phonological representations. When the model has been trained to criterion, the choice of a point on the input plane leads to the choice of a location in the output plane that is very close to the appropriate target point. If our only goal were a feasibility study, to show that the model can satisfactorily pair orthographic and phonological strings for regularly and irregularly spelled words, this would be satisfactory. However, our goals are more ambitious: to be able to emulate the brain's performance when given novel input (e.g., pronounceable nonwords) or network damage; and, more fundamentally, to emulate the brain's way of handling this problem. Introducing novel input or creating network damage also creates a very pragmatic problem: Now picking a point in the input orthographic plane yields a locus in the output phonological plane that is not very close to the target point. If it is closer to an alternate point, we may choose to call it a paralexical error. If it is beyond a criterion distance from any point in the target plane, we may choose to call it an anomic error. However, it seems unlikely that the brain uses distance from the target point as its operating criterion—and from a purely pragmatic point of view, how does one translate such distances into the operational grist of human experiments in this genre: naming latency?

An innovative solution to these problems is reflected in the network in Figure 12.18 (Plaut et al., 1996). This network differs from that in Figure 12.17 in that there are feedback connections from each unit in the output layer to each hidden unit, and there are connections between each of the units in the output layer. This network can be trained in a manner similar to the network in Figure 12.17 by using a modification of the backpropagation algorithm called "backpropagation over time." The recurrent connections and the interconnections give this network the capability for settling into the best answer over a period of time in precisely the same manner as the room descriptor model gradually settles into a state corresponding to a particular room. To return to the metaphor of points in a plane, the extra connections have transformed the points in the output plane into basins of various size, shape, and depth. When the network generates a moderate miss (because of novel input or network damage), the output will land in one of these basins and, over time,

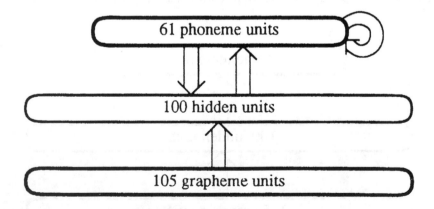

FIGURE 12.18. An adaptation of the backpropagation network model depicted in Figure 12.17, employing feedback connections from the output units to the hidden units and interconnections between hidden units. These additional connections give the network the capabilities of an attractor network (see text). From Plaut, D. C., McClelland, J. L., Seidenberg, M. S., & Patterson, K. (1996). Understanding normal and impaired word reading: Computational principles in quasi-regular domains. *Psychological Review, 103,* 56–115. Copyright © 1996 by the American Psychological Association. Reprinted with permission.

settle to the bottom of the basin. The time to settle provides a natural measure of naming latency. The forces in the network that drive it to settle in the bottom of basins have led to the term "attractor network" to describe this type of model.

To fully demonstrate the significance of this innovation, it is necessary to add a degree of complexity to the metaphor of points and basins in planes: The basins do not correspond to actual words, but to clusters of phonemic features that the model has learned through experience are associated with each other to one degree or another. If the output layer corresponds to semantic features, these clusters will correspond to features that are associated with each other to the extent that they define discrete concepts (again as in the room descriptor model). By limiting the possible outcomes on the basis of the structure it has imputed from the learning experience, the model is exerting top-down influence on the interpretation of novel input or input rendered noisy by network damage. Thus this model not only has allowed a pragmatically desirable outcome, but has incorporated one of the single most appealing features of IAMs and the heuristic value of being able to utilize the backpropagation algorithm to wire a network containing thousands of connections (26,582 in the network depicted in Figure 12.18). Were this type of network applied to acoustic–phonological processing, nearly all the various phonological clumping effects instantiated in the Dell-derived model (Chapter 3) or the alternative depicted in Figure 12.16 might well be captured in the implicit structure in the single network, exactly analogous to the grapheme-to-phoneme network discussed here.

NEURAL PLAUSIBILITY OF COMPUTATIONAL MODELS

PDP models have been developed in the context of a long history of computational models, many extraordinarily sophisticated and capable (see, e.g., the review by Carpenter, Miyake, & Just, 1995). The standard for judging computational models has been primarily, if not exclusively, their ability to account for empirical data (i.e., their heuristic value). PDP models are held to this same standard, but their particular value derives from their ability to meet a second standard, that of neural plausibility. To the extent that a model is neurally plausible, the assumptions built into that model represent testable hypotheses about neural structure and function, not just about brain function.

The neural plausibility of a particular model is difficult to judge, because we have only very vague ideas about the precise ways in which neuronal networks actually function. However, we can identify some features of PDP models that are absolutely characteristic of neural networks: (1) behavior as an emergent property of large numbers of relatively simple units extensively interconnected with each other; (2) processing through the spread of activation; (3) schemas defined by distributed representations; (4) knowledge represented in the strength of interunit connections; (5) bottom-up and top-down flow of information via the reciprocal connections that are ubiquitous in the brain; and (6) networks that support both memory and processing. That a great deal remains to be learned about the detailed basis of these features does not reduce our certainty that they are indeed characteristics of neural microstructure.

It is common these days to see various computational models held up as viable if not superior alternatives to PDP models, or to see one PDP model touted as superior to another. How does one judge their neural plausibility? A few examples may help to answer this question. Coltheart and colleagues (Coltheart, Curtis, Atkins, & Haller, 1993; Coltheart & Rastle, 1994) have developed a three-route reading model (letter-to-phoneme conversion, lexical, and semantic routes) as an alternative to the two-route model developed by

Plaut et al. (1996) (see "Dyslexia" under "A Synopsis of PDP Studies of Language," below). Their letter-to-phoneme conversion route employs, in essence, a look-up table to derive the correct phoneme from a particular letter or combination of letters. As a digital computer device, this is not neurally plausible; also, if damaged by a lesion, it would clearly fail catastrophically, not gracefully. Furthermore, the lexical route of this model employs entirely local representations. Although local representations have been used extensively in PDP models and have served many good purposes (simplification, clarification, demonstration of bottom-up and top-down processing effects, the effects of spreading activation), the distributed representations employed in the Plaut et al. (1996) PDP model clearly represent a substantial advance in neural plausibility over the model of Coltheart and colleagues.

Just and Carpenter (1992) have developed a model of syntactic processing that accounts remarkably well for performance on ambiguous sentences such as the sentences with reduced relative clauses discussed earlier. However, the structure of the model is inspired by phrase structure rules, not by principles of neural network architecture. Thus, although the model provides a powerful account for brain behavior, it tells us nothing about how that behavior arises out of neural network function, and it does not allow us to test any hypotheses about neural network function.

In PDP models, graceful degradation is a natural outcome of the facts that memory and processing take place in the same network and that both are distributed throughout the network. Partial damage anywhere in the network can thus cause only modest declines in the reliability of knowledge recovery and processing efficiency. Knowledge and processing are intrinsically always a matter of degree. Networks that separate knowledge from processing (e.g., Haarman & Kilk, 1991; Just & Carpenter, 1992) must resort to loss of abstract resources that are not tied to specific brain structures or processes; cannot account for why these resources, but not the knowledge and processes themselves, are affected by lesions; cannot account for graded degradation of knowledge and processes; and rely on transfer of symbolic entities, rather than spread of activation, to provide input to their models. Thus, in the final analysis, however great their heuristic value, they do not help us to understand how neural microstructure generates behavior.

A SYNOPSIS OF PDP STUDIES OF LANGUAGE

Context Effects in Letter Perception

In an early study, McClelland and Rumelhart (McClelland & Rumelhart, 1981; Rumelhart & McClelland, 1982) constructed a three-level IAM. This model consisted of a bottom feature level made up of units corresponding to each of the various line segments required to construct upper-case letters; an intermediate level of letter units; and a top level of four-letter word units. There was free flow of excitatory and inhibitory activity between levels, and units were mutually inhibitory within levels, providing the basis for winner-take-all effects (the greater the activity of a unit, the greater its ability to squelch its same-level neighbors). McClelland and Rumelhart were able to simulate a variety of effects already demonstrated experimentally in human studies, including better letter perception when a letter is part of a word or of a nonword sharing many letters with real words. Such effects result from the top-down spread of activation from words to their component letters, and in the case of nonwords, top-down ramifications of competition between the various words that resemble the nonword. The model was able to identify letters that were ambiguous because of missing features by utilizing word knowledge. Finally, the model was used to test a variety of effects that had not previously been tested in human subjects. This investigation was very influential because it demonstrated the ability of a relatively simple IAM to account for an enormous body of experimental data, and to do so via fairly transparent and neurophysiologically appealing mechanisms.

Dyslexia

Printed-to-Spoken-Word Encoding and Surface Dyslexia

Seidenberg, McClelland, and Patterson (Patterson, Seidenberg, & McClelland, 1989; Seidenberg & McClelland, 1989) developed a three-layer model composed of orthographic input units, phonological output units, and an intermediate layer of hidden units. Wickelfeatures were encoded by output units, and analogous coarsely coded three-grapheme clusters (i.e., with some overlap in their distributed representations) were used for input units. Regular and irregular words were handled in similar fashion. The model was trained on a large corpus of single-syllable English words, and a standard back-propagation algorithm was used to adjust connection weights. This model recapitulated a number of phenomena observed in normal human subjects, including faster naming of high-frequency words and little impact of degree of regularity in spelling on the latency of naming of high-frequency words; slow naming of low-frequency words whose spelling–sound correspondence is truly exceptional (e.g., "pint," "sew")(highly inconsistent); somewhat faster naming of low-frequency words whose spelling–sound correspondence is ambiguous (e.g., "gown," "down," "brown" vs. "blown," "shown," "grown") (moderately inconsistent); still shorter latencies for low-frequency mildly inconsistent words (e.g., "mint," "lint," "print," where the single exception is "pint"); and the shortest latencies (only slightly longer than for higher-frequency words) for low-frequency regular words (e.g., "must").

When the model was damaged (thus modeling acquired dyslexia), errors increased for all types of words in proportion to extent of damage. However, the difference in error score between correct and alternative pronunciations was always less for inconsistent words. Thus substitutions of the alternative (regularized) form of inconsistent words were relatively more likely than substitutions for regular words, generally emulating the pattern of surface dyslexia.

Plaut et al. (1996) have since refined this model in important ways. By changing to a straightforward representation of graphemes and phonemes (in lieu of Wickelfeatures), they have developed a model that acquires a better implicit knowledge of grapheme-to-phoneme correspondences. This improvement is reflected in a performance on pronounceable nonwords (poor in the 1989 model) that is precisely as good as that of human subjects. This model also captures the frequency–consistency interactions observed in the original model. By adding recurrent connections between hidden unit and output unit layers and interconnections between the output units, Plant et al. endowed this model with the features of an attractor network (see "PDP Models and Neural Structure," above). Finally, they revisited the problem of surface and phonological dyslexia. To do this, they modified the training of the model by incorporating progressive input to phoneme layer units from an external source (conceived as semantics) that was proportional to word frequency but conveyed no word-specific information. Thus, in this new model, part of the information—a part that was purely frequency-dependent—was derived from this external input rather than from learned grapheme–phoneme correspondences. Pronounceable nonwords and highly consistent words were relatively immune to the effects of lesions to this outside, "semantic" source, because their grapheme–phoneme correspondence patterns were unambiguously represented in the network. However, inconsistent words, even in the isolated orthographic–phonological network, were less redundantly represented in the orthographic–phonological correspondence patterns because these patterns conflicted (e.g., "brown" vs. "shown"). When the network was trained with semantic input, these conflicting correspondence patterns were even less well learned to the extent that the outside semantic input contributed to the target activation patterns of the words involved. When semantic input to the network was reduced (by increasing noise in the connections), these inconsistent patterns were particularly likely to be dominated by the correspondence patterns most unambiguously entrenched in the orthographic–phonological network, leading to regularization errors. Thus a lesion that preferentially damaged semantic input to the network reproduced the pattern of surface dyslexia (in which lexical–semantic dysfunction is characteristically severe). By inference (this was not actually tested), a lesion that preferentially damages the orthographic–phonological network itself will lead to particular impairment in applying grapheme–phoneme correspondence patterns, and hence maximal impairment in pronounceable nonword reading; however, it will relatively spare (in a frequency-dependent fashion) real words, whether consistent or inconsistent—the pattern of phonological dyslexia.

Thus the interactive semantic–orthographic–phonological network can account for the two dyslexias without the requirement of a separate lexical route, in fact incorporating a single reading pathway linked to graded (albeit vastly simplified) semantic influence. This connectionist model accounts for the data much better than the traditional two-route model: Unlike the two-route model, which dichotomizes words into regular (consistent) and irregular (inconsistent), the connectionist model provides a logical accounting for the *graded* consistency that actually exists. It also offers a logical accounting for the different performance of persons with various developmental and acquired dyslexias in terms of individual differences in the relative tradeoffs between phonology and semantics during the network development of reading skills. These differences interact, in turn, with differences in the distribution of damage in acquired lesions.

Printed-Word-to-Concept Encoding and Deep Dyslexia

Hinton and Shallice (1991) constructed a network consisting of an input graphemic layer, a layer of hidden units, and an output sememe layer. Local representations were used in the grapheme layer. There were four groups of units corresponding to the four positions of each of the three- or four-letter input words, and within each group was a place for each of the letters that could appear in that word position, using the 40 words in the model's vocabulary (8 each of indoor objects, animals, body parts, foods, and outdoor objects). Distributed representations were used in the sememe layer, each unit corresponding to a given semantic feature. Thus the meaning of a word was defined by a particular pattern of on-and-off units in the sememe layer. Sememe units were heavily interconnected (largely via an additional set of hidden units), providing the model with attractor network properties. The entire network was trained via the backpropagation procedure, and then it was damaged at various points by randomly eliminating a percentage of units, setting some connection weights to zero, or adding noise. Lesions induced semantic errors (e.g., "mud" → "bog"), visual errors (e.g., "bun" → "rum"), mixed semantic–visual errors (e.g., "cat" → "rat"), and "other" errors (visually and semantically unrelated). Noise in connections from grapheme units to intermediate units was particularly likely to lead to visual errors, and disconnection of intermediate units from sememe units was especially likely to lead to semantic errors. Depending on criteria set for response strength, the network was variably "anomic" (i.e., failed to make any response at all).

Plaut and Shallice (1991, 1993) subsequently modified this model in several ways in an effort to simulate specific aspects of deep dyslexia. Most importantly, they added another layer of intermediate units followed by a phonological unit layer after the semantics layer (trained separately) in order to enable the semantics layer to provide phonological output, and they changed the vocabulary to include a mix of concrete and abstract words. The operational difference between these two word types was the average number of semantic features defining them: 18.2 for concrete, 4.7 for abstract. The model was trained to criterion and then damaged in the same ways as the model already discussed. In general, there were more correct responses to concrete than to abstract words except when the lesion involved the semantic level itself (the usual finding in deep dyslexia), in which case abstract words enjoyed an advantage (the finding in one reported case). Also as in deep dyslexia, visual errors were more common with abstract than with concrete words. The susceptibility of abstract words to visual errors reflected their relative paucity of semantic features. Consequently, they were supported by fewer links within the semantic level—links that would tend to bind near-misses to their semantic schemas (creating correct responses or semantic paraphasias), and thus to resist slips originating between orthographic and semantic levels that produce a high frequency of visual errors. Visual errors involving abstract words were thus less likely to be cleaned up.

Rehabilitation Effects in a Model of Deep Dyslexia

Plaut (1996) employed a three-layer model consisting of input units providing the basis for distributed representations of three- to four-letter word orthography; intermediate units; and output units providing the basis for distributed representations of words over semantic features. Semantic units were partially interconnected, providing the basis for attractor network features. This model was tested in prior extensive modeling studies of deep dyslexia (see the discussion just above). After it was trained to criterion on 40 words, the network was damaged by randomly destroying connections at certain levels, and then it was retrained on the entire 40 words or on a randomly chosen subset of 20. Regardless of lesion locus, the model relearned at a far higher rate than it learned in the first place, reflecting the extensive information that remained in the network connections despite the damage. Retraining after damage to semantic interconnections produced a rapid return to nearly perfect performance on the trained items and a pronounced improvement on untrained items—indicating substantial generalization of learning. However, retraining after lesions of the orthographic-to-intermediate-unit connections produced somewhat more modest improvement in trained items (still much faster learning than during the original training) but no generalization. The reason for the differential effect of lesion locus on generalization was that there was substantial overlap in semantic representations of words. Thus improvement in the generation of trained semantic representations contributed to improvement in untrained but partially overlapping representations. However, relationships between orthography and semantics are arbitrary. As a result, they are completely orthogonal: Retraining of one word-to-meaning correspondence contributes nothing to the retraining of another word-to-meaning correspondence. This investigation serves to emphasize differences in the behavior of overlapping and orthogonal representations, as noted earlier in the chapter.

Neglect and Attentional Dyslexia

Mozer and Behrman (1992) developed an IAM of reading that incorporated an attentional mechanism. The attentionally lesioned model successfully accounted for a number of attributes of neglect dyslexia: the tendency to neglect the left side of words; the tendency to extinguish the left word of word pairs; improvement in performance proportional to the distance a stimulus is moved into right hemispace; improvement with directed attention to left hemispace; better performance with words than with nonwords; better performance with word pairs that can combine (e.g., "cow boy" as opposed to "sun fly"); and tendency to exhibit left-sided neglect with words that contain embedded words on the right (e.g., "peanut," "triangle"), but to exhibit incorrect backward completion with words that do not contain such embedded words (e.g., "Irish" or "Polish" for "Parish"). They were also able, with different adjustment of model parameters, to simulate the behavior of normal subjects whose attention is directed to the right (Behrmann, Moscovitch, & Mozer, 1991). The model, lesioned in a different fashion, accounted for the problems of attentional dyslexia, including inability to read words letter by letter; difficulty in identifying a letter surrounded by other letters; and tendency of letters to migrate from one word to another, yielding anticipatory or perseverative paralexical errors.

A Programmable Blackboard Model of Reading

McClelland (1986) attempted to deal with the problem of simultaneous processing of multiple sequential items in a serial stream, as in reading or listening to spoken language—in this case, in a reading model. The essence of the problem is that actual reading reflects the combined effects of knowledge about letter–word correspondences, interactions between adjacent words, and serial position effects (i.e., the letter string at the center of foveation enjoys primacy, even though it may be influenced by preceding and following letter strings). McClelland achieved these effects through a model consisting of a "central module" in which knowledge of letter–word correspondences was stored in connection strengths, and a series of "programmable modules," each of which processed a letter cluster in the input stream. The programmable modules derived their knowledge about letter–word correspondences through connection strengths that were transiently defined, as needed, by the central module. At the same time, programmable modules influenced each other via their simultaneous projections to the central module. This model also partially separated working memory (the pattern of connection strengths in the programmable modules) from long-term memory (the pattern of connection strengths in the central module).

Phrase Analysis

Wermter and Lehnert (1992) developed a PDP model to interpret the relationships between noun phrases in sequences of prepositional phrases, such as "symposium on hydrodynamics in the ionosphere." The most reasonable interpretation of this sequence is that "hydrodynamics in the ionosphere" is the subject of the symposium, as it is unlikely that the symposium itself would take place in the upper levels of the atmosphere. The constraints in the Wermter and Lehnert model included the plausibility of prepositional relationships, the physical distance between noun phrases, and the presence or absence of a violation of the "no-crossing" constraint (e.g., "influence of the temperature on the electrons in Fahren-heit," in which "influence" relates to electrons and "Fahrenheit" relates to temperature—i.e., the relationships "cross"). The plausibility of prepositional relationships was learned by separate pattern associator networks developed for each preposition, which were exposed to large corpuses of plausible (e.g., "hydrodynamics in ionosphere") and implausible (e.g., "symposium in ionosphere") noun pairs, each noun represented as clusters of semantic features. This work provides a plausible explanation for the acquisition and representa-tion of our knowledge of the various semantic relationships between nouns that define the selection of prepositions. It also illustrates how different linguistic constraints can be brought to bear simultaneously to support natural language interpretation (i.e., parallel-constraint satisfaction).

Sentence Comprehension

St. John and McClelland (McClelland, St. John, & Taraband, 1989; St. John & McClelland, 1992) developed a model designed to comprehend single-clause sentences (i.e., to make the appropriate thematic role assignments). Sentences included active- and passive-voice forms as well as ambiguous words. For example, in the sentence "The pitcher threw the ball," "pitcher" can refer to a baseball player or a container, "threw" to propelling or hosting, and "ball" to a sphere or a dance. Only the combination of words succeeds in disambiguating these terms. As the model was fed each succeeding word of the sentence, it updated its thematic role assignments according to the new semantic and syntactic informa-tion it had just received, and narrowed the inferences it had made from prior information. The model learned to interpret sentences through extended training using a backpropagation algorithm. Thus it approached sentence comprehension as a problem in parallel-constraint satisfaction, in which multiple semantic and syntactic pieces of information competed in defining the ultimate interpretation of the sentence. The authors also applied a similar model to story comprehension (St. John, 1992; St. John & McClelland, 1992).

Lexical Ambiguity

Kawamoto (1988, 1993) developed a network of 216 units over which 12 pairs of ambiguous four-letter words were mapped as distributed representations (e.g., "fine" (adjective—adequate), "fine" (noun—money payment); "rose" (noun—flower), "rose" (adjective—hue); "dove" (noun—bird), "dove" (verb—went in head first). Forty-eight of the units were used to represent graphemic features, 48 for phonemic features, 24 for syntactic features, and 96 for semantic features. Every unit was connected to every other unit, forming an autoassociator network (like the room descriptor model). The network was then trained so that the presentation of the graphemic portion of a word would elicit a pattern of activity in the remaining 168 units corresponding to the appropriate phonemic, syntactic, and semantic features. Word frequency was captured by the amount of exposure the network was given to a particular version of a word. Once trained, the network would reliably end up with the most common form when there was a large frequency disparity, but some-times, depending on the exact training history, it would end up with a less common form when the frequency of the two forms differed only slightly. When the network was seman-tically or syntactically primed (by activating the appropriate units ahead of time), activation patterns corresponding to both forms of the word would initially grow; eventually, however, the activation of the primed form would accelerate to a maximum, and the activation corresponding to the unprimed form would die out. Context and frequency competed in this process, but context tended to win. This experiment exactly replicated findings from priming experiments in humans that, regardless of context, all available meanings of a word are initially accessed but only the primed form is retained after sufficient time has elapsed. Kawamoto was also able to demonstrate priming effects latent in word sequence by building in a buffer module that "remembered" the last word processed. The syntactic units of the word in the buffer were then linked to the autoassociator module in such a way that only certain syntactic transitions were allowed (e.g., adjective $\rightarrow$ adjective or noun; noun $\rightarrow$ preposition or verb). Despite the ambiguity of syntactic priming provided in this way, the network successfully arrived at syntactically acceptable sequences—an exercise in parallel-constraint satisfaction. The importance of this model lies in its demonstration of the ease with which different senses of a word can be generated from variously competing semantic, syntactic, frequency, and contextual influences, given linked distributed representations; the way in which frequency can be represented as a natural attribute of this system (connection weights); and the faithful replication of the time course of events observed in human lexical priming experiments.

Phonological Processing

Dell, Julian, and Govindjee (1993) constructed a three-level model of phonological processing comprised of an input lexical layer, an intermediate hidden-unit layer, and an output phonological feature layer. In addition, the model had feedback from the hidden-unit layer that was delayed one time step and projected back to the hidden-unit layer, and feedback from the output layer that was projected back to the hidden-unit layer. These recurrence features provided the hidden-unit layer with information about prior performance that enabled it to perform sequential processing. An input lexical representation consisted of a random distribution of 30 0's and 1's (in effect, a distributed representation over 30 semantic feature units of one of the 50 three-phoneme words on which the model was trained), and the output phonological representations consisted of 18 units corresponding to English phonological distinctive features. As a new input word was provided, activation flowed, and a representation of the first phoneme of the output appeared in the output layer. The feedback of this output and the hidden-unit pattern though the recurrent pathways then triggered the second phoneme of the word in the output. Repeated feedback then triggered the third phoneme and finally a null pattern signaling the end of the word. As each output pattern was produced, the network was trained using a backpropagation algorithm. After the network was trained to criterion, it achieved 90% correct performance. Of the errors, 92.6% involved phonotactically legal strings (compared with 99% in natural error collections from normal subjects). Consonants substituted for consonants and vowels for vowels 97.6% of the time (compared with at least 99.5% in natural error corpuses). Of the substitutions, 5.6% were vowel–consonant substitutions and 2.1% were consonant–vowel (compared with 6% and 2% in natural error corpora). Since most of the words were consonant–vowel–consonant, this corresponds to relative preservation of the rhyme constituent. Single-consonant errors involved syllable (word) onsets 61.6% of the time (compared with 62% in natural error corpora). These various effects reflect the degree to which the model had learned the patterns of phonological sequences in the 50-word training set. The high substitution rate on the first phoneme reflects the fact that the model was selecting this phoneme without any context provided by the recurrent links. Finally, the phonemic substitutions tended to be near-misses in terms of number of distinctive features.

With certain lesions of the model (e.g., noise added to connections between hidden units and output units), the number of errors increased only modestly, and the pattern of errors remained the same. However, with other lesions (e.g., noise added to the recurrent connections), the model's performance declined sharply: Phonotactic violations rose to 18.9%, and errors no longer tended to involve initial consonants, doing so only 24.3% of the time. The question arises as to whether the model would degrade more gracefully if lesions involved both direct and recurrent pathways (as would probably be the case in the brain).

Deep Dysphasia

Martin, Dell, Saffran, and Schwartz (1994) extended their prior (Martin & Saffran, 1992), in-depth neuropsychological study of a patient with deep dysphasia by reporting the results of their efforts to simulate this patient's behavior with an IAM. Their patient, NC, experienced a left middle cerebral artery aneurysmal subarachnoid and intracerebral hemorrhage that left him with what would traditionally be defined as Wernicke's aphasia. His spontaneous speech was fluent but contained numerous formal verbal paraphasias, semantic paraphasias, phonological paraphasias, and neologisms (most target-related). Comprehension was poor. Digit span was profoundly reduced (0.65). Naming was characterized by a high frequency of formal verbal paraphasias (20%), some semantic paraphasias (3%), and many neologisms (21%), as well as occasional neologisms and formal paraphasias on semantic paraphasias. He was able to repeat 58% of concrete words, 17% of abstract words, 21% of closed-class words, and 3% of nonwords. Repetition errors were dominated by formal paraphasias (38%), semantic paraphasias (12%), and neologisms (3%). The semantic paraphasias in repetition were what defined this patient as having deep dysphasia rather than routine Wernicke's aphasia.

Martin et al. (1994) utilized a three-level IAM derived from Dell's 1986 model (Dell, 1986; Dell & O'Seaghdha, 1991) and composed of semantic, lexical, and phonological units (see Chapter 3). Words were input as distributed representations across semantic feature units, and output was defined by activation of specific phoneme units after activation had spread through the network. Minor adjustments to the model led to a very faithful replication of performance by normal subjects. The model was then damaged by variously accelerating the rate of decay in the activation levels of the units. With an appropriately selected decay rate, the model replicated NC's distribution of errors in naming with extraordinary accuracy. Unfortunately, this tour de force depended on the fact that semantic units were activated only at the beginning of each run, rather than throughout each run (as would probably be the case if one had a concept or image in mind that one was naming). As long as activation decay was minimal, the activated semantic units maintained their influence throughout the run, successfully suppressing competing phonological influences. However, with accelerated decay, semantic and phonological activation patterns competed on equal terms, and phonological influences were prominently manifested in a high rate of formal paraphasias and neologisms. The model's weakness, however, highlights the limits of our knowledge regarding the interface between lexical–phonological systems on the one hand and both the semantic field and phonological representations on the other. Martin, Saffran, and Dell (1996) subsequently explored the ability of the lesioned model to simulate NC's repetition performance.

CONCLUSION

I have sought first and foremost in this chapter to develop a basic understanding of PDP models in their particular applications to language processes. In the course of this discussion, however, I hope that several other things have become clear. First, it should be evident that PDP does have the potential to account for complex behavior in terms of neural microstructure. Failures of simulations to account for observed behavior clearly stem from the inadequacies of particular models, even as they often further validate the general approach. Even at this early stage, the science of PDP has given us a glimpse of how we will ultimately understand the brain—in terms of the mathematics of stochastic processing.

Second, it should be clear that the basic structure of neural networks and their intrinsic behavioral properties have profound implications for the behaviors that emanate from these networks. Inference, generalization, graceful degradation, bottom-up and top-down processing effects, content-addressable memory, a capability for extracting the essential elements from variously redundant data sets, parallel-constraint satisfaction, and a capability for capturing complex relationships between various collections of sequences (a problem almost paradigmatic of language development)—all of these are functions intrinsic to PDP networks that have powerful explanatory power for the entire spectrum of behavior exhibited by neural net organisms, from mosquitoes to humans. What is particularly startling is that heretofore we have had to posit largely ad hoc explanations for most of these phenomena.

Third, it should be clear that PDP models provide enormous opportunities to test our assumptions about neural microstructure for their ability to account for observed phenomena. However, we will avail ourselves of this opportunity only if we strive to develop models that have neural plausibility.

There are still many issues to be addressed by PDP models. In fact, the field is only now coming to maturity as a science. The reading model developed by Plaut et al. (1996) demonstrates the power of a network that employs both distributed representations and recurrent connections, giving it attractor properties. It also shows quite clearly that many phenomena heretofore explained in cognitive processing models on the basis of different processing routes can be more compellingly explained on the basis of the interactions of two or more network systems (in the Plaut et al. model, an orthographic–articulatory pattern associator and an orthographic–semantic–articulatory pattern associator). Further progress will depend not only on further developing such models but also on applying them to sentences. The work by St. John and colleagues (McClelland et al., 1989; St. John, 1992; St. John & McClelland, 1992) has shown how a PDP model can deal with sentence comprehension as a problem of parallel-constraint satisfaction, availing itself not only of knowledge about general associations between things it has learned in order to make inferences, but also of information about specific instances. These models do not, however, employ the knowledge of causality that is so essential to our understanding of what we hear and read, but also goes to the heart of the syntax problem. Linguistics has led us to view syntactic processing as a complex sequential and hierarchical process substantially constrained by verbs and their predicate argument structures and phrase structure rules. However, an alternative approach that lends itself to PDP (and plausibly neural) instantiation may be to view a verb as a peculiar form of adjective that nuances the meaning of the agent, patient, recipient, or the like. PDP networks employing distributed representations have shown virtually limitless powers to capture nuance. For example, "The man hit the woman" may be translated as "The man [hitter] the woman [hittee]," capturing causality, our inferences about the nature of this transformed man and woman, and the associative links between them. Thus nuance captured by distributed representations, coupled with the capabilities for parallel-constraint satisfaction (another PDP strength), may be capable of solving much of the syntax problem. Major problems remain, however, such as binding (e.g., binding a pronoun to its antecedent) and, most seriously, sequence. PDP models have barely explored, let alone offered, compelling solutions for the problem that much of what we do—language in particular—is serially ordered over time. PDP models, although they employ a variety of heuristically very powerful learning algorithms, have yet to successfully capture the all-at-once learning achieved by the hippocampal system, the actual learning mechanism underlying acquisition of procedural memory, or the differences in network structure that may perhaps underlie the representations of declarative and procedural knowledge. Finally, there remains a large gap between the simplistic and highly artificial units of PDP models and the operational units of neural microstructure. This owes to our lack of understanding of the microscopic organization and function of cerebral cortex. However, PDP is generating hypotheses that may inspire specific lines of investigation into the function of neural microstructure (e.g., Chappell & Humphreys, 1994; O'Reilly & McClelland, 1994).

ACKNOWLEDGMENT

I am deeply indebted to James L. McClelland for his generous guidance and his many helpful suggestions.

NOTE

1. More recent models utilize an intermediate layer of hidden units between input and output layers that are able to capture regularities in the input data, such as acceptable relationships between phonemes in a particular position in a word and surrounding phonemes, and obviate the need for such contrivances as the Wickelphone. These hidden-unit layer models are also much better at relating regularities in the input data to regularities in the output data (e.g., in relating orthographic to phonological word forms). This is a nice example of how a network can use a simple device to perform a complicated computation and concurrently achieve greater overall computational power. The use of hidden units in learning networks, however, did not truly become feasible until mathematical techniques were developed to transmit learned information back through the multiple layers of the network. The most popular of these is backpropagation (see below) (Rumelhart, Hinton, & Williams, 1986).

REFERENCES

Bates, E., Friederici, A., & Wulfeck, B. (1987). Grammatical morphology in aphasia: Evidence from three languages. *Cortex, 23,* 545–574.

Behrmann, M., Moscovitch, M., & Mozer, M. C. (1991). Directing attention to words and nonwords in normal subjects and in a computational model: Implications for neglect dyslexia. *Cognitive Neuropsychology, 8,* 213–248.

Bybee, J. L., & Slobin, D. I. (1982). Rules and schemas in the development and use of the English past tense. *Language, 58,* 265–289.

Carpenter, P. A., Miyake, A., & Just, M. A. (1995). Language comprehension: Sentence and discourse processing. *Annual Review of Psychology, 46,* 91–120.

Chappell, M., & Humphreys, M. S. (1994). An auto-associative neural network for sparse representations: Analysis and application to models of recognition and cued recall. *Psychological Review, 101,* 103–128.

Coltheart, M., Curtis, B., Atkins, P., & Haller, M. (1993). Models of reading aloud: Dual-route and parallel-distributed-processing approaches. *Psychological Review, 100,* 589–608.

Coltheart, M., & Rastle, K. (1994). Serial processing in reading aloud: Evidence for dual-route models of reading. *Journal of Experimental Psychology: Human Perception and Performance, 20,* 1197–1211.

Daugherty, K., & Seidenberg, M. S. (1992). Rules or connections?: The past tense revisited. In *Proceedings of the Fourteenth Annual Conference of the Cognitive Science Society* (pp. 259–264). Hillsdale, NJ: Erlbaum.

Dell, G. S. (1986). A spreading-activation theory of retrieval in sentence production. *Psychological Review, 93,* 283–321.

Dell, G. S., Juliano, C., & Govindjee, A. (1993). Structure and content in language production: A theory of frame constraints in phonological speech errors. *Cognitive Science, 17,* 149–195.

Dell, G. S., & O'Seaghdha, P. G. (1991). Mediated and convergent lexical priming in language production: A comment on Levelt et al. (1991). *Psychological Review, 98,* 604–614.

Elman, J. L., Bates, E. A., Johnson, M. H., Karmiloff-Smith, A., Parisi, D., & Plunkett, K. (1996). *Rethinking innateness: A connectionist perspective on development.* Cambridge, MA: MIT Press.

Farah, M. J., & McClelland, J. L. (1991). A computational model of semantic memory impairment: Modality-specificity and emergent category-specificity. *Journal of Experimental Psychology: General, 120*(4), 339–357.

Finkel, L. H. (1990). A model of receptive field plasticity and topographic map reorganization in the somatosensory cortex. In S. J. Hanson & C. R. Olson (Eds.), *Connectionist modeling and brain function: The developing interface* (pp. 164–192). Cambridge, MA: MIT Press.

Granger, R., Ambros-Ingerson, J., Antón, P., & Lynch, G. (1990). Unsupervised perceptual learning: A paleocortical model. In S. J. Hanson & C. R. Olson (Eds.), *Connectionist modeling and brain function: The developing interface* (pp. 105–131). Cambridge, MA: MIT Press.

Haarman, J. J., & Kilk, H. H. J. (1991). A computer model of the temporal course of agrammatic sentence understanding: The effects of variation in severity and sentence complexity. *Cognitive Science, 15,* 49–87.

Hebb, D. O. (1949). *The organization of behavior.* New York: Wiley.

Hinton, G. E. (1989). Connectionist learning procedures. *Artificial Intelligence, 40,* 185–234.

Hinton, G. E., McClelland, J. L., & Rumelhart, D. E. (1986). Distributed representations. In D. E. Rumelhart, J. L. McClelland, & the PDP Research Group (Eds.), *Parallel distributed processing: Explorations in the microstructure of cognition. Vol. 1. Foundations* (pp. 77–109). Cambridge, MA: MIT Press.

Hinton, G. E., & Shallice, T. (1991). Lesioning an attractor network: Investigations of acquired dyslexia. *Psychological Review, 98,* 74–95.

Hoeffner, J. (1992). Are rules a thing of the past?: The acquisition of verbal morphology by an attractor network. In *Proceedings of the Fourteenth Annual Conference of the Cognitive Science Society* (pp. 861–866). Hillsdale, NJ: Erlbaum.

Jaeger, J. J., Lockwood, A. H., Kemmerer, D. L., Van Valin, R. D., Murphy, B. W., & Khalak, H. G. (1996). A positron emission tomographic study of regular and irregular verb morphology in English. *Language, 72,* 451–497.

Just, M. A., & Carpenter, P. A. (1992). A capacity theory of comprehension: Individual differences in working memory. *Psychological Review, 99,* 122–149.

Kawamoto, A. H. (1988). Distributed representations of ambiguous words and their resolution in a connectionist network. In S. L. Small, G. W. Cottrell, & M. K. Tanenhaus (Eds.), *Lexical ambiguity resolution: Perspectives from psycholinguistics, neuropsychology, and artificial intelligence* (pp. 195–228). San Mateo, CA: Morgan Kauffman.

Kawamoto, A. H. (1993). Nonlinear dynamics in the resolution of lexical ambiguity: A parallel distributed processing account. *Journal of Memory and Language, 32,* 474–516.

MacDonald, M. C., Pearlmutter, N. J., & Seidenberg, M. S. (1994). Lexical nature of syntactic ambiguity resolution. *Psychological Review, 101,* 676–703.

MacWhinney, B., & Leinbach, J. (1991). Implementations are not conceptualizations: Revising the verb learning model. *Cognition, 40,* 121–153.

Marr, D. (1971). Simple memory: A theory for archicortex. *Philosophical Transactions of the Royal Society of London, Series B, 262,* 23–81.

Martin, N., Dell, G. S., Saffran, E. M., & Schwartz, M. F. (1994). Origins of paraphasias in deep dysphasia: Testing the consequences of a decay impairment to an interactive spreading activation model of lexical retrieval. *Brain and Language, 47,* 609–660.

Martin, N., & Saffran, E. M. (1992). A computational account of deep dysphasia: Evidence from a single case study. *Brain and Language, 43,* 240–274.

Martin, N., Saffran, E. M., & Dell, G. S. (1996). Recovery in deep dysphasia: Evidence for a relation between auditory–verbal STM capacity and lexical errors in repetition. *Brain and Language, 52,* 83–113.

McClelland, J. L. (1986). The programmable blackboard model of reading. In J. L. McClelland, D. E. Rumelhart, & the PDP Research Group (Eds.), *Parallel distributed processing: Explorations in the microstructure of cognition. Vol. 2. Psychological and biological models* (pp. 122–169). Cambridge, MA: MIT Press.

McClelland, J. L., & Elman, J. L. (1986). Interactive processes in speech perception: The TRACE model. In J. L. McClelland, D. E. Rumelhart, & the PDP Research Group (Eds.), *Parallel distributed processing: Explorations in the microstructure of cognition. Vol. 2. Psychological and biological models* (pp. 58–121). Cambridge, MA: MIT Press.

McClelland, J. L., & Kawamoto, A. H. (1986). Mechanisms of sentence processing: Assigning roles to constituents of sentences. In J. L. McClelland, D. E. Rumelhart, & the PDP Research Group (Eds.), *Parallel distributed processing: Explorations in the microstructure of cognition. Vol. 2. Psychological and biological models* (pp. 272–325). Cambridge, MA: MIT Press.

McClelland, J. L., McNaughton, B. L., &, O'Reilly, R. C. (1995). Why there are complementary learning systems in the hippocampus and neocortex: Insights from the successes and failures of connectionist models of learning and memory. *Psychological Review, 102,* 419–457.

McClelland, J. L., & Plaut, D. C. (1993). Computational approaches to cognition: Top-down approaches. *Current Opinion in Neurobiology, 3,* 209–216.

McClelland, J. L., & Rumelhart, D. E. (1981). An interactive activation model of context effects in letter perception: Part 1. An account of basic findings. *Psychological Review, 88,* 375–407.

McClelland, J. L., Rumelhart, D. E., & Hinton, G. E. (1986). The appeal of parallel distributed processing. In D. E. Rumelhart, J. L. McClelland, & the PDP Research Group (Eds.), *Parallel distributed processing: Explorations in the microstructure of cognition. Vol. 1. Foundations* (pp. 3–44). Cambridge, MA: MIT Press.

McClelland, J. L., Rumelhart, D. E., & the PDP Research Group. (Eds.). (1986). *Parallel distributed processing: Explorations in the microstructure of cognition. Vol. 2. Psychological and biological models.* Cambridge, MA: MIT Press.

McClelland, J. L., St. John, M., & Taraban, R. (1989). Sentence comprehension: A parallel distributed processing approach. *Language and Cognitive Processes, 4,* 287–335.

McCloskey, M., & Cohen, N. J. (1989). Catastrophic interference in connectionist networks: The sequential learning problem. In G. H. Bower (Ed.), *The psychology of learning and motivation: Advances in research and theory* (pp. 109–165). San Diego: Academic Press.

Miller, K. D., & Stryker, M. P. (1990). The development of ocular dominance columns: Mechanisms and models. In S. J. Hanson & C. R. Olson (Eds.), *Connectionist modeling and brain functions: The developing interface* (pp. 255–350). Cambridge, MA: MIT Press.

Montague, P. R., Gally, J. A., & Edelman, G. M. (1991). Spatial signaling in the development and function of neural connections. *Cerebral Cortex, 1,* 199–220.

Mozer, M. C., & Behrmann, M. (1992). Reading with attentional impairments: A brain-damaged model of neglect and attentional dyslexias. In R. G. Reilly & N. E. Sharkey (Eds.), *Connectionist approaches to natural language processing* (pp. 409–460). Hillsdale, NJ: Erlbaum.

Norris, D. (1992). Connectionism: A new breed of bottom-up model. In R. G. Reilly & N. E. Sharkey (Eds.), *Connectionist approaches to natural language processing* (pp. 351–371). Hillsdale, NJ: Erlbaum.

O'Reilly, R. C., & McClelland, J. L. (1994). Hippocampal conjunctive encoding, storage, and recall: Avoiding a trade-off. *Hippocampus, 4,* 661–682.

Patterson, K. E., Seidenberg, M. S., & McClelland, J. L. (1989). Connections and disconnections: Acquired dyslexia in a computational model of reading processes. In R. G. M. Morris (Ed.), *Parallel distributed processing: Implications for psychology and neurobiology* (pp. 131–181). Oxford: Clarendon Press.

Pinker, S. (1991). Rules of language. *Science, 253,* 530–534.

Pinker, S., & Prince, A. (1988). On language and connectionism: Analysis of a parallel distributed processing model of language acquisition. In S. Pinker & J. Mehler (Eds.), *Connections and symbols* (pp. 73–193). Cambridge, MA: MIT Press.

Plaut, D. C. (1996). Relearning after damage in connectionist networks: Toward a theory of rehabilitation. *Brain and Language, 52,* 25–82.

Plaut, D. C., McClelland, J. L., Seidenberg, M. S., & Patterson, K. (1996). Understanding normal and impaired word reading: Computational principles in quasi-regular domains. *Psychological Review, 103,* 56–115.

Plaut, D. C., & Shallice, T. (1991). Effects of word abstractness in a connectionist model of deep dyslexia. In *Proceedings of the Thirteenth Annual Conference of the Cognitive Science Society* (pp. 73–78). Hillsdale, NJ: Erlbaum.

Plaut, D. C., & Shallice, T. (1993). Deep dyslexia: A case study of connectionist neuropsychology. *Cognitive Neuropsychology, 10,* 377–500.

Plunkett, K., & Marchman, V. (1991). U-shaped learning and frequency effects in a multi-layered perceptron: Implications for child language acquisition. *Cognition, 38,* 43–102.

Plunkett, K., & Marchman, V. (1993). From rote learning to system building: Acquiring verb morphology in children and connectionist nets. *Cognition, 48,* 21–69.

Price, C., Wise, R., Ramsay, S., Friston, K., Howard, D., Patterson, K., & Frackowiak, R. (1992). Regional response differences within the human auditory cortex when listening to words. *Neuroscience Letters, 146,* 179–182.

Quinlan, P. (1991). *Connectionism and psychology: A psychological perspective on new connectionist research.* Chicago: University of Chicago Press.

Ramón y Cajal, S. (1923). *Recuerdos de mi vida.* Madrid: Pueyo.

Rolls, E. T., & Treves, A. (1998). *Neural networks and brain function.* New York: Oxford University Press.

Rumelhart, D. E., Hinton, G. E., & McClelland, J. L. (1986). A general framework for parallel distributed processing. In D. E. Rumelhart, J. L. McClelland, & the PDP Research Group (Eds.), *Parallel distributed processing: Explorations in the microstructure of cognition. Vol. 1. Foundations* (pp. 45–76). Cambridge, MA: MIT Press.

Rumelhart, D. E., Hinton, G. E., & Williams, R. J. (1986). Learning internal representations by error propagation. In D. E. Rumelhart, J. L. McClelland, & the PDP Research Group (Eds.), *Parallel distributed processing: Explorations in the microstructure of cognition. Vol. 1. Foundations* (pp. 318–362). Cambridge, MA: MIT Press.

Rumelhart, D. E., & McClelland, J. L. (1982). An interactive activation model of context effects in letter perception: Part 2. The contextual enhancement effect and some tests and extensions of the model. *Psychological Review, 89,* 60–94.

Rumelhart, D. E., & McClelland, J. L. (1986). On learning the past tenses of English verbs. In J. L. McClelland, D. E. Rumelhart, & the PDP Research Group (Eds.), *Parallel distributed processing: Explorations in the microstructure of cognition. Vol. 2. Psychological and biological models* (pp. 216–271). Cambridge, MA: MIT Press.

Rumelhart, D. E., McClelland, J. L., & the PDP Research Group. (Eds.). (1986). *Parallel distributed processing: Explorations in the microstructure of cognition. Vol. 1. Foundations.* Cambridge, MA: MIT Press.

Rumelhart, D. E., Smolensky, P., McClelland, J. L., & Hinton, G. E. (1986). Schemata and sequential thought processes in PDP models. In J. L. McClelland, D. E. Rumelhart, & the PDP Research Group (Eds.), *Parallel distributed processing: Explorations in the microstructure of cognition. Vol. 2. Psychological and biological models* (pp. 7–57). Cambridge, MA: MIT Press.

Sadato, N., Ibañez, V., Deiber, M.-P., Campbell, G., Leonardo, M., & Hallet, M. (1996). Frequency-dependent changes of regional cerebral blood flow during finger movements. *Journal of Cerebral Blood Flow and Metabolism, 16,* 23–33.

Seidenberg, M. S. (1997). Language acquisition and use: Learning and applying probabilistic constraints. *Science, 275,* 1599–1603.

Seidenberg, M. S., & McClelland, J. L. (1989). A distributed, developmental model of word recognition and naming. *Psychological Review, 96,* 523–568.

Singer, W. (1994). Putative functions of temporal correlations in neocortical processing. In C. Koch & J. L. Davis (Eds.), *Large-scale neuronal theories of the brain* (pp. 201–237). Cambridge, MA: MIT Press.

Small, S. L. (1994). Connectionist networks and language disorders. *Journal of Communicative Disorders, 27,* 305–323.

Smith, S., & Bates, E. (1987). Accessibility of case and gender contrasts for agent–object assignment in Broca's aphasics and fluent anomics. *Brain and Language, 30,* 8–32.

Smith, S. D., & Mimica, I. (1984). Agrammatism in a case-inflected language: Comprehension of agent–object relations. *Brain and Language, 21,* 274–290.

Smolensky, P. (1986). Neural and conceptual intrpretations of PDP models. In J. L. McClelland, D. E. Rumelhart, & the PDP Research Group (Eds.), *Parallel distributed processing: Explorations in the microstructure of cognition. Vol. 2. Psychological and biological models* (pp. 390–431). Cambridge, MA: MIT Press.

Squire, L. R. (1992). Declarative and non-declarative memory: Multiple brain systems supporting learning and memory. *Journal of Cognitive Neuroscience, 4*, 232–243.

Squire, L. R., & Zola-Morgan, S. (1991). The medial temporal lobe memory system. *Science, 253*, 1380–1386.

St. John, M. F. (1992). The story Gestalt: A model of knowledge-intensive processes in text comprehension. *Cognitive Science, 16*, 271–306.

St. John, M. F., & McClelland, J. L. (1992). Parallel constraint satisfaction as a comprehension mechanism. In R. G. Reilly & N. E. Sharkey (Eds.), *Connectionist approaches to natural language processing* (pp. 97–136). Hillsdale, NJ: Erlbaum.

Tanzi, E. (1893). I fatti e le induzioni nell'odierna istologia del sistema nervoso. *Riv Sper Freniatr Med Leg Alienazioni Ment, 19*, 419–472.

Trueswell, J. C., Tanenhaus, M. K., & Garnsey, S. M. (1994). Semantic influences on parsing: Use of thematic role information in syntactic ambiguity resolution. *Journal of Memory and Language, 33*, 285–318.

Ullman, M. T., Corkin, S., Coppola, M., Hickok, G., Growdon, J. H., Koroshetz, W. J., & Pinker, S. (1997). A neural dissociation within language: Evidence that the mental dictionary in part of declarative memory, and that grammatical rules are processed by the procedural system. *Journal of Cognitive Neuroscience, 9*, 266–276.

Ungerleider, L. G. (1995). Functional brain imaging studies of cortical mechanisms of memory. *Science, 270*, 769–775.

Warrington, E. K., & McCarthy, R. (1983). Category specific access dysphasia. *Brain, 106*, 859–887.

Warrington, E. K., & Shallice, T. (1984). Category specific semantic impairments. *Brain, 107*, 829–854.

Wermter, S., & Lehnert, W. G. (1992). Noun phrase analysis with connectionist networks. In R. G. Reilly & N. E. Sharkey (Eds.), *Connectionist approaches to natural language processing* (pp. 75–95). Hillsdale, NJ: Erlbaum.

Zipser, D., & Andersen, R. (1988). Back propagation learning simulates response properties of a subset of posterior parietal neurons. *Nature, 332*, 679–684.

13

ATTENTION, RESOURCE ALLOCATION, AND LANGUAGE

IRA FISCHLER

Effective use of language requires the coordination of a remarkable range of cognitive processes. Whether we are conversing idly with our children or engaging in a scholarly debate in the pages of scientific journals, comprehension depends on the appropriate engagement of systems for processing phonological (or orthographic), lexical, syntactic, semantic, and discourse information, from a spoken or written message. Production depends on a complementary array of processes leading from an intended message to a sequence of articulatory (or praxic) movements that give form to the idea.

Intuitively, attentional mechanisms appear to play a significant role in many language tasks. If our attention drifts as we listen or read, we may realize that we haven't been comprehending any of the message. As we speak, we hesitate and pause at points that demand generation of particular morphological or lexical items, syntactic forms, or pragmatic tone. Some of the earliest work on auditory attention, in fact, demanded selective listening to one of two competing verbal messages presented dichotically (Cherry, 1953), and demonstrated how profoundly attention to one linguistic source can limit processing of other concurrent messages. In large part, though, experimental studies of attention and of language have followed relatively independent paths (Fischler, 1998). Indeed, it is still possible to find volumes on attention that include no references to language in the index (e.g., Pashler, 1998), and texts on language with little or no consideration of attention (e.g., Harley, 1995). Recently, however, there has been growing interest in how, and to what extent, the engagement and control of various language processes depend on attentional mechanisms and skills. This interest has been shared by cognitive psychologists (e.g., see Logan, 1995), cognitive neuroscientists (e.g., see Fischler, 1998), neuropsychologists (e.g., see Eviatar, 1998; Crosson, Chapter 14, this volume), aphasiologists, and clinicians in practice (e.g., see McNeil, Odell, & Tseng, 1991; Murray, Holland, & Beeson, 1998).

COMPONENTS OF ATTENTION

Part of the difficulty in studying the role of "attention" in language stems from the diversity of attentional constructs, and the wide variety of processes and measures, that have fallen under its rubric. Despite William James's (1890, Vol. 1, p. 403) claim that "Everyone knows what attention is," the term has been used historically to refer to a great variety of potentially independent processes and mechanisms, including selectivity for one of several competing external or internal sources of information (with facilitation of selected sources and/or inhibition of others); division of attention among tasks, and executive control over the allocation of attentional resources to those tasks; orienting to unexpected or task-relevant stimuli and events; vigilance, or maintenance of attention to one source of input in anticipation of rare events; and the overall level of activation or arousal of the organism, which may have an impact on the efficiency of information processing. There are also phenomenological senses of attention, which stress the role of awareness and conscious experience; and motivational senses stressing the goals and choices that guide overt and covert behavior and help to determine what captures our interest. Even the seemingly distinct processes of working memory may share certain dimensions with attention. For example, many studies of working memory, coming from the tradition of Baddeley's (1986) multicomponent model of short-term memory, deal with the same kinds of dual-task paradigms that are common to the study of attention. Baddeley (1993) has discussed the "fuzzy bounds" between the constructs of attention and short-term memory.

Not surprisingly, there is a corresponding diversity in the ways that attention has been operationalized and manipulated. These include simple instructions to attend "more" to one stimulus or task than another (e.g., Gopher, Brickner, & Navon, 1982); variations in the difficulty of some aspect of a single task, such as the syntactic complexity of sentences (e.g., King & Kutas, 1995); and the unexpected presentation of stimuli in the visual periphery during visual search tasks (e.g., Theeuwes, Kramer, Hahn, & Irwin, 1998).

In their critical review of the concept of attention as both cause and effect in cognition, Johnston and Dark (1986) were pessimistic that a unitary construct is useful at all in cognitive theory. Similarly, Pashler and Carrier (1996) responded to James's claim by adding that "when the goal is to understand mental phenomena at a mechanistic level, it may be better to assume that no one knows what attention is, and even to assume that there probably is no 'it' to be understood" (p. 14). Most theorists acknowledge the diversity of processes being described and the multidimensional nature of attention (e.g., Barkley, 1996), but then go on to specify those components of attention in the context of an information-processing (e.g., Pashler & Carrier, 1996), factor-analytic (e.g., Mirsky, Anthony, Duncan, & Ahearn, 1991) or brain systems (e.g., Posner, 1995) framework, and subsequently focus on a more narrowly defined domain.

Attention as Resource Allocation

One popular definition of attention, which stresses both its limited capacity and its selective nature, is the dynamic allocation of a limited pool of cerebral processing resources to the various tasks at hand, both internal and external. Kahneman's (1973) classic work on attention and effort formalized a resource-based view of attention and applied it to a wide range of information-processing tasks. Norman and Bobrow (1975) contrasted data-limited and resource-limited processes in cognition, and rigorously developed the idea of a common pool of attentional resources that can be allocated in graded fashion between tasks.

Over the years, this view of attention as the allocation of a common, limited resource pool has been subjected to rather strong criticism. Based on the pattern of performance obtained under dual-task conditions (when subjects must deal with two concurrent discrete or continuous tasks), Wickens (e.g., 1984) proposed a "multiple-resource theory," distinguishing among resources based on dimensions of modality (auditory vs. visual), processing stages (encoding vs. central processing vs. response), and processing codes (spatial vs. verbal). The basic notion is that, rather than a single pool of resources, there are sets of relatively independent resources. To the extent that two tasks or processes make demands on different resource sets, they can be performed concurrently. To be fair, both Kahneman (1973), in his notion of structural interference between tasks, and Norman and Bobrow (1975), in their analysis of data-limited aspects of processing, anticipated that there may be specific limits or sources of interference in any complex of tasks that are not due simply to limits on "general resources."

Multiple-resource theory in turn was criticized as being too unconstrained. Navon (1984) argued that patterns of tradeoffs between concurrent tasks may be due to compliance with experimenter demands, and that dual-task interference may be caused by "crosstalk" or outcome conflicts between concurrent tasks (Navon & Miller, 1987). The very assumption that resources can be allocated in a graded fashion, when we take a finer-grained look at performance, was questioned by Pashler (1994). Noting the pattern of slowing of the second of two responses made to two slightly asynchronous stimuli (the "psychological refractory period"; Welford, 1952), Pashler argued that graded resource allocation could not explain the distribution of latencies within a block of trials in which subjects were asked to "divide" attention between the two stimuli. His view was that the stage of processing subject to capacity limitations is that of response preparation, selection, and perhaps execution, and that attention in this sense is an all-or-none phenomenon. (Meyer & Kieras, 1997, present a somewhat less rigid view of how limited capacity in perceptual–motor and working memory systems may be flexibly allocated in two-response tasks; see below.) Furthermore, whereas some investigators have tried to identify different brain regions with different resource pools (see, e.g., Pribram & McGuiness, 1975), others suggest that a search for brain regions that are responsible for selectively engaging appropriate linguistic and other cognitive functions may be more fruitful than a search for various "resource pools" (Nadeau & Crosson, 1997; see Crosson, Chapter 14, this volume).

Despite this controversy, the notion of resource limits and allocation remains a useful heuristic for understanding limited capacity and selectivity in human performance, whether we think of the limit in terms of resources, structures, or processes. By analogy, the distinction between short-term and long-term memory has been hotly debated theoretically (see, e.g., Nairne, 1996), but it has remained perhaps the most common, important, and useful organizing principle for thinking about memory in the laboratory as well as in the clinic. Wickens (e.g., Sarno & Wickens, 1995) and others have continued to make effective use of the multiple-resource approach, for example, in both theoretical and applied areas (see especially Wickens, 1992, Ch. 9). An excellent discussion of the historical development and controversies of resource theory, alternative "structural" approaches to dual-task interference, and the use of central and autonomic approaches to measure resource allocation can be found in Kramer and Spinks (1991).

The remainder of this chapter considers, in a highly selective manner, how attention as resource allocation can be seen in various language tasks. I begin with studies of how attentional allocation modulates the recognition and production of individual words and their attributes. I then briefly consider work on the attentional demands of syntactic processing, and conclude with studies of attention to higher-level discourse comprehension and planning. In each case, the focus is on behavioral and electrophysiological measures, and reflects an information-processing perspective.

Measuring Resource Allocation in Language Tasks

The resource allocation view of attention leads to several basic questions that can be asked about performance. The first question (or set of questions) concerns what the total quantity of resources is; how this quantity may change with maturation, aging, disease, and injury; and how it may be affected by variations in alertness and arousal.

Second, task difficulty can be viewed as a particular level of resource demand or "mental workload." The demands of a given task will vary at different stages of its execution. One of the first methods used to measure the momentary demands of a task was the secondary-probe task of Posner and Boies (1971). In this method, the reaction time to an auditory tone presented during execution of a "primary" task was taken as a measure of the attentional load of the primary task at the point of tone presentation. In studies using dual-task procedures, it is critical that variations in momentary demands be considered, particularly if subjects appear to be able to perform a second task with little overall cost to the first.

Third, success for a given task and individual will depend on how well resources can be appropriately allocated to task components over time. Figure 13.1, from Meyer and Kieras (1997), illustrates how fine-grained this allocation may need to be in even the simple task of responding to each of two consecutive stimuli. The ability to allocate resources appropriately (modeled by Meyer & Kieras as the controlled access to a single-channel executive process) over the course of such tasks will depend on a number of factors, including the complexity of the task components, and the person's familiarity with these components and their combination (see Damos & Wickens, 1980). The general level of arousal can affect the allocation as well as the amount of resources: As arousal becomes too high, the ability to coordinate what Easterbrook (1959) called "central" and "peripheral" task cues may be compromised.

Fourth is the relation of practice and task demands. As a given task becomes highly practiced, demands on limited resources decrease, to the point where performance takes on the characteristics of automaticity: It requires few if any resources, occurs quickly, and can "capture" focal attention regardless of a person's intent. A classic example comes from the selective listening task, in which Neville Moray, a pioneer in the study of selective attention, was found to be far better than the average Oxford undergraduate at "shadowing" one auditory message and concurrently detecting occasional digits in an auditory stream in the other ear (Underwood, 1974). A more recent example in the imaging domain was the demonstration by Petersen, Fox, Posner, Mintun, and Raichle (1989) that repeatedly asking subjects to generate verbs to go with particular nouns (e.g., "hit" to go with "hammer") eliminated the activity seen in the anterior cingulate and other frontal regions.

The notion of automaticity has been a controversial one, largely because of early claims that posed the issue as a dichotomy between automatic and attentional processes (e.g., Posner & Snyder, 1975; Hasher & Zacks, 1979). Finer techniques have shown that even so-called "automatic" processes require at least some attentional resources (see Allport, 1993; Carr, 1992). Also, automatic processes were thought to be in some ways qualitatively different from the controlled, effortful approaches to performance of that task. In some cases, this is clearly true: Contrast the process of searching memory for the product of two two-digit numbers that might result from constant practice, with the more conventional processes involved in calculating the product via algorithms learned in elementary school. (See Logan, 1988, for a theoretical account of this sense of automaticity; and see Staszewski, 1988, for a remarkable demonstration of how effortless some problems can

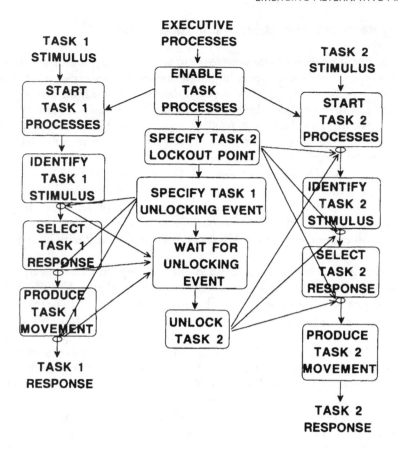

FIGURE 13.1. The component and executive processes for an adaptive model of executive control, showing how subtasks in a dual-choice reaction time task may be flexibly scheduled. From Meyer, D. E., & Kieras, D. E. (1997). A computational theory of executive cognitive processes and multiple-task performance: Part 2. Accounts of psychological refractory-period phenomena. *Psychological Review, 104,* 749–791. Copyright 1997 by the American Psychological Association. Reprinted with permission of the authors.

become with intensive training.) In other cases, though, such as the way in which lexical and semantic information is activated by a spoken or written word, the issue is less clear. Yehene and Tzelgov (1996) have argued that in many tasks, both "algorithmic" and "retrieval" factors contribute to automaticity. In any case, the notion that as tasks are more highly practiced, they may become relatively automatic and less demanding of resources seems beyond dispute.

ATTENTIONAL RESOURCES AND LEXICAL PROCESSING

Most of the work on language and attention that I consider here concerns one or more of the various aspects of attentional resource allocation considered in the preceding section. In such work, it is important to specify as precisely as possible just what aspect of attention is being studied. For example, the imposition of a "memory load"—a small number of words, numbers, or letters that must be maintained during performance of a primary task—is a commonly used means to attempt to decrease the resources available for a primary task. The maintenance of such a load appears to demand little attention, and thus has little effect on choice reaction time (Logan, 1978). Initiating or refreshing the load, however, may be highly attention-demanding (e.g., Naveh-Benjamin & Jonides, 1984; see Pashler & Carrier, 1996, p. 17, for a discussion). Even so, subjects may find a way to effectively "time-share" refreshing the memory load with execution of the primary task, alternating the two in such a fashion that there is little resultant interference.

A number of studies using memory load as a concurrent task have failed to find changes in concurrent retrieval of words from long-term memory (e.g., Baddeley, Lewis, Eldridge, & Thomson, 1984; Craik, Govoni, Naveh-Benjamin, & Anderson, 1996), leading some investigators to conclude that "episodic retrieval" of words does not require attention. However, a closer look at the dynamics of retrieval has shown that if the opportunities for time sharing are minimized, episodic retrieval appears to be resource-demanding (Carrier & Pashler, 1995; Naveh-Benjamin, Craik, Guez, & Dori, 1998). My colleagues and I found that when subjects were required to monitor a sequence of spoken digits for a pattern of three consecutive odd numbers (a dual task introduced by Craik, 1982), the speed and accuracy of concurrent recognition memory for word pairs were substantially impaired, despite the infrequent rate of overt responses required in the digit-monitoring task (Fischler, Howland, & Besson, 1994). The impairment for semantically related word pairs was less than that for unrelated pairs, suggesting that episodic memory for strong associations may be more resistant to distraction. Figure 13.2 shows the pattern of impairment observed.

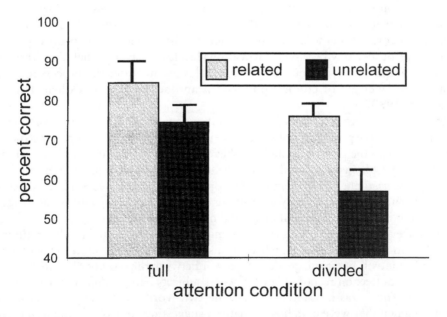

FIGURE 13.2. Effects of divided attention on speed and accuracy of episodic recognition for semantically related and unrelated word pairs. From Fischler, I., Howland, B., & Besson, M. (1994, November). *Divided attention and recognition memory: An ERP analysis.* Paper presented at the meeting of the Psychonomic Society, St. Louis, MO. Reprinted with permission of the authors.

Allocation of Attention and Sublexical Attributes of Words

In both visual and auditory modalities, the activation of various lexical attributes of words in normal adults would seem to be highly overlearned and relatively immune to attentional manipulations. Demonstrations of how irrelevant aspects of words can influence decisions about other attributes have been taken as evidence for the automatic nature of attribute activation. For example, irrelevant orthographic information can hinder phonological decisions about auditorily presented words (e.g., Tanenhaus, Flanigan, & Seidenberg, 1980). Conversely, irrelevant phonological information can hinder semantic decisions about visually presented words (e.g., Luo, Johnson, & Gallo, 1998).

Nevertheless, there is evidence that attentional demands play a role in activation of various attributes of words. Chiarello, Maxfield, Richards, and Kahan (1995) used a "crossword" format that combined vertical and horizontal letter strings presented to the left or right of a fixation point. The task was to read one string out loud and to ignore the other. When subjects were asked to pronounce the horizontal string and to ignore the vertical string, there was some distraction effect compared to a no-crossword control string. However, it made little difference whether the distractor string consisted of random letters, a pseudoword, or a word unrelated or related to the target. Furthermore, there was only a modest facilitation when the distractor was the identical word. One interpretation of this pattern is that since normal reading is so highly practiced, the less automatic processing of the vertical distractor had little impact on performance. However, when the vertical word was the target, the horizontal word had a substantial distraction effect. Also, there was a modest facilitation when the distractor and target words were semantically related.

The general implication of these results is that when the primary language task is made more difficult (e.g., by making the vertical word the target), there is greater opportunity for the intrusion of other processes, particularly if they are themselves highly practiced and automatic (here, the unintended reading of the horizontal words). Chiarello et al. (1995) interpreted their results in the context of a connectionist model of word processing in which attentional resources may be directed to various levels or "layers," including very "early" sensory and graphemic levels and "late" semantic layers, and influence processing efficiency by biasing the weights of connections within and across layers (Cohen, Dunbar, & McClelland, 1990).

Attention has been manipulated in a number of ways in further efforts to determine how it modulates the processing of various lexical attributes. For example, instructions to direct attention to the first or second syllable of spoken words enhanced detection of an embedded target phoneme located nearer the attended syllable (Pallier, Sebastian-Galles, Felguera, & Christophe, 1993). Finney, Protopapas, and Eimas (1996) later showed that this effect occurred in English only with words receiving second-syllable stress, suggesting an interaction between attentional focus and natural prosody.

Bates, Devescovi, Hernandez, and Pizzamiglio (1996) presented modifier–noun word pairs in Italian that were either matched or mismatched in gender marking. Compared to a noun-only control condition, gender agreement between the modifier and the noun target had its greatest effect on response latency when subjects had to indicate the gender of the target noun. There was interference when the two words were mismatched, as well as facilitation when they were matched—a pattern suggesting controlled attentional processing. However, even when gender was irrelevant (in a target noun repetition task), there was still an effect of gender agreement. This pattern of priming—with evidence both for processes that rely little on attentional resources, and for those that depend on attention—is typical of the literature on word priming.

The impact of attention on lexical processing has also been examined by comparing populations that are believed to vary in the quantity of available cognitive resources. Elderly individuals are often considered to have reduced attentional capacity compared to younger persons, in part because of the slowing and/or weakening of a broad spectrum of processes. MacKay and Abrams (1998), for example, found that older adults made more errors producing irregular spellings (i.e., words that contained unusual phoneme–grapheme mappings, such as "calendar" vs. "waiter"), but did not differ from younger adults for regularly spelled words. MacKay and Abrams suggest that with age, activation paths between and within levels of representation weaken. For regularly spelled words, correct spelling is supported both by "top-down" links from the lexical–semantic representation of the words, and by "lateral" links from the phonological representation for such words. For irregularly spelled words, however, the weakened top-down links may sometimes fail to inhibit the incorrect phonological priming of orthography (/ka/ /len/ /dêr/). Since the task allowed the spellers to inspect and correct their output, the failure of the older subjects to detect their own errors also suggests a decreasing ability to shift attention from the phonological to the semantic routes as older adults monitor their output.

Allocation of Attention and Lexical Access

For visual presentation, "lexical access"—the retrieval of a word's representation in the mental lexicon—would appear to require little effort or attention. Supportive results have been obtained in a range of behavioral studies of visual word recognition. For example, if a "prime" word is searched for a target letter (sublexical focus), lexical decision to an immediately subsequent target word is speeded if prime and target are identical. The effect is lexical rather than orthographic, since there is no identity priming for letter search of nonwords (i.e., orthographically and phonologically legal strings with no lexical status) (Besner, Smith, & MacLeod, 1990).

The evidence for effortless activation of words presented auditorally is less consistent, and several studies have demonstrated that, at least for attention to one of two ears, lexical access may fail for words presented to the unattended ear. Okita and Jibu (1998) made use of the finding that the N400 component of event-related potentials (ERPs) to words is significantly reduced with immediate repetition. Words and occasional nonwords were concurrently presented to both ears, and subjects were instructed to signal the occurrence of nonwords in one ear (the attended ear). The N400 for a word delivered to the *attended* ear was reduced if that word had just been presented to that ear. However, if the word had just been presented to the *unattended* ear, the N400 to its subsequent presentation on the attended ear was *not* reduced. This result is particularly striking since the repetition was immediate, and the relation between prime and test was one of identity, rather than a semantic association (see below). One important difference between this finding and those of Besner et al. (1990) in the visual domain is that the identity "prime" in Besner et al.'s task was in the same approximate spatial location as the target, but the prime and target were in different spatial locations in the dichotic listening task of Okita and Jibu (1998). Since other studies suggest an early spatial filtering for words presented in unattended visual locations (see, e.g., McCann, Folk, & Johnston, 1992), it would be interesting to see whether unattended words presented in the same auditory "space" can prime lexical access of subsequent repetitions.

Allocation of Attention and Semantic Attributes of Words

The most widely studied aspect of word recognition and attention concerns the semantic priming effect, in which a preceding "prime" word influences processing of subsequent words that are semantically related to the prime. Neely (1977), in the framework of the Posner and Snyder (1975) view of attention and automaticity, first demonstrated that priming of lexical decisions has both attentional and automatic components. Prime words were category names (e.g., "bird"). In his "shift" condition, primes were likely to be followed by target words from a specific, different category (e.g., tools). When there was sufficient time to shift attention to the expected category—700 milliseconds (ms) or greater stimulus onset asynchrony (SOA), between prime and target—the shifted-category targets (e.g., "hammer") showed facilitation, and the same-category targets (e.g., "robin") showed inhibition, compared to a no-prime condition. This was consistent with an attentional bias toward the expected test words. With only 250 ms between prime and target word onset, however, the pattern was strikingly different: Same-category targets showed facilitation, despite their being unexpected, while shifted-category targets showed no effect of the prime. The facilitation of same-category targets at short latencies was taken as evidence for automatic semantic priming of same-category exemplars that persisted until there was sufficient time to shift attention, according to expectancies, to different-category exemplars.

The impact of attentional factors on the presence or magnitude of semantic priming, for a variety of semantic decisions, is well established, as a recent review by Maxfield (1997) demonstrates. Even when lexical access is highly practiced, activation and "spread" of semantic information may be attention-bound. Maxfield (1995) showed effects of strategic factors on the amount of priming under the short-SOA conditions thought to minimize attentional factors. Searching the prime word for a target letter decreased the amount of semantic priming seen with short-SOA (300-ms) lexical decision priming, and performing a concurrent secondary task eliminated priming altogether even when the prime word was read (Maxfield, 1995).

Similar attentional effects have been shown in studies using the N400 component of the ERPs elicited by familiar words. Kutas and Hillyard (1980) first showed that the N400 was substantially reduced by preceding the word with a sentence context that made the word very predictable (e.g., "He spread warm butter on his . . ." preceding "toast" as opposed to "socks"). Later studies found similar reductions in N400 amplitude by single-word primes that were semantic associates (e.g., Bentin, 1987).

Attentional manipulations that have altered the N400 semantic priming effect include changing the proportion of pairs containing related words (Holcomb, 1988); presenting prime words in the unattended ear during a selective listening task (e.g., Bentin, Kutas, & Hillyard, 1995); requiring decisions about graphemic rather than semantic attributes of the word pair (e.g., Besson, Fischler, Boaz, & Raney, 1992); and requiring decisions about semantic relatedness rather than animateness of the word pair, and adding a demanding concurrent task (e.g., Fischler, Howland, Sikkema, & Besson, 1999). Figure 13.3 shows the reduction in the N400 semantic priming effect for graphemic decision (upper portion) and semantic decision (lower portion) observed in the Besson et al. (1992) study.

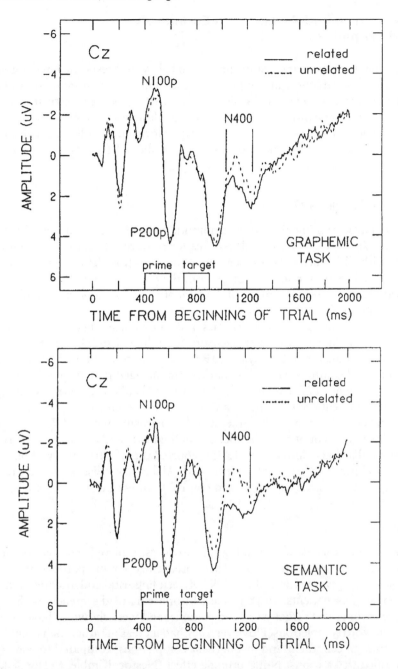

FIGURE 13.3. Effects of "level of processing" on the N400 component of the ERPs to semantically related and unrelated words. Top portion shows the N400 for a graphemic decision comparing the pattern of vowels and consonants of the two words. Bottom portion shows the N400 for a semantic decision comparing animateness of the two words. When words are semantically related and a subject attends to a shared semantic feature (animateness), a stronger N400 effect is produced than when the words are semantically related but the subject attends to a shared orthographic feature. From Besson, M., Fischler, I., Boaz, T., & Raney, G. (1992). Effects of automatic associative activation on explicit and implicit memory tests. *Journal of Experimental Psychology: Learning, Memory, and Cognition, 18,* 89–105. Copyright 1992 by the American Psychological Association. Reprinted with permission of the authors.

Semantic Priming and Attention in Cognitively "Stressed" Populations

It is thought that the effects of semantic primes on behavioral response latency and on N400 amplitude reflect a reduction in the processing demands of comprehension of the target word in that linguistic context (see Fischler & Raney, 1991). Some investigators have looked, therefore, for smaller semantic priming effects in populations of subjects in whom attentional resources in general appear to be reduced. I first review some evidence for this hypothesis, but then argue that the outcome depends on a number of factors that are not typically separated in this research.

Aging and Alzheimer's Disease

Studies of semantic priming and N400 amplitude have been carried out with a variety of populations characterized by reduced resources or resource allocation capabilities, including patients with Alzheimer's disease, schizophrenia, attention-deficit/hyperactivity disorder (ADHD), and a variety of aphasias. In general, the pattern of results supports the notion of decreased ability to take advantage of the semantic context, as seen in diminished effects of context on N400 amplitude.

In healthy aged subjects, several studies have shown a smaller effect of semantic context on N400 amplitude (e.g., Gunter, Jackson, & Mulder, 1992; Iragui, Kutas, & Salmon, 1996; Miyamoto, Katayama, & Koyama, 1998). This pattern of diminished context effects on N400 amplitude is often even more marked among aged patients with Alzheimer's disease (e.g., Iragui et al., 1996; Castaneda, Ostrosky-Solis, Perez, Bobes, & Rangel, 1997).

A decline in attentional resources and control has been found to be an early consequence of Alzheimer's disease (see Greenwood & Parasuraman, 1997, for a recent overview), and this may account for other deficits in linguistic and cognitive performance. For example, Neils, Roeltgen, and Greer (1995) reported that the frequency of phonologically implausible spellings in a group of patients with Alzheimer's disease was correlated more strongly with tests of visual attention and control than with tests of language abilities.

Schizophrenia

Among the various classes of psychological disorders, schizophrenia is notable for both attentional and language disturbances. Therefore, schizophrenic patients are of particular interest in scientific investigation of the link between linguistic and attentional phenomena. In two recent studies, patients with chronic schizophrenia read sentences with semantically congruent or incongruent target word completions, and were shown to have delayed N400 latencies to all word completions. However, they had increased rather than diminished N400 amplitudes to both congruent and incongruent completions, compared to control subjects, and so demonstrated a robust N400 priming effect (Nestor, Kimble, O'Donnell, & Smith, 1997; Niznikiewicz, O'Donnell, Nestor, & Smith, 1997). Consistent with these results are demonstrations that semantic priming of word recognition among schizophrenic patients is comparable to that found in normal controls (see Henik, Nissimov, Priel, & Umansky, 1995).

Exploring Group Differences

Many of the preceding studies have simply compared the size of priming effects on behavioral and electrophysiological measures in normal and impaired groups. However striking the overall differences between groups may be, there is little we can conclude from these studies about the source or specific nature of the differences. How should priming effects be changed by a general reduction in processing resources, for example? Should we expect larger priming effects, as the diminished ability to process the target words provides a greater opportunity for the prime to facilitate performance? But the prime may be harder to process as well, and may therefore provide less support for dealing with the target words. This may result in smaller priming effects. Of course, both prime and target processing may be impaired, potentially resulting in no differences in priming between groups. With respect to the N400 ERP, should we expect an increased N400 amplitude in the context of reduced cognitive resources (as found by Nestor et al., 1997; see above), reflecting the increased impact a prime may have on a degraded target representation? Or should we expect a reduced N400 amplitude, reflecting further depletion of already degraded resources by processing of the prime itself, which substantially mitigates prime–target interactions?

Overall differences between groups therefore cannot be ascribed to specific linguistic processes or to more general attentional mechanisms without more systematic manipulations—either manipulations of linguistic factors that are known to place demands on one or another component of attentional allocation, use of dual tasks involving linguistic and/ or nonlinguistic demands, or some independent assessment of attentional abilities in the groups. Studies that add these kinds of manipulations to the group comparisons in an attempt to identify the source of group differences are becoming more frequent. One approach has been to vary the level or strength of the semantic relationship between the prime and target stimuli, the rationale being that if the impairment is due to dysfunction within the semantic system, it should show up as an interaction between group and the prime–target relationship. Schwartz, Kutas, Butters, and Paulsen (1996), for example, compared ERPs to visually presented words in patients with Alzheimer's disease and age-matched subjects. Target words were primed with an auditory category name. Related primes could be at either a superordinate or a subordinate level. Although patients with Alzheimer's disease showed diminished overall priming effects (see above), the category manipulation had similar effects on both reaction time and the N400 effect in the two groups. This suggested to the authors that the attenuation of the N400 effect was due more to changes in "top-down" attentional control of language than to impairment in the "bottom-up" structure of semantic networks (but cf. Iragui et al., 1996).

An alternative investigative approach is the introduction of secondary or dual tasks to determine whether two groups are differentially affected by the increased load on attentional resources. This has become an increasingly popular strategy to evaluate the claim that at least some of the language problems seen in aphasic patients are due to problems in resource availability or allocation, as opposed to damage to linguistic structures (e.g., Blackwell & Bates, 1995; Tseng, McNeil, & Milenkovic, 1993; see also Crosson, Chapter 14, this volume).

In a series of papers, Murray and colleagues have used this approach to study the resource allocation and attentional capacity of aphasic patients. Murray, Holland, and Beeson (1997a) compared aphasic patients to normal control subjects on several tasks involving auditory processing, one nonverbal (tone discrimination) and two verbal (lexical decision and semantic categorization). When the tasks were presented in isolation (primary task only), the aphasic patients performed as well as the control subjects. However, when the stimuli for the secondary task were present, the aphasic patients were slower and less accurate than the control subjects, in both a focused-attention condition (in which only the primary task had to be performed) and a divided-attention condition (in which both the primary and secondary tasks had to be performed). This was true when the two verbal tasks were combined, as well as for the two verbal–nonverbal combinations. The aphasic patients, but not the control subjects, showed interference in the focused-attention conditions, and in the divided-attention conditions they had greater difficulty following instructions as to which stimulus to respond to first. Since both aphasic patients and control subjects showed greater interference for the verbal–verbal combination, Murray et al. (1997a) concluded that the aphasic patients' difficulty with the dual-task environment was not due to a linguistic impairment, but due to impairment in evaluating the demands of the dual tasks and/or deploying resources appropriately. Interestingly, the pattern of dual-task impairment was no different in patients with anterior lesions than in patients with posterior lesions, consistent with the view that the successful allocation of attention requires the coordination of frontal and parietal attentional systems (cf. Posner, 1995; Crosson, Chapter 14, this volume).

Murray et al. (1997a) also observed that whereas estimates of the degree of language impairment did not significantly predict dual-task deficits in the aphasic group, degree of language impairment was significantly associated with the variability of performance across dual-task trials. This suggests that the aphasic patients were selectively impaired at maintaining an appropriate attentional set across as well as within dual-task trials, and that the allocation and control of attention in this particularly demanding context required more resources than they had available. (See Tseng et al., 1993; see also Barkley, 1996, p. 50, for a discussion of how variability of performance can illuminate impairments of attentional control in patients with ADHD.)

Summary: Attention and Lexical Processing

Even for language tasks that appear to be relatively "automatic" and effortless, we have seen how the successful allocation of attentional resources is involved in the processing of words and their attributes (both in production and in comprehension), and how various types of impairments may disrupt this allocation. Let us turn now to language tasks that would seem to be more demanding of resources—namely, comprehension or production of the syntactic and semantic structure of sentences, and of the integrative, intersentence structures that capture the overall meaning of the discourse.

THE ATTENTIONAL DEMANDS OF SENTENCE PROCESSING

Sentences vary widely in syntactic structure and complexity. As complexity increases, we might expect that for both comprehension and production, resources will be more heavily taxed. One way to show this in comprehension tasks is to vary the syntactic complexity of sentences and to observe the real-time effects of this on performance. In a lexical decision task involving priming for sentence-final words, a colleague and I (Fischler & Bloom, 1980) presented syntactically simple (e.g., "The hungry bear ate some stale . . .") or complex (e.g., "George couldn't believe his son stole a . . .") sentences, one word at a time, at rates varying from 4 to 28 words/second. At the end of each sentence, a word or nonword appeared and remained visible until a lexical decision was made. As can be seen in Figure 13.4, at the slower rates (4 and 12 words/second), both simple and complex contexts speeded lexical decision to sentence-final words that were semantically congruent and expected, compared to semantically incongruent final words (e.g., ". . . some stale bread" as opposed to "brick")"; ". . . stole a car" as opposed to "pride)." As sentence processing was made

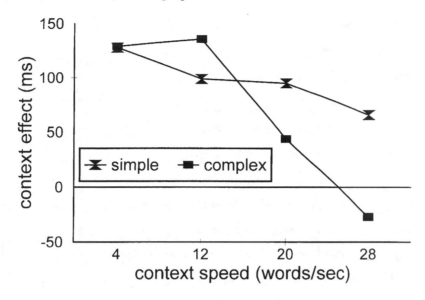

FIGURE 13.4. Effects of syntactically simple and complex sentence contexts on lexical decision speed to sentence-final words, as a function of the rate at which the words of the contexts were shown. The "context effect" is the mean lexical decision latency for semantically incongruent completions, minus that for semantically congruent ones (see text). From Fischler, I., & Bloom, P. A. (1980). Rapid processing of the meaning of sentences. *Memory and Cognition, 8,* 216–225. Copyright 1980 by the Psychonomic Society. Adapted with permission.

more difficult by increasing the presentation rate, the amount of priming decreased for both sentence types, but this decrease was greater for the syntactically complex sentences.

Sentences that place more demands on resources, by increasing the load that must be maintained and manipulated in working memory, also influence the N400 priming effect. Gunter, Jackson, and Mulder (1995) compared the effect of sentence contexts with low or high "working memory demands." They found that for young adults, the difference between the N400 amplitude evoked by sentences with semantically congruent completions and that evoked by sentences with incongruent completions was reduced by high working memory demands. Among middle-aged subjects, high working memory demands eliminated the N400 priming effect altogether.

One popular way to vary syntactic complexity is to compare "subject-relative" with "object-relative" sentences. Consider these examples:

> *Subject-relative:* "The reporter who harshly attacked the senator admitted the error."
> *Object-relative*: "The reporter who the senator harshly attacked admitted the error."
> (Strictly speaking, of course, this sort of sentence is grammatically incorrect—"who" should be "whom"—but it is a type of error that is firmly entrenched in everyday discourse.)

Object-relative sentences are more difficult for aphasic patients to process (e.g., Hickok, Zurif, & Canseco-Gonzalez, 1993). They are also more difficult for normal subjects, when those subjects are engaged in a secondary task (e.g., King & Just, 1991). The relative demands of the more complex sentences have been shown "on-line" in an ERP study by King and Kutas (1995). Figure 13.5 shows the averaged ERPs to sequences of words

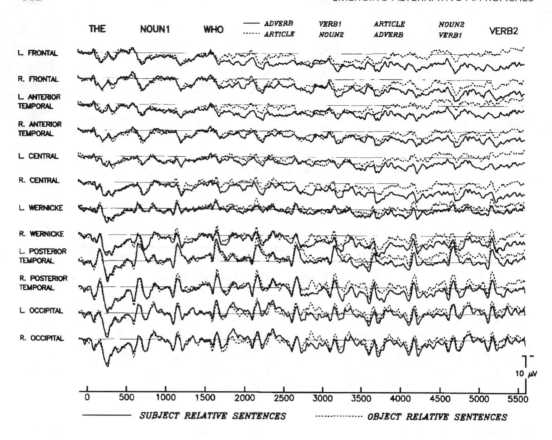

FIGURE 13.5. ERPs to visually presented sentences with object-relative versus subject-relative clauses (see text). From King, J. W., & Kutas, M. (1995). Who did what and when? Using word-level and clause-level ERPs to monitor working-memory usage in reading. *Journal of Cognitive Neuroscience, 7*, 376–395. Copyright 1995 by the MIT Press. Reprinted with permission.

presented a word at a time at 500 ms/word. Within 300 ms of the point at which the sentences diverge—at the article indicating that an object-relative clause is beginning (e.g., "The reporter who *the . . .*")—the ERP associated with the object-relative sentence shows a greater positivity that continues through the clause. The differences appear over both left and right frontal locations, as well as the left anterior temporal location, suggesting that the more complex sentences are more demanding of both general and language-specific processes.

Two recent studies show how dual-task procedures can reduce the attentional resources available for sentence processing. One examined syntactic comprehension of spoken sentences by normal subjects (Blackwell & Bates, 1995), and the second examined the production of sentences to describe visually presented pictures by mildly aphasic patients (Murray et al., 1998). In both studies, the authors argued forcefully that some rather specific patterns of impairment in morphosyntactic analysis can result from what Blackwell and Bates (1995) call "global stress" of resource reduction.

Blackwell and Bates (1995) review the impact of what they term the "global stress" factor in language function and impairment. Previous work had shown that a variety of

Italian patients with presumably reduced attentional resources, including patients with anomia, elderly patients with brain lesions but no language impairment, and elderly patients with orthopedic impairments (see discussion above of aging and resources), displayed an "agrammatical profile" on judgments of verb–noun agreement that was typical of Italian patients with Broca's aphasia (Bates, Friederici, & Wulfeck, 1987). Stressing normal subjects by presenting words of sentences at a rapid rate (cf. Fischler & Bloom, 1980, described above) can produce a similar "agrammatical profile" in their grammaticality judgments (Miyake, Carpenter, & Just, 1994).

In the study of Blackwell and Bates (1995), normal undergraduates judged the grammaticality of sentences presented auditorily. On some trials, two-, four-, or six-digit numbers had to be kept in mind as subjects listened to sentences and made their judgments. Grammatical errors to be detected included transposition errors ("She selling is books"), omission errors ("She selling books"), and agreement errors ("She are selling books").

Figure 13.6 shows the effects of increased memory load on accuracy of detecting these errors, as assessed by differences in A-prime scores (a standardized signal detection measure based on the proportions of correct detections and false alarms) compared to the no-load baseline. Detection of agreement errors was impaired with a memory load of as little as two digits, whereas the detection of omission or transposition errors was not significantly impaired until the memory load rose to six digits. These data are to a large extent in accord with observations of both language comprehension and production by patients with Broca's aphasia: Agreement errors are most common in these patients, whereas transposition errors are rare. Detection of omission errors, which are common in the language production of patients with nonfluent aphasia, is as impaired as the detection of agreement errors, at least when the memory load is six digits.

Maintenance of a subspan memory load has also been shown to impair sentence comprehension by normal subjects and by patients with Alzheimer's disease, with the latter

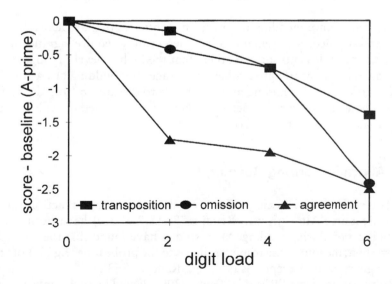

FIGURE 13.6. Accuracy of detection for three types of grammatical errors in spoken sentences, as a function of concurrent digit load. From Blackwell, A., & Bates, E. (1995). Inducing agrammatic profiles in normals: Evidence for the selective vulnerability of morphology under cognitive resource limitation. *Journal of Cognitive Neuroscience, 7*, 228–257. Copyright 1995 by MIT Press. Reprinted with permission.

more impaired than the former (Waters, Caplan, & Rochon, 1995). In this study, the informational complexity of the sentence (in terms of the number of propositions) was a better predictor of dual-task interference than was syntactic complexity.

As part of their study of the effects of dual-task conditions on the language performance of patients with mild aphasia, Murray, Holland, and Beeson (1997b; see above) examined the accuracy of grammaticality judgments in isolation and under various conditions of focused and divided attention. They found that although aphasic and normal individuals were indistinguishable in the isolation condition, aphasic patients showed greater impairment under all the dual-task conditions.

Murray et al. (1998) explored the expressive language of individuals with mild fluent aphasia under single- and dual-task conditions. As before, one task was linguistic and the other involved tone discrimination. Quality of verbal descriptions of pictures was examined in the absence of the tone discrimination task, in the presence of tones that were to be ignored (focused attention), or in the presence of tones that were to be discriminated (divided attention). Increased resource demands had little effect on the quality of picture descriptions by control subjects, indicating that they could deal with the demands of both tasks effectively. However, with comparable increases in resource demands, the aphasic patients showed increased impairment of expressive language as reflected by a variety of measures. Sentences became less syntactically complex and more likely to be ill formed or incomplete, suggesting that at least the larger-scale aspects of syntactic generation are resource-limited. Impairments in lexical retrieval became more common, with fewer total words generated and more word selection errors produced. As predicted, one aspect of production that is thought to be relatively automatic—the morphological complexity of verb phrases—showed no greater impairment with increased demands.

THE ATTENTIONAL DEMANDS OF DISCOURSE PROCESSING

We have seen how comprehending or producing sentences that are lexically appropriate, synactically well formed, and semantically coherent may require significant attentional resources and control. It is no surprise, then, that the highest level of language use—connecting sentences into a meaningful, coherent passage, and building or creating a coherent message—is particularly demanding and vulnerable to disruption from distraction. I provide examples here of how various methodologies have been used to evaluate the resource demands of reading and writing discourse.

Resource Allocation during Reading

Variants of the Posner and Boeis (1971) secondary-probe tone reaction time task (see "Measuring Resource Allocation in Reading Tasks," above) have been used to study attentional allocation during reading. Most studies have found that the more demanding or difficult the text, the longer the response time is to the probe tone (e.g., Inhoff & Fleming, 1989), although there are exceptions (see, e.g., Raney, 1993).

Early components of the ERPs (N100 and P200) elicited by such probe tones have also been used to assess the attentional demands of text comprehension. Since no overt response needs to be made to the probe tone, this technique allows subjects to focus purely on the task of understanding the material, and avoids problems related to how different subjects might prioritize the two tasks. It has been shown that N100 amplitude is reduced when a concurrent stimulus is attended to (e.g., Picton & Hillyard, 1974). Raney (1993) found that when a passage was read a second time, the amplitude of the N100 and P200 ERPs associated with the probe tone increased (suggesting less early competition for attention to the probe tone). In contrast, rereading produced a reduction in the amplitude of a later positive component of the probe tone ERP, as well as increases in overt reaction time to the probe (in a companion study). This pattern suggested that during the second reading, attention shifted from lower-level processes, which might compete with early probe tone analysis, to the level of more integrative processes, which might compete with late probe tone analysis.

These ideas were recently confirmed in a study using a very different approach to evaluating resource allocation during reading. Millis, Simon, and tenBroek (1998) had undergraduates read challenging text from scientific publications, twice through. Silent reading time was measured either sentence by sentence (Experiment 1), or word by word via a moving-window technique (Experiment 2). Resource "consumption" by particular processes was estimated during each reading by the slope of the regression lines associated with specific predictor variables; a steeper slope implied greater demands through that process. For lexical access, the investigators used word frequency; for "propositional assembly," they used the number of propositions and number of new arguments introduced in each sentence; for the highest level of "text integration," they used ratings of thematic importance for each sentence. For immediate rereading, the contribution of lexical access to reading times either remained stable or decreased slightly, suggesting little change in this relatively automatic process. In contrast, the slope for the two measures of propositional assembly consistently decreased across readings, while that for the importance measure increased, suggesting again a shift in the kind and level of information being attended to during a second reading. When the second reading was delayed by 1 week, these changes were for the most part attenuated.

The Attentional Demands of Writing

More than many other tasks involving language, the psychology of writing approaches the psychology of thinking: Language is the means to bringing form to the writer's mental model of the material, and recreating it in the mind of the reader. I close this section of the chapter with a brief look at some recent work demonstrating the high attentional demands of the writing process.

Using the Posner and Boeis (1971) probe tone reaction time method (see "Measuring Resource Allocation in Reading Tasks," above), Kellogg (1994) assessed the cognitive effort demanded by the three primary stages of writing—discourse planning, translating into text, and reviewing. Each of these produced an increase in probe tone reaction time (compared to the time required to respond to the probe tone alone) that was twice that observed during a word-list-learning task or one involving reading difficult material. In fact, the only comparable increase in probe tone reaction time was found among chess experts during tournament games. Clearly, planning and composing prose are among the most effortful and attention-demanding language tasks that people are faced with.

ATTENTION, RESOURCE ALLOCATION, AND LANGUAGE IMPAIRMENT

I hope that this chapter has shown the usefulness, in both normal and impaired populations, of viewing attention as the allocation of limited processing resources to the tasks involved in language comprehension and production. Even without a fine-grained analysis of the particular resources that may be demanded by a particular process, the notions of resource limitations and resource allocation are proving to be helpful in understanding at least some consequences of the damage that results in aphasia.

Several theoretical points made in the foregoing discussion seem worth highlighting in trying to bridge resource theory and clinical evaluation and rehabilitation. First, both the single-resource and multiple-resource approaches seem to have value in elucidating the pattern of interference produced by increasing attentional demands. The single-resource view suggests that a common attentional resource or limit cuts across a wide range of specific tasks. This helps us in understanding how very dissimilar tasks may produce substantial amounts of dual-task interference. Stressing the system through additional tasks, through increases in task complexity, or through a variety of neurological impairments will compromise performance across a wide range of tasks.

The multiple-resource view of attention is supported by the greater interference that is observed when tasks or component processes compete for similar resources; hence greater dual-task interference is seen with the combination of two verbal tasks than with a combination of a verbal and a nonverbal task. In evaluating any impairment in attentional resources or allocation in a patient population, it seems critical not just to show that the patients are particularly impaired in dual-task relative to single-task conditions, as compared to normal controls, but to investigate the extent of impairment across various task combinations. By showing that both normal and aphasic subjects did worse on the verbal–verbal task combinations, for example, Murray et al. (1997a) were able to argue that the attentional impairment was general rather than specific to resources that support language. Only if the patients showed a *greater relative* impairment on similar compared with dissimilar competing tasks could domain-specific attentional impairment be inferred.

Second, what looks like a rather specific impairment to a language process may in fact be due to more general stress on attentional resources (Blackwell & Bates, 1995). Even instances of very specific dissociations in performance on syntactic tasks by different groups of patients may not be evidence for damage to specific language structures or modules, and only a systematic examination of how attentional demands interact with functional impairments can settle the issue. As Blackwell and Bates (1995) put it,

> While the data show that there are certainly some impairments that appear to be unique to either Broca's or Wernicke's [aphasia], there are also others that have been traditionally ascribed to these syndromes alone, and often to the specific tissue sites involved, which in fact may be explicable by more general mechanisms. (p. 244) . . . Apparent damage to a "syntax module" may be due to the particular vulnerability of those aspects of syntax implicated. (p. 245)

Third, it is critical for studies of patients with aphasia (or, indeed, any patients in whom it is suspected that attentional resources have been compromised) to include more than just a comparison of the patients' performance with that of normal subjects on some attention-demanding task. The investigation must also include manipulations of both specific linguistic functions and global stress, combined in a variety of dual-task conditions. Only in this way is it possible to specify not only (1) whether the impairment is in a specific process or in the attentional control of that process, but (2) if it is attentional, what aspect of attentional control is impaired (the overall available resources, the dynamic allocation of resources to specific processes, or the use of self-monitoring to evaluate performance and alter the allocation as appropriate). For example, Murray et al. (1997a) suggest that since aphasic patients as a group are slower and more variable in responses to various tasks than are control subjects, and since degree of linguistic impairment predicts variability of performance across tasks, "the aphasic individuals may have greater difficulty promptly initiating and shifting attentional resources rather than evaluating resource demands" (p. 805) of the dual tasks.

A more fine-grained analysis of the attentional abilities or shortcomings of aphasic individuals should also lead to improved intervention. At the very least, as suggested by Murray et al. (1998), this could involve testing and training under conditions that better capture the everyday potential for distraction, and the demands for task coordination, in the patients' social environment. Second, to the extent that there has been damage to automatic aspects of specific language processes and skills, so that what was once automatic now demands more attentional effort than before, the goal should be to reestablish the automaticity of those processes.

Some basis for optimism regarding the potential for establishing new procedural knowledge, despite catastrophic impairment in the ability to acquire new declarative knowledge, comes from recent attempts to teach new computer-based word-processing skills to patients with profound amnesia. Although it may take an amount of training that is orders of magnitude greater than that for normal subjects, and although qualitatively different strategies for task performance may be required (e.g., because of the inability of these patients to monitor and remember their errors), at least some patients can reach a level of skill allowing professional employment (Van der Linden & Coyette, 1995).

Finally, specific training on attentional focus and resource management in some individuals may prove helpful. Wickens (e.g., 1992), among others, has suggested that coordinating the multiple resources demanded by several ongoing tasks or processes is itself a skill that can be developed and modified (see Damos & Wickens, 1980). This should be done within the language domain to the extent possible, since clearly much time-sharing skill lies in learning how to coordinate two or more specific tasks or processes. But there may also be a role for "general attentional skill" to play, particularly if we believe that there is a general attentional system that cuts across tasks and domains. It is conceivable that dual-task training on nonverbal task combinations might generalize to improved ability in coordinating the processes and resources needed for speaking, listening, and understanding.

ACKNOWLEDGMENTS

Preparation of this chapter was supported by the Center for the Study of Emotion and Attention at the University of Florida, and by Grant No. P50-MH52384 from the National Institute of Mental Health. Discussions about language and attention with the members of the Center for Neuropsychological Studies at the University of Florida—in particular, those with the editors of this volume—were especially helpful in framing the issues discussed here. I am grateful to Stephen Nadeau, whose extensive comments on an earlier version of the chapter improved the clarity and logic of the presentation significantly.

REFERENCES

Allport, A. (1993). Attention and control: Have we been asking the wrong questions? A critical review of twenty-five years. In D. E. Meyer & S. Kornblum (Eds.), *Attention and performance XIV: Synergies in experimental psychology, artificial intelligence, and cognitive neuroscience* (pp. 183–218). Cambridge, MA: MIT Press.
Baddeley, A. D. (1986). *Working memory*. Oxford: Clarendon Press.

Baddeley, A. D. (1993). Working memory or working attention? In A. D. Baddeley & L. Weiskrantz (Eds.), *Attention: Selection, awareness, and control. A tribute to Donald Broadbent* (pp. 152–170). Oxford: Oxford University Press.

Baddeley, A., Lewis, V., Eldridge, M., & Thomson, N. (1984). Attention and retrieval from long-term memory. *Journal of Experimental Psychology: General, 113,* 518–540.

Barkley, R. A. (1996). Critical issues in research on attention. In G. R. Lyon & N. A. Krasnegor (Eds.), *Attention, memory, and executive function* (pp. 45–56). Baltimore: Brookes.

Bates, E., Devescovi, A., Hernandez, A., & Pizzamiglio, L. (1996). Gender priming in Italian. *Perception & Psychophysics, 58,* 992–1004.

Bates, E., Friederici, A., & Wulfeck, B. (1987). Comprehension in aphasia: A cross-linguistic study. *Brain and Language, 32,* 19–67.

Bentin, S. (1987). Event-related potentials, semantic processes, and expectancy factors in word recognition. *Brain and Language, 31,* 308–327.

Bentin, S., Kutas, M., & Hillyard, S. A. (1995). Semantic processing and memory for attended and unattended words in dichotic listening: Behavioral and electrophysiological evidence. *Journal of Experimental Psychology: Human Perception and Performance 21,* 54–67.

Besner, D., Smith, M. C., & MacLeod, C. M. (1990). Visual word recognition: A dissociation of lexical and semantic processing. *Journal of Experimental Psychology: Learning, Memory, and Cognition, 16,* 862–869.

Besson, M., Fischler, I., Boaz, T., & Raney, G. (1992). Effects of automatic associative activation on explicit and implicit memory tests. *Journal of Experimental Psychology: Learning, Memory, and Cognition, 18,* 89–105.

Blackwell, A., & Bates, E. (1995). Inducing agrammatic profiles in normals: Evidence for the selective vulnerability of morphology under cognitive resource limitation. *Journal of Cognitive Neuroscience, 7,* 228–257.

Carr, T. H. (1992). Automaticity and cognitive anatomy: Is word recognition "automatic"? *American Journal of Psychology, 105,* 201–237.

Carrier, L. M., & Pashler, H. (1995). Attentional limits in memory retrieval. *Journal of Experimental Psychology: Learning, Memory, and Cognition, 21,* 1339–1348.

Castaneda, M., Ostrosky-Solis, F., Perez, M., Bobes, M. A., & Rangel, L. E. (1997). ERP assessment of semantic memory in Alzheimer's disease. *International Journal of Psychophysiology, 27,* 201–214.

Cherry, C. (1953). Some experiments on the recognition of speech with one and with two ears. *Journal of the Acoustical Society of America, 25,* 975–979.

Chiarello, C., Maxfield, L., Richards, L., & Kahan, T. (1995). Activation of lexical codes for simultaneously presented words: Modulation by attention and pathway strength. *Journal of Experimental Psychology: Human Perception and Performance, 21,* 776–808.

Cohen, J. D., Dunbar, K., & McClelland, J. L. (1990). On the control of automatic processes: A parallel distributed processing account of the Stroop effect. *Psychological Review, 97,* 332–361.

Craik, F. I. M. (1982). Selective changes in encoding as a function of reduced processing capacity. In F. Klix, J. Hoffman, & E. van der Meer (Eds.), *Cognitive research in psychology* (pp. 152–161). Berlin: Deutscher Verlag der Wissenschaffen.

Craik, F. I. M., Govoni, R., Naveh-Benjamin, M., & Anderson, N. D. (1996). The effects of divided attention on encoding and retrieval processes in human memory. *Journal of Experimental Psychology: General, 125,* 159–180.

Damos, D. L., & Wickens, C. D. (1980). The identification and transfer of timesharing skills. *Acta Psychologica, 46,* 15–39.

Easterbrook, J. A. (1959). The effect of emotion on cue utilization and the organization of behavior. *Psychological Review, 66,* 183–201.

Eviatar, Z. (1998). Attention as a psychological entity and its effects on language and communication. In B. Stemmer & H. A. Whitaker (Eds.), *Handbook of neurolinguistics* (pp. 275–287). New York: Academic Press.

Finney, S. A., Protopapas, A., & Eimas, P. D. (1996). Attentional allocation to syllables in American English. *Journal of Memory and Language, 35,* 893–909.

Fischler, I. (1998). Attention and language. In R. Parasuraman (Ed.), *The attentive brain* (pp. 381–399). Cambridge, MA: MIT Press.

Fischler, I., & Bloom, P. A. (1980). Rapid processing of the meaning of sentences. *Memory & Cognition, 8,* 216–225.

Fischler, I., Howland, B., & Besson, M. (1994, November). *Divided attention and recognition memory: An ERP analysis*. Paper presented at the meeting of the Psychonomic Society, St. Louis, MO.

Fischler, I., Howland, B., Sikkema, R., & Besson, M. (1999). *Attention, semantic priming and memory for word pairs: An ERP analysis*. Unpublished manuscript, University of Florida.

Fischler, I., & Raney, G. E. (1991). Language by eye: Behavioral and psychophysiological approaches to reading. In J. R. Jennings & M. G. H. Coles (Eds.), *Handbook of cognitive psychophysiology: Central and autonomic nervous system approaches* (pp. 511–574). Chichester, England: Wiley.

Gopher, D., Brickner, M., & Navon, D. (1982). Different difficulty manipulations interact differently with task emphasis: Evidence for multiple resources. *Journal of Experimental Psychology: Human Perception and Performance, 8,* 146–158.

Greenwood, P. M., & Parasuraman, R. (1997). Attention in aging and Alzheimer's disease: Behavior and neural systems. In J. A. Burack & J. T. Enns (Eds.), *Attention, development, and psychopathology* (pp. 288–317). New York: Guilford Press.

Gunter, T. C., Jackson, J. L., & Mulder, G. (1992). An electrophysiological study of semantic processing in young and middle-aged academics. *Psychophysiology, 29,* 38–54.

Gunter, T. C., Jackson, J. L., & Mulder, G. (1995). Language, memory, and aging: An electrophysiological exploration of the N400 during reading of memory-demanding sentences. *Psychophysiology, 32,* 215–229.

Harley, T. A. (1995). *The psychology of language: From theory to data.* Hove, England: Psychology Press.

Hasher, L., & Zacks, R. T. (1979). Automatic and effortful processes in memory. *Journal of Experimental Psychology: General, 108,* 356–388.

Henik, A., Nissimov, E., Priel, B., & Umansky, R. (1995). Effects of cognitive load on semantic priming in patients with schizophrenia. *Journal of Abnormal Psychology, 104,* 576–584.

Hickok, G., Zurif, E., & Canseco-Gonzalez, E. (1993). Structural description of agrammatic comprehension. *Brain and Language, 45,* 371–395.

Holcomb, P. J. (1988). Automatic and attentional processing: An event-related brain potential analysis of semantic priming. *Brain and Language, 35,* 66–85.

Inhoff, A. W., & Fleming, K. (1989). Probe-detection times during the reading of easy and difficult text. *Journal of Experimental Psychology: Learning, Memory, and Cognition, 15,* 339–351.

Iragui, V., Kutas, M., & Salmon, D. P. (1996). Event-related brain potentials during semantic categorization in normal aging and senile dementia of the Alzheimer's type. *Electroencephalography and Clinical Neurophysiology: Evoked Potentials, 100,* 392–406.

James, W. (1890). *The principles of psychology* (2 vols.). New York: Holt.

Johnston, W. A., & Dark, V. J. (1986). Selective attention. *Annual Review of Psychology, 37,* 43–75.

Kahneman, D. (1973). *Attention and effort.* Englewood Cliffs, NJ: Prentice-Hall.

Kellogg, R. T. (1994). *The psychology of writing.* New York: Oxford University Press.

King, J., & Just, M. A. (1991). Individual differences in syntactic processing: The role of working memory. *Journal of Memory and Language, 30,* 580–602.

King, J. W., & Kutas, M. (1995). Who did what and when? Using word-level and clause-level ERPs to monitor working-memory usage in reading. *Journal of Cognitive Neuroscience, 7,* 376–395.

Kramer, A., & Spinks, J. (1991). Capacity views of human information processing. In J. R. Jennings & M. G. H. Coles (Eds.), *Handbook of cognitive psychophysiology: Central and autonomic nervous system approaches* (pp. 179–249). Chichester, England: Wiley.

Kutas, M., & Hillyard, S. A. (1980). Reading senseless sentences: Brain potentials reflect semantic incongruity. *Science, 207,* 203–205.

Logan, G. D. (1978). Attention in character-classification tasks: Evidence for the automaticity of component stages. *Journal of Experimental Psychology: General, 107,* 32–63.

Logan, G. D. (1988). Automaticity, resources, and memory: Theoretical controversies and practical implications. *Human Factors, 30,* 583–598.

Logan, G. D. (1995). Linguistic and conceptual control of visual spatial attention. *Cognitive Psychology, 28,* 103–174.

Luo, C. R., Johnson, R. A., & Gallo, D. A. (1998). Automatic activation of phonological information in reading: Evidence from the semantic relatedness decision task. *Memory & Cognition, 26,* 833–843.

MacKay, D., & Abrams, L. (1998). Age-linked declines in retrieving orthographic knowledge: Empirical, practical, and theoretical implications. *Psychology and Aging, 13,* 647–662.

Maxfield, L. (1995). *Turning down the semantic noise: The interaction of prime processing demands and activation of semantic information.* Unpublished doctoral dissertation, Syracuse University.

Maxfield, L. (1997). Attention and semantic priming: A review of prime task effects. *Consciousness and Cognition: An International Journal, 6,* 204–218.

McCann, R. S., Folk, C. L., & Johnston, J. C. (1992). The role of spatial attention in visual word processing. *Journal of Experimental Psychology: Human Perception and Performance, 18,* 1015–1029.

McNeil, M. R., Odell, K., & Tseng, C. H. (1991). Toward the integration of resource allocation into a general theory of aphasia. *Clinical Aphasiology, 20,* 21–39.

Meyer, D. E., & Kieras, D. E. (1997). A computational theory of executive cognitive processes and multiple-task performance: Part 2. Accounts of psychological refractory-period phenomena. *Psychological Review, 104,* 749–791.

Millis, K. K., Simon, S., & tenBroek, N. S. (1998). Resource allocation during the rereading of scientific texts. *Memory & Cognition, 26,* 232–246.

Mirsky, A. F., Anthony, B. J., Duncan, C. C., & Ahearn, M. B. (1991). Analysis of the elements of attention: A neuropsychological approach. *Neuropsychology Review, 2,* 109–145.

Miyake, A., Carpenter, P. A., & Just, M. A. (1994). A capacity approach to syntactic comprehension disorders: Making normal adults perform like aphasic patients. *Cognitive Neuropsychology, 11,* 671–717.

Miyamoto, T., Katayama, J., & Koyama, T. (1998). ERPs, semantic processing and age. *International Journal of Psychophysiology, 29,* 43–51.

Murray, L. L., Holland, A. L., & Beeson, P. M. (1997a). Auditory processing in individuals with mild aphasia: A study of resource allocation. *Journal of Speech, Language, and Hearing Research, 40,* 792–808.

Murray, L. L., Holland, A. L., & Beeson, P. M. (1997b). Grammaticality judgments of mildly aphasic individuals under dual-task conditions. *Aphasiology, 11,* 993–1016.

Murray, L. L., Holland, A. L., & Beeson, P. M. (1998). Spoken language of individuals with mild fluent aphasia under focused and divided-attention conditions. *Journal of Speech, Language, and Hearing Research, 41,* 213–227.

Nadeau, S. E., & Crosson, B. (1997). Subcortical aphasia. *Brain and Language,* 355–402.

Nairne, J. S. (1996). Short-term/working memory. In E. L. Bjork & R. A. Bjork (Eds.), *Handbook of perception and cognition: Memory* (2nd ed., pp. 101–126). San Diego, CA: Academic Press.

Naveh-Benjamin, M., Craik, F. I. M., Guez, J., & Dori, H. (1998). Effects of divided attention on encoding and retrieval processes in human memory: Further support for an asymmetry. *Journal of Experimental Psychology: Learning, Memory, and Cognition, 24,* 1091–1104.

Naveh-Benjamin, M., & Jonides, J. (1984). Maintenance rehearsal: A two-component analysis. *Journal of Experimental Psychology: Learning, Memory, and Cognition, 10,* 369–385.

Navon, D. (1984). Resources: A theoretical soup stone? *Psychological Review, 91,* 216–234.

Navon, D., & Miller, J. (1987). Role of outcome conflict in dual-task interference. *Journal of Experimental Psychology: Human Perception and Performance, 13,* 435–448.

Neely, J. H. (1977). Semantic priming and retrieval from lexical memory: Roles of inhibitionless spreading activation and limited-capacity attention. *Journal of Experimental Psychology: General, 106,* 226–254.

Neils, J., Roeltgen, D. P., & Greer, A. (1995). Spelling and attention in early Alzheimer's disease: Evidence for impairment of the graphemic buffer. *Brain and Language, 49,* 241–262.

Nestor, P. G., Kimble, M. O., O'Donnell, B. F., & Smith, L. (1997). Aberrant semantic activation in schizophrenia: A neurophysiological study. *American Journal of Psychiatry, 154,* 640–646.

Niznikiewicz, M. A., O'Donnell, B. F., Nestor, P. G., & Smith, L. (1997). ERP assessment of visual and auditory language processing in schizophrenia. *Journal of Abnormal Psychology, 106,* 85–94.

Norman, D. A., & Bobrow, D. G. (1975). On data-limited and resource-limited processes. *Cognitive Psychology, 7,* 44–64.

Okita, T., & Jibu, T. (1998). Selective attention and N400 attenuation with spoken word repetition. *Psychophysiology, 35,* 260–271.

Pallier, C., Sebastian-Galles, N., Felguera, T., & Christophe, A. (1993). Attentional allocation within the syllabic structure of spoken words. *Journal of Memory and Language, 32,* 373–389.

Pashler, H. (1994). Dual-task interference in simple tasks: Data and theory. *Psychological Bulletin, 116,* 220–244.

Pashler, H. (Ed.). (1998). *Attention.* Hove, England: Psychology Press.

Pashler, H., & Carrier, M. (1996). Structures, processes, and the flow of information. In E. L. Bjork & R. A. Bjork (Eds.), *Handbook of perception and cognition: Memory* (2nd ed., pp. 3–29). San Diego, CA: Academic Press.

Petersen, S. E., Fox, P. T., Posner, M. I., Mintun, M., & Raichle, M. E. (1989). Positron emission tomographic studies of the processing of single words. *Journal of Cognitive Neuroscience, 1,* 153–170.

Picton, T. W., & Hillyard, S. A. (1974). Human auditory evoked potentials: II. Effects of attention. *Electroencephalography and Clinical Neurophysiology, 36,* 191–200.

Posner, M. I. (1995). Attention in cognitive neuroscience: An overview. In M. S. Gazzaniga (Ed.), *The cognitive neurosciences* (pp. 615–624). Cambridge, MA: MIT Press.

Posner, M. I., & Boies, S. J. (1971). Components of attention. *Psychological Review, 78,* 391–408.

Posner, M. I., & Snyder, C. R. R. (1975). Attention and cognitive control. In R. Solso (Ed.), *Information processing and cognition* (pp. 55–85). Hillsdale, NJ: Erlbaum.

Pribram, K. H., & McGuinness, D. (1975). Arousal, activation, and effort in the control of attention. *Psychological Review, 82,* 116–149.

Raney, G. E. (1993). Monitoring changes in cognitive load during reading: An event-related brain potential and reaction time analysis. *Journal of Experimental Psychology: Learning, Memory, and Cognition, 19,* 51–69.

Sarno, K. J., & Wickens, C. D. (1995). Role of multiple resources in predicting time-sharing efficiency: Evaluation of three workload models in a multiple-task setting. *International Journal of Aviation, 5,* 107–130.

Schwartz, T. J., Kutas, M., Butters, N., & Paulsen, J. S. (1996). Electrophysiological insights into the nature of the semantic deficit in Alzheimer's disease. *Neuropsychologia, 34,* 827–841.

Staszewski, J. J. (1988). Skilled memory and expert mental calculation. In M. T. H. Chi & R. Glaser (Eds.), *The nature of expertise* (pp. 71–128). Hillsdale, NJ: Erlbaum.

Tanenhaus, M. K., Flanigan, H. P., & Seidenberg, M. S. (1980). Orthographic and phonological activation in auditory and visual word recognition. *Memory & Cognition, 8,* 513–520.

Theeuwes, J., Kramer, A. F., Hahn, S., & Irwin, D. E. (1998). Our eyes do not always go where we want them to: Capture of the eyes by new objects. *Psychological Science, 9,* 379–385.

Tseng, C. H., McNeil, M. R., & Milenkovic, P. (1993). An investigation of attention allocation deficits in aphasia. *Brain and Language, 45,* 276–296.

Underwood, G. (1974). Moray vs. the rest: The effects of extended shadowing practice. *Quarterly Journal of Experimental Psychology, 26,* 368–372.

Van der Linden, M., & Coyette, F. (1995). Acquisition of word-processing knowledge in an amnesic patient: Implications for theory and rehabilitation. In R. Campbell & M. A. Conway (Eds.), *Broken memories: Case studies in memory impairment* (pp. 54–76). Oxford: Blackwell.

Waters, G. S., Caplan, D., & Rochon, E. (1995). Processing capacity and sentence comprehension in patients with Alzheimer's disease. *Cognitive Neuropsychology, 12,* 1–30.

Welford, A. T. (1952). The 'psychological refractory period' and the timing of high-speed performance: A review and a theory. *British Journal of Psychology, 43,* 2–19.

Wickens, C. D. (1984). Processing resources in attention. In R. Parasuraman & D. R. Davies (Eds.), *Varieties of attention* (pp. 63–102). New York: Academic Press.

Wickens, C. D. (1992). *Engineering psychology and human performance.* New York: HarperCollins.

Yehene, V., & Tzelgov, J. (1996). Towards a two-factor model of automaticity: A transfer test of the algorithmic factor. *Psychologia: Israel Journal of Psychology, 5,* 121–136.

14

SYSTEMS THAT SUPPORT LANGUAGE PROCESSES: ATTENTION

BRUCE CROSSON

At the risk of oversimplification, it is worth stating that this chapter and the following chapter about working memory deal with brain systems and cognition. When functional systems approaches to brain functions (e.g., Luria, 1962/1966, 1973) replaced strict localization on the one hand and mass action on the other, the idea was advanced that different brain regions work together to perform a cognitive activity, each making a unique contribution to the function of the collective system. A single brain structure may be incorporated into systems for several cognitive activities, performing a similar function in each of the systems. The brain possesses some flexibility in composing functional systems, particularly for complex cognitive activities that can be approached in more than one way. Systems approaches have offered useful heuristics for conceptualizing many aspects of brain functions and are relied upon heavily in the current chapter and the chapter on working memory.

Nonetheless, functional systems models have demonstrated some limitations, and if they are to remain viable, they will have to incorporate concepts from other models. Connectionist models such as parallel distributed processing (PDP; McClelland, Rumelhart, & the PDP Research Group, 1986; Rumelhart, McClelland, & the PDP Research Group, 1986) can explain some aspects of brain functions that functional systems approaches leave unresolved. For example, the concept of "graceful degradation" explains how damaged systems frequently arrive at correct resolution of cognitive stimuli and problems in a parsimonious fashion that escapes systems models. The challenge of the future, and therefore of this chapter, is to integrate functional systems concepts with other models to offer plausible, parsimonious explanations of how the brain performs various cognitive activities.

From a functional systems standpoint, we know that simple cognitive activities provide the foundation for more complex operations. In order to understand language, it is necessary to focus on one source of linguistic information to the exclusion of other, distracting sources of sensory input. Furthermore, in order to understand a conversation, it is necessary not only to hold "on-line" certain contextual information, but also to maintain a temporary record of previous linguistic information from the conversation in order to interpret current input. Speaking also requires that one engage in the assimilation of linguistic output to the exclusion of potential competing activities. Thus the abilities to focus attention, to prioritize one activity among several possibilities, and to maintain a temporary record of contextual and linguistic information, though not strictly linguistic activities, are necessary for the efficient operation of linguistic processes. The purpose of the present chapter is to address attentional mechanisms and how they support language, including current knowledge regarding neural substrates of attention.

The chapter is divided into a section on psychological constructs, a section on anatomical substrates, and a section on clinical applications. In all these areas, conceptual linkages between language models on the one hand, and attention models on the other hand, are desparately needed to further our understanding of language and related systems. With this knowledge, we can begin to design assessments and treatments that address the attentional aspects of language systems.

COGNITIVE CONSTRUCTS

In 1890 William James claimed, "Everyone knows what attention is. It is the taking possession by the mind, in clear and vivid form, one out of what seem several simultaneously possible objects or trains of thought" (Vol. I, pp. 403–404). Posner and Boies (1971) later proposed three components of attention: "arousal," "selective attention," and "vigilance." In their paradigm, "arousal" is a general facilitation of cognitive processing for any source of information, but "selective attention" is facilitation of cognitive processing for a specific source of information, frequently to the exclusion of other sources. "Vigilance" is the ability to sustain arousal and selective attention over time. Thus, for Posner and Boies (1971), "selective attention" is very similar to James's (1890) use of the word "attention." This chapter focuses on how attention to language processes is established and maintained; that is, it addresses primarily selective attention.

Frequently, psychological theories have treated attention as a resource that can be allocated to processing information from certain sources or to certain activities. This conceptualization has led to the formulation of questions that have been difficult to answer. For example, is attention a single resource, or is it multiple resources? Can an attentional resource be divided among multiple information sources or activities, or is it indivisible? Considerable research has led to no clear answers on these subjects (e.g., Ballesteros, Manga, & Coello, 1989; Friedman, Polson, & Dafoe, 1988; Gladstones, Regan, & Lee, 1989; Pashler, 1991; Pashler & O'Brien, 1993). (See also Fischler, Chapter 13, this volume.)

I favor a view similar to that of Cohen (1993). That is, attention and intention are natural processes that arise out of various cognitive activities, and to some degree are inseparable from those activities. The need to attend selectively to one source of information over another or to prioritize one activity at the expense of others arises from the bottlenecks created by competition for use of the same processing, planning, and execution mechanisms by different potential stimuli and activities. This conceptualization of attention and intention has the advantage of focusing on processes rather than on a specific resource. It allows us to focus on how brain systems operate to direct attention to the appropriate source of information or activity, as opposed to searching for the neural equivalent of an attentional resource.

Heilman, Watson, and Valenstein (1993) have cited evidence for two types of attention: attention to sensory stimuli and attention to action. I refer to the former as "selective attention," and, in keeping with Heilman et al., I refer to the latter as "intention." The term "attention" is used here as a superordinate construct to encompass both selective attention and intention. From the viewpoint of language, selective attention is relevant to focusing on a particular source of information (e.g., a particular speaker), as well as deciding what incoming linguistic information to process further. In actuality, however, attention can be focused on internal as well as external sources of information. Obviously, the ability to turn the focus of attention inward to thoughts plays a role in the formulation of language sequences to communicate the thoughts.

Intention is the form of attention necessary to formulate and carry out actions. It is separate in some respects from selective attention to sensory information; at least, it can be isolated in some experimental paradigms from selective attention to sensory cues (e.g., Watson, Miller, & Heilman, 1978). Thus, in cognitive activities that require the formulation and execution of a response, a subject must intend to respond. Intention to act can be generated in two ways (Heilman, Watson, & Valenstein, 1993): (1) A response to an external stimulus is exogenously evoked (or "exo-evoked"), and (2) a response to an internal motivation or need is endogenously evoked (or "endo-evoked"). As applied to language, intention refers to the readiness to speak or produce some other form of linguistic output. Language can be evoked by external stimuli or can be brought about by internal motivations.

In spite of our ability to separate selective attention and intention in some experimental paradigms or other instances, intention and selective attention are frequently interrelated. In our everyday endeavors, the actions or plans we intend to carry out will determine the internal or external stimuli to which we attend. Furthermore, our perceived needs will influence both our intentions and the stimuli to which we choose to attend. Thus, as noted by Heilman et al. (1993), attention and intention are intertwined with motivation and brain structures that subserve motivation (i.e., parts of the limbic system).

To this point, I have discussed directing attention to a specific source of information or preparing to perform an activity to meet a specific goal. It is also necessary to focus on the selection of specific actions or concepts among the array of possible actions that could meet a particular motivational constraint. For example, from the possible ways to express a particular idea, we must make choices regarding particular lexical items that will most precisely and efficiently convey the idea. How we select one from a number of competing lexical items to convey an idea is also within the realm of attention and is a critical point of interface between attentional and language systems. Drawing on a number of lines of evidence and conceptual work, including connectionist models, a colleague and I (Nadeau & Crosson, 1997) have postulated a "selective engagement" mechanism that serves to engage those brain mechanisms necessary to perform a given cognitive activity, while holding other mechanisms in a state of relative disengagement. Engagement of the various brain mechanisms facilitates the activation of neural nets in which various types of cognitive representations reside. In the realm of lexical retrieval, we (Crosson & Nadeau, 1998; Crosson, 1999) have suggested that selective engagement serves to heighten differences in activation levels between a target lexical item and semantically related items through feedback and feedforward with semantic features. When differences in activation levels are amplified, the selection of the target item over semantically related competitors is facilitated.

Competition within cognitive systems may occur not only at the level of lexical retrieval, but also at the level of motivations driving the system. When two or more motivations are competing to direct attentional and/or intentional processes, one or more mechanisms for prioritizing motivations are necessary in order to control attentional and intentional processes. This mechanism has been referred to as the "supervisory attentional system" (Norman & Shallice, 1986) or the "central executive" (e.g., Baddeley, 1990; Cowan, 1988). Cowan uses the term "central executive" to refer to a conglomeration of related processes that direct attention and control voluntary action. As related to language, executive processes may direct attention to certain internal or external sources of linguistic or semantic information, or may direct intention toward producing linguistic communication in the service of some goal. For example, a worker may need to solve a problem involving mental arithmetic. He or she may have to direct attention to a coworker who is giving pertinent information, and, intermittently, to internal manipulations of that information in the process of problem solving. When a solution has been derived, the worker must prepare to communicate to others in order to implement the solution.

For the sake of completeness, it must be noteed that automatic mechanisms also capture attention—for example, orienting responses. Such automatic mechanisms do not involve executive processes, since they do not require a conscious direction of attention or intention; however, automatic processes may compete with or supersede voluntary direction of attention through executive processes.

The interface between attention and language is summarized in Figure 14.1. Attentional processes arise naturally out of the use of language to accomplish various goals. Three types of attentional processes have been identified: "selective attention," "intention," and "selective engagement." "Selective attention" refers to the ability to focus on a source of linguistic information to the exclusion of other information sources, and the ability to select specific linguistic information for further processing. "Intention" refers to the preparation to use language and is necessary for the formulation of verbal output. Intention affects attention because the intention to perform a particular activity determines the external and internal sources of information to which we attend. "Selective engagement" refers to the process of engaging specific brain regions needed for cognitive tasks and enables efficient selection

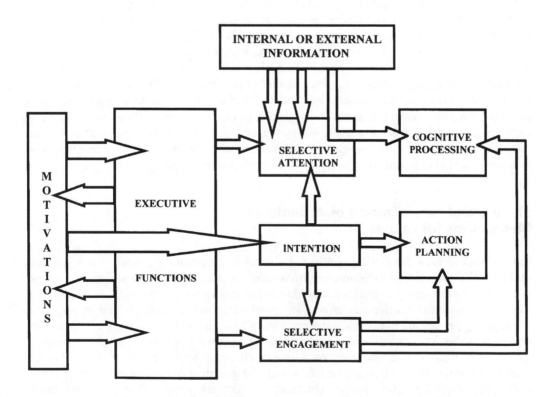

FIGURE 14.1. Schematic representation of relationships among selective attention, intention, selective engagement, motivation, and executive functions.

of competing lexical alternatives. Intention influences selective engagement because the intention to perform an activity must determine what brain systems are brought on-line through selective engagement. The ability to selectively engage appropriate brain systems affects the efficiency of cognitive processing and action planning. Selective attention, intention, and selective engagement are all driven by motivational processes involving limbic structures. Executive functions prioritize the competing motivations, so that the influence of one motivation on selective attention, intention, and selective engagement predominates. The predominant motivation influences the sources of information to which we attend, the actions and activities that we intend, and the brain mechanisms that we engage during language processes.

ANATOMICAL SUBSTRATES

As we consider the anatomical substrates for attentional processes that have an impact on language, two questions arise: What structures are involved in regulating attentional processes that subserve language? And are the structures that regulate attention for language processes shared with systems that perform different cognitive functions? The questions can be addressed at a number of different levels. At the most global, we might simply ask whether attentional mechanisms are shared between language and other cognitive systems, or whether attentional mechanisms for language reside primarily in the language-dominant hemisphere. At a greater level of specificity, we might ask exactly which structures contribute to the attentional substrates of language. Currently, these questions are difficult to answer because of a lack of good experimental paradigms for studying the neurobiological substrates of attention for language. As the reader will probably note in reading the following paragraphs, it is often difficult to experimentally separate language from the attentional mechanisms that support it. In dealing with the neurobiological substrates of attention and language, I draw selectively upon both empirical studies and theoretical treatments of attention and the attention–language interface. The following discussion, then, addresses two questions: (1) At the most general level, are attentional mechanisms shared between language and other cognitive systems, and do attentional systems affecting language reside within the language-dominant hemisphere? (2) What specific mechanisms from an anatomical standpoint may be involved in attention to language?

Sharing and Lateralization of Attentional Mechanisms for Language

In our laboratory, Petry (1995) conducted a study to determine whether or not language and spatial monitoring share common attentional mechanisms, and, if so, whether or not such mechanisms reside in the language-dominant hemisphere. She used a dual-task paradigm to explore the interference effects on visual selective attention created by two types of language processing in normal subjects. Figure 14.2 shows the sequence of stimuli presented to subjects. The covert-orientation-of-visual-attention task (COVAT; Posner & Cohen, 1980) involved responding to a lateralized target appearing after a cue. The cue was the brightening of a box to the left or right of a central fixation point. Either 100 or 800 milliseconds (ms) after the cue, the target (an asterisk) appeared in one of the boxes. On valid trials, the target appeared in the box that brightened; on invalid trials, the target appeared in the opposite box. On some trials (uncued trials), the target appeared in one of

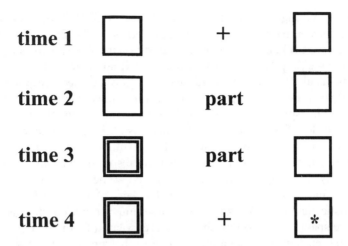

FIGURE 14.2. Sequence of stimuli for Petry's (1995) study. At time 1, two boxes are positioned to the left or right of a central fixation point (crosshairs). At time 2, the central fixation point is replaced by a word. The subject either reads the word aloud (reading task) or generates a semantic associate of the word (semantic associate task). At time 3, one of the boxes brightens, and at time 4, a target (asterisk) appears either in the box that brightened (valid trial) or in the opposite box (invalid trial). When the target appears, the subject presses a key as quickly as possible.

the boxes without a cue. In the dual-task paradigm, a word was presented either 100 or 250 ms before the COVAT cue. Subjects either had to read the word or had to generate a semantic associate for it. Normally, a cue in one visual field will shorten reaction times to targets on valid trials, but will delay responses to targets on invalid trials. Damage to structures in one hemisphere has a varying impact on responses to cues or targets presented in contralesional space, depending on the location of the lesion within the hemisphere (Posner, Walker, Friedrich, & Rafal, 1984, 1987; Rafal & Posner, 1987); this suggests that spatial attentional mechanisms are lateralized. Based on previous research with normal subjects (Posner, Early, Reiman, Pardo, & Dhawan, 1988), the expectation was that subjects would be unaffected by cues presented in the right visual field while performing a language task. In other words, subjects would be unable to use cues presented in their right visual field because left-hemisphere mechanisms were engaged in processing linguistic stimuli. Thus it was thought that this pattern would represent the interference of the language task on left-hemisphere spatial processing mechanisms.

No such effect was found. Instead, the reading and the semantic tasks both generated interference without respect to the visual field of the target or cue, as indicated by delays in responding to targets. Furthermore, the semantic task generated massive delays relative to the reading task. Finally, as expected, responses were faster to valid trials under single-task conditions, but this validity effect was lost under most dual-task conditions. If language and spatial attention shared no common attentional mechanisms, the language tasks should have interfered relatively little with the spatial attention task. Instead, the interference effects indicated a common attention mechanism, regardless of the visual field for target or cue. The hypothesis that was based on the assumption of lateralization of attentional mechanisms for language was not confirmed; responding to stimuli in both visual fields was affected. Thus these findings do not suggest any specific location of the common mechanism for attention to language and space.

It is worth examining the earlier results of Posner et al. (1988), since they could lead to a different conclusion from the one reached by Petry (1995). They also used a dual-task paradigm with the COVAT, but their language condition involved having subjects "shadow" a literary passage (i.e., repeat a literary passage that they heard). There were 20 normal subjects (18 right-handed). Under the shadowing condition, subjects responded more slowly on the COVAT, as in Petry's experiment. However, subjects showed a validity effect in the right visual field, responding more quickly to valid than to invalid trials. They lost this validity effect in the left visual field. In a later analysis of the experiment, Posner and Early (1990) suggested that this lack of a validity effect resulted from the fact that invalid cues in the right visual field did not distract subjects from responding to targets in the left visual field. The generally slower responding again suggests some attentional mechanisms common to language and visual–spatial functions. The lack of an effect for invalid cues only from the right visual field further suggests that under interference conditions from language, right-hemisphere spatial attention mechanisms are isolated from left-hemisphere input to some extent. The left hemisphere cannot isolate itself from the distracting effects of invalid cues in the left visual field. In other words, when the left hemisphere is occupied with language processing, its automatic spatial processing no longer affects the right hemisphere. It follows from this analysis that although each hemisphere contains mechanisms for attending to contralateral space, under normal conditions these attentional mechanisms interact in complex ways.

How can the results of Posner et al. (1988) be reconciled with those of Petry (1995)? First, one should note that subjects in both studies showed significant delays in the spatial processing task when performing language tasks, indicating attentional mechanisms common to spatial processing and language. Regarding the lack of a validity effect in the left visual field found during language processing by Posner et al. and not by Petry, three differences may be important. First, Petry's language tasks were tightly time-locked to presentation of the COVAT cue, whereas the task of Posner et al. was more or less continuous. Longer intervals between the language stimulus and the COVAT cues in Petry's experiment might have led to different results. Second, the nature of language processing was different in the two experiments. In Petry's experiment, subjects were processing lexical stimuli, whereas in Posner et al.'s experiment, subjects were reproducing narrative discourse. Perhaps these different types of language processing require different attentional mechanisms. Third, Petry's stimuli were presented visually, while the stimuli used by Posner et al. were auditory. Perhaps the demands for visual processing of linguistic stimuli in Petry's study led to greater interference with processing of visual–spatial stimuli.

Attempts have been made to explore the interface between language and attention in patients with various forms of brain injury or disease, and these studies have some bearing on intrahemispheric attentional mechanisms. That is, the difficulties in attention demonstrated by aphasic patients would suggest that attentional mechanisms reside, at least in part, in the language-dominant hemisphere. For example, Tseng, McNeil, and Milenkovic (1993) presented a dual-task paradigm using linguistic stimuli to aphasic and control subjects. Subjects had to listen to words in order to identify both phonemic targets and semantic targets embedded in a list, with the number of foils being equal to the number of targets. Subjects were required to press one button on a computer keyboard if the word appearing was a target, and another if the word appearing was not a target. The ratio of phonemic to semantic targets varied from 2:8 to 5:5 to 8:2 in different sessions. In an explicit condition, subjects were given information about the ratio of phonemic to semantic targets and a strategy with which to respond, whereas in an implicit condition no information was given. Normal subjects improved reaction times to phonemic targets when the density of phonemic targets increased, whether or not they were explicitly given information about target density. For semantic targets, their reaction times improved with increased semantic target density only when information about target density was explicitly given. For aphasic patients, neither reaction times nor accuracy improved with changes in target density. The authors concluded that the aphasic patients either could not evaluate the attentional demands of the task or could not adequately allocate attentional resources. One problem with this interpretation is that one cannot distinguish whether the aphasic patients' reaction times reflected attentional factors or primary difficulties in linguistic processing of the stimuli in accordance with task demands. Such difficulties are evident from the high error rates for aphasic subjects (4–40%) as compared to control subjects (0–1.4%). Thus the processing difficulties of aphasic individuals may entirely override any attentional considerations, and such studies do not provide definitive information regarding lateralization mechanisms.

The conundrum of how to measure effects of attentional problems on language deficits in aphasic patients can be resolved to some extent if a simple assumption is made. To the extent that attentional mechanisms for language are shared with other cognitive processes (as indicated by Petry, 1995, and Posner et al., 1988), it may be possible to devise tasks that can demonstrate the relationship between attention and language in aphasia. One way to do this would be to manipulate attention through nonlanguage channels and to record the effects on language. A second approach would be to correlate nonlinguistic measures of attention with language performance in aphasic patients.

Murray, Holland, and Beeson (1997) studied semantic judgments and lexical decision tasks in mildly aphasic and normal individuals. Tasks were presented under three conditions: (1) no distraction present; (2) target stimuli for a secondary task present, but performance of only the primary task required; and (3) target stimuli for a secondary task present, and simultaneous task performance required. Secondary-task stimuli were either verbal or nonverbal. The semantic judgment task required subjects to determine whether a word was a member of a specific category; the lexical decision task required subjects to determine whether a stimulus was a real word. In the verbal distraction condition, the two verbal tasks (semantic judgment and lexical decision) served as distractors for one another. The nonverbal distraction task required subjects to discriminate whether a tone was of high or low frequency. Aphasic patients were more susceptible than controls to the presence of a distractor for both the semantic judgment and lexical decision tasks. Although the effects of distraction were especially severe if the distractor was verbal, it is unclear whether such effects were due to attentional or to language deficits. However, the presence of the nonverbal stimuli also degraded language performance to a greater extent in the aphasic patients than in the control subjects. This finding suggests that attention deficits were present in the patients with aphasia. There were no significant correlations between aphasia severity and performance under either the verbal or nonverbal distraction conditions. This finding indicates that severity of aphasia could not account for the attention deficits, and suggests some independence of the two phenomena. The authors had predicted greater deterioration of performance during distraction and dual-task conditions in patients with frontal as opposed to posterior lesions, because the frontal lobes are involved in executive functions that control and direct attention. No consistent differences were found between patients with frontal versus posterior lesions. At least two factors may have contributed to the lack of differences between these two lesion types. First, the tasks involved both significant attentional and significant intentional components. Although patients with both types of lesions showed disruption of performance with distraction or in dual-task conditions, this disruption may have occurred at different points in processing. That is, patients with posterior lesions may have exhibited disrupted performance in simultaneous processing of incoming stimuli, while patients with frontal lesions may have shown disrupted performance in simultaneous preparation of outputs. Second, as noted by the authors, the structural imaging scans (computerized tomography [CT] or magnetic resonance imaging [MRI]) used to locate lesions may give an incomplete picture of structural damage and functional implications. We (Nadeau & Crosson, 1997) have discussed this problem extensively.

The second approach, correlating nonlinguistic measures of attention with language functions, has also been used in patients with language deficits. We (Petry, Crosson, Rothi, Bauer, & Schauer, 1994) used the COVAT, described above (Posner & Cohen, 1980), to explore attention in right-handed patients who had aphasia after left-hemisphere stroke. The task was done alone, without any interference conditions. At a 100-ms cue-to-target interval, normal age-matched controls demonstrated the expected validity effect in both visual fields (i.e., faster responding on valid than on invalid trials). In comparison, aphasic subjects responded significantly more slowly than controls on all trials. Furthermore, aphasic patients did not show a validity effect for targets in the left visual field, with responses to invalid targets in the left visual field being significantly faster than responses to invalid targets in the right visual field. Patients with larger validity effects on the right than on the left side also had more significant impairments in language comprehension and expression. One explanation for these findings is similar to that noted above for subjects in the dual-task paradigm of Posner et al. (1988): Right-hemisphere spatial attention mechanisms are not affected by invalid cues presented to the damaged left hemisphere, whereas left-hemisphere spatial attention mechanisms are still affected by invalid cues presented to the intact right hemisphere. There was a correlation between the spatial attention tasks and language performance, such that a larger difference in validity effects between the right and left visual fields was seen in patients with greater language impairment. It should also be noted that the generally slowed responses of aphasic patients are like the responses of normal subjects in dual-task conditions (Petry, 1995; Posner et al., 1988) and suggest a general sharing of language and spatial attention mechanisms. The fact that these effects are seen in patients with left-hemisphere lesions suggests that the left hemisphere participates in the common mechanism for attention to language and spatial attention. However, the fact that cues in the right visual field do not distract patients from responding to a target in the left visual field leads to the inescapable conclusion that attentional mechanisms in the two hemispheres normally interact.

Massman et al. (1993) studied the relationship of a different form of spatial attention to language deficits and constructional apraxia in patients with Alzheimer's disease (AD). It is known that in early stages, AD may affect one hemisphere more than the other in some patients. Massman et al. located three groups of patients with AD: patients whose Boston Naming Test scores were significantly worse than their Wechsler Adult Intelligence Scale—Revised (WAIS-R) Block Design scores; patients whose Block Design scores were significantly worse than their Boston Naming Test scores; and patients whose Block Design and Boston Naming Test scores were comparable. Subjects were presented with stimuli on a computer monitor that included large 1's composed of either small 1's or small 2's, and large 2's composed of either small 1's or 2's. Subjects were instructed to attend either to the small numbers (local condition) or to the large configuration (global condition), and to press one key for 1's and another key for 2's. Accuracy of response was measured for stimuli in which the global configuration was in conflict with the local characters (i.e., a large 1 consisting of small 2's or a large 2 consisting of small 1's). Patients with spatial (Block Design) impairments were significantly less accurate when asked to attend to the global as compared to the local features, and patients with naming impairments were significantly less accurate when asked to attend to the local as compared to the global features. Reaction times were analyzed for stimuli in which global and local information were congruent (and error rates were low). It was found that patients with more severely impaired naming responded more quickly on trials during which they attended to the global as opposed to the local features. Patients with impaired spatial abilities showed the reverse pattern. The authors concluded that poor attention to the local configuration reflected disruption of left-hemisphere attentional mechanisms, while poor attention to the global configuration reflected disruption of right-hemisphere attentional mechanisms. Thus the two hemispheres appear to be specialized for attending to different kinds of spatial information. Although previous research has shown that acquired lesions of the left hemisphere tend to lead to a greater advantage in processing global over local stimuli than is present in normal controls (Lamb, Robertson, & Knight, 1989), the relationship of this phenomenon to language deficits in these patients is not known. It is possible that the findings reflect common mechanisms for spatial attention and language, but it is also possible that mechanisms for spatial attention and language are distinct but both dysfunctional in these patients. Furthermore, it is unclear how attention to global or local features is related to other attentional measures, such as those discussed above (i.e., Petry et al., 1994).

The findings of Coslett and his colleagues are more definitive, both with respect to attentional mechanisms common to spatial and language processing, and with respect to localization of at least one attentional mechanism. Coslett, Schwartz, Goldberg, Haas, and Perkins (1993) described a patient with left temporo-parietal and left anterior cingulate lesions who showed "profound and disabling posturing and involuntary movement" (p. 529). of the right arm when he attempted to use it in his right hemispace. Yet when he used the right hand in his left hemispace, the involuntary movements were minimized or even eliminated. Experimental tasks demonstrated a powerful effect of hemispace in which movements were performed with the right hand, but movements performed with the left hand were also affected by hemispace. Motor performance was also improved to some degree by orienting the patient's head to the left as opposed to the right. The patient was noted to have language deficits. On a variety of tasks including auditory comprehension, visual naming, oral reading, narrative language production, and verbal fluency, the patient was noted to perform much better when stimuli were presented from the left as opposed to the right side, or when he oriented to the left as opposed to the right side. In a subsequent study, Coslett (1999) found some patients (4 of 29, using conservative criteria) who performed significantly more poorly on one or more language tasks when orienting attention to the hemispace contralateral to their cerebrovascular accident. No subjects performed significantly better when attending to the contralateral hemispace. All subjects demonstrating this hemispatial effect had parietal lobe lesions. Thus the hemispatial effects found in the patient described above (Coslett et al., 1993) were not unique. Coslett (1999) has suggested that parietal lobe attentional mechanisms serve to hold stimuli in contralateral hemispace in registration with the appropriate processing systems.

Like some of the studies discussed above (i.e., Petry et al., 1994; Posner et al., 1988), the studies by Coslett and colleagues suggest that right- and left-hemisphere attentional mechanisms interact. Furthermore, their data suggest that if right-hemisphere attentional mechanisms can be engaged by manipulating spatial attention, they can substitute, at least in part, for dysfunctional left-hemisphere mechanisms in aphasic patients with left parietal lesions.

A study by Anderson (1996) demonstrated effects similar to those found by Coslett and colleagues. Anderson described an aphasic patient with left temporo-parietal and right parietal infarctions who had disproportionate difficulty canceling pictures (e.g., of a pen-cil) in the right side of space relative to the left side of space when the pictures he was asked to cancel were named by the experimenter. Cancellation of lines and of meaningful objects when the target was presented visually was relatively unimpaired. The author con-cluded that the patient had a form of neglect for lexical–semantic processing in the right side of space. However, this study also demonstrated that the patient's ability to detect and cancel pictures on the basis of lexical–semantic input improved when pictures were presented in the left hemispace (i.e., the hemispace ipsilateral to the language-dominant hemisphere). This finding, which is similar to those of Coslett (1999), suggests that shift-ing the patient's hemispatial attention in such a way that right-hemisphere mechanisms were engaged improved his ability to use lexical-semantic input to guide selection of visual stimuli. Apparently, the right parietal lesion did not damage the critical right-hemisphere attentional mechanism.

Some tentative conclusions can be drawn from these studies. First, attentional processes subserving language share at least some mechanisms with attention for other cognitive processes (Petry, 1995; Posner et al., 1988). One probable purpose of these common mecha-nisms is to prioritize the use of limited processing resources for linguistic and nonlinguistic functions. Second, the left hemisphere appears to participate in these common attentional mechanisms for language and other processes (Anderson, 1996; Coslett, 1999; Petry et al., 1994). However, under normal circumstances, there appear to be complex interactions between left- and right-hemisphere attentional processes. In some circumstances with apha-sic patients, undamaged attentional mechanisms in the nondominant hemisphere can be engaged to compensate for damaged attentional mechanisms in the dominant hemisphere (Coslett et al., 1993; Coslett, 1999). Because tasks in most of these studies involved both processing of incoming stimuli and generation of a response, it is difficult to separate selective attention and intentional processes.

Specific Left-Hemisphere Mechanisms Involved in Attention for Language

Although the literature cited above suggests attentional mechanisms common to language and other cognitive functions, and also suggests that at least some of these mechanisms rely on left-hemisphere structures, the question remains as to which specific left-hemisphere structures may be involved. In order to answer this question, we can turn to the model of Heilman et al. (1993). Although developed primarily in the arena of spatial attention, this model can be adapted as a starting point to address the interface of attention and language. Recent functional neuroimaging literature supports this application.

Heilman et al. (1993) reviewed the literature on attentional systems. In particular, with respect to selective attention, they concluded that frontal cortex and perhaps sensory association cortex can influence transmission of information to the cortex through con-nections with the nucleus reticularis. The nucleus reticularis is a thin shell of neurons sur-rounding the thalamus that sends inhibitory fibers to thalamic nuclei. The nucleus reticularis in turn regulates the transmission mode of primary sensory relay nuclei of the thalamus (i.e., the medial geniculate, lateral geniculate, and ventral posterior nuclei). These effects are prelinguistic in nature, in that information that is not transmitted to primary sensory cortex via primary thalamic relay nuclei is not available for further processing at a linguis-tic level. In other words, the impact on language comprehension has to do with whether or not certain information becomes available for linguistic processing. Heilman et al. noted that the anterior cingulate cortex connects with lateral frontal cortex, providing frontal cortex with information about the motivational state of the organism. To the extent that goal-directed mechanisms of the frontal cortex then influence attention (e.g., see the discussion of Nadeau & Crosson, 1997, below), the anterior cingulate cortex may affect this process. There is also evidence, which I discuss below, that the pre-supplementary motor area (pre-SMA) and related structures in the adjacent Brodmann's area (BA) 32 are involved in some aspect of initiating language output. Pre-SMA and apparently adjacent BA 32 are connected to lateral prefrontal and premotor cortex (Luppino, Matelli, Camarda, & Rizzolatti, 1993; Matsuzaka, Aizawa, & Tanji, 1992; Picard & Strick, 1996). Studies of similar, though not identical, cortex in monkeys suggest that BA 32 has connections with the cingulate gyrus (Morecraft & Van Hoesen, 1998). On the sensory side, posterior cingulate cortex communicates with polymodal and supramodal sensory association cortex, providing the anatomical substrate by which motivational state influences sensory processes. The relationship of posterior cingulate cortex to language processing has been worked out less well than the relationship of medial frontal cortex; however, some functional neuroimaging evidence suggests that posterior cingulate cortex influences processing of language input. At the level of the thalamus, the evidence suggests that the pulvinar is involved somehow in lexical–semantic processing, consistent with the anatomical connections of this nucleus (for a review, see Crosson, 1992). As in the proposal of Heilman et al. (1993), it is possible that attention for language processing is influenced by the cortical input to the nucleus reticularis, which in turn influences the pulvinar. The relationships among these structures are shown in Figure 14.3.

Functional imaging studies of semantic monitoring can also give us some insights into selective attention mechanisms. Particularly relevant to this issue was a study accomplished

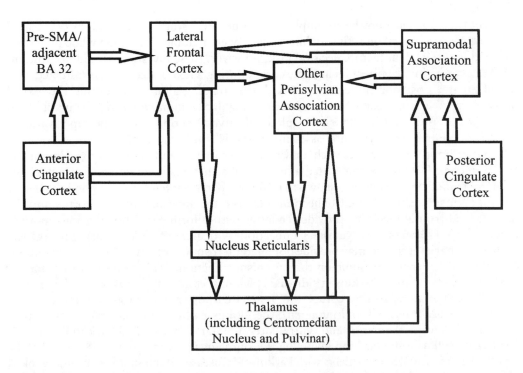

FIGURE 14.3. Connections among structures thought to be involved in selective attention for language.

by Demonet, Price, Wise, and Frackowiak (1994). In this study, subjects performed a semantic monitoring task that involved listening to nouns (animal names) paired with adjectives. They had to press a button when the animal was small and the adjective was a positive attribute. Subjects also performed a phonemic task in which they monitored nonwords for the phoneme /b/ preceded by a /d/ in the previous syllable. Subjects pressed a button when the target occurred; target density was 30% in both tasks. When the positron emission tomography (PET) image acquired during the phonemic task was subtracted from the image acquired during the semantic task, an area of increased activity was seen in the left posterior cingulate cortex in addition to left dorsolateral frontal cortex (an area different from that noted by Petersen, Fox, Posner, Mintun, & Raichle, 1988, or McCarthy, Blamire, Rothman, Gruetter, & Shulman, 1993). Additional areas of activation included left and right angular gyrus and left middle temporal gyrus. Thus the findings of Demonet et al. (1994) support the participation of the posterior cingulate and inferior parietal cortices in a task that involves attending to the semantic properties of heard words, but other studies indicate that the role of the posterior cingulate cortex is not unique to semantic analysis.

For example, when Frith, Friston, Liddle, and Frackowiak (1991a) subtracted PET images acquired during word repetition from images acquired during word generation, they found that the posterior cingulate cortex and an area in the posterior superior temporal gyrus demonstrated greater activity during word repetition than during word generation. Subjects of Frith, Friston, Liddle, and Frackowiak (1991b) showed increased blood flow to the left and right posterior cingulate areas during a lexical decision task. Other areas of increased activity during the lexical decision task included the auditory association cortex, left frontal pole, and right ventral prefrontal cortex. One component that semantic monitoring, repetition, and lexical decision tasks have in common is a need for accurate analysis of heard words. In other words, selective attention to the incoming linguistic stimuli is necessary.

Yet the story may not be so simple. In another PET study, Price et al. (1994) found greater posterior cingulate activity while subjects were reading aloud than while they were engaged in a false-font feature decision task; however, these investigators did not find increased activity in the posterior cingulate cortex during a lexical decision task. In fact, they found greater posterior cingulate activity during reading aloud than during the lexical decision task. It is unclear why the posterior cingulate region would not be involved in lexical decision tasks if its job is to regulate selective attention based upon motivational constraints. Further experimental assessment of this issue is needed.

Based upon their own research as well as their review and analysis of the literature, Heilman et al. (1993) also implicated a number of structures in intentional systems. Dorsolateral frontal areas have been shown to be involved in the intention to respond to sensory stimuli (Watson et al., 1978). Connections between the anterior cingulate cortex and the dorsolateral frontal lobe may provide the latter with information about various motivations and need states of the organism. Connections with areas of multisensory convergence, such as the parietal cortex, may provide dorsolateral frontal cortex with information about external stimuli that may summon the organism to action. Making inferences from the type of akinesia seen in Parkinson's disease, Heilman et al. (1993) suggested that a loop from the dorsolateral frontal cortex and associated posterior cortices through the neostriatum (caudate nucleus and putamen), the globus pallidus and substantia nigra pars reticulata, the ventral anterior and ventral lateral thalamic nuclei, and back to the frontal cortex, as well as a similar loop involving the supplementary motor area (SMA), may be involved in intention. Since patients with Parkinson's disease exhibit more of an endo-evoked akinesia, one might conclude that these structures are more involved in endo-evoked intention. The caudal intralaminar nuclei (centromedian–parafascicular) may be involved in intentional activity by virtue of two types of connectivity. First, these nuclei project heavily to the neostriatum, providing a means for affecting endo-evoked intention. Second, these nuclei project to the dorsolateral frontal cortex, providing a means for affecting intentional activities involving the dorsolateral frontal cortex. (See Mennemeier et al., 1997, for further discussion of the role of the caudal intralaminar nuclei in intention.) The nucleus reticularis may modulate activity of the ventral anterior, ventral lateral, and centromedian–parafascicular nuclei through its inhibitory gamma-aminobutyric acid-ergic connections with these nuclei. Finally, the midbrain reticular formation affects tonic activity in both the centromedian–parafascicular complex and the nucleus reticularis. The relationships among these structures have been diagrammed in Figure 14.4.

Goldberg (1985) presented a similar hypothesis regarding endo-evoked and exo-evoked intentions, based upon his extensive analysis of the literature. He suggested that the SMA plays an important role in intentional processes when internal context influences the elaboration of action (i.e., endo-evoked actions). Since the SMA is the recipient of basal ganglia projections via the thalamus, this hypothesis is consistent with the analysis of Heilman et al. (1993). Goldberg also suggested that the lateral premotor system is involved in actions guided by external circumstances (i.e., exo-evoked actions). Since the reviews of Goldberg (1985) and Heilman et al. (1993), the division of medial BA 6 into SMA proper and pre-SMA has become common. SMA is connected to lateral motor and premotor systems, and pre-SMA is connected to lateral prefrontal and premotor systems (Luppino et al., 1993;

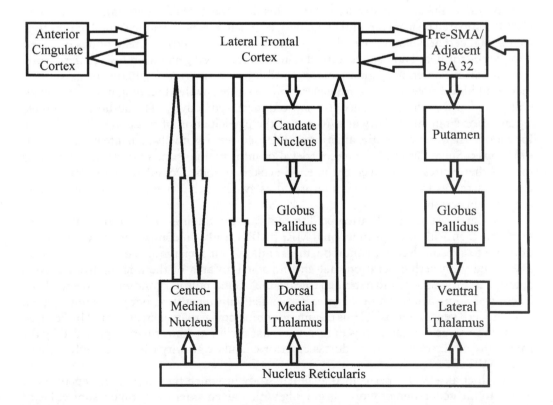

FIGURE 14.4. Connections among structures thought to be involved in the intentional aspects of language.

Matzusaka et al., 1992; Picard & Strick, 1996). The most recent literature has implicated pre-SMA and, to some degree, SMA in initiation of language output. A recent study in our laboratory found some evidence of a shift in the balance of activity from pre-SMA to lateral frontal cortex as word generation tasks become more driven by external stimuli than by internal mechanisms (Sadek et al., 1999). This finding is generally consistent with Goldberg's (1985) hypothesis, except that pre-SMA and not SMA was implicated in initiation of internally driven word generation.

Language disturbances resulting from damage to the mesial frontal cortex (SMA and anterior cingulate cortex), or connections between mesial frontal cortex and anterior perisylvian language cortex in the dominant hemisphere, probably reflect disruption of the intention to communicate. Patients with these lesions are initially mute, but their speech and language output evolves to become slow (nonfluent) and hypophonic. In general, output improves with repetition (Barris & Schuman, 1953; Benson, 1993; Jonas, 1981; Nielson & Jacobs, 1951). The relative sparing of repetition raises a question regarding endo- versus exo-evoked responses, suggesting that when the response is highly constrained by the input, output is less impaired; this is consistent with Goldberg's (1985) hypothesis.

Early functional neuroimaging studies implicated the anterior cingulate gyrus and dorsolateral prefrontal cortex in language processes. One process in which these areas of cortex seemed to be involved is the generation of language (i.e., the internal processes necessary to access internally stored information to generate responses). Two studies have compared language generation tasks to repetition, using PET. In these designs, internally generated language involves endo-evoked intention. Repetition, on the other hand, involves responding on the basis of an external stimulus (i.e., exo-evoked intention). Petersen et al. (1988) compared regional cerebral blood flow while subjects were reading aloud or repeating to regional cerebral blood flow while they were generating verbs for read nouns or generating verbs for heard nouns, respectively. In both the word generation tasks, inferior prefrontal cortex, anterior cingulate cortex, and inferior anterior cingulate cortex showed increased blood flow. In the word generation task that involved reading nouns, dorsolateral and lateral prefrontal cortex also showed increased activity. The authors interpreted the anterior cingulate activity as evidence of the participation of this cortex in "selection for action." In other words, the anterior cingulate cortex was involved in intentional aspects of the task. Since this task involves retrieval of information from an internal database, it may further represent involvement in endo-evoked actions. Dorsolateral and lateral prefrontal increases in activity were interpreted as evidence that these areas are involved in semantic processing.

McCarthy et al. (1993) attempted to replicate the findings of Petersen et al. (1988), using the identical task in a functional MRI (fMRI) study. In comparing the verb generation task to a resting baseline condition, these authors found a large area of increased activity associated with verb generation that encompassed an area of the inferior frontal gyrus anterior to Broca's area and extended toward the frontal pole in the dominant hemisphere. There was some activation in this area associated with repetition, but it was not as great as in the verb generation task. Thus the inferior prefrontal activity increase found by Petersen et al. (1988) was replicated. It is unfortunate that the limited information provided by the McCarthy et al. study did not address anterior cingulate activity (they used only a single axial fMRI slice).

Frith et al. (1991a) performed a similar study in which they compared repetition of words to the generation of words beginning with a given letter every time a subject heard the word "next." It should be noted that in contrast to the study of Petersen et al. (1988), the generation task of Frith et al. did not involve a strong semantic component; it could be performed by accessing lexical items without attention to their semantic associations. During generation of words, the anterior cingulate cortex showed increased blood flow, as did a large region in the left dorsolateral prefrontal cortex. In a separate experiment, the authors also had subjects move fingers that an experimenter touched and compared resulting images to those from a condition in which they had subjects select the finger to be moved every time a finger was touched. When subjects had to select which finger to move, an area of anterior cingulate cortex (smaller than in the word generation experiment) showed increased blood flow, and a region of dorsolateral frontal cortex (somewhat different from the area in the word generation experiment) showed increased blood flow. Although Petersen et al. (1988) had interpreted increased blood flow in the dorsolateral frontal region to indicate involvement of this cortex in semantic processes, Frith et al. suggested that the dorsolateral frontal cortex is involved in generation of responses through willed action. It is of interest that in these studies, there was overlap in anterior cingulate activity changes, and to some degree dorsolateral frontal activity changes, between language and motor tasks; this suggests that neural mechanisms related to endo-evoked intention may be shared between the two tasks.

Frith et al. (1991b) as well as Friston, Frith, Liddle, and Frackowiak (1991) also compared changes in brain activity for internal generation and external generation in a slightly different study. Tasks performed in this study included an initial and ending resting baseline, counting, a lexical decision task in which subjects said "correct" for words and "incorrect" for nonwords (extrinsic generation), saying as many words as a subject could think of beginning with the letter "a" (intrinsic generation), and saying as many jobs as a subject could think of (intrinsic generation). When the intrinsic generation conditions were compared with all other conditions, small areas of increased activity were seen in the left and right anterior cingulate gyrus. Larger increases were seen in the left dorsolateral prefrontal cortex and parahippocampal gyrus. Such an increase in anterior cingulate activity was not seen for the lexical decision task. These findings strengthen the conclusion that anterior cingulate and dorsolateral frontal participation are necessary in language tasks that require internal generation.

However, the more recent data of Warburton et al. (1996) suggest that the original studies may have been in error regarding the location of medial frontal activity during language generation. Using PET imaging, these authors found that the peak of medial frontal activity change during word generation was located either in what appears to be the paracingulate sulcus between supracallosal BA 32 and pre-SMA, or above the paracingulate sulcus in pre-SMA. The considerable dispersion of activity that PET acquisitions and subsequent smoothing algorithms create makes it difficult to resolve the exact location of activity. On the other hand, in a recent fMRI study in our laboratory (Crosson, Sadek, et al., 1999), we plotted activity of individual subjects during word generation alternating with repetition. Results were generally consistent with the findings of Warburton et al. For individual subjects, we consistently found activity in a medial frontal region occupied by pre-SMA and adjacent BA 32, with somewhat more activity in pre-SMA than in BA 32 (Figure 14.5). Activity was also seen in SMA, but for fewer subjects than in pre-SMA/BA 32. In none of our 28 subjects was significant activity seen in the anterior cingulate gyrus. This finding is consistent with group analyses of our word generation data (Crosson, Radonovich, et al., 1999; Sadek et al., 1999). Thus, regarding initiation during word generation, more recent studies indicate that cortex in the cingulate gyrus has not been active, while cortex in pre-SMA and adjacent BA 32 has been consistently active.

A difference in tasks engaging SMA and pre-SMA should also be noted. In their review of the literature, Picard and Strick (1996) noted that "simple" language tasks (e.g., repetition)

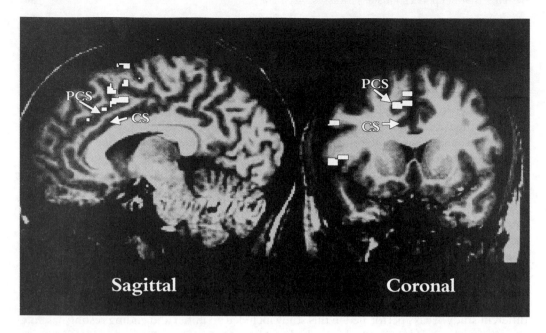

FIGURE 14.5. Images from word generation experiment. Sagittal (left) and coronal (right) fMRI images of medial frontal activity for a single subject. The subject generated as many words as he could for a given category (e.g., "birds" or "weather events"); 17.4-second periods of word generation were alternated with 17.4-second periods of rest for 6.4 cycles. The white areas represent correlations ($r \geq .50$) between the acquired fMRI signal and a sinusoidal reference waveform that is time-locked to the alternating cycles of word generation and rest. Some activity lies within the paracingulate sulcus (PCS), which is thought to be the dividing line between pre-SMA and adjacent BA 32, but activity also lies above the PCS in pre-SMA. Activity rarely extends into the cingulate sulcus (CS) if a PCS is prominent. The PCS was prominent in 75% of our subjects and absent or not prominent in 25% of our subjects. In no case did activity extend into the cingulate gyrus.

tended to be associated with activity peaks in SMA, and that "complex" language tasks tended to be associated with activity peaks in pre-SMA. This observation is generally consistent with our own observations (Crosson, Radonovich, et al., 1999; Crosson, Sadek, et al., 1999; Sadek et al., 1999), although we would rephrase the difference as follows: For repetition, activity seems to be confined to SMA, but for word generation, both SMA and pre-SMA are involved.

Furthermore, both medial frontal cortex (SMA, pre-SMA, cortex anterior to pre-SMA in the medial frontal gyrus, BA 32, and sometimes cingulate gyrus) and dorsolateral frontal regions have shown increased activity during semantic monitoring tasks that do not involve verbal output (Binder et al. 1997; Petersen, Fox, Posner, Mintun, & Raichle, 1989; Demonet et al., 1994). For example, Petersen et al. (1989) engaged a small number of subjects in a semantic monitoring task. Subjects were required to monitor visually presented animal names for dangerous animals. Target density was varied: 1 in 40 for the low-target-density condition and 20 in 40 for the high-target-density condition. Some degree of lateral frontal activation was seen in both cases; the authors suggested that this area is involved in semantic aspects of monitoring. Of further importance for the present discussion was a higher level of activity in the anterior cingulate cortex in the high-target-density condition. Since more frequent responding was required in the high-density condition, this finding implies that the anterior cingulate area is involved in some aspect of generating individual responses.

We recently performed an fMRI experiment in working memory, in which we found that as long as subjects treated words as lexical units, pre-SMA demonstrated greater activity than during a control, nonlexical, orthographic task that made no demands on working memory (Crosson, Rao, et al., 1999). However, when stimuli were not treated as lexical units (i.e., when phonological working memory or orthographic working memory were used to process only parts of words), pre-SMA did not show greater activity than during the control task. One possible explanation is that SMA plays a role in lexical retrieval or processing. Some support can be found for this position in other functional imaging studies. For example, Price et al. (1994) found increased medial frontal activity in a lexical decision task. On the other hand, preliminary data from a study under way in our laboratory indicate that generation of nonwords engages medial frontal cortex as much as generation of words. It suffices to say that the role of medial frontal cortex in language appears to involve intention, but the complete story on how pre-SMA and adjacent BA 32 facilitate language has yet to be fully elucidated.

Finally, we (Nadeau & Crosson, 1997) suggested a process by which cortical mechanisms necessary to perform a particular cognitive activity are selectively engaged. In part, the theory was based on the observation that the inferior thalamic peduncle and the nucleus reticularis regulate cortical responses to external stimuli and resulting behavior (Skinner & Yingling, 1977; Yingling & Skinner, 1977). It was also based upon our own analysis of lesion location in four cases of thalamic aphasia. In two instances, the lesion extended from the dominant thalamus into the portion of the nucleus reticularis that the inferior thalamic peduncle pierces. In the other two cases, the lesion included the centromedian nucleus. Naming was extensively evaluated in one case with nucleus reticularis involvement and in one case with centromedian involvement (Raymer, Moberg, Crosson, Nadeau, & Rothi, 1997). Deficits were very similar, affecting the lexical–semantic interface. This similarity suggested that the centromedian nucleus is involved in a system with the nucleus reticularis and the inferior thalamic peduncle. According to the theory, the frontal lobes, inferior thalamic peduncle, nucleus reticularis, and centromedian nucleus are involved in selectively engaging cortical mechanisms needed for a particular cognitive activity. Activation of nets that link semantic attributes to lexical items results in selection of the appropriate lexical item corresponding to the desired concept. In a sense, selective engagement can be conceptualized as improving the efficiency and accuracy of lexical selection. The anatomical relationships in this system are diagrammed in Figure 14.6.

To recapitulate, the data regarding anatomical systems supporting attentional processes for language are evolving; however, some tentative conclusions about these systems can be drawn. With respect to intention (Figure 14.4), recent studies suggest that pre-SMA is involved in aspects of language generation that include initiation of language. Although pre-SMA is a part of medial BA 6 (like SMA), its connectivity is different. Pre-SMA is anterior to SMA and is connected to lateral frontal cortex that is involved in action planning, while SMA is more connected to the lateral motor system (Luppino et al., 1993; Matzusaka et al., 1992; Picard & Strick, 1996). Although early PET studies (Frith et al., 1991a, 1991b; Petersen et al., 1988) suggested that supracallosal area 24 (i.e., the anterior cingulate gyrus) is involved in language initiation, recent PET (Warburton et al., 1996) and fMRI (Crosson, Radonovich, et al., 1999; Crosson, Sadek, et al., 1999; Sadek et al., 1999) investigations have failed to find any evidence of involvement of the anterior cingulate gyrus in language initiation. Pre-

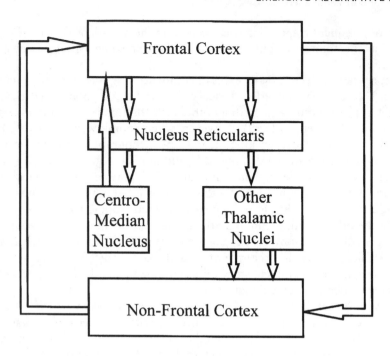

FIGURE 14.6. Connections among structures thought to be involved in selective engagement of cortical mechanisms for language.

SMA may also be involved in some aspects of language generation. As suggested more generally by Heilman et al. (1993), anterior cingulate cortex may be involved in the motivations that drive language generation and formulation. Unfortunately, motivational context has not been addressed in these studies, and functional imaging paradigms to explore motivational aspects of language are needed. It may be that motivational manipulations applied to word generation paradigms will produce activity changes in the cingulate gyrus. With respect to emotional factors in language generation, we recently explored semantic processing of emotional connotation during word generation (Crosson, Radonovich, et al., 1999). Comparison of fMRI images acquired during generation of words with emotional connotations to images acquired during generation of emotionally neutral words did not demonstrate significant differences in the medial frontal cortex, although activity changes were noted near the frontal and temporal poles. Thus medial frontal cortex does not seem to be involved in processing emotional connotation.

The dorsolateral frontal cortex also receives information from posterior cortex responsible for processing sensory-perceptual information. Because dorsolateral frontal cortex also projects to the anterior cingulate area (Pandya & Yeterian, 1985), it can influence the strength of motivations based upon analysis of environmental information. Thus the strength of motivations may be influenced by, and reprioritized on the basis of, environmental constraints. The reciprocal influence of motivations and action plans may occur via mechanisms implicit in connectionist and PDP models (Figure 14.7). In keeping with analyses of working memory by Goldman-Rakic and her colleagues (Funahashi, Bruce, & Goldman-Rakic, 1989; Wilson, Scalaidhe, & Goldman-Rakic, 1993), the region of dorsolateral frontal cortex involved in initiating and planning an activity may depend on the type of information needed.

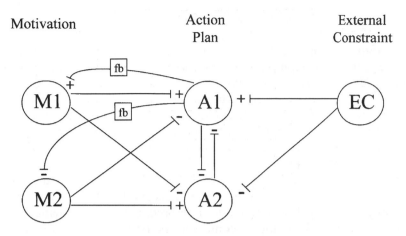

FIGURE 14.7. Two motivations (M1 and M2) begin at equal strengths but are mutually exclusive, in that M1 enhances one competing action plan (A1) and inhibits another competing action plan (A2), while M2 inhibits A1 and enhances A2. An external constraint (EC) is favorable to (i.e., enhances) A1 but will prevent (i.e., inhibit) A2. After EC influences A1 and A2, feedback from A1 tends to enhance M1 but inhibit M2. Thus M1 will tend to prevail, barring other influences. +, enhancement; –, inhibition; fb, feedback from action plan to motivation.

The role of posterior cingulate cortex in supporting language functions appears to be more in the realm of selective attention (Figure 14.3). Demonet et al. (1994) found greater activity in posterior cingulate cortex during a semantic monitoring task than during a phonemic monitoring task. Binder et al. (1997) reported a similar finding for posterior cingulate cortex when comparing semantic monitoring with tone pitch monitoring. Frith et al. (1991a) found greater posterior cingulate activity during repetition of words than during internally driven generation of words, suggesting that attending to the external stimuli requires the participation of the posterior cingulate cortex. Furthermore, these authors found that posterior cingulate activity was greater during a task involving finger movement in response to tactile stimuli than during a similar task in which the decision as to which fingers to move was internally mediated. Thus posterior cingulate cortex appears to play a role in attention to nonlinguistic as well as linguistic external stimuli. The role of more lateral cortex, such as temporal or parietal cortex, in selective attention is less secure. The exact location of lateral posterior cortex involved in attention, like that of lateral frontal cortex, may depend partly upon the type of stimuli being processed. Frith et al. (1991a) showed greater superior temporal gyrus activation during word repetition than during word generation. For the generation task, subjects heard the word "next" every time they were to generate a word; therefore, the differences between the generation task and the repetition task could not be a simple matter of auditory stimulation. The temporal cortex would have to be engaged in attention to and/or analysis of the lexical information necessary to perform the repetition task. Future studies will be helpful in addressing issues of attention if they are designed to separate attention from processing; this problem will be a significant challenge in the design of studies. Finally, the frontal lobes, inferior thalamic peduncle, nucleus reticularis, and centromedian nucleus appear to be involved in selectively engaging cortical mechanisms necessary for language activities. This selective engagement process allows the speaker to activate the appropriate lexical item for an intended concept. Selective engagement improves the efficiency at which the language system operates.

CLINICAL APPLICATIONS

Application of the current model to assessment and treatment of patients with attentional and language problems is a complicated issue. Because application to the treatment setting depends upon adequate assessment, I cover this topic first. From the standpoint of selective attention, the first issue to be noted is the inadequacy of traditional neuropsychological assessment in dealing with selective attention. Typically, attention has been considered a unitary construct, and there is a long-honored but highly inaccurate clinical lore that digit span is a good measure of attention. I have noted elsewhere (Crosson, 2000) that patients with significant attention problems may do well on digit span measures. The typical factor-analytic approach to interpreting specific WAIS subtests as tapping attention is also problematic, in part because WAIS subtests are multifaceted. Indeed, the multifaceted nature of most neuropsychological tests precludes interpretation of performance as exclusively tapping attention. Although versions of continuous-performance tests are becoming popular as measures of vigilance, such measures do not address selective attention.

A good place to start a discussion of assessment of attentional mechanisms is with generalized mechanisms. By "generalized," I mean those mechanisms that are capable of enhancing or prioritizing information processing in multiple cognitive systems (e.g., language, spatial processing, memory) or across the cerebral hemispheres. Evidence from neurologically normal subjects suggests that language shares attentional mechanisms with other cognitive functions, such as simple spatial analysis. For example, delayed responding to a spatial attention task has been found when subjects must concurrently process words, especially the meaning of words (Petry, 1995). Delayed responding to the same spatial attention task also occurs when subjects are required to shadow text (Posner et al., 1988). Although subjects showed differences between visual fields during concurrent shadowing of text, the elevation of reaction times in both visual fields when subjects were shadowing text or processing words suggests that the common attentional mechanism affects reaction times to spatial targets without respect to the hemisphere in which the information is initially processed. It makes a certain amount of sense that some supraordinate mechanism is needed to coordinate the activity between hemispheres. The nature of this coordinating mechanism is not entirely clear—for example, whether it involves selective attention to the sensory input, the intention to respond, and/or selective engagement of the appropriate mechanisms. It is most likely that all of these forms of attention must be involved to coordinate activity between systems and across hemispheres. From an anatomical standpoint, the question arises as to whether this common mechanism is located in the left hemisphere or the right hemisphere. Luria (1966, 1973) suggested that via its role in language processing, the language-dominant hemisphere functions to control cognitive processing in other domains.

How to measure dysfunction in such a generalized attention mechanism for clinical purposes is a difficult question. One possible way to measure the involvement in patients with aphasia would be to administer the spatial task used by Posner et al. (1988) and Petry (1995) to patients with aphasia, and to assess whether reaction times are increased above the normal range. This is exactly what we (Petry et al., 1994) did, and we found generally increased reaction times for patients with aphasia, in addition to differences in the pattern of response between the right and the left visual fields. However, the reliability and validity of this task for individual clinical assessment remain to be established. Thus considerable work is needed before this problem can be addressed clinically.

Another level at which to consider the interface between language and attention is whether or not attentional mechanisms specific to language or other left-hemisphere processes exist. Differences in responses to stimuli in different visual fields for subjects shadowing text (Posner et al., 1988) or for aphasic patients (Petry et al., 1994), differences in attention to global and local features (Massman et al., 1993), and changes in performance when the visual field of presentation is switched (Coslett et al., 1993; Coslett, 1999) are all suggestive of specfic left-hemisphere mechanisms of attention. Again, whether or not the spatial attention task used by Posner et al. (1988) or Petry (1995), or the global–local task used by Massman et al. (1993), would have adequate validity or reliability for routine clinical usage has yet to be determined. The repetition of different, already standardized language tasks from both sides of a patient's hemispace, as accomplished by Coslett and colleagues (Coslett et al., 1993; Coslett, 1999), is an intriguing idea. If the patient consistently performs better when the stimuli are presented from a particular side, there may be implications for treatment, which I discuss shortly. The findings of Coslett (1999) suggest that changing to the "good" hemispace is an effective way of improving language performance for patients with parietal lesions.

In the preceding discussion, I have implicated pre-SMA and the posterior cingulate cortex in intentional and attentional processes related to language. It seems likely that the anterior cingulate cortex is involved in the motivational and emotional aspects of language. The bulk of the evidence comes from functional neuroimaging studies of normal subjects, although patients with medial frontal lesions do exhibit language symptoms. Language in these patients is characterized by nonfluent verbal output and echolalia, with relatively good comprehension and repetition (Benson, 1993). Although Benson called this syndrome "supplementary motor aphasia," he noted that the damage typically occurs in the anterior cingulate cortex as well as in the SMA. Damasio and Anderson (1993) have referred to the same syndrome as "mutism" and noted that it is generally associated with some degree of akinesia and bradykinesia (thus the classical term "akinetic mutism"). These authors also noted that the mutism syndrome occurs with unilateral (left or right) or bilateral lesions, and that patients usually recover from unilateral lesions within weeks. These observations suggest that the left and right medial frontal cortices may be more functionally interchangeable than the perisylvian cortices. From the standpoint of clinical assessment, a clinician would see the syndrome described by Benson in severe cases, in which the symptoms are quite obvious. After some degree of recovery or in milder cases, the clinician might see significant delays in initiating verbal as well as other responses. It has generally been assumed that damage to language and speech programming mechanisms in the lateral, anterior language cortex may also cause nonfluent symptoms, such as difficulty in initiation. Thus the clinician may have to rely in part on an anatomical description of lesion location (i.e., from CT or MRI scans) to distinguish intentional disorders from other causes of nonfluent output.

The impact of posterior cingulate lesions on cognition is less certain. Memory problems have been reported with retrosplenial lesions, but language symptoms have not been prominent (Valenstein et al. 1987). As noted above, some evidence from PET studies suggests the involvement of posterior cingulate cortex in semantic monitoring of words (Demonet et al., 1994; Frith et al., 1991a, 1991b). If the role of posterior cingulate cortex in attention proposed by Heilman et al. (1993) is correct, patients with lesions to this cortex should show attentional deficits in multiple domains of processing within the hemisphere in question.

With regard to rehabilitation, the literature addressing the interface of attentional and language mechanisms does not offer much guidance. Thus there is a considerable need for research. If Coslett and colleagues (Coslett et al., 1993; Coslett, 1999) are correct, attentional problems related to parietal dysfunction may be amenable to treatments that engage attention in the unaffected (i.e., ipsilesional) hemispace. There are two possible ways in which this strategy may be used. The first is in a "vicariative" fashion (Rothi, 1995). That is, treatment can be initiated by presenting stimuli for various language tasks in the unaffected hemispace as a way of engaging selective attention mechanisms in the intact hemisphere and substituting them for dysfunctional selective attention mechanisms in the damaged hemisphere. Once the attentional mechanisms in the unaffected hemisphere seem consistently engaged when stimuli are presented in the ipsilesional hemispace, the hemispatial manipulation can be gradually faded out by moving stimuli successively closer to the midline, and eventually even into the contralesional hemispace. The objective will be to make the engagement of selective attention mechanisms in the intact hemisphere automatic whenever the patient uses language. The second possible way to use this strategy is as a permanent compensatory mechanism (Rothi, 1995) if the patient cannot learn to automatically engage attentional mechanisms from the intact hemisphere whenever language is used. The key to success of either treatment would be to select the patients who are most likely to benefit. The research by Coslett and colleagues suggests that patients whose performance improves when stimulation is moved to the ipsilesional hemispace may be the optimal recipients of such a treatment. Similar strategies may be developed for intentional systems, such that performing or directing actions into the ipsilesional hemispace may be contemplated as a way of engaging intentional mechanisms in the intact hemisphere during language tasks.

Indeed, we are in the process of applying such treatments to naming deficits in our lab. The rationale for the attention treatment comes directly from the research of Coslett and colleagues, as described above. It requires patients to attend to and name a picture on their left side during treatment. We expect to have preliminary data regarding the effectiveness of this treatment in the next few months. The intentional treatment involves initiating an action with the left arm in the left hemispace as a patient names a picture.

Studies that combine the use of symbolic gesture (American Indian Sign Language) with naming treatment provide evidence relevant to the intention treatment. When symbolic gesture and naming are performed simultaneously, there is a beneficial effect on naming. The patients in such studies usually have severe motor programming difficulties in speech (so-called "apraxia of speech"). Since these patients ordinarily also have significant motor impairment of the dominant hand, the production of symbolic gestures is usually adapted to the nondominant hand. Several case studies and small-group studies indicate that simultaneous training of oral object naming and symbolic gesture improves oral naming (e.g., Hoodin & Thompson, 1983; Kearns, Simmons, & Sisterhen, 1982; Pashek, 1998; Skelly, Schinsky, Smith, & Fust, 1974), although some studies have noted more limited improvement (e.g., Raymer & Thompson, 1991). Because gesture training alone does not increase oral naming skills (Hoodin & Thompson, 1983; Kearns et al., 1982), and oral naming training alone does not increase oral naming skills (Hoodin & Thompson, 1983), it is the simultaneous training of oral naming with symbolic gesture that increases naming skills. In a recent study, Pashek (1998) trained a nonfluent patient without hemiplegia to name objects (1) while simultaneously using symbolic gesture with the right hand, (2) while simultaneously using symbolic gesture with the left hand, and (3) while using no symbolic gesture. The patient consistently performed better on words trained with left- than with right-hand gestures, and consistently performed better with words trained with simultaneous symbolic gesture of either hand than with words trained with no gestures. Thus, even when the dominant right hand could be used for symbolic gestures, training with the left hand appeared to have some advantage.

Why should simultaneous training of symbolic signs, especially with the left hand, facilitate oral naming for trained words? One possibility is that the initiation of a manual gesture with the left hand primes intention mechanisms in the right hemisphere that facilitate initiation and relearning of the oral names. If this hypothesis is true, then initiation of nonsymbolic movements with the left hand should also facilitate relearning words and naming objects . As noted above, an experimental treatment devised in our laboratory combines the use of nonsymbolic movements of the left hand with object naming. Three patients with nonfluent aphasia who received this treatment showed significant improvement in naming during treatment, compared to a stable baseline (see Richards, Singletary, Koehler, Crosson, & Rothi [2000] for a brief case report.) A follow-up study is being designed to ascertain whether the nonsymbolic movements are the active component of the treatment.

Finally, functional neuroimaging techniques offer a promising tool not only for looking at normal brain functioning, but also for understanding how intact elements in brain systems function when other elements are damaged. Functional neuroimaging may be used to identify intact areas that do or do not respond normally to language tasks in patients with aphasia. It may also be used to identify how elements in systems respond to different manipulations, which may in turn predict whether certain treatments will be successful. Such information should be valuable in rehabilitation planning. For example, if residual language function is dependent on left-hemisphere mechanisms, treatments addressing intention may be contraindicated. On the other hand, if right lateral frontal and left medial frontal cortices are involved in language generation, then various manipulations may be tried during functional neuroimaging to ascertain whether the medial frontal cortex of the right hemisphere can be activated to substitute for that of the damaged hemisphere. Strategies that do so may then be used in treatment, under the assumption that using lateral and medial frontal mechanisms from the same hemisphere will lead to superior language performance.

In summary, the study of specific brain components involved in the interface of attention and language is a field with great promise. Functional neuroimaging techniques may be useful in examining attentional and intentional systems in normal brains. If attentional mechanisms are to be addressed as rehabilitation targets in aphasic patients, the success of the endeavor will depend upon being able to specify the nature of the attentional deficit(s), the underlying neuroanatomical causes, and strategies for vicariation or compensation.

ACKNOWLEDGMENTS

Work on this chapter was supported in part by Grant No. DC03455 from the National Institute on Deafness and Other Communication Disorders, and by a grant from the Brooks Health Foundation, Jacksonville, Florida.

REFERENCES

Anderson, B. (1996). Semantic neglect? *Journal of Neurology, Neurosurgery and Psychiatry, 60,* 349–350.

Baddeley, A. D. (1990). *Human memory: Theory and practice.* Needham Heights, MA: Allyn & Bacon.

Ballesteros, S., Manga, D., & Coello, T. (1989). Attentional resources in dual-task performance. *Bulletin of the Psychonomic Society, 27,* 425–428.

Barris, R. W., & Schuman, H. R. (1953). Bilateral anterior cingulate gyrus lesions: Syndrome of the anterior cingulate gyri. *Neurology, 3,* 44–52.

Benson, D. F. (1993). Aphasia. In K. M. Heilman & E. Valenstein (Eds.), *Clinical neuropsychology* (pp. 17–36). New York: Oxford University Press.

Binder, J. R., Frost, J. A., Hammeke, T. A., Cox, R. W., Rao, S. M., & Prieto, T. (1997). Human brain language areas identified by functional magnetic resonance imaging. *Journal of Neuroscience, 17,* 353–362.

Cohen, R. A. (1993). *The neuropsychology of attention.* New York: Plenum Press.

Coslett, H. B. (1999). Spatial influences on motor and language function. *Neuropsychologia, 37,* 695–706.

Coslett, H. B., Schwartz, M. F., Goldberg, G., Hass, D., & Perkins, J. (1993). Multi-modal hemispatial deficits after left hemisphere stroke. *Brain, 116,* 527–554.

Cowan, N. (1988). Evolving conceptions of memory storage, selective attention, and their mutual constraints within the human information processing system. *Psychological Bulletin, 104,* 163–191.

Crosson, B. (1992) *Subcortical functions in language and memory.* New York: Guilford Press.

Crosson, B. (1999). Subcortical mechanisms in language: Lexical–semantic mechanisms and the thalamus. *Brain and Cognition, 40,* 414–438.

Crosson, B. (2000). Application of neuropsychological assessment results. In R. D. Vanderploeg (Ed.), *Clinician's guide to neuropsychological assessment* (pp. 195–244). Mahwah, NJ: Erlbaum.

Crosson, B., & Nadeau, S. E. (1998). The role of subcortical structures in linguistic processes: Recent developments. In B. Stemmer & H. A. Whitaker (Eds.), *Handbook of neurolinguistics* (pp. 431–445). San Diego, CA: Academic Press.

Crosson, B., Radonovich, K., Sadek, J. R., Gökçay, D., Bauer, R. M., Fischler, I. S., Cato, M. A., Maron, L., Auerbach, E. J., Browd, S. R., & Briggs, R.W. (1999). Left-hemisphere processing of emotional connotation during word generation. *NeuroReport, 10,* 2449–2455.

Crosson, B., Rao, S. M., Woodley, S. J., Rosen, A. C., Bobholz, J. A., Mayer, A., Cunningham, J. M., Hammeke, T. A., Fuller, S. A., Binder, J. R., Cox, R. W., & Stein, E. A. (1999). Mapping of semantic, phonological, and orthographic verbal working memory in normal adults with functional magnetic resonance imaging. *Neuropsychology, 13,* 171–187.

Crosson, B., Sadek, J. R., Bobholz, J. A., Gökçay, D., Mohr, C. M., Leonard, C. M., Maron, L., Auerbach, E. J., Browd, S. R., Freeman, A. J., & Briggs, R. W. (1999). Activity in the paracingulate and cingulate sulci during word generation: An fMRI study of functional anatomy. *Cerebral Cortex, 9,* 307–316.

Damasio, A. R., & Anderson, S. W. (1993). The frontal lobes. In K. M. Heilman & E. Valenstein (Eds.), *Clinical neuropsychology* (pp. 409–460). New York: Oxford University Press.

Demonet, J.-F., Price, C., Wise, R., & Frackowiak, R. S. J. (1994). Differential activation of right and left posterior sylvian regions by semantic and phonological tasks: A positron-emission tomography study in normal human subjects. *Neuroscience Letters, 182,* 25–28.

Friedman, A., Polson, M. C., & Dafoe, C. G. (1988). Dividing attention between the hands and the head: Performance trade-offs between rapid finger tapping and verbal memory. *Journal of Experimental Psychology: Human Perception and Performance, 14,* 60–68.

Friston, K. J., Frith, C. D., Liddle, P. F., & Frackowiak, R. S. J. (1991). Investigating a network model of word generation with positron emission tomography. *Proceedings of the Royal Society of London Series B, 244,* 101–106.

Frith, C. D., Friston, K., Liddle, P. F., & Frackowiak, R. S. J. (1991a). Willed action and the prefrontal cortex in man: A study with PET. *Proceedings of the Royal Society of London, Series B, 244,* 241–246.

Frith, C. D., Friston, K. J., Liddle, P. F., & Frackowiak, R. S. J. (1991b). A PET study of word finding. *Neuropsychologia, 29,* 1137–1148.

Funahashi, S., Bruce, C. J., & Goldman-Rakic, P. S. (1989). Mnemonic coding of visual space in the monkey's dorsolateral prefrontal cortex. *Journal of Neurophysiology, 61,* 331–349.

Gladstones, W. H., Regan, M. A., & Lee, R. B. (1989). Division of attention: The single-channel hypothesis revisited. *Quarterly Journal of Experimental Psychology, 41A,* 1–17.

Goldberg, G. (1985). Supplementary motor area structure and function: Review and hypotheses. *Behavioral and Brain Sciences, 8,* 567–616.

Heilman, K. M., Watson, R. T., & Valenstein, E. (1993). Neglect and related disorders. In K. M. Heilman & E. Valenstein (Eds.), *Clinical neuropsychology* (3rd ed., pp. 279–336). New York: Oxford University Press.

Hoodin, R. B., & Thompson, C. K. (1983). Facilitation of verbal labeling in adult aphasia by gestural, verbal or verbal plus gestural training. In R. H. Brookshire (Ed.), *Clinical Aphasiology Conference Proceedings* (pp. 62–64). Minneapolis, MN: BRK Publishers

James, W. (1890). *The principles of psychology* (2 vols.). New York: Holt.

Jonas, S. (1981). The supplementary motor region and speech emission. *Journal of Communication Disorders, 14,* 349–373.

Kearns, K. P., Simmons, N. N., & Sisterhen, C. (1982). Stural sign (Amer-Ind) as a facilitator of verbalization in patients with aphasia. In R. H. Brookshire (Ed.), *Clinical Aphasiology Conference Proceedings* (pp. 183–191). Minneapolis, MN: BRK Publishers.

Lamb, M. R., Robertson, L. C., & Knight, R. T. (1989). Attention and interference in the processing of global and local information: Effects of unilateral temporal–parietal junction lesions. *Neuropsychologia, 27,* 471–483.

Luppino, G., Matelli, M., Camarda, R. M., & Rizzolatti, G. (1993). Corticocortical connections of area F3 (SMA-proper) and area F6 (pre-SMA) in the macaque monkey. *Journal of Comparative Neurology, 338,* 114–140.

Luria, A. R. (1966). *Higher cortical functions in man* (B. Haigh, Trans.). New York: Basic Books. (Original text published by Moscow University Press, 1962)

Luria, A. R. (1973). *The working brain: An introduction to neuropsychology* (B. Haigh, Trans.). New York: Basic Books.

Massman, P. J., Delis, D. C., Filoteo, V., Butters, N., Salmon, D. P., & Demadura, T. L. (1993). Mechanisms of spatial impairment in Alzheimer's disease subgroups: Differential breakdown of directed attention to global–local stimuli. *Neuropsychology, 7,* 172–181.

Matsuzaka, Y., Aizawa, H., & Tanji, J. (1992). A motor area rostral to the supplementary motor area (presupplementary motor area) in the monkey: Neuronal activity during a learned motor task. *Journal of Neurophysiology, 68,* 653–662.

McCarthy, G., Blamire, A. M., Rothman, D. L., Gruetter, R., & Shulman, R. G. (1993). Echoplanar magnetic resonance imaging studies of frontal cortex activation during word generation in humans. *Proceedings of the National Academy of Sciences USA, 90,* 4952–4956.

McClelland, J. L., Rumelhart, D. E., & the PDP Research Group. (Eds.). (1986). *Parallel distributed processing: Explorations in the microstructure of cognition. Vol. 2. Psychological and biological models.* Cambridge, MA: MIT Press.

Mennemeier, M., Crosson, B., Williamson, D. J., Nadeau, S. E., Fennell, E., Valenstein, E., & Heilman, K. M. (1997). Tapping, talking and the thalamus: Possible influence of the intralaminar nuclei on basal ganglia function. *Neuropsychologia, 35,* 183–193.

Morecraft, R. J., & Van Hoesen, G. W. (1998). Convergence of limbic input to the cingulate motor cortex in the rhesus monkey. *Brain Research Bulletin, 45,* 209–232.

Murray, L. L., Holland, A. L., & Beeson, P. M. (1997). Auditory processing in individuals with mild aphasia: A study of resource allocation. *Journal of Speech, Language, and Hearing Research, 40,* 792–808.

Nadeau, S. E., & Crosson, B. (1997). Subcortical aphasia. *Brain and Language, 58,* 355–402.

Nielsen, J. M., & Jacobs, L. L. (1951). Bilateral lesions of the anterior cingulate gyri: Report of case. *Bulletin of the Los Angeles Neurological Society, 16,* 231–234.

Norman, D. A., & Shallice, T. (1986). Attention to action: Willed and automatic control of behavior. In R. J. Davidson, G. E. Schwartz, & D. Shapiro (Eds.), *Consciousness and self-regulation* (Vol. 4, pp. 1–18). New York: Plenum Press.

Pandya, D. N., & Yeterian, E. H. (1985). Architecture and connections of cortical association areas. In A. Peters & E. G. Jones (Eds.), *Cerebral cortex: Vol. 4. Association and auditory cortices* (pp. 3–62). New York: Plenum Press.

Pashek, G. V. (1997). A case study of gesturally cued naming in aphasia: Dominant versus nondominant hand training. *Journal Communication Disorders, 30,* 349–366.

Pashler, H. (1991). Shifting visual attention and selecting motor responses: Distinct attentional mechanisms. *Journal of Experimental Psychology: Human Perception and Performance, 17,* 1023–1040.

Pashler, H., & O'Brien, S. (1993). Dual-task interference and the cerebral hemispheres. *Journal of Experimental Psychology: Human Perception and Performance, 19,* 315–330.

Petersen, S. E., Fox, P. T., Posner, M. I., Mintun, M., & Raichle, M. E. (1988). Positron emission tomographic studies of the cortical anatomy of single-word processing. *Nature, 331,* 585–589.

Petersen, S. E., Fox, P. T., Posner, M. I., Mintun, M., & Raichle, M. E. (1989). Positron emission tomographic studies of the processing of single words. *Journal of Cognitive Neuroscience, 1,* 153–170.

Petry, M. C. (1995). *The effects of lexical and semantic processing on visual selective attention.* Unpublished doctoral dissertation. University of Florida.

Petry, M. C., Crosson, B., Rothi, L. J. G., Bauer, R. M., & Schauer, C. A. (1994). Selective attention and aphasia in adults: Preliminary findings. *Neuropsychologia, 32,* 1397–1408.

Picard, N., & Strick, P. L. (1996). Motor areas of the medial wall: A review of their location and functional activation. *Cerebral Cortex*, 6, 342–353.

Posner, M. I., & Boies, S. W. (1971). Components of attention. *Psychological Review*, 78, 391–408.

Posner, M. I., & Cohen, Y. (1980). Attention and the control of movements. In G. G. Stelmach & J. Requin (Eds.), *Tutorials in motor behavior* (pp. 243–258). Amsterdam: North Holland.

Posner, M. I., & Early, T. S. (1990). In reply to "What is left of attention in schizophrenia?" *Archives of General Psychiatry*, 47, 394–395.

Posner, M. I., Early, T. S., Reiman, E., Pardo, P. J., & Dhawan, M. (1988). Asymmetries in hemispheric control of attention in schizophrenia. *Archives of General Psychiatry*, 45, 814–821.

Posner, M. I., Walker, J. A., Friedrich, F. A., & Rafal, R. D. (1984). Effects of parietal injury on covert orienting of attention. *Journal of Neuroscience*, 4, 1863–1874.

Posner, M. I., Walker, J. A., Friedrich, F. A., & Rafal, R. D. (1987). How do the parietal lobes direct covert attention? *Neuropsychologia*, 25, 135–145.

Price, C. J., Wise, R. J., Watson, J. D., Patterson, K., Howard, D., & Frackowiak, R. S. (1994). Brain activity during reading. The effects of exposure duration and task. *Brain*, 117, 1255–1269.

Rafal, R. D., & Posner, M. I. (1987). Deficits in human visual spatial attention following thalamic lesions. *Proceedings of the National Academy of Sciences USA*, 84, 7349–3753.

Raymer, A. M., Moberg, P., Crosson, B., Nadeau, S., & Rothi, L. J. G. (1997). Lexical–semantic deficits in two patients with dominant thalamic infarction. *Neuropsychologia*, 35, 211–219.

Raymer, A. M., & Thompson, C. K. (1991). Effects of verbal plus gestural treatment in a patient with aphasia and severe apraxia of speech. In T. E. Prescott (Ed.), *Clinical aphasiology* (Vol. 20, pp. 507–519). Austin, TX: Pro-Ed.

Richards, K., Singletary, F., Koehler, S., Crosson, B., & Rothi, L. J. G. (2000). Treatment of nonfluent aphasia through the pairing of a nonsymbolic movement sequence and naming. *Journal of the International Neuropsychological Society*, 6, 241.

Rothi, L. J. G. (1995). Behavioral compensation in the case of treatment of acquired language disorders resulting from brain damage. In R. A. Dixon & L. Backman (Eds.), *Compensating for psychological deficits and declines* (pp. 219–230). Mahwah, NJ: Erlbaum.

Rumelhart, D. E., McClelland, J. L., & the PDP Research Group. (Eds.). (1986). *Parallel distributed processing: Explorations in the microstructure of cognition. Vol. 1. Foundations.* Cambridge, MA: MIT Press.

Sadek, J. R., Maron, L. M., Crosson, B., Auerbach, E. J., Browd, S., Leonard, C. M., & Briggs, R. W. (1999). Medial and lateral frontal cortex: An fMRI investigation of internally versus externally guided language. *Journal of the International Neuropsychological Society*, 5, 135.

Skelly, M., Schinsky, L., Smith, R. W., & Fust, R. S. (1974). American Indian sign (Amerind) as a facilitator of verbalization for the oral verbal apraxic. *Journal of Speech and Hearing Disorders*, 39, 445–456.

Skinner, J. E., & Yingling, C. D. (1977). Central gating mechanisms that regulate event-related potentials and behavior. In J. E. Desmedt (Ed.), *Attention, voluntary contraction and event related potentials* (pp. 30–69). Basel: Karger.

Tseng, C. H., McNeil, M. R., & Milenkovic, P. (1993). An investigation of attention allocation deficits in aphasia. *Brain and Language*, 45, 276–296.

Valenstein, E., Bowers, D., Verfaellie, M., Heilman, K. M., Day, A., & Watson, R. T. (1987). Retrosplenial amnesia. *Brain*, 110, 1631–1646.

Warburton, E., P., Wise, R. J. S., Price, C. J., Weiller, C., Hadar, U., Ramsay, S., & Frackowiak, R. S. J. (1996). Noun and verb retrieval by normal subjects: Studies with PET. *Brain*, 119, 159–179.

Watson, R. T., Miller, B. D., & Heilman, K. M. (1978). Nonsensory neglect. *Annals of Neurology*, 3, 505–508.

Wilson, F. A. W., Scalaidhe, S. P. O., & Goldman-Rakic, P. S. (1993). Dissociation of object and spatial processing domains in primate prefrontal cortex. *Science*, 260, 1955–1958.

Yingling, C. D., & Skinner, J. E. (1977). Gating of thalamic input to cerebral cortex by nucleus reticularis thalami. In J. E. Desmedt (Ed.), *Attention, voluntary contraction and event related potentials* (pp. 70–96). Basel: Karger.

15

SYSTEMS THAT SUPPORT LANGUAGE PROCESSES: VERBAL WORKING MEMORY

BRUCE CROSSON

"Working memory" refers to the capacity to hold information "on-line" for imminent use in the service of some goal. Thus working memory allows us to keep incoming information available until we need it for some purpose. For example, when a waiter tells us about several special items not on the restaurant's regular menu, we hold them in working memory until we choose the selection we wish to order. However, we can also retrieve information from long-term memory into working memory when we need that information for some reason. As an illustration, when my spouse tells me that we must be in Jacksonville by 9:00 A.M. tomorrow, I can retrieve the information from my long-term memory into working memory that it takes approximately an hour and a half to drive to Jacksonville. Then I can calculate when we will need to leave in order to arrive on time. While verbal working memory uses language in order to hold information on-line, it also acts as a supporting system in complex language usage. To understand a conversation, it is often necessary to hold previous statements in mind in order to understand current remarks. Thus working memory is a substrate for complex language usage. This is why verbal working memory has been classified as a process subserving language.

The relationship between working memory and "short-term memory" varies, depending upon the particular theorist; thus it is necessary to comment on the use of these terms. Shiffrin (1993) endorsed three "widely accepted" principles of short-term memory. First, it relies upon the temporary activity of neural structures. Some theories discuss the activation of various units (e.g., lexical items) above some presumed baseline level. This activation decays relatively rapidly in the absence of some effort to maintain it; therein lies the temporary nature of short-term memory. Second, operations to control cognition are carried out in short-term memory. According to Shiffrin, such operations include deciding where to direct attention, choosing what information to rehearse and how to rehearse it to maintain it in short-term memory, or choosing strategies to access information in short-term or long-term memory. Third, short-term memory is limited in capacity. In other words, we can hold only a certain number of items in our immediate attention. Essentially, the present definition of working memory can be considered synonymous with Shiffrin's conceptualization of short-term memory. Although the concept of working memory places an emphasis on cognitive control in the service of some goal, working memory can also be assumed to decay when we cease to make an effort to maintain it, and it can be considered to have a limited capacity.

This chapter first covers cognitive models of working memory. The threads mentioned by Shiffrin (1993) can be seen in the various theories of verbal working memory discussed here. A good place to start is Baddeley's model of verbal working memory, which operates as a phonological system. Because of the limitations of a model based solely on phonological information, I then turn to alternative views that take lexical, semantic, and syntactic information into account. Finally, I discuss a parallel-distributed-processing (PDP) account of working memory, which assumes temporary activation of phonological, lexical, and semantic information. After discussing these theories, I turn to the anatomical substrates of working memory, discussing both animal models and functional neuroimaging studies of verbal working memory. Finally, I consider rehabilitation of deficits that include significant declines in working memory.

COGNITIVE MODELS OF WORKING MEMORY

The Baddeley Model

In 1974, Baddeley and Hitch first wrote about a model that has had a profound influence on the study of verbal working memory. The model is reasonably simple, yet elegant. According to these authors, verbal working memory consists of three components (Figure 15.1). The first is a phonological store, in which phonological information can be held for very brief periods of time (i.e., 1.5 to 2.0 seconds) (Baddeley, 1990). Without some sort of process to refresh the phonological store, information fades rapidly. The second component is articulatory control processes, which allow for covert (i.e., inner) as well as overt speech. Covert speech can be used for subvocal rehearsal, through which information can be maintained in the phonological store for longer periods of time. For example, when you look up a phone number, you may rehearse it to yourself until you have dialed it so that you do not forget it. The third component of the model is a central executive. The central executive sets priorities for attention and action, thereby determining what information needs to be maintained in working memory to support the pursuit of current goals.

Evidence supporting this phonological rehearsal model of verbal working memory has been reviewed in detail elsewhere (Baddeley, 1990; Baddeley & Hitch, 1994). Briefly, some of the supporting data are as follows. The phonological nature of verbal working memory is demonstrated by the fact that immediate serial recall is impaired in neurologically normal subjects when items are similar in sound or articulatory characteristics (Conrad & Hull, 1964; Baddeley, 1966). Salamé and Baddeley (1987) demonstrated that spoken words and nonsense syllables interfered equally with immediate recall of visually presented digits. Since nonsense syllables have no meaning or lexical representations, we must assume that the phonological nature of these stimuli interferes with the phonological processing of digits. Finally, when normal subjects utter an irrelevant sound during immediate serial recall, performance deteriorates (Baddeley, Lewis, & Vallar, 1984). Presumably, the deterioration in performance is caused by the fact that producing the irrelevant utterance interferes with subvocal rehearsal.

In spite of considerable support for Baddeley's model of phonological rehearsal in verbal working memory, there are significant flaws in this position. Most notably, the concept that working memory depends *only* on phonological processes cannot be recon-

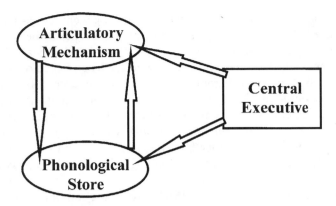

FIGURE 15.1. Schematic of Baddeley's phonological loop used in verbal working memory. According to Baddeley (1990), this is the primary mechanism used in verbal working memory. The phonological loop used in simple rehearsal consists of the articulatory mechanism and the phonological store. The phonological store is the mechanism that holds phonological information on line temporarily. When the articulatory mechanism initiates subvocal rehearsal of information that is in the phonological store, the phonological store is refreshed, preventing excessive decay. The central executive exercises control over the phonological loop (1) by selecting what information will be held in the phonological store, and (2) by initiating rehearsal through the articulatory mechanism to prevent decay.

ciled with our ability to understand an extended conversation. The continuous need to attend to new phonological input would not allow us to keep previous information in phonological working memory, because the old information would be constantly replaced by the new input. This viewpoint has been bolstered by studies of complex syntax comprehension in patients with extremely limited memory spans. Complex syntactic constructions are presumed to require working memory, because the meaning of the sentence is not immediately obvious, and items must be held in working memory until comprehension of the syntactic structures determines the proper relationship between the items. Whereas early evidence suggested that patients with limited memory spans performed poorly on comprehension of complex syntax (Caramazza, Basili, Koller, & Berndt, 1981; Saffran & Marin, 1975), later studies have indicated that patients with severe limitations in phonological rehearsal may perform at relatively normal levels on comprehension of complex syntax (e.g., R. C. Martin, Blossom-Stach, Yaffee, & Wetzel, 1995; Vallar & Baddeley, 1984). It is this problem that has caused investigators to look for alternatives to a single, phonological store subserving verbal working memory.

A Model of Multiple Verbal Working Memories

R. C. Martin and Romani (1994) have reviewed the evidence on verbal working memory and have suggested that in addition to phonological working memory, lexical–semantic and syntactic working memories exist. Their arguments were based primarily upon analysis of three patients; each patient's major impairment was in a different one of these three processes. The patients were given two tasks involving lexical working memory. One involved presenting a list of words and determining whether a subsequent probe rhymed with any words on the list. The other involved presenting a list of words and determining whether a subsequent probe was in the same semantic category as any words on the list.

For the rhyming task, thought to tap phonological working memory, patient AB performed better than patient EA. On the category probe task, patient EA performed better than patient AB. A third patient, MW, performed better than AB and EA—at normal or near-normal levels—on both the category and rhyming probe tasks. When tested on sentences, patient AB (who was impaired on the category probe task) had greater difficulty distinguishing semantically anomalous sentences (i.e., longer reaction times) than either MW or EA. On a grammaticality judgment task, MW performed worse than other subjects in judging verb agreement, and performed worse when intervening words required maintenance of syntactic information in working memory for short times. The authors concluded that EA, AB, and MW exemplified impairment of phonological, semantic, and syntactic working memory, respectively.

Although R. C. Martin and Romani (1994) have made convincing arguments in favor of lexical–semantic and syntactic working memories, a few aspects remain to be addressed. First, their patients appeared to experience other language problems besides those involving working memory, and it is unclear what bearing these other deficits may have had on their working memory. For example, should a deficit in syntactic working memory be accompanied by a deficit in processing syntax, or can the two be dissociated? Second, the authors did not elaborate upon whether rehearsal impacts lexical–semantic and syntactic working memory in the same way that it affects phonological working memory. Can lexical–semantic working memory be enhanced by rehearsal, and if so, how? Third, it is possible that other manipulations affect lexical–semantic working memory—for example, whether or not a subject attends to semantic or phonological information when words are presented. Finally, it is unclear how various decision-making processes (i.e., the central executive) may affect lexical–semantic and syntactic short-term stores.

A review of the literature on long-term memory may yield some potential answers to these questions. For example, Craik and Lockhart (1972) demonstrated that processing semantic information about a lexical item led to better long-term memory retention than processing phonological or orthographic features did. This effect has been replicated many times. Related to this effect of semantic processing is the concept of "elaborative rehearsal." Elaborative rehearsal involves the reorganization of incoming material to fit in with information that is already in long-term memory. Evidence suggests that elaborative rehearsal also leads to better long-term memory than simple repetition of an item does. Semantic processing and elaborative rehearsal have usually been taken to affect long-term memory (e.g., see Baddeley, 1990, or Saffran & Marin, 1975, for a discussion). Indeed, it has been proposed that short-term memory operates on the basis of phonological (phonemic) information, while long-term memory operates on the basis of semantic information (McCarthy & Warrington, 1990; Shallice & Warrington, 1970). This architecture of short-term and long-term memory has been used to explain patients who cannot repeat words or sentences verbatim but who maintain adequate long-term memory (e.g., Saffran & Marin, 1975). Thus proponents suggest that information can be put into long-term memory without first going through short-term memory, as proposed by Atkinson and Shiffrin (1968) and others.

A logical extension of R. C. Martin and Romani's (1994) conclusions suggests that lexical–semantic working memory can be enhanced by attending to the semantic properties of words or by elaborative rehearsal. Indeed, it is plausible that the favorable impact of these processes on long-term memory is mediated by lexical–semantic working memory mechanisms. In other words, long-term verbal memory may be accessed via working memory, but it is lexical–semantic working memory through which this access is achieved. Many studies addressing the relationship of short-term and long-term memory have used tests of phonological working memory; without a means for testing semantic working memory, it is premature to discard models that purport working memory to be the gateway to long-term storage. It is of interest, in this regard, that patients who have relatively intact long-term memory but cannot repeat sentences verbatim can paraphrase the sentences (e.g., Saffran & Marin, 1975). Shiffrin (1993) has clearly stated that our conceptualizations of short-term memory must accommodate many different kinds of information, which each have their own short-term memory processes. Yet he notes that the relationship between short-term and long-term memory is unclear. Although these may be different forms of memory, others have advocated that they are simply different manifestations of the same processes. For example, Cowan (1988) conceptualized short-term memory as the subset of items from long-term memory that is currently at a heightened state of activation. PDP models can resolve some of these issues and account for data that are problematic for other models.

A PDP Model

N. Martin and her colleagues (N. Martin, Dell, Saffran, & Schwartz, 1994; N. Martin & Saffran, 1992; N. Martin, Saffran, & Dell, 1996) have proposed a model of working memory based on Dell's (Dell, 1986; Dell & O'Seaghdha, 1991) interactive spreading-activation theory of language processing. This model is similar in framework to other PDP models. Detailed explanation of the fundamentals of PDP is beyond the scope of this chapter, but the reader is referred to Farah (1997) for a brief explanation, or Rumelhart, McClelland, and the PDP Research Group (1986) for more detailed explanations (see also Nadeau, Chapter 12, this volume). Basically, in PDP models there are different levels of processing. A simple reading model (Figure 15.2) described by McClelland and Rumelhart (1981) involves three levels of processing: a feature level (letters are made up of visual features), a letter level, and a word level. At each level, there are units (nodes) representing individual features, letters, or words, respectively. When the correct features are activated, their connections with letter units will activate the representation for the corresponding letter. When the correct letters are activated, the corresponding word will be activated. Connections can be formed within levels or between levels; they may either facilitate or inhibit activation of their target. Activation of units decays (i.e., activation tends to diminish over time unless it is maintained by input). Although a target word is activated by input of its corresponding features, visually similar words will also be activated at the same time (usually to a lesser degree), because of the features and letters they share with the target word.

N. Martin et al. (1996) have proposed three levels of information in lexical working memory: phonological, lexical, and semantic (Figure 15.3). A sequence of processing steps takes place in the neurologically normal brain when a person hears a word. After the word is heard, the phonological characteristics are processed, activating the appropriate phonological units. The activated phonological units in turn activate various lexical units. At the next step in processing, activated lexical units activate various semantic nodes, but also feed back activation to associated phonological units. Then the semantic and phonological units feed back activation to units at the lexical level. Multiple passes through this processing sequence may be necessary to identify the spoken word, but eventually the pattern of activity in the lexical nodes sharpens, causing the node representing the correct word to achieve a level of activation above that of competitors and adequate to trigger release into the output stream.

N. Martin and her colleagues (N. Martin & Saffran, 1992; N. Martin et al., 1994, 1996) have used this model to explain the pattern and evolution of deficits in a patient, NC, who had severe difficulties with repetition of words and nonwords. When first tested 2 months

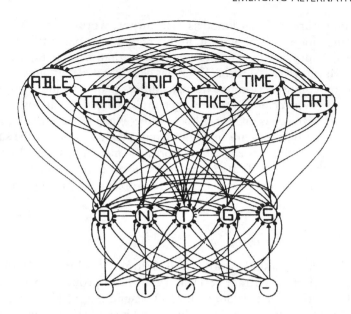

FIGURE 15.2. Schematic diagram demonstrating a PDP model for word reading. The facilitation and inhibition patterns shown are for the letter "T" in the initial position of a four-letter word. Shown are the feature, letter, and lexical levels of processing. Arrowheads at the end of a line indicate facilitation; dots at the end of a line indicate inhibition. Those features that make up "T" facilitate the "T" node, but other features inhibit it if they are activated. Once activation of the lexical nodes is initiated, words that begin with "T" will feed back facilitation to the "T" node at the letter level when activated; other words feed back inhibition if activated. Note that within the letter level, the "T" node, when activated, inhibits its neighboring competitors for the initial position. Likewise, when a competitor is activated, it inhibits the "T" node. From McClelland, J. L., & Rumelhart, D. E. (1981). An interactive activation model of context effects in letter perception: Part I. An account of basic findings. *Psychological Review, 88,* 375–407. Copyright 1981 by the American Psychological Association. Reprinted with permission of the authors.

after his stroke (N. Martin & Saffran, 1992), NC's single-word repetition was severely impaired, and his memory span for digits or words was less than one item with auditory presentation and a pointing response. Repetition of single words was only 30% correct. His errors included semantic paraphasias, formal paraphasias (real words that sounded like the targets), phonemic paraphasias, and neologisms. The authors explained this pattern of deficits by hypothesizing an abnormally high rate of decay at all levels of processing affecting auditory lexical memory. After activation by phonological nodes, lexical nodes in turn activate both semantic and phonological nodes. At the same time, the activation of the lexical nodes decays rapidly, such that the original activation of lexical nodes has little influence by the time lexical nodes are reactivated by semantic and phonological nodes. This being the case, activation from semantic and phonological nodes is likely to activate semantically and phonologically related items, respectively. Thus the rapid decay of the original activation at the lexical nodes accounts for the pattern of semantic and phonological errors, because the semantic and phonological nodes have been more recently primed and are more likely to influence lexical selection. N. Martin et al. (1994) subsequently showed that by accelerating decay rates in a computer model, they could reproduce NC's pattern of deficits.

When NC was retested 20 months after his stroke (N. Martin et al., 1996), his digit and word span improved to two to three items for auditory presentation with a pointing response. Single-word repetition improved to 85% correct. Errors still included formal paraphasias and neologisms, but he no longer produced semantic paraphasias. In a computer simulation, the authors found that they could reproduce this error pattern by using the previous model with a reduced rate of node activation decay. They further showed that semantic errors would reemerge for both NC and the computer model with an increased time between word presentation and repetition, which allowed decay to reach greater levels. In short, the model, as originally conceptualized, can account for the pattern of recovery as well as for the original deficits.

This model, with its multiple levels of auditory–verbal working memory and PDP processes, may have applicability to other deficits as well. For example, the cases discussed

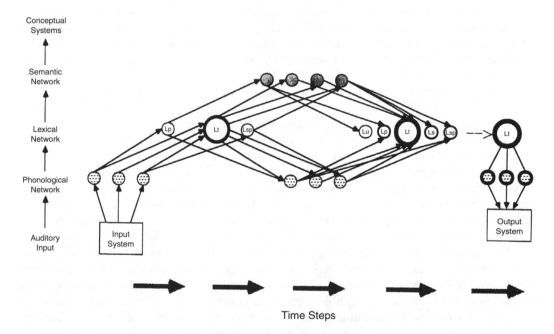

Time Steps

FIGURE 15.3. Diagram illustrating the time steps in the PDP model of repetition used by N. Martin et al. (1996). At the first time step, auditory input activates nodes at the phonological level. The activation of these phonological nodes in turn propagates activation to lexical nodes at the second time step. The lexical target (Lt) receives greater activation than lexical competitors that are phonologically related (Lp) or competitors that are both phonologically and semantically related (Lsp); however, these competitors are activated to some degree by input from the phonological nodes. Once the lexical nodes are activated, they feed forward activation to semantic nodes and feed back activation to phonological nodes at time step 3. At time step 4, the activation achieved at the semantic and phonological nodes feeds back to the lexical nodes, which in turn facilitate lexical selection. At this time, active semantic nodes may propagate activity to lexical nodes for competitors that are semantically related (Ls), to nodes for competitors that are both phonologically and semantically related to the target (Lsp), and even to nodes for items that are unrelated to the target (Lu). Iterations of this process continue until, at the final time step, the lexical target achieves an activation level sufficiently above that of competitors to trigger release of the lexical target into the output stream. N. Martin and colleagues (N. Martin & Saffran, 1992; N. Martin et al., 1994, 1996) have manipulated activation decay rates at these nodes to explain the error patterns and recovery patterns in a case of deep dyslexia. From Martin, N., Saffran, E. M., & Dell, G. S. (1996). Recovery in deep dysphasia: Evidence for a relation between auditory–verbal STM capacity and lexical errors in repetition. *Brain and Language*, *52*, 83–113. Copyright 1996 by Academic Press. Reprinted with permission.

by R. C. Martin and Romani (1994) did not have deficits entirely isolated to a single aspect of verbal working memory. Although EA had greater impairment of phonological than of semantic working memory, her semantic working memory was not at normal levels. While AB had greater impairment of semantic than phonological working memory, his phonological working memory was impaired. The interconnection of phonological and semantic units with lexical units in the model of N. Martin and colleagues suggests that because of semantic–lexical–phonological interactions, the loss of semantic working memory capacity may have a negative impact on phonological working memory, and vice versa.

In summary, Baddeley's working memory model (Baddeley, 1990; Baddeley & Hitch, 1974, 1994) has received considerable support in the literature. Nonetheless, it is entirely dependent on phonological mechanisms. In a typical conversation, the long string of phonological units that are input one after another will make it virtually impossible to keep track of content via phonological mechanisms alone. Some have solved this conundrum by proposing that semantic information is the purview solely of long-term memory, and that long-term memory may be used to track the content of a conversation (e.g., McCarthy & Warrington, 1990; Saffran & Marin, 1975; Shallice & Warington, 1970). This viewpoint has been increasingly challenged. First, the pattern of deficits in patients who cannot repeat sentences verbatim but who can repeat the essential meaning of a sentence (e.g., Saffran & Marin, 1975) can be as easily explained by the existence of semantic working memory as it can by the use of a semantically based long-term memory. Furthermore, N. Martin et al. (1994) have provided evidence of dissociation of semantic and phonological working memory, and perhaps of syntactic working memory as well. Nonetheless, the data of this group are not adequately explained by a model that relies upon entirely separate phonological and semantic working memories, because their patient with a deficit in semantic working memory had some impairment of phonological working memory, and their patient with a deficit in phonological working memory had some impairment of semantic working memory. N. Martin and her colleagues (N. Martin & Saffran, 1992; N. Martin et al., 1994, 1996) have proposed a model that addresses this problem. They have used a spreading-activation (PDP) model in which phonological and semantic working memory both interact with and enhance lexical working memory. This reasoning suggests an interdependence of phonological, semantic, and lexical working memory representations in a way that can explain the incomplete separation of phonological and semantic working memory found by R. C. Martin and Romani (1994). Because of its explanatory power, the model of N. Martin and colleagues seems preferable to the other models at this time.

THE NEUROANATOMY OF WORKING MEMORY

The lesion literature has not provided extensive evidence regarding the neural substrates of verbal working memory. However, there are two sources of studies that can shed some light on verbal working memory. The first is the literature on animal models of working memory. Because nonhuman species do not communicate using elaborate symbols in the way humans do, animal models cannot give us direct information about verbal working memory. Nonetheless, this research can provide a general framework that can be applied to questions about verbal working memory. The second source of information regarding the anatomy of human working memory is the functional neuroimaging literature. The intricacies of task design, limitations in localization, and individual differences in structural and functional anatomy suggest that functional neuroimaging studies must be approached with some caution (Nadeau & Crosson, 1995). On the other hand, when used appropriately, functional neuroimaging can provide a powerful tool to assist in mapping functions of the human brain.

Animal Models

Studies with animal models have piqued interest in the neural substrates for working memory, especially regarding the role of the frontal lobes (e.g., Fuster, 1973; Goldman-Rakic, Funahashi, & Bruce, 1990). One area of interest is the dissociation of different forms of working memory in the frontal lobes of monkeys. Ungerleider and Mishkin (1982) had previously shown two streams for processing visual information in the posterior cortex: a dorsal stream for processing spatial location, and a ventral stream for processing visual object identity. More recently, Goldman-Rakic and her colleagues (Funahashi, Bruce, & Goldman-Rakic, 1989; Wilson, Scalaidhe, & Goldman-Rakic, 1993) have used single-unit recording methods to show that visual working memory for spatial location and object identity can be dissociated in the frontal cortex of monkeys, with frontal areas connected to the dorsal visual stream processing working memory for spatial location, and frontal areas connected to the ventral visual stream processing working memory for object identity. This research has some implications for verbal working memory. As noted previously, R. C. Martin and Romani (1994) have suggested different forms of verbal working memory (i.e., phonological, semantic, and syntactic). The work of Goldman-Rakic and colleagues raises the question of whether different frontal locations may subserve phonological, semantic, and syntactic working memory. The concept of dissociated frontal regions for various domains of working memory is also at odds with the theory of a single central executive for all forms of working memory; it raises the possibility of multiple control processes, one for each type of working memory.

A different issue is the question of what frontal neurons are contributing to working memory. Goldman-Rakic et al. (1990) have demonstrated frontal neurons that stay active during a delay between stimulus offset and actions based on information contained in the stimulus. Indeed, this type of neuron was among the most prevalent in the populations of frontal neurons responding to working memory tasks. Is the information actually held on-line frontally? Goldman-Rakic et al. (1990) reported that frontal neurons active during delays coded spatial information needed for performance of the working memory task, and that neurons that coded spatial information could be dissociated from those that coded the response at the end of the delay. A colleague and I (Nadeau & Crosson, 1997) have suggested that frontal activity serves to selectively engage neural networks representing working memories, temporarily keeping them on-line. This selective engagement may be achieved via direct cortico-cortical connections, or via a thalamic pathway involving the inferior thalamic peduncle, the nucleus reticularis thalami, and specific thalamic nuclei. For verbal working memory, the thalamic nuclei involved may be those most heavily connected with areas of cortex involved in language processing, such as the pulvinar and the lateral posterior nucleus.

There are limitations to the single-cell recording methods used by Goldman-Rakic and her colleagues. One is that they can only be used in animal models, for which the study of language processing (and therefore verbal working memory) is impossible. A second disadvantage is that it has been difficult to study multiple parts of a brain system at one time (though this limitation is rapidly being overcome through multiple-electrode recording techniques). A third is the difficulty in distinguishing the nature of changes in neuronal activity. For example, it would be difficult to ascertain on the basis of the activity changes described by Goldman-Rakic et al. (1990) whether frontal neurons are involved in continuing to selectively engage the specific neural nets to facilitate holding information online, or whether the information may be temporally stored in the frontal cortex. The first two of these problems can be solved by using functional neuroimaging techniques to study verbal working memory; that is, operation of the whole brain can be studied in neurologically normal humans. Unfortunately, functional imaging is no more successful than single-neuron recording in telling us the specific nature of the information implicit in the firing of single neurons or aggregates of neurons.

Functional Neuroimaging Studies

Functional neuroimaging of normal language and working memory has most commonly been done with positron emission tomography (PET) or functional magnetic resonance imaging (fMRI). These techniques measure changes in blood flow, metabolism, or blood oxygenation that accompany changes in neural synaptic activity in various brain structures. To image normal cognition, the most commonly used PET techniques provide measures of changes in regional cerebral blood flow, which are in turn dependent on underlying metabolic changes. The most commonly used fMRI technique at the current time measures blood oxygenation changes that are correlated with changes in regional cerebral blood flow. The metabolic activity that drives these hemodynamic changes occurs primarily at the level of the synapse. The reader who wishes more details on functional neuroimaging techniques is referred to the Nadeau and Crosson (1995) article.

It is of some interest that functional neuroimaging research in humans has generally confirmed the participation of some frontal structures in visual working memory, along with more posterior areas (Jonides et al., 1993; McCarthy et al., 1994; Petrides, Alivisatos, Evans, & Meyer, 1993; Swartz, Halgren, Fuster, & Mandelkern, 1994; Swartz et al., 1995). Indeed, in their functional imaging studies, Courtney and colleagues (Courtney, Ungerleider, Keil, & Haxby, 1996; Courtney, Petit, Maisog, Ungerleider, & Haxby, 1998) demonstrated separation within the frontal lobes of areas related to spatial location and facial identity, presumably related to working memory and corresponding to the dorsal ("where") and ventral ("what") visual processing streams. Smith et al. (1995) also found evidence of separate spatial and object working memory systems in the frontal lobes, although the areas implicated were not the same as those in the studies of Courtney and colleagues. The dissociation of frontal as well as posterior cortical regions for spatial and object identity working memory raises some interesting possibilities for verbal working memory. As noted above, R. C. Martin and Romani (1994) provided evidence for partially separable verbal working memory systems for processing phonological characteristics of words, semantic characteristics of words, and syntactic relationships between words in sentences. One would expect that these different forms of working memory would have different neuroanatomical substrates as well.

However, most of the functional imaging research on verbal working memory has applied the model of Baddeley (Baddeley, 1990; Baddeley & Hitch, 1974, 1994), which only addresses phonological working memory. The reader will recall that in this model, verbal working memory is presumed to consist of a central executive and a phonological loop. The phonological loop in turn consists of an acoustic store and an articulatory mechanism for subvocal rehearsal. Paulesu, Frith, and Frackowiak (1993) performed a working memory experiment in which neurologically normal subjects performed four tasks during

$H_2{}^{15}O$ PET: briefly remembering visually presented letter strings, judging whether or not letters rhymed, remembering nonsense visual characters, or judging the visual similarity of nonsense characters. Subjects were instructed to rehearse letter strings silently during the verbal working memory task. The critical comparison was between remembering letter strings and making rhyme judgments, because both tasks involved visual and phonological processing, but only the working memory task involved short-term storage of information. For this comparison, activity increases were found in the left supramarginal gyrus. Broca's area was also somewhat more activated in the working memory task than in the rhyme judgment task. On the basis of their findings, the authors concluded that Broca's area was responsible for phonological rehearsal, while the left supramarginal gyrus was the location of the phonological store. Subsequently, Paulesu et al. (1995) replicated their earlier findings with respect to the involvement of Broca's area and the supramarginal gyrus in an experiment involving verbal working memory for letters. It should be noted that letters have a phonological code and perhaps some lexical identity as well, but they have little semantic value. Therefore, these experiments tested primarily phonological but not semantic working memory.

Petrides, Alivisatos, Meyer, and Evans (1993) had subjects perform a self-ordered working memory task (saying digits 1 through 10 in random order without repeating a digit) and an externally ordered working memory task (listening to an experimenter repeat digits 1 through 10 in random order to determine the missing digit) during $H_2{}^{15}O$ PET scanning. Although rehearsal itself may not have been a large factor in this study, subjects were saying digits aloud. During both the self-ordered and the externally ordered tasks (as compared to a counting control task), there was increased activity bilaterally in dorsolateral frontal cortex and premotor cortex, greater on the left than the right. There was also bilaterally increased activity in posterior parietal cortex (in or around Brodmann's area [BA] 40 and/or BA 7). It is of interest that there was increased activity in an anterior cingulate area only in the self-ordered task, and in right frontal polar cortex only in the externally ordered task. When images from the externally ordered task were "subtracted" from images from the self-ordered task, there was increased activity in the supplementary motor area (SMA), motor face area, Broca's area, cerebellum, and brainstem, which probably represented the greater motor activity required in repeating numbers than in listening to them. When images from the self-ordered task were subtracted from images from the externally ordered task, there was increased activity bilaterally in the temporal lobe (three areas in the left hemisphere, two areas in the right hemisphere). Activity in some of these areas was probably due to the greater auditory processing demands in the externally ordered task relative to the internally ordered task. Again, it should be noted that isolated numbers have little semantic value; thus this study primarily tested phonological working memory.

Cohen et al. (1994) used fMRI to explore activity in the frontal cortex in a working memory task that involved tracking letter sequences. Subjects were instructed not to subvocalize. These authors also found increased activity widely distributed in the frontal cortex (in or around BAs 9, 44, 45, 46, and 10) in the left and/or right hemispheres of some subjects. Some activity changes in or around BA 47 were found as well. Eleven of 12 subjects showed increased activity in at least one of these areas.

Fiez et al. (1996) have been among the few investigators to use words as opposed to digits or letters during functional neuroimaging of verbal working memory. They employed separate working memory tasks in which normal subjects were asked to remember related words, unrelated words, or pseudowords silently for 55 seconds during $H_2{}^{15}O$ PET scanning. It is highly probable that subjects used rehearsal as a memory maintenance strategy in these tasks. Areas of increased activity elicited by the combined verbal working memory tasks (relative to a fixation control task) included SMA, left and right dorsolateral pre-frontal cortex (in or around BA 9), Broca's area, and areas in the left and right cerebellum. There was no overlap with areas activated during counting. No differences were found when working memory for related and unrelated words was compared directly. When working memory for pseudowords was compared to working memory for real words, the only area of increased activity was in the posterior left frontal area near its junction with the insula.

We (Crosson et al., 1999) designed a study based in part on the distinction by R. C. Martin and Romani (1994) between phonological and semantic working memory. We had subjects perform three working memory tasks and one control task. On each working memory task, subjects saw three "memory" words presented together, followed by eight "test" words presented one at a time. On the semantic working memory task, subjects had to remember the memory words and respond affirmatively when the test word was a member of a cate-gory represented by any of the three memory words. On the phonological working memory task, subjects had to respond affirmatively when the test word rhymed with any memory word. On the orthographic working memory task, subjects had to respond affirmatively when the test word had the same three or more last letters as any memory word. On the control task, subjects identified consonant strings with the same first and last letters.

It is of interest that subjects used phonological or visual strategies in the orthographic working memory task, but processed whole lexical items in the semantic and phonologi-cal working memory tasks. Compared to the control task, all areas of increased activity in all verbal working memory tasks were in the left hemisphere. No areas of increased activ-ity were found in the right cerebral hemisphere. All three working memory tasks activated cortex in or near Broca's area and some area in the lateral premotor cortex. The activation of Broca's area was consistent with subjects' report that they used subvocal rehearsal in all working memory tasks. SMA and the anterior thalamus were activated in both the seman-tic and phonological working memory tasks. Since subjects processed entire lexical items in these tasks but not in the orthographic working memory task, SMA and anterior thalamic activity may have been due to lexical processing. The anterior thalamus may be involved in extended selective engagement of the neural nets in which preexisting lexical items reside, consistent with our theory (Nadeau & Crosson, 1997; Crosson & Nadeau, 1998; Crosson, 1999). Areas of activation unique to the semantic task included frontal cortex outside Broca's area and premotor cortex, the posterior thalamus, and inferior posterior temporal cortex. These areas may be involved in the semantic processing unique to the semantic task (e.g., Binder et al., 1997 [frontal cortex]; Crosson, 1992 [thalamus]; Raymer et al., 1997 [posterior temporal lobe]). Areas of activity unique to the phonological working memory task were in the inferior temporo-occipital junction, the right cerebellum, and the brainstem. The activity at the temporo-occipital junction may involve the transformation of written words into sounds (Rapcsak, Rothi, & Heilman, 1987), while the cerebellar and brainstem activations may be related to the close relationship between speech sounds and motor patterns (e.g., Liberman, 1993). An area of increased activity in the extrastriate visual cortex during the orthographic working memory task may represent visual processing, consistent with the findings of Petersen, Fox, Snyder, and Raichle (1990). Thus there were some com-mon but many separate cortical mechanisms involved in the different forms of working memory. Unfortunately, this experiment does not enable us to separate brain regions in-volved in basic semantic, phonological, and visual processes from the regions uniquely engaged in working memory.

Thus a majority of functional neuroimaging studies of verbal working memory to date have used stimuli (letters or numbers), that lend themselves to phonological processing.

Such stimuli may be represented as unique lexical items as well, but they have little semantic value when used in the absence of contextual information. Findings from working memory tasks involving numbers and letters are generally supportive of Baddeley's model, with Broca's area and the left supramarginal gyrus involved in a phonological rehearsal loop. Broca's area may be responsible for rehearsal, and cortex in the left supramarginal gyrus may be responsible for the phonological store. The conclusion that the supramarginal gyrus is involved in storage of phonological information during working memory is consistent with evidence that this structure is needed for multiple aspects of phonological processing (Alexander, 1997). A lesion of the supramarginal gyrus may be the necessary and sufficient structural abnormality for conduction aphasia (Alexander, 1997); conduction aphasia involves disproportionate difficulties in repetition, often accompanied by predominantly phonological paraphasias in naming and spontaneous language (see also Nadeau, Chapter 3, this volume). Reduction in short-term storage of verbal (phonological) information has been used as an explanation for conduction aphasia (e.g., Saffran & Marin, 1975; Caramazza et al., 1981). There is evidence that Broca's area is involved in phonological processing, including but not limited to motor and articulatory processes (e.g., Ojemann, 1983). Thus this view of Broca's area and the supramarginal gyrus of the left hemisphere is consistent with previous literature regarding these areas. However, it should be pointed out that Broca's area and the left supramarginal gyrus are not exclusively involved in the phonological loop. It is probably more accurate to conceptualize them as being recruited for this function because their more basic information-processing capacities support it. For example, increased activity has been observed in Broca's area, even when rehearsal was discouraged (Cohen et al., 1994); this indicates that it may be involved in other aspects of phonological processing. With respect to working memory for letters and numbers, it should also be noted that activity changes in lateral premotor cortex (around BA 6) and sometimes in left frontal cortex outside Broca's area have been noted. Areas of inconsistently increased activity in the medial frontal cortex have included the SMA (or often the portion of medial BA 6 currently thought to be pre-SMA) and anterior cingulate cortex, the latter appearing only in a self-ordered task.

Application of the model of R. C. Martin and Romani (1994) to verbal working memory has only begun. In our recent study (Crosson et al., 1999), performed at the Medical College of Wisconsin, we showed some fractionation of posterior left-hemisphere systems involved in semantic, phonological, and orthographic working memory. Our study of phonological working memory did not replicate prior studies implicating the left supramarginal gyrus in this function. The fact that we did not elicit activity in this region may have been due to the use of consonant strings in our control task. Since previous studies of phonological working memory showing activity in the supramarginal gyrus involved letters, our control task may also have activated this region, thus eliminating potential differences in the activity generated by the control and experimental tasks. Some evidence suggests that the posterior temporal activity noted on the semantic tasks is in an area that may be involved in semantic processing, and that the extrastriate visual cortex involved in orthographic working memory is involved in visual processing of written material. It seems probable either that areas involved in semantic or orthographic processing are recruited as temporary storage sites for working memory, or that the temporary storage sites for these kinds of information are anatomically adjacent to cortex used to process the information. Indeed, the pattern of activity associated with semantic working memory in our study appears to be very similar to that described by Binder et al. (1997) in their study of semantic monitoring.

Interpretation of frontal activity in semantic, phonological, and orthographic working memory tasks is more difficult. All our tasks elicited activation in or near Broca's area, which may be due to rehearsal or to other processes. Likewise, some lateral premotor regions were active in every task. SMA and anterior thalamic activity may be necessary for continuing activation of preexisting lexical forms. Lateral frontal activity outside of Broca's area, premotor cortex, and adjacent regions was evident only on the semantic task. Again, Broca's area appears to be involved in multiple activities. It is unclear what other frontal activities may be specific to working memory. In short, the anatomy of working memory systems other than the phonological loop is still under investigation.

EVALUATION AND TREATMENT OF WORKING MEMORY DEFICITS

With the exception of language treatment, cognitive rehabilitation is a discipline in its infancy. Most treatments based upon an understanding of the cognitive structure of language are also relatively recent innovations. Several early studies of cognitive rehabilitation have provided rather disappointing results. Various mistakes have been made in these endeavors, including the use of a single treatment for patients with heterogeneous cognitive impairments. Such an approach may obscure benefits for a subset of patients with a treatable deficit, because they are mixed with patients for whom the treatment may not be appropriate. In other words, one must carefully evaluate patients and base treatment on detailed individual cognitive profiles. Rather than outlining a specific program of assessment and treatment for different types of verbal working memory, I discuss a general approach that emphasizes recent models of working memory.

Assessment of Verbal Working Memory

The literature reviewed in this chapter suggests that a useful evaluation of verbal working memory will involve two dimensions: the kind of working memory being assessed, and the particular processes that contribute to working memory. Regarding type of working memory, R. C. Martin and Romani (1994) have proposed three types of verbal working memory: phonological, semantic, and syntactic. These authors and their colleagues have tested phonological memory span by presenting word lists of varying length to patients, followed by a rhyme probe (i.e., subjects are given a word and asked whether one of the list words rhymes with the probe word). Span is determined by calculating the percentage of accurate responses for lists of various lengths. Semantic span is tested in a similar way, except that subjects must decipher whether the probe is a member of the same category as any of the list words. Syntax span is determined by having subjects make grammaticality judgments about sentences in which the critical elements determining the grammatical correctness of each sentence are separated by varying numbers of additional words.

N. Martin and colleagues (N. Martin & Saffran, 1992; N. Martin et al., 1994, 1996) used a PDP (spreading-activation) model, which includes phonological, semantic, and lexical nodes that interact with feedforward and feedback processes. In this system, the memory span task with semantic probes discussed by R. C. Martin and Romani (1994) would best be thought of as lexical–semantic, because it involves the semantic features of real words. Likewise, the memory span task with phonological probes can be conceptualized as lexical–phonological. A way of testing more purely phonological memory would be to use span for nonwords. Indeed, the inability to repeat nonwords has been considered to be one of the hallmarks of deep dysphasia (e.g., Katz & Goodglass, 1990).

The second dimension on which verbal working memory should be evaluated is the component procedures that are necessary to hold information on line for impending use. Shiffrin's (1993) assessment of the characteristics of short-term memory offers a good guideline for such assessment. Based on his analysis, three component procedures can be evaluated. The first procedural variable is storage capacity: Shiffrin has noted that short-term memory has a limited capacity. Tests of memory span are constructed to determine the capacity limitations for working memory. For example, the semantic and phonological memory span measures discussed by R. C. Martin and Romani (1994) are also designed to measure capacity limitations.

The second procedural variable is the capacity to hold information in memory across time, without refreshing the short-term store with operations such as rehearsal. In other words, the short-term store should be assessed for abnormal rate of decay. N. Martin and colleagues (N. Martin & Saffran, 1992; N. Martin et al., 1994, 1996) have successfully shown the impact of abnormal rates of decay on working memory. In order to do so, patients' accuracy in maintaining multiple bits of information in the short-term store for progressively longer intervals can be measured. To prevent rehearsal, patients can perform an alternative activity during delays. Essentially, this is the Brown–Peterson, or Peterson and Peterson, paradigm (Brown, 1958; Peterson & Peterson, 1959). In assessing rate of decay, the evaluator should remain mindful that some investigators believe short-term and long-term storage procedures can be fractionated from one another. If this is true, then in patients with increased rates of decay, long-term memory may be invoked to compensate for increasingly rapid decay within the short-term store. This may make it difficult to assess rate of decay, especially in cases of milder deficits. The findings of N. Martin and colleagues (N. Martin & Saffran, 1992; N. Martin et al., 1994, 1996) indicate that in some instances of more severe impairment, abnormal rate of decay can cause the pattern of deficits in deep dysphasia (i.e., difficulty repeating nonwords, with semantic as well as phonological errors in repetition and other speech).

The final procedural variable to be investigated is the ability to perform operations on the information in order to maintain it in the short-term store, or to modify or use it in various cognitive operations. If Baddeley has been correct, one primary operation for maintaining information in short-term phonological stores is simple repetition of the information (i.e., rehearsal). Earlier in this chapter, I have suggested that elaborative rehearsal may be a procedure that refreshes short-term semantic stores. The ability to manipulate information in short-term storage may affect a patient's ability to consolidate the information into long-term memory or to use it for problem solving. One interesting question is to what degree working memory problems contribute to difficulties in problem solving. Goldman-Rakic (1994) has suggested that this contribution may be substantial.

Theoretically at least, it is possible that capacity limitations, decay rate, and the ability to perform various operations on information in short-term storage may vary according to the type of information being stored. For example, R. C. Martin and Romani (1994) have purported to show differential impairment of short-term capacity for semantic and phonological information. On the other hand, feedforward and feedback processes of spreading-activation models imply an interdependency of different levels of processing, such that, for example, changes in semantic working memory may affect phonological working memory and vice versa. N. Martin and her colleagues (N. Martin & Saffran, 1992; N. Martin et al., 1994, 1996) have shown that abnormal rates of decay in lexical, semantic, or phonological information may have implications for patterns of deficits in multiple domains of working memory. This factor may account for the mixed patterns of deficits in the patients observed by R. C. Martin and Romani (1994), as noted previously in this chapter. However, it seems prudent to assess capacity limitations, decay rate, and ability to manipulate information for phonological, lexical, semantic, and perhaps syntactic information.

Treatment of Deficits in Verbal Working Memory

Treatment of working memory deficits should flow from the conceptual framework and the deficits found during assessment, as detailed above. Before I discuss rehabilitation of working memory per se, it is worth noting that attentional deficits may have a significant adverse impact on working memory. If working memory impairment is suspected, patients should also be assessed for an attentional disturbance; if problems in attention are discovered, they should ordinarily be addressed before treating working memory problems (or at least addressed concomitantly with working memory problems), because alleviation of attentional problems may mitigate working memory deficits. I have discussed a conceptual framework for, evaluation of, and treatment of attention deficits in Chapter 14 of this volume.

Treatment that directly addresses working memory impairment should be focused on those kinds of working memory and those processes in working memory that assessment procedures have shown to be impaired. Rothi (1995) has suggested that three different kinds of treatment strategies can be used:

1. "Restitution" is an attempt to reconstruct the system in its original form. Restitutive treatments are generally appropriate for the earliest stages of rehabilitation and capitalize on normal biological mechanisms of recovery.

2. "Vicariation" is an attempt to reconstruct the system in a way that substitutes intact cognitive mechanisms for damaged ones. Vicariation can be started early in the rehabilitation process, especially when structural images of the brain strongly suggest that the neurological mechanism subserving the target cognitive function is permanently damaged. However, it can also be used in the later stages of rehabilitation when restitution is no longer appropriate. The assumption is that intact cognitive mechanisms have viable neurological substrates that can be used in reconstructing the cognitive system, bypassing the damaged substrates of the impaired cognitive mechanisms.

3. When attempts at restitution and vicariation have not been entirely successful in achieving nearly normal function, "substitution" can be used. Substitution involves attempting to compensate for impaired cognition by an entirely different means.

One restitutive strategy for treating capacity limitations in working memory is stimulation. Stimulation involves having the patient attempt to store larger and larger amounts of the appropriate information (phonological, semantic, or syntactic). The assumption is that the patient's attempts at temporary storage of the information will stimulate and optimize normal biological recovery mechanisms. It must be cautioned that stimulation should not be viewed like exercise to "build the brain muscle." Often it will not be effective in restoring function, because the underlying conditions are not favorable. Once it is ascertained that stimulation will produce no further improvement, therapy should turn to vicariative and substitutive strategies.

Theoretically, vicariative strategies can be used in rehabilitation of working memory when one type of working memory is more affected by brain damage than another. Suppose, for example, that a patient shows impairment of semantic working memory with relative preservation of phonological working memory. Furthermore, the patient may have significant difficulty in verbal problem solving because he or she cannot hold the meaning of information in mind while trying to solve the problem. One method for confronting this problem may be to teach the patient to use intact phonological working memory to substitute for impaired semantic working memory. To enhance phonological working memory, the therapist may teach the patient to rely upon simple rehearsal of important information, while extracting semantic information as necessary. Note that the attempt is still to reconstruct a working memory system, but one using some different cognitive components.

The limitations of this approach should be immediately apparent to the reader. First, the patient's ability to use semantic information may be closely linked to difficulties in working memory. In this case, the patient may not be able to extract the necessary semantic information because of a more fundamental deficit in processing semantic information, even though he or she may be able to use rehearsal to keep the basic content available. However, if it can be established that the patient has the ability to extract needed semantic information appropriately, the strategy will be useful. Second, the use of rehearsal will prevent the patient from processing further incoming information efficiently. Thus the strategy is most useful when there is not a relatively long stream of incoming information.

Finally, when restitutive and vicariative approaches are unavailable or have not produced the desired functional results, substitutive strategies can be tried. A number of substitutive approaches may be tried to compensate for impaired verbal working memory. For example, the patient described above may be taught to write information on a note pad, so that the necessary information is in front of him or her instead of in working memory. The patient may also be taught to have others repeat themselves if long-term stores are more viable than short-term stores. Repetition will help the information be placed into long-term stores, which may then be used as a substitute to some degree for a limited capacity in short-term storage. The experienced clinician has probably noted that the application of these strategies will require some awareness on the patient's part that there is a deficit for which compensation may be useful. The relationship between awareness and compensation has been discussed elsewhere (Barco, Crosson, Bolesta, Werts, & Stout, 1991; Crosson et al., 1989).

SUMMARY

In summary, this chapter has attempted to break working memory down along two dimensions. Evidence is beginning to suggest multiple kinds of verbal working memory (i.e., phonological, lexical, semantic, and syntactic), and it is possible for one form of working memory to be impaired while others remain relatively intact (R. C. Martin & Romani, 1994). Some kinds of verbal working memory seem to be interdependent (e.g., phonological, lexical, and semantic), and a PDP modeling approach may have considerable explanatory value (N. Martin & Saffran, 1992; N. Martin et al., 1994, 1996). Assessment and rehabilitation approaches will follow from such a conceptual understanding of verbal working memory. As we understand more about the cognitive processes and the underlying anatomical systems, we will be more prepared to engage in rehabilitation of working memory deficits.

REFERENCES

Alexander, M. P. (1997). Aphasia: Clinical and anatomic aspects. In T. E. Feinberg & M. J. Farah (Eds.), *Behavioral neurology and neuropsychology* (pp. 133–149). New York: McGraw-Hill.

Atkinson, R. C., & Shiffrin, R. M. (1968). Human memory: A proposed system and its control processes. In K. W. Spence & J. T. Spence (Eds.), *The psychology of learning and motivation: Advances in research and theory* (Vol. 2, pp. 90–195). New York: Academic Press.

Baddeley, A. D. (1966). Short-term memory for word sequences as a function of acoustic, semantic and formal similarity. *Quarterly Journal of Experimental Psychology, 18*, 362–365.

Baddeley, A. D. (1990). *Human memory: Theory and practice.* Needham Heights, MA: Allyn & Bacon.

Baddeley, A. D., & Hitch, G. J. (1974). Working memory. In G. H. Bower (Ed.), *The psychology of learning and motivation: Advances in research and theory* (Vol. 8). New York: Academic Press.

Baddeley, A. D., & Hitch, G. J. (1994). Developments in the concept of working memory. *Neuropsychology, 8*, 485–493.

Baddeley, A. D., Lewis, V. J., & Vallar, G. (1984). Exploring the articulatory loop. *Quarterly Journal of Experimental Psychology, 36*, 233–252.

Barco, P. P., Crosson, B., Bolesta, M. M., Werts, D., & Stout, R. (1991). Levels of awareness and compensation in cognitive rehabilitation. In J. S. Kreutzer & P. Wehman (Eds.), *Cognitive rehabilitation for persons with traumatic brain injury: A functional approach* (pp. 129–146). Baltimore: Brookes.

Binder, J. R., Frost, J. A., Hammeke, T. A., Cox, R. W., Rao, S. M., & Prieto, T. (1997). Human brain language areas identified by functional magnetic resonance imaging. *Journal of Neuroscience, 17*, 353–362.

Brown, J. (1958). Some tests of the decay theory of immediate memory. *Quarterly Journal of Experimental Psychology, 10*, 12–21.

Caramazza, A., Basili, A. G., Koller, J., & Berndt, R. S. (1981). An investigation of repetition and language processing in a case of conduction aphasia. *Brain and Language, 14*, 235–271.

Cohen, J. D., Forman, S. D., Braver, T. S., Casey, B. J., Servan-Schreiber, D., & Noll, D. C. (1994). Activation of the prefrontal cortex in a nonspatial working memory task with Functional MRI. *Human Brain Mapping, 1*, 293–304.

Conrad, R., & Hull, A. J. (1964). Information, acoustic confusion and memory span. *British Journal of Psychology, 55*, 429–432.

Courtney, S. M., Petit, L., Maisog, J. M., Ungerleider, L. G., & Haxby, J. V. (1998). An area specialized for spatial working memory in the human frontal cortex. *Science, 279*, 1347–1351.

Courtney, S. M., Ungerleider, L. G., Keil, K., & Haxby, J. V. (1996). Object and spatial visual working memory activate separate neural systems in human cortex. *Cerebral Cortex, 6*, 39–49.

Craik, F. I. M., & Lockhart, R. S. (1972). Levels of processing: A framework for memory research. *Journal of Verbal Learning and Verbal Behavior, 11*, 671–684.

Crosson, B. (1992). *Subcortical functions in language and memory.* New York: Guilford Press.

Crosson, B. (1999). Subcortical mechanisms in language: Lexical–semantic mechanisms and the thalamus. *Brain and Cognition, 40*, 414–438.

Crosson, B., Barco, P. P., Velozo, C. A., Bolesta, M. M., Cooper, P.V., Werts, D., & Brobeck, T. C. (1989). Awareness and compensation in postacute head injury rehabilitation. *Journal of Head Trauma Rehabilitation, 4*(3), 46–54.

Crosson, B., & Nadeau, S. E. (1998). The role of subcortical structures in linguistic processes: Recent developments. In B. Stemmer & H. A. Whitaker (Eds.), *Handbook of neurolinguistics* (pp. 431–445). San Diego, CA: Academic Press.

Crosson, B., Rao, S. M., Woodley, S. J., Rosen, A. C., Bobholz, J. A., Mayer, A., Cunningham, J. M., Hammeke, T. A., Fuller, S. A., Binder, J. R., Cox, R. W., & Stein, E. A. (1999). Mapping of semantic, phonological, and orthographic verbal working memory in normal adults with functional magnetic resonance imaging. *Neuropsychology, 13*, 171–187.

Dell, G. S. (1986). A spreading-activation theory of retrieval in sentence production. *Psychological Review, 93*, 283–321.

Dell, G. S., & O'Seaghdha, P. G. (1991). Mediated convergent lexical priming in language production: A comment on Levelt, et al. (1990). *Psychological Review, 98*, 604–614.

Farah, M. J. (1997). Computational modeling in behavioral neurology and neuropsychology. In T. E. Feinberg & M. J. Farah (Eds.), *Behavioral neurology and neuropsychology* (pp. 121–130). New York: McGraw-Hill.

Fiez, J. A., Raife, E. A., Balota, D. A., Schwarz, J. P., Raichle, M. E., & Petersen, S. E. (1996). A positron emission tomography study of the short-term maintenance of verbal information. *Journal of Neuroscience, 16*, 802–822.

Funahashi, S., Bruce, C. J., & Goldman-Rakic, P. S. (1989). Mnemonic coding of visual space in the monkey's dorsolateral prefrontal cortex. *Journal of Neurophysiology, 61*, 331–349.

Fuster, J. M. (1973). Unit activity in prefrontal cortex during delayed-response performance: Neuronal correlates of transient memory. *Journal of Neurophysiology, 36*, 61–78.

Goldman-Rakic, P. S. (1994). Working memory dysfunction in schizophrenia. *Journal of Neuropsychiatry and Clinical Neurosciences, 6*, 348–357.

Goldman-Rakic, P. S., Funahashi, S., & Bruce, C. J. (1990). Neocortical memory circuits. *Cold Spring Harbor Symposium on Quantitative Biology, 55*, 1025–1038.

Jonides, J., Smith, E. E., Koeppe, R. A., Awh, E., Minoshima, S., & Mintun, M. A. (1993). Spatial working memory in humans as revealed by PET. *Nature, 363*, 623–635.

Katz, R., & Goodglass, H. (1990). Deep dysphasia: An analysis of a rare form of repetition disorder. *Brain and Language, 39*, 153–185.

Liberman, A. M. (1993). In speech perception, time is not what it seems. *Annals of the New York Academy of Sciences, 682*, 264–271.

Martin, N., Dell, G. S., Saffran, E. M., & Schwartz, M. F. (1994). Origins of paraphasias in deep dysphasia: Testing the consequences of a decay impairment to an interactive spreading activation model of lexical retrieval. *Brain and Language, 47*, 609–660.

Martin, N., & Saffran, E. M. (1992). A computational account of deep dysphasia: Evidence from a single case study. *Brain and Language, 43*, 240–274.

Martin, N., Saffran, E. M., & Dell, G. S. (1996). Recovery in deep dysphasia: Evidence for a relation between auditory–verbal STM capacity and lexical errors in repetition. *Brain and Language, 52*, 83–113.

Martin, R. C., Blossom-Stach, C., Yaffee, L., & Wetzel, F. (1995). Consequences of a motor programming deficit foor rehearsal and written sentence comprehension. *Quarterly Journal of Experimental Psychology, 48A*, 536–572.

Martin, R. C., & Romani, C. (1994). Verbal working memory and sentence comprehension: A multiple-components view. *Neuropsychology, 8*, 506–523.

McCarthy, G., Blamire, A. M., Puce, A., Nobre, A. C., Bloch, G., Hyder, F., Goldman- Rakic, P., & Shulman, R. G. (1994). Functional magnetic resonance imaging of human prefrontal cortex activation during a spatial working memory task. *Proceedings of the National Academy of Sciences USA, 91*, 8690–8694.

McCarthy, R. A., & Warrington, E. K. (1990). *Cognitive neuropsychology: A clinical introduction.* New York: Academic Press.

McClelland, J. L., & Rumelhart, D. E. (1981). An interactive activation model of context effects in letter perception: Part I. An account of basic findings. *Psychological Review, 88*, 375–407.

Nadeau, S. E., & Crosson, B. (1995). A guide to the functional imaging of cognitive processes. *Neuropsychiatry, Neuropsychology, and Behavioral Neurology, 8*, 143–162.

Nadeau, S. E., & Crosson, B. (1997). Subcortical aphasia. *Brain and Language, 58*, 355–402.

Ojemann, G. A. (1983). Brain organization for language from the perspective of electrical stimulation mapping. *Behavioral and Brain Sciences, 2*, 189–230.

Paulesu, E., Connelly, A., Frith, C. D., Friston, K. J., Heather, J., Myers, R., Gadian, D. G., & Frackowiak, R. S. J. (1995). Functional MR imaging correlations with positron emission tomography: Initial experience using a cognitive activation paradigm on verbal working memory. *Functional Neuroimaging, 5*, 207–225.

Paulesu, E., Frith, C. D., & Frackowiak, R. S. J. (1993). The neural correlates of the verbal component of working memory. *Nature, 362*, 342–345.

Petersen, S. E., Fox, P. T., Snyder, A. Z., & Raichle, M. E. (1990). Activation of extrastriate and frontal cortical areas by visual words and work-like stimuli. *Science, 249*, 1041–1044.

Peterson, L. R., & Peterson, J. J. (1959). Short-term retention of individual verbal items. *Journal of Experimental Psychology, 58*, 193–198.

Petrides, M., Alivisatos, B., Evans, A. C., & Meyer, E. (1993). Dissociation of human mid-dorsolateral from posterior dorsolateral frontal cortex in memory processing. *Proceedings of the National Academy of Sciences USA, 90*, 873–877.

Petrides, M., Alivisatos, B., Meyer, E., & Evans, A. C. (1993). Functional activation of the human frontal cortex during the performance of verbal working memory tasks. *Proceedings of the National Academy of Sciences USA, 90*, 878–882.

Rapcsak, S. Z., Rothi, L. J. G., & Heilman, K. M. (1987). Phonological alexia with optic and tactile anomia: A neuropsychological and anatomical study. *Brain and Language, 31*, 109–121.

Raymer, A. M., Foundas, A., Maher, L. M., Greenwald, M. R., Morris, M., Rothi, L. J. G., & Heilman, K. M. (1997). Cognitive neuropsychological analysis and neuroanatomic correlates in a case of acute anomia. *Brain and Language, 58*, 137–156.

Rothi, L. J. G. (1995). Behavioral compensation in the case of treatment of acquired language disorders resulting from brain damage. In R. A. Dixon & L. Backman (Eds.), *Compensating for psychological deficits and declines* (pp. 219–230). Hillsdale, NJ: Erlbaum.

Rumelhart, D. E., McClelland, J. L., & the PDP Research Group. (Eds.). (1986). *Parallel distributed processing: Explorations in the microstructure of cognition. Vol. 1. Foundations.* Cambridge, MA: MIT Press.

Saffran, E. M., & Marin, O. S. M. (1975). Immediate memory for word lists and sentences in a patient with deficient auditory short-term memory. *Brain and Language, 2,* 420–423.

Salamé, P., & Baddeley, A. D. (1987). Noise, unattended speech and short-term memory. *Ergonomics, 30,* 1185–1193.

Shallice, T., & Warrington, E. K. (1970). Independent functioning of verbal memory stores: A neuropsychological study. *Quarterly Journal of Experimental Psychology, 22,* 261–273.

Shiffrin, R. M. (1993). Short-term memory: A brief commentary. *Memory and Cognition, 21,* 193–197.

Smith, E. E., Jonides, J., Koeppe, R. A., Awh, E., Schumacher, E., & Minoshima, S. (1995). Spatial vs. object working memory: PET investigations. *Journal of Cognitive Neuroscience, 7,* 337–358.

Swartz, B. E., Halgren, E., Fuster, J., & Mandelkern, M. (1994). An [18]FDG-PET study of cortical activation during a short-term visual memory task in humans. *NeuroReport, 5,* 925–928.

Swartz, B. E., Halgren, E., Fuster, J., Simpkins, F., Gee, M., & Mandelkern, M. (1995). Cortical metabolic activation in humans during a visual memory task. *Cerebral Cortex, 3,* 205–214.

Ungerleider, L. G., & Mishkin, M. (1982). Two cortical visual systems. In D. J. Ingle, M. A. Oodale, & F. J. W. Mansfield (Eds.), *Analysis of visual behavior* (pp. 549–586). Cambridge, MA: MIT Press.

Vallar, G., & Baddeley, A. D. (1984). Phonological short-term store, phonological processing and sentence comprehension: A neuropsychological case study. *Cognitive Neuropsychology, 1,* 121–141.

Wilson, F. A. W., Scalaidhe, S. P. O., & Goldman-Rakic, P. S. (1993). Dissociation of object and spatial processing domains in primate prefrontal cortex. *Science, 260,* 1955–1958.

PART V

Practical Considerations

16

SINGLE-SUBJECT EXPERIMENTAL DESIGNS IN APHASIA

KEVIN P. KEARNS

The clinical science of aphasiology is replete with suggestions for treating aphasic persons. Novel intervention approaches have been based on a variety of rationales, including psychosocial considerations (Lyon, Cariski, Keisler, et al., 1997), neurobehavioral issues (Sparks, Helms, & Albert, 1974), psycholinguistic models of normal language (Thompson, Shapiro, & Roberts, 1993; Schwartz, Saffran, Fink, Myers, & Martin, 1994; Mitchum, Haendiges, & Berndt, 1993), cognitive-neurobehavioral issues (McNeil, Odell, & Tseng, 1991), and pragmatic considerations (Aten, Caliguiri, & Holland, 1982; Springer, 1991). Importantly, the applied literature supports the conclusion that treatment of aphasic individuals is indeed efficacious (Holland et al., 1996; Robey, 1994, 1998, 1999).

The positive outlook for clinical aphasiology must, however, be tempered by the fact that to date there have been few well-controlled treatment studies of aphasia. Furthermore, large-scale efforts to investigate treatment efficacy have not frequently given due consideration to statistical power and related issues (Schoonen, 1991).

Additional data are needed to demonstrate the effectiveness of our interventions. This need has become particularly acute because of the current realities of clinical practice, and because of pressures from the U.S. government and other funding agencies to demonstrate beneficial and cost-effective treatments. The overall impact of the proliferation of managed care organizations and changes in reimbursement levels has been to reduce hospital lengths of stay, and in some cases access to rehabilitation services. In addition, clinicians are facing burgeoning caseloads, an increasing number of medically complex patients, and pressure for accountability and documentation of all aspects of patient care.

There has also been increasing pressure to provide efficacy and outcome data to the federal government and third-party agencies. Clinicians are anxious for data that will guide decisions regarding the type and intensity of treatment for aphasic patients. It is important for researchers and clinicians alike to gather objective data about the treatment process. The purpose of this chapter is to describe basic principles of single-subject experimental research designs and their use is studying treatment effectiveness and generalization in aphasia. Specifically, a brief overview of basic principles of single-subject research methodologies is presented, and specific design options are discussed. The need for programmatic research that is methodologically sound, conceptually salient, and based on a series of systematic, replicated studies is also emphasized.

BASIC CONSIDERATIONS

Single-subject experimental designs have evolved within the tradition of the applied behavioral analysis branch of experimental psychology (Baer, Wolf, & Risley, 1968, 1987; Barlow, Hayes, & Nelson, 1984; Barlow & Hersen, 1984; Hersen & Barlow, 1976; Iwata et al, 1989; Kazdin, 1982). The primary purpose of this approach to treatment research is to explore functional relationships between an independent variable, such as aphasia treatment, and change in a socially significant dependent variable, such as communicative effectiveness. These designs have alternately been called "single-case" or "within-subject" designs, and they are frequently used to evaluate the effectiveness of and generalization of aphasia treatment (Kearns & Thompson, 1991a, 1991b). The basic premises of this tradition of single-subject methodologies are that treatment research should be applied, conceptual, analytic, and generalizable (Baer, et al., 1968, 1987).

The "applied" aspect refers to the fact that single-subject research focuses on pragmatic rather than theoretical considerations. In particular, the goal of single-subject studies is often to facilitate clinically significant treatment outcomes, such as improving the functional communication ability of aphasic individuals. This emphasis on quality-of-life issues and the need to maintain a pragmatic focus does not imply that single-subject research is atheoretical. Indeed, more often than not, researchers have attempted to take advantage of single-subject methodologies to investigate theoretically motivated treatment issues in aphasia (Raymer, Thompson, Jacobs, & LeGrand, 1993; Loverso, Prescott, & Sellinger, 1988; Schwartz et al., 1994; Thompson, Raymer, & LeGrand, 1992; Thompson et al., 1993). Moreover, as a colleague and I (Kearns & Thompson, 1991a) have pointed out, the advancement of clinical aphasiology through single-subject research is inextricably linked to our ability to relate experimental questions, outcomes, and rationales to basic theoretical issues.

The "analytic" facet of single-subject research stresses the fact that these designs are experimental in nature and that careful attention is given to the factors contributing to internal validity. For example, attention is given to the need for operational specificity, reliability, and the careful sequencing of experimental conditions in a manner that demonstrates experimental control (Connell & McReynolds, 1986; Kearns, 1986a; McReynolds & Kearns, 1983; McReynolds & Thompson, 1986). In single-subject experimental research, each individual serves as his or her own control. That is, each subject is exposed to every condition of the study, and data are collected repeatedly over time to measure the impact of the presence or absence of each intervention on performance. Careful manipulation and juxtaposition of treatment and no-treatment (baseline) conditions is conducted in a way that changes only a single variable at a time while keeping all other relevant variables constant.

Examination and measurement of performance during each treatment and no-treatment phase provide data that can be analyzed for temporal patterns of change through ongoing visual inspection of graphically displayed data. Visual analysis of level, slope, trend, and variability within and across treatment and no-treatment conditions provides the basis for determining whether changes in the dependent measures covary with the application and removal of treatment. Single-subject experimental designs are experimental rather than correlational or descriptive in nature. Therefore, careful application of these designs can be used to establish a functional relationship between treatment variables and changes in socially significant behaviors.

Researchers who employ single-subject experimental designs are typically interested in establishing the generalizability of treatment effects. The investigation of treatment principles that can be used to facilitate generalization has increasingly been emphasized in the aphasia literature (Davis, 1986; Doyle & Goldstein, 1985; Doyle, Goldstein, & Bourgeois, 1987; Doyle, Goldstein, Bourgeois, & Nakles, 1989; Doyle, Oleyar, & Goldstein, 1989; Kearns & Potechin-Scher, 1988; Kearns & Yedor, 1991; Raymer & Thompson, 1991; Thompson et al., 1993). Aphasia treatment studies that examine the efficacy or efficiency of aphasia treatment interventions without addressing generalization issues can also make significant contributions to the literature. However, clinical researchers have increasingly examined generalization of treatment effects across stimuli, people, settings, and time.

A final basic consideration of single-subject methodology involves the manner in which variability is viewed and controlled. Unlike group researchers, who typically attempt to control intersubject variability statistically, single-subject investigators focus on within-subject variability and the discovery of means to control it. It is assumed that variability is a component of individual performance that can be brought under experimental control. Investigators typically go to great lengths to expose measurement and other sources of variability, and to minimize their influence on the experimental process. This variability assumption has led to the development of flexible experimental procedures that can be applied, often without relying on statistical inference testing (Kearns, 1986a; Thompson & McReynolds, 1986; Connell & McReynolds, 1986; Schoonen, 1991).

Although many single-subject experimental studies in aphasia rely solely on the visual analysis of data, appropriate statistical methods have been proposed to examine treatment effectiveness within this paradigm (Kazdin, 1982; Willmes, 1990; Huitema, 1986). When statistical procedures are used, it is particularly important to consider the statistical independence of within-subject replications. Although the amount of serial dependence present in behavioral treatment studies is debatable (Huitema, 1986b), the use of specialized statistical analytic procedures may be necessary when assumptions of statistical independence cannot be met (Robey, 1999; Suen & Ary, 1989).

DESIGN OPTIONS AND EXPERIMENTAL CONTROL

As noted above, the logic underlying single-subject experimental designs is that each subject acts as his or her own control by receiving both baseline (no-treatment) and treatment conditions over time. The systematic juxtaposition of treatment and no-treatment conditions over time, if properly designed and implemented, can result in a high degree of internal validity and experimental control. The judicious use of untreated conditions or untreated subjects is also a critical element in designing single-subject experimental studies. Furthermore, within- and across-subject replications are critical to controlling the influences of extraneous variables and enhancing the believability of the investigators' conclusions that treatment is solely responsible for improvements in their aphasic subjects' language and communication.

An important assumption inherent in single-subject research is that performance during baseline conditions can be used to predict future performance in the absence of treatment. In other words, it is assumed that there is an equal probability that extraneous influences on language and communication are present during both baseline and treatment conditions. Thus data from the baseline phase represent the effects of extraneous variables on communicative abilities prior to the intervention, and data from the experimental or treatment phase reflect these influences, as well as the impact of treatment. An important caveat to these assumptions is that a sufficiently long and stable period of baseline observation is necessary before investigators can confidently predict whether the level and trend of baseline data will continue without treatment. Once established, a stable base rate of performance can serve as a standard against which subsequent treatment effects can be evaluated.

The baseline or no-treatment phase of a single-subject experimental study is often referred to as the "A phase." Similarly, the experimental or treatment phase is generally referred to as the "B phase." These notations are frequently used as a convenience to label graphically presented single-subject data. Of course, other notations are also employed, such as the use of the term "C phase" to designate a second treatment phase that differs from the original treatment condition.

Baseline

During the baseline phase (A phase) of a study, the target behavior is observed and scored prior to intervention, to establish the pretreatment rate of responding. Baseline data are frequently obtained on nonstandardized probes that the investigator has determined to be representative of the functional behavior under study. The use of nonstandardized probes as primary dependent measures in single-subject research requires careful definition and specificity of target behaviors. In addition, it is necessary to obtain independent interrater reliability on the observation and scoring of such behaviors. The development and use of nonstandardized probes in aphasia treatment studies places an additional responsibility on the investigators to demonstrate that word lists, sentences, and conversational samples are selected from a homogeneous pool of items, which are carefully controlled for factors that might influence or contaminate subject responding.

Another consideration in baseline testing is that the period of assessment should be sufficiently long so that trends in the data can be established prior to intervention. At a minimum, three baseline probes, and often many more, are required to establish a stable baseline. It is worth noting that individual baseline testing sessions are usually conducted within a restricted period of time, so that any extraneous variables influencing performance are evident throughout the baseline phase. In practice, this often means that pretreatment sessions are conducted within a matter of days before the treatment phase of the study is initiated.

Treatment

The experimental or treatment phase of the study (B phase) is often applied in a manner that reflects the clinical reality of the type of treatment being administered. That is, depending on the nature of the experimental questions and the type of treatment being applied, intervention may be administered on a daily or biweekly basis, just as it is in clinical practice. At a minimum, the frequency and intensity of treatment should be sufficient to allow treatment effects to be demonstrated. As in the baseline phase, sessions during the treatment phase must occur at regular intervals, to ensure that any extraneous factors that influence performance are present throughout this phase of the investigation.

In order to compare performance data obtained during the baseline and treatment phases, it is essential that performance on dependent variables be measured on the same tasks under the same conditions for both phases. That is, behavioral probes used to assess improvements in communicative abilities of aphasic individuals during the treatment phase should be the same as those used to assess pretreatment performance during the baseline phase. Investigators may, of course, use different probe items selected from the same general pool of homogenous probe items used during the baseline phase. In addition to taking care to ensure that the dependent measure is the same during all phases of the study, it is important to ensure that probe data are not scored during the treatment phase in a manner that is contaminated by feedback, reinforcement, or other types of investigator input. To ensure comparability of baseline and treatment phase probe data, investigators often readminister baseline probes during the treatment phase as the primary means of monitoring the influence of treatment on the dependent measure. Thus, for studies designed to facilitate word retrieval in aphasia, a pool of randomized word lists used to establish baseline rates of word retrieval performance may be readministered throughout the treatment phase prior to one or more of the weekly treatment sessions. The important issue is that performance data obtained during treatment sessions may be contaminated by the treatment process itself, and care needs to be taken to equate the testing conditions across both baseline and treatment sessions.

As is true in the baseline phase, the length of the intervention phase is determined by the investigators on a study-by-study basis. Quite often, investigators will establish a behavioral criterion—for example, 90% correct performance on a measure of the targeted behavior—and will continue treatment until that criterion is met or until a preestablished maximum number of treatment sessions has been conducted. Criteria used to determine the length of the treatment phase of a single-subject study should be made as explicit as possible, and they should be made on an a priori basis. Failure to establish criteria for guiding methodological decisions prior to making procedural changes in single-subject studies provides a serious threat to the internal validity of an investigation (Kearns, 1992). Although the flexibility inherent in the use of single-subject methodologies is an important aspect of these designs (Thompson & McReynolds, 1986), on-line decisions about the length of baseline and treatment phases can result in biased manipulations of the data and should be avoided whenever possible.

EVALUATION STRATEGIES AND DESIGN OPTIONS

Before I discuss specific single-subject experimental design options for aphasia treatment studies, it may be useful to discuss descriptive case studies briefly. Intensive study of aphasic individuals over time has contributed significantly to the aphasia literature, beginning with the case descriptions of Broca (1861) and Wernicke (1874). Despite their potential for contribution to the literature, case studies of individuals undergoing aphasia treatment do not provide the level of scientific rigor necessary to determine treatment effectiveness. Regardless of the level of insight reflected in the observations, or the operational specificity entailed, descriptions of a baseline phase followed by a treatment phase (i.e., AB designs) do not enable a demonstration of experimental control. Even if there are marked improvements in performance during the treatment phase, case studies are insufficient to rule out the possibility that non-treatment-related variables are responsible for the observed changes in performance. Extraneous variables that can affect performance during the treatment phase of a case study of an aphasic person include spontaneous physiological recovery and concurrent pharmacological treatments. To rule out the effects of these and other possible confounding variables, within- and across-subject replications of the treatment effect are necessary.

Even the most elemental forms of single-subject experimental designs require a minimum of two demonstrations that changes in performance are related to the application or removal of treatment. In addition, additional experimental control is demonstrated when it can be shown that only directly treated communicative behaviors change with the application or removal of treatment, while untreated control behaviors remain relatively unchanged. These additional control elements distinguish true single-subject experimental designs from case studies.

The basic means of increasing internal validity for single-subject studies is to combine multiple A and B phases across time, behaviors, subjects, and/or settings. Elsewhere (Kearns, 1986a), I have summarized relevant evaluation strategies, clinical research questions, selected design options, and basic considerations in implementing single-subject designs. Although a comprehensive review of all single-subject experimental design options is not within the scope of this chapter, those that are most germane are reviewed in subsequent sections. Prototypical design options are also considered, and examples are provided to demonstrate their use to develop and evaluate novel treatments for aphasia.

Before deciding on an experimental design, clinical researchers often begin with a general evaluation strategy and a related clinical research question (Kazdin, 1982). The four evaluation strategies listed in Table 16.1 relate logically to the research questions and design options available. For example, the treatment–no-treatment comparison strategy is, as the name implies, used to assess the effectiveness of treatment by comparing it to a no-treatment (baseline) condition. In essence, this strategy relates to the clinical research question of whether or not a treatment package, with all of its steps and components, facilitates improved performance relative to a no-treatment (baseline) condition. The primary single-subject experimental design options associated with this evaluation strategy are withdrawal and reversal designs, such as the ABAB design, and multiple-baseline designs and their variants.

Although the withdrawal and reversal designs are not often selected for aphasia treatment research, there are instances in which this option may be appropriate (Kearns & Salmon, 1984). In the ABAB withdrawal design, a treatment package is alternately applied and withdrawn across successive experimental phases, to determine whether changes in the dependent measure are strongly correlated with the presence or absence of treatment. The aphasia treatment under study is considered to be efficacious (1) if there is a stable or a deteriorating performance during baseline phases when treatment is not available, (2) if the targeted communication behavior improves during treatment phases, and (3) if withdrawal of treatment is correlated with a change in behavior toward base rate levels of responding (i.e., a return to baseline). As shown in Figure 16.1, there are essentially three points of proof for demonstrating experimental control and treatment effectiveness with this design. A between-phase comparison of the baseline phase with the first treatment phase provides initial information that improvements have occurred in the target behavior, and that treatment may have been one factor responsible for these improvements. In the withdrawal (second A) phase, the dependent measures are evaluated but treatment is withdrawn. That is, the withdrawal phase represents a second period of baseline testing. If withdrawing treatment during this phase results in a return toward the initial level of baseline responding, additional support is provided for the argument that treatment has been responsible for the changes in behavior. Logically, if one can assume that extraneous factors have been present during all phases, and that only one variable (treatment) has been manipulated during the initial treatment and withdrawal phases, then treatment would appear to be the primary cause for performance change. The third and final point of proof for demonstrating that changes in performance have been caused by treat-

TABLE 16.1. Evaluation Strategies, Research Questions, Design Options, and Considerations for Single-Subject Experimental Designs

Evaluation strategy	Clinical research question	Selected design options	Basic considerations
Treatment–no-treatment comparison	Does treatment, with all of its components, result in improved performance relative to no treatment?	Withdrawal and reversal designs ABAB BAB ABA	Is the therapeutic effect likely to reverse following the withdrawal of treatment?
		Multiple-baseline designs (MB) Across behaviors Across settings Across subjects	Are functionally independent behaviors or settings available? Are homogeneous subjects available?
		Multiple-probe technique (variation of MB) (Horner & Baer, 1978)	Are functionally independent behaviors available? Are long or continuous baselines impractical?
Component assessment	Relative to a treatment package, to what degree do separate components of treatment contribute to improvement?	Interaction (reduction) BC-B-BC-B BC-B-BC-A-BC-B-BC	Can the components be examined alone and in combination with the treatment package? Can replication be obtained across subjects?
	Does the addition of a component to a treatment package facilitate treatment effectiveness?	Interaction (additive) B-BC-B-BC B-BC-B-A-B-BC-B	Can the components be examined alone and in combination with the treatment package? Can replication be obtained across subjects?
Treatment–treatment comparison	What is the relative effectiveness of two or more treatments?	Alternating-treatments design	Can treatments be rapidly alternated for each subject?
		Replicated-crossover design (Barlow, Hayes, & Nelson, 1984)	Are multiple subjects or target behaviors available? Can treatment be "crossed over"? Are nearly equal phase lengths possible?
Successive-level analysis	Does treatment result in acquisition of successive steps in a chaining sequence?	Multiple-probe technique	Are steps in the treatment sequence independent? Are earlier steps prerequisite to acquiring later steps?
	Does treatment effectively modify a single, gradually acquired behavior?	Changing criterion design	Will changes in the dependent variable correspond to changes in the criterion level? Will the dependent variable stabilize at successively more stringent criterion levels?

Note. From Kearns, K. P. (1986a). Within-subject experimental designs: II. Design selection and arrangement of experimental phases. *Journal of Speech and Hearing Disorders, 51,* 204–214. Copyright 1986 by American Speech–Language Hearing Association. Reprinted with permission.

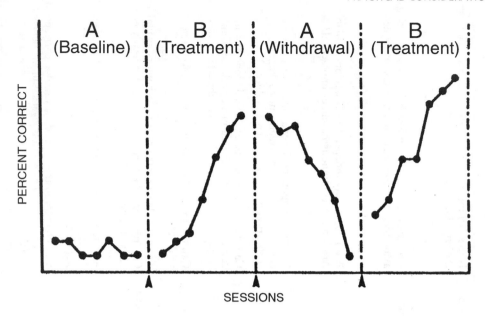

FIGURE 16.1. An ABAB withdrawal design with alteration of no treatment and treatment phases. From McReynolds, L. V., & Thompson, G. K. (1986). Flexibility of single-subject experimental designs. Part I: Review of the basics of single-subject designs. *Journal of Speech and Hearing Disorders, 51*, 194–203. Copyright 1986 by American Speech–Language Hearing Association. Reprinted with permission.

ment rather than extraneous factors comes in the final phase of the ABAB withdrawal design, when treatment is reinstated. If, as shown in Figure 16.1, effects seen in the first treatment phase are replicated in the final treatment phase, then further evidence is provided that the change in performance is probably due to treatment.

A close variant of the ABAB withdrawal design is an ABAB reversal design. The primary distinction between these two designs is that additional experimental manipulations are used to facilitate decreases in the level of performance on the target behavior during the second A phase of a study. When a reversal design is employed, the return toward baseline is undertaken by applying the independent variable to a second behavior that is incompatible with the initial target behavior (Kearns & Salmon, 1984).

The use of ABAB withdrawal designs is often not desirable in aphasia research, where language and other nonreversible behaviors are typically targeted for improvement. Furthermore, some have argued that reversing the effects of improved communication performance may be ethically untenable, even if the reversal is temporary. Finally, many researchers and clinicians apply treatment packages in the hopes that the improvements not only will be maintained but will generalize to other communication situations and conditions. Therefore, studies in which investigators are interested in examining the effects of generalization of treatment results may have less use for withdrawal and reversal designs.

The second prototypical design used for treatment–no-treatment comparison is the multiple-baseline design. Whereas the ABAB withdrawal and its variants are used to determine treatment effectiveness by applying and removing treatment to a single behavior, various multiple-baseline designs incorporate control conditions across behaviors, subjects, or settings. The most common form of the multiple-baseline design is a multiple-baseline-across-behaviors design. With this design, baselines are obtained for two or more similar but independent behaviors in a single subject. Following baseline testing, treatment is individually and sequentially applied to one target behavior at a time, and baseline measurement continues for the remaining untreated behaviors. After criterion is met for the first behavior, treatment is sequentially applied to the remaining behaviors. All behaviors not currently in treatment during a multiple-baseline study remain in baseline testing (Figure 16.2).

There are two points of control with multiple-baseline-across-behaviors designs. First, for each behavior under study, the base rate of responding should remain relatively stable until that behavior is directly treated. Thus an across-phase comparison between the baseline and treatment conditions should show a marked improvement with treatment, and this response pattern should be replicated across all the target behaviors and treatments. The second means of demonstrating experimental control with the multiple-baseline-across-behaviors design is that with each subsequent application of treatment, the remaining untreated (control) behaviors should remain relatively stable. As is true with the ABAB design, repeated replication of treatment effects within the same subject is crucial to demonstrating that intervention, rather than extraneous variables in the environment, is responsible for improvement in an aphasic individual's communicative abilities.

The multiple-baseline-across-behaviors design has become the standard for aphasia treatment research. This design option is particularly attractive when target behaviors are unlikely to be reversible or when it is not desirable to reverse treatment effects. It should also be noted that once treatment has begun with the multiple-baseline-across-behaviors design, it is continued across behaviors. Therefore, the use of this design raises fewer ethical objections than withdrawal or reversal designs do.

Multiple-baseline designs are particularly useful for targeting multiple communication behaviors for change within an individual. However, caution should be used when targeting three or more behaviors with this design, since additional control issues relating to the order of delivery of treatment to the various behaviors may arise. In addition, judi-

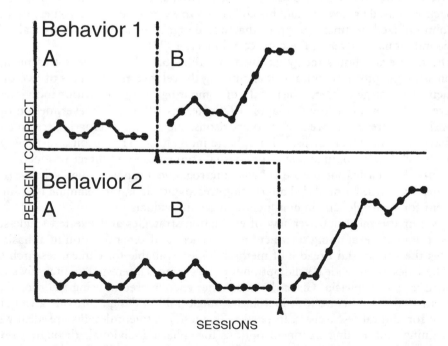

FIGURE 16.2. Prototypical graph of data from a fictitious multiple-baseline-across-behaviors design. From McReynolds, L. V., & Thompson, C. K. (1986). Flexibility of single-subject experimental designs. Part I: Review of the basics of single-subject designs. *Journal of Speech and Hearing Disorders, 51,* 194–203. Copyright 1986 by American Speech–Language Hearing Association. Reprinted with permission.

cious selection of the multiple target behaviors is necessary with a multiple-baseline-across-behaviors design, because generalization of treatment effects from trained to untrained behaviors results in a lack of experimental control. Finally, investigators may choose to use multiple-baseline designs across individuals or settings, rather than behaviors.

In addition to treatment–no-treatment comparisons, single-subject experimental designs can be used to evaluate the specific contributions of various components to a treatment package (component assessment), to examine the relative effectiveness of two or more treatments (treatment–treatment comparison), and to evaluate successive levels or steps in a treatment sequence (successive-level analysis). For the most part, the design options associated with these evaluation strategies incorporate the same control procedures used in the basic withdrawal and multiple-baseline designs outlined above. For example, the interaction designs used to evaluate components of a treatment package involve a withdrawal strategy. However, rather than comparing baseline and treatment conditions in an ABAB sequence, investigators compare individual components of treatment to a multicomponent treatment package. Thus an interaction design may be conducted in which the effect of a treatment package with two primary components (BC) is compared to that of a treatment package with one major component. This type of interaction design is designated as a BC-B-BC-B design. Similarly, a multicomponent treatment package can be compared to the entire package, in an interaction single-subject experimental design (e.g., BC-ABC-BC-ABC). Simmons (1980) provides one of the few examples of the use of an interaction design to explore the relative effectiveness of components of a treatment package in aphasia.

The evaluation strategy of a successive-level analysis uses single-subject experimental designs, such as the multiple-probe technique and the changing-criterion design, which are adaptations of the multiple-baseline design format. The multiple-probe technique permits objective examination of the acquisition of sequential steps in a treatment program. This approach was used by Loverso and his colleagues to examine the effectiveness of a multi-step computerized treatment program that was designed to facilitate the verbal skills of aphasic individuals (Loverso, Prescott, & Sellinger, 1992).

The final evaluation strategy outlined in Table 16.1, the treatment–treatment comparison strategy, provides a means of examining the relative effectiveness of two or more treatments for a single subject. The pitfalls of comparing treatments within individual subjects are well known (Barlow & Hayes, 1979; Kearns, 1986a); however, design options appropriate for treatment–treatment comparisons, such as the alternating-treatments design, have been modified for use with aphasic individuals. Thompson and McReynolds (1986), for example, compared auditory–visual stimulation and direct production treatment methods of facilitating the use of "wh" interrogatives in aphasia. Similarly, we (Kearns & Yedor, 1991) used a modified alternating-treatments design to examine two forms of treatment for verbal deficits in nonfluent aphasic individuals.

In summary, this brief overview of evaluation strategies and selected single-subject design options for examining treatment effectiveness and generalization in aphasia demonstrates the variety and breadth of methodologies available for clinical research in this area. These designs provide a valid option for investigators interested in intensely studying treatment issues in aphasia. Given the difficulties encountered in using traditional group designs to study treatment effects in aphasia, single-subject designs provide a valuable alternative for clinical researchers. In particular, these treatment designs are ideally suited for designing and refining treatment options for aphasic individuals through a series of studies that incorporate both direct and systematic replications. Single-subject experimental designs are particularly well suited to studying patterns of individual improvements over time, in a controlled manner that permits analysis of cause-and-effect relationships between treatment variables and functional target behaviors. This emphasis on individual performance, which is graphically displayed and analyzed, allows investigators to uncover sources of variability and to refine treatment procedures. In addition, the emphasis on providing detailed information on individual subjects and then replicating effects in other aphasic persons and under different conditions allows clinicians to make strong logical generalizations about how individual patients with similar characteristics might respond to the treatment under study. The empirical demonstration of the effects of treatment, and of the degree to which these effects generalize to more natural settings and conditions is consonant with both clinicians' and third-party payers' concern with the functional impact of intervention.

Although single-subject designs are being used with increasing frequency to study the effectiveness of treatment in aphasia, there have been relatively few systematic attempts to use this methodology to investigate novel treatment packages through replicated series of treatment studies that define the limits of the intervention (Kearns & Thompson, 1991a, 1991b). Although there are notable exceptions (Thompson & McReynolds, 1986; Thompson et al., 1993, 1997; Schwartz et al., 1994), there have been relatively few attempts to conduct a series of systematic replications of a given aphasia treatment by varying the subjects, settings, and other conditions necessary to define the limits of success of intervention. The final section of this chapter is used to emphasize the need for systematic replication of single-subject aphasia treatment studies in an effort to build and refine our clinical interventions.

TECHNIQUE BUILDING IN APHASIA

My colleagues and I conducted a series of single-subject studies to examine the effectiveness and generalization of a specific form of aphasia treatment (Kearns, 1986b; Kearns and Potechin-Scher, 1988; Kearns & Yedor, 1992). The purpose of this series was to examine a method of treatment called "response elaboration training" (RET). This form of treatment was originally designed to facilitate an increase in verbal elaboration skills in nonfluent aphasic patients (Kearns, 1985, 1986b). It had been previously observed that overly didactic training may inhibit flexible and creative language use, and may limit the generalization of improvements in language abilities in aphasia. RET was designed as a departure from highly structured, clinician-directed therapy. In essence, it is an attempt to facilitate generalized improvement in aphasic individuals' ability to elaborate conversational topics. The emphasis in RET is on shaping and chaining patient-initiated, rather than clinician-selected, responses.

The chief dependent measure in this series of studies was the amount of information content produced in response to simple line drawings, which were devoid of context. Other measures used to evaluate treatment progress included the number of novel responses produced and the efficiency of verbal production.

The pictures used to elicit responding in these studies were intended as means of eliciting patient-initiated responses to such themes as sports and activities of daily living. Following an initial spoken response to a given stimulus picture, a series of "wh" questions was orally presented by the experimenter to elicit more elaborate responding. The "wh" questions were used to prompt subjects to provide additional information not depicted in, but relevant to, the general themes in the pictures. For example, in response to a simple line drawing of someone kicking a football, one aphasic subject chose to discuss a recent game played by the local professional football team. In contrast, a second subject elaborated on his grandson's role on the local high school football team.

To summarize, RET involves eliciting elaboration of spontaneously initiated responses to simple line drawings, which are systematically chained together into longer responses over a number of trials, using a verbal cueing strategy. The ultimate goals of this technique are to facilitate an increase in the amount of verbal content produced by subjects and to promote a generalized increase in their verbal skills. Throughout the investigations described here, the emphasis was on facilitating a generalized increase in the amount of information content provided, regardless of the form of a patient's response. Thus an agrammatical response that contained three content words was given equal weighting to a more syntactically correct sentence having the same amount of information.

The scoring procedures used throughout these studies were similar to those detailed by Nicholas and Brookshire (1993). In addition, independent interobserver reliability rates were obtained for the scoring of subject responses in each investigation. Reliability rates generally ranged from 85% to 95%.

Our initial study of RET examined treatment effectiveness for individuals with Broca's aphasia through a series of direct replications. In subsequent studies, systematic replications were obtained with fluent aphasic patients to determine the usefulness of the treatment procedure with this population. In subsequent studies, the procedure was compared to a more traditional, syntactically based, verbal treatment program, as well as to a contextually richer, more animated picture-based treatment program. Finally, RET principles were extended for use with nonverbal aphasic patients, in an effort to promote functional communicative drawing.

Various single-subject experimental designs were used to evaluate the effectiveness of RET and its utility for various types of language impairment, including multiple-baseline-across-behaviors designs with a multiple-probe component and combined alternating-treatments–multiple-baseline designs. As noted earlier, descriptive analyses were also developed to examine the qualitative aspects of communicative performance. Since multiple-baseline designs and their variants are the single-subject study options most frequently employed in clinical aphasiology, I begin with an example using this methodology. The second example chosen for demonstration purposes highlights the need to modify treatments flexibly and to employ treatment combinations to maximize experimental control in single-subject designs. Finally, a third example is provided to demonstrate how single-subject experimental designs can be used to obtain information about important issues such as generalization.

Example 1: A Multiple-Baseline Study

We (Kearns & Potechin-Scher, 1988) examined the effectiveness and generality of RET for three aphasic individuals. One of the individuals, a patient with Broca's aphasia, was included to replicate earlier results, which had indicated that this treatment procedure was effective in increasing the amount of verbal information produced by nonfluent aphasic patients. Two fluent aphasic patients, one with conduction aphasia and one with anomic aphasia, were studied to provide information about the value of RET for fluent patients. Extensive generalization data were obtained on all subjects, to help establish the extent to which treatment might benefit language production in the full range of natural contexts.

The specific purposes of the study were to determine whether RET would facilitate an increase in the number of content words produced, and to assess whether generalization to untrained stimuli, conversational partners, different settings, and spontaneous discussions would occur. Finally, follow-up probes were also included, to determine whether improvements in verbal elaboration skills would be maintained over time.

The experimental design used in this study was a multiple-baseline design across treatment sets, with periodic probes sampling multiple behaviors during all treatment phases. Stimuli consisted of pictures that were presented in the absence of any specific context. Thirty stimulus pictures were divided into two training sets of 10 items each and a set of 10 items never used during training that were used to test generalization. Weekly probe sessions were held to assess performance with pictures that were not included in treatment sessions.

The data that follow are for RW, a 59-year-old man. RW was is a college-educated man who had experienced a single left-hemisphere stroke 20 months prior to initiation of the study. His profile on the Western Aphasia Battery (WAB; Kertesz, 1979), was consistent with Broca's aphasia, and his Aphasia Quotient (AQ) on the WAB was 34.8. His performance during the study is graphically displayed in a typical multiple baseline design format in Figure 16.3.

The top of Figure 16.3 shows performance on the first training set during baseline (B'ln in the figure; A) treatment (RET; B), and maintenance phases of this study. The middle portion of the figure displays RW's performance on the second set of training items during baseline (A) and treatment (B) phases. Performance on generalization items (never used in treatment) is shown at the bottom of the figure. The graphed data represent mean numbers of content words produced during probe sessions conducted throughout the study. Data to the right of the graphs (×'s) represent performance during probe sessions conducted 2.5, 3, and 5 months after the conclusion of treatment. They provide a measure of the extent to which treatment effects were maintained.

As indicated previously, multiple-baseline designs require that the initial baseline be established for both behaviors prior to the initiation of the study. Treatment is subsequently begun on the first set of items until a predetermined criterion is met, while baseline measurement is continued for the second, untreated set of items. Upon achievement of criterion for the first set of items, training is then initiated on the second set.

Examination of the top graph in Figure 16.3 reveals that RW produced fewer than one content word per baseline session on the 10 items in the first set. After the initiation of treatment for that set of items, there was a gradual increase in performance until he produced a mean of five content words per session on these items. Examination of the bottom graph reveals that the mean number of content words produced on the second set of items remained relatively steady at approximately two per session throughout the extended baseline phase. Subsequent initiation of treatment on the second set of pictures replicated the results achieved with the first set of training items, in that RW rapidly met the training criterion for these items following the intervention. Finally, gains made during treatment were largely maintained on probes obtained up to 5 months after the completion of the study.

Overall, the results of the multiple-baseline study for this subject demonstrate that there was a relatively steady low level of performance prior to treatment on both training sets, and that an obvious increase in performance occurred once training was initiated for each of the two sets of items. Importantly, the training effects were specific to the items trained, and the baseline level of responding was maintained prior to the initiation of treatment for a particular set of items (the second set). Although not shown in this graph, performance was similar when probes were administered by a clinician not involved in the study or by RW's spouse. In addition, RW performed at similar high levels when probes were administered by his spouse at home. Thus treatment effects generalized to other conversational partners and conversational circumstances. Data for this subject provided direct replication of previous findings regarding the effectiveness and generalizability of RET

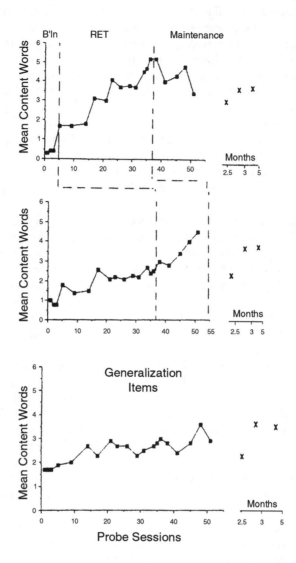

FIGURE 16.3. Mean number of content words produced before, during, and after treatment on two sets of trained items (top, middle), and on generalization (untrained) items (bottom), for a patient with Broca's aphasia (RW). Baseline performance before training is plotted for the first 4 sessions in each graph. The first set of items was trained between sessions 5 and 37. Performance on these items rapidly improved during this time period (top graph). Some generalization effects were seen for the second (not yet trained) set of items during this time (middle graph). Training ceased on the first set of items at week 37 and was conducted on the second set of items from weeks 38 to 52. A modest dropoff in performance on the first set of items was noted during this time (top graph), while rapid improvement was noted for the second set of items (middle graph). Modest generalization effects were noted on untrained items throughout training of both the first and second sets of items (bottom graph). The graphs to the right document performance on follow-up probes from 2.5 to 5 months after completion of all therapy. Data from Kearns, K. P., & Potechin-Scher, G. (1988). The generalization of response elaboration training effects. In T. E. Prescott (Ed.), *Clinical Aphasiology Conference proceedings* (Vol. 18). San Diego, CA: College-Hill Press. Copyright 1989 by Thomas E. Prescott.

for patients with Broca's aphasia. Importantly, previous results for patients with Broca's aphasia were also replicated with the two fluent patients who participated in the study, providing some evidence that the treatment was of potential value for fluent as well as nonfluent patients.

Example 2: An Alternating-Treatments Comparison

In an attempt to explore the value of this therapeutic technique further, we (Kearns & Yedor, 1991) compared RET with a highly structured, convergent treatment program for aphasia. The primary purpose of this study was to determine whether the "loose training" paradigm of RET had any inherent advantages over a structured sentence-training approach. The structured approach required subjects to produce preselected sentences in response to picture stimuli corresponding to each targeted lexical items (subject, verb, object, etc.). This contrasted sharply with the RET format, which, as noted earlier, is based on the elicitation and scaffolding of spontaneous responses into patient-directed conversational descriptions. The design used to study this issue was an alternating-treatments design in which the two treatments (employing different stimulus sets) were simultaneously presented to individual subjects in a rapidly alternating fashion. Care must be taken with this type of design to ensure that the subjects discriminate between the two treatments and that all efforts are made to minimize the potential for treatment interference effects. Although logistically difficult, this design has the potential for providing information about the relative effectiveness of two or more treatments in an individual subject. Since the basic AB format of the alternating-treatments design does not in itself control for extraneous factors that might influence the results of a study, a multiple-baseline component was added to the alternating-treatments design to provide additional experimental control in this study. Data from this combined alternating-treatments–multiple-baseline comparison of RET and convergent therapy are presented for subject NS in Figure 16.4. NS was a 61-year-old woman who was treated 37 months after a left-hemisphere stroke. Her AQ on the WAB was 61, and the pattern of deficits was consistent with the diagnosis of Broca's aphasia.

The data graphed in Figure 16.4 represent the mean number of content words produced on probe measurement sets during RET treatment (open squares) and convergent therapy (CT in the figure; filled circles). Data are displayed over time for probes obtained during baseline, alternating-treatments (ATD in the figure), and maintenance phases. During the baseline phase, the subject was asked to describe picture stimuli subsequently used during RET and convergent training. Figure 16.4 shows that prior to intervention, NS produced a mean of approximately 1.5 content words per session, both for items used during RET and for items used during convergent treatment. A similar level of baseline performance was documented with two other sets of training items used in a second phase of the study, which was designed to test the replicability of results achieved in the first phase (bottom graph). Examination of results achieved with the first two sets of treated items (top graph) reveals that there was a rapid and pronounced increase in the mean number of content words produced to the pictures used during RET (open squares), while there was a more modest gain in responses to the pictures used during convergent therapy (filled circles). The difference in the effects of these two types of therapy was maintained in probes obtained a month after completion of the study. The results of treatment with the second sets of items replicated those achieved with the first sets (bottom graph), in that there was a more rapid and greater increase in the mean number of content words produced to the items used in RET than to the items used during convergent therapy (probe sessions 13–15).

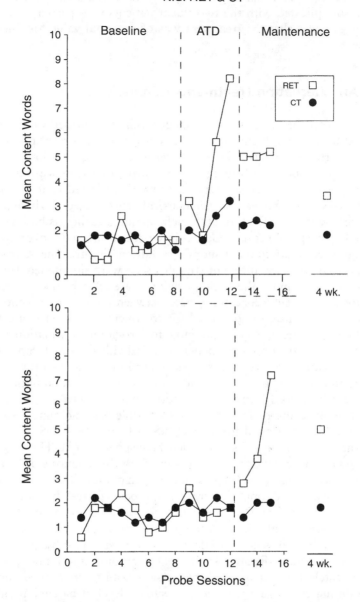

FIGURE 16.4. Mean number of content words produced during RET probes (open squares) and convergent treatment (CT) probes (filled circles) during baseline, alternating-treatments (ATD), and maintenance phases. Data from Kearns, K. P., & Yedor, K. (1991). An alternating treatments comparison of loose training and a convergent treatment strategy. In T. H. Prescott (Ed.), *Clinical aphasiology* (Vol. 20). Austin, TX: Pro-Ed. Copyright 1991 by Pro-Ed.

These results graphically show the potential benefits of using an alternating-treatments design with the added control of the multiple-baseline component. Subject NS appeared to respond more favorably to the RET treatment format than to the more structured convergent therapy, and these differences were replicated across different sets of training items for the same subject. Results achieved with a second subject in this study did not clearly favor one form of treatment over the other. In any event, a treatment–treatment comparison, using single-subject experimental designs, has the potential to provide information about the relative effectiveness of treatment options for aphasic individuals.

Example 3: Systematic Replication across Modalities

In an effort to determine whether the principles underlying RET could be extended and used with other communication modalities, we (Kearns & Yedor, 1992) adapted this training format to attempt to facilitate functional communicative drawing in individuals with severe aphasia and apraxia of speech who had no other functional means of communication. The two subjects in this study had previously unsuccessfully been enrolled in therapy to facilitate verbal responding, and attempts had also been made to use alternative and augmentative communication modes with these patients. That is, in addition to traditional therapy, the subjects had either rejected or did not gain functional competence with supplemental aids such as communication boards or computers. A nonverbal form of RET was developed and tested in a multiple-baseline-across-behaviors study (responses to sets of picture items). The treatment paradigm was similar to that employed with verbal RET. However, spontaneously initiated subject *drawings* were sequentially shaped and chained into more elaborate and functional graphic representations of the themes in the pictures. Again, a verbal cueing strategy was used to prompt the aphasic individuals to refine and add more content in successive attempts to elaborate on the stimulus pictures.

Multiple-baseline data for WG, one of our two subjects, are presented in Figure 16.5. A diagnosis of severe Broca's aphasia and apraxia of speech was made on the basis of his performance on the Boston Diagnostic Aphasia Examination (Goodglass & Kaplan, 1983) and additional testing of motor speech abilities. A reliable scoring procedure was developed to measure drawing content, and the graph depicts the mean number of "content units" drawn for stimulus pictures depicting activities of daily living (ADLs; top graph) and stimulus pictures (depicting sports bottom graph). Consistent with the multiple-baseline format, pretreatment baseline data were obtained for both sets of picture stimuli, and then treatment was initiated for the first set of items (ADLs) while baseline testing continued for the second set of items (sports). Treatment for the second set of items was not initiated until criterion was met for the first set of items.

Examination of the figure reveals that low and relatively stable rates of pretreatment drawing content were produced during the baseline phase for both sets of items. Treatment for the ADL (top graph) resulted in rapid and clinically significant improvement in the mean number of drawing content units for the stimulus pictures. This was true whether the subject was administered the probes by the treatment clinician (filled squares) or a second clinician not involved in the study (x's).

Examination of the bottom of the graph reveals that a relatively low and stable drawing content was maintained during the extended baseline period for this set of items. Improvement in the mean number of drawing content units produced to these items did not occur until the items were specifically treated. Thus it would appear that the training effects were specific to each treatment set and unlikely to be due to extraneous variables. This conclusion was reinforced by the fact that these results were replicated with a second subject.

An interesting aspect of this study was that despite the success of the RET treatment for facilitating functional drawing content on structured probes during treatment, probes of the subject's use of drawing for functional purposes at an adult day health care facility revealed that he did not spontaneously use this method of communication, despite its availability to him. As a result, a second phase of treatment was initiated, in which WG was required to use

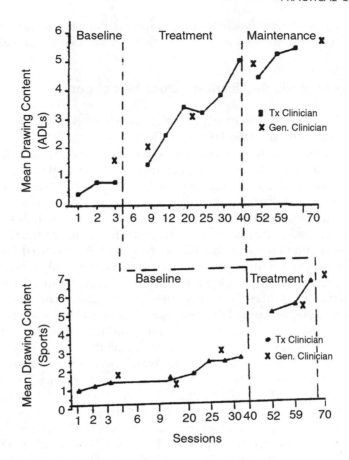

FIGURE 16.5. Mean drawing content produced during probes for baseline, treatment, and maintenance phases of a multiple-baseline-across-behaviors study. Generalization of performance to a clinician not involved in the study is also presented (×). From Kearns, K. P., & Yedor, K. (1992). *Artistic activation therapy: Drawing conclusions.* Paper presented at the Clinical Aphasiology Conference, Durango, CO. Reprinted with permission of the authors.

his drawing ability to communicate functional requests at mealtime. This more functional treatment milieu ultimately resulted in the spontaneous use of communicative drawing for such purposes. Thus, as a result of the controlled manner in which the effectiveness and generalization of training was examined via a single-subject experimental format, we were able to identify the limits of generalization and flexibly adapt the training to meet the individual needs of the aphasic persons in the study. Importantly, these results also challenged our assumptions about generalization and highlighted a need for increasingly powerful treatment packages for facilitating functional responding by aphasic patients in natural settings.

SUMMARY

The purpose of this chapter has been to outline basic principles and components of single-subject experimental designs for evaluating treatment effectiveness in aphasia. A brief discussion of basic principles has been followed by an overview of evaluation strategies and design options that can be employed to study efficacy issues. I have stressed that some design options, such as the multiple-baseline design, are more readily adapted to the development and refinement of treatment packages. The final section of this chapter has been used to emphasize the need for direct and systematic replications of novel aphasia treatments using single-subject designs, and to demonstrate basic principles of technique building, using examples from our research into one approach to aphasia intervention.

As with all methods of research, there are both advantages and limitations to using the types of designs outlined in this chapter. Single-subject experimental designs are uniquely suited to examining treatment issues, because they use subjects as their own controls. Careful incorporation of basic scientific components, such as reliability, operational specificity, and experimental control, combined with within- and across-subject replication (readily achieved with these designs), make them a useful addition to our clinical research armamentarium. Moreover, investigators who adapt these research strategies often emphasize clinical significance over the statistical significance of treatment research findings. The search for large and functional improvements in our aphasic patients invites us to study the pattern of individual improvement over time, while uncovering sources of variability that may weaken our treatment packages. Overall, the judicious use of single-subject experimental designs to examine conceptually salient treatment issues has much to contribute to our clinical science, as well as to the patients we serve.

REFERENCES

Aten, J., Caligiuri, M., & Holland, A. (1982). The efficacy of functional communication therapy for chronic aphasic patients. *Journal of Speech and Hearing Disorders, 47,* 93–96.

Baer, D. M., Wolf, M. M., & Risley, T. R. (1968). Some current dimensions of applied behavior analysis. *Journal of Applied Behavior Analysis, 1,* 91–97.

Baer, D. M., Wolf, M. M., & Risley, T. R. (1987). Some still-current dimensions of applied behavior analysis. *Journal of Applied Behavior Analysis, 20,* 313–328.

Barlow, D. H., & Hayes, S. C. (1979). Alternating treatments design: One strategy for comparing the effects of two treatments in a single subject. *Journal of Applied Behavior Analysis, 12,* 199–210.

Barlow, D. H., Hayes, S. C., & Nelson, R. D. (1984). *The scientist practitioner: Research and accountability in clinical and educational settings.* New York: Pergamon Press.

Barlow, D. H., & Hersen, M. (1984). *Single case experimental designs: Strategies for studying behavior change* (2nd ed.). New York: Pergamon Press.

Broca, P. (1861). Remarques sur le de la faculte du langage articule sur[??] d'une observation d'aphemie. *Bulletin of the Society of Anthropology Paris, 2,* 219.

Connell, P. J., & McReynolds, L. V. (1986). Flexibility of single-subject experimental designs: Part III. Using flexibility to design or modify experiments. *Journal of Speech and Hearing Disorders, 51,* 214–225.

Davis, G. A. (1986). Questions of efficacy in clinical aphasiology. In R. H. Brookshire (Ed.), *Clinical Aphasiology Conference proceedings* (Vol. 16). Minneapolis, MN: BRK.

Doyle, P., & Goldstein, H. (1985). Experimental analysis of acquisition and generalization of syntax in Broca's aphasia. In R. H. Brookshire (Ed.), *Clinical Aphasiology Conference proceedings* (Vol. 15). Minneapolis, MN: BRK.

Doyle, P., Goldstein, H., & Bourgeois, M. S. (1987). Experimental analysis of syntax training in Broca's aphasia: A generalization and social validation study. *Journal of Speech and Hearing Disorders, 52,* 143–155.

Doyle, P., Goldstein, H., Bourgeois, M. S., & Nakles, K. O. (1989). Facilitating generalized requesting behavior in Broca's aphasia: An experimental analysis of a generalization training procedure. *Journal of Applied Behavior Analysis, 22,* 157–170.

Doyle, P., Oleyar, K. S., & Goldstein, H. (1989). Facilitating functional conversational skills in aphasia: An experimental analysis of a generalization training procedure. In T. E. Prescott (Ed.), *Clinical Aphasiology* (Vol. 19). San Deigo, CA: College-Hill Press.

Goodglass, H., & Kaplan, E. (1983). *The assessment of aphasia and related disorders* (2nd Ed.). Philadelphia: Lea and Febiger.

Hersen, M., & Barlow, D. H. (1976). *Single case experimental designs: Strategies for studying behavior change.* New York: Pergamon Press.

Holland, A. L., Fromm, D. S., De Ruyter, F., & Stein, M. (1996). Treatment efficacy: Aphasia. *Journal of Speech and Hearing Research, 39,* S27–S36.

Homer, R. D., & Baer, D. M. (1978). Multiple-probe technique: A variation on the multiple baseline. *Journal of Applied Behavior Analysis, 11,* 189–196.

Huitema, B. (1986a). Autocorrelation in behavioral research: Wherefore art thou? In A. Poling & R. W. Fugua (Eds.), *Research methods in applied behavior analysis.* New York: Plenum Press.

Huitema, B. (1986b). Statistical analysis and single-subject designs: Some misunderstandings. In A. Poling & R. W. Fugua (Eds.), *Research methods in applied behavior analysis.* New York: Plenum Press.

Iwata, B., Bailey, J., Fuqua, R. W., Neef, N., Page, T., & Reid, D. (1989). *Methodological and conceptual issues in applied behavior analysis.* Lawrence, KS: Society for the Experimental Analysis of Behavior.

Kazdin, A. E. (1982). *Single-case research designs: Methods for clinical and applied settings.* New York: Oxford University Press.

Kearns, K. P. (1985). Response elaboration training for patient-initiated utterances. In R. H. Brookshire (Ed.), *Clinical Aphasiology Conference proceedings* (Vol. 15). Minneapolis, MN: BRK.

Kearns, K. P. (1986a). Within-subject experimental designs: II. Design selection and arrangement of experimental phases. *Journal of Speech and Hearing Disorders, 51,* 204–214.

Kearns, K. P. (1986b). Systematic programming of a pragmatic approach to aphasia management. In R. O. C. Marshall (Ed.), *Case studies in aphasia rehabilitation.* Austin, TX: Pro-Ed.

Kearns, K. P. (1992). Methodological issues in aphasia treatment research: A single-subject perspective. In J. A. Cooper (Ed.), *Aphasia treatment: Current approaches and opportunities.* Bethesda, MD: NIH-NIDCD Monograph 93-3424.

Kearns, K. P., & Potechin-Scher, G. (1989). The generalization of response elaboration training effects. In T. E. Prescott (Ed.), *Clinical Aphasiology* (Vol. 18). San Diego, CA: College-Hill Press.

Kearns, K. P., & Salmon, S. (1984). An experimental analysis of auxiliary and copula verb generalization in aphasia. *Journal of Speech and Hearing Disorders, 49,* 152–163.

Kearns, K. P., & Thompson, C. K. (1991a). Analytical and technical directions in applied aphasia analysis: The Midas touch. In T. E. Prescott (Ed.), *Clinical aphasiology* (Vol. 19). Austin, TX: Pro-Ed.

Kearns, K. P., & Thompson, C. K. (1991b). Technical drift and conceptual myopia: The Merlin effect. In T. H. Prescott (Ed.), *Clinical aphasiology* Vol. 19. Austin, TX: Pro-Ed.

Kearns, K. P., & Yedor, K. (1991). An alternating treatments comparison of loose training and a convergent treatment strategy. In T. E. Prescott (Ed.), *Clinical aphasiology,* (Vol. 20). Austin, TX: Pro-Ed.

Kearns, K. P., & Yedor, K. (1992). *Artistic activation therapy: Drawing conclusions.* Paper presented at the Clinical Aphasiology Conference, Durango, CO.

Loverso, F. L., Prescott, T. E., & Sellinger, M. (1988). Cueing verbs: A treatment strategy for aphasic adults (CVT). *Journal of Rehabilitation Research and Development, 25,* 47–60.

Lyon, J., Cariski, D., Keisler, L., et al. (1997). Communication partners: Enhancing participation in life and communication for adults with aphasia in natural settings. *Aphasiology, 11,* 693–708.

McNeil, M. R., Odell, K., & Teng, C. H. (1991). Toward the integration of resource allocation into a general theory of aphasia. In T. E. Prescott (Ed.), *Clinical aphasiology* (Vol. 20). Austin, TX: Pro-Ed.

McReynolds, L.V., & Kearns, K.P. (1983). *Single-subject experimental designs in communicative disorders.* Austin, TX: Pro-Ed.

McReynolds, L. V., & Thompson, C. K. (1986). Flexibility of single-subject experimental designs: Part I. Review of the basics of single-subject designs. *Journal of Speech and Hearing Disorders, 51,* 194–203.

Mitchum, C. C., Haendiges, A. N., & Berndt, R. S. (1993). Model-guided treatment to improve written sentence production: A case study. *Aphasiology, 7,* 71–109.

Nicholas, L. E., & Brookshire, R. H. (1993). A system for socring main concepts in the discourse of non-brain damaged and aphasic speakers. In M. L. Lemme (Ed.), *Clinical aphasiology* (Vol. 21). Austin, TX: Pro-Ed.

Raymer, A., & Thompson, C. K. (1991). Effects of verbal plus gestural treatment in a patient with aphasia and severe apraxia of speech. In M. L. Lemme (Ed.), *Clinical aphasiology* (Vol. 20). Austin, TX: Pro-Ed.

Raymer, A., Thompson, C. K., Jacobs, B., & LeGrand, H. R. (1993). Phonological treatment of naming deficits in aphasia: Model-based generalization analysis. *Aphasiology, 7,* 27–53.

Robey, R. R. (1994). The efficacy of treatment for aphasic persons: A meta-analysis. *Brain and Language, 47,* 582–608.

Robey, R. R. (1998). A meta-analysis of clinical outcomes in the treatment of aphasia. *Journal of Speech and Hearing Research, 14,* 172–187.

Robey, R. R. (1999). Single-subject clinical outcome research: Designs, data, effect sizes, and analyses. *Aphasiology, 13,* 445–473.

Schoonen, R. (1991). The internal validity of efficacy studies: Design and statistical power in studies of language therapy for aphasics. *Brain and Language, 41,* 446–464.

Schwartz, M. F., Saffran, E. M., Fink, R. B., Myers, J. L., & Martin, N. (1994). Mapping therapy: A treatment program for agrammatism. *Aphasiology, 8,* 19–54.

Simmons, N. N. (1980). Choice of stimulus modes in treating apraxia of speech: A case study. In R. H. Brookshire (Ed.), *Clinical aphasiology conference proceedings.*

Sparks, R., Helms, N., & Albert, M. (1974). Aphasia rehabilitation resulting from melodic intonation therapy. *Cortex, 10,* 303–316.

Springer, L. (1991). Facilitating group rehabilitation. *Aphasiology, 5,* 563–566.

Suen, H. K., & Ary, D. (1989). *Analyzing quantitative behavioral observation data.* Hillsdale, NJ: Erlbaum.

Thompson, C. K. (1989). Generalization in the treatment of aphasia. In J. Sparadin & L. V. McReynolds (Eds.), *Generalization strategies in the treatment of communication disorders.* New York: Decker.

Thompson, C. K., & McReynolds, L. V. (1986). Wh- interrogative production in agrammatic aphasia: An experimental analysis of auditory–visual stimulation and direct-production treatment. *Journal of Speech and Hearing Research, 29,* 193–206.

Thompson, C. K., Raymer, A., & LeGrand, H. (1992). Effects on phonologically based treatment on aphasic naming deficits: A model-driven approach. In T. E. Prescott (Ed.), *Clinical aphasiology* (Vol. 20). Austin, TX: Pro-Ed.

Thompson, C. K., Shapiro, L. P., & Roberts, M. M. (1993). Treatment of sentence production deficits in aphasia: A linguistic-specific approach to wh- interrogative training and generalization. *Aphasiology, 7,* 111–133.

Thompson, C. K., Shapiro, L. P., Tait, M., Jacobs, B., & Schneider, S. (1997). Training and generalized production of wh-questions and NP movement structures in agrammatic aphasia. *Journal of Speech and Hearing Research, 40,* 228–244.

Wernicke, C. (1874). *Der aphasische symptomkomplex.* Breslau: Cohn and Wergert.

Willmes, K. (1990). Statistical methods for single-case study approach to aphasia therapy research. *Aphasiology, 4,* 415–456.

INDEX

443